COMPLEMENTARY AND INTEGRATIVE THERAPIES FOR MENTAL HEALTH AND AGING

COMPLEMENTARY AND INTEGRATIVE THERAPIES FOR MENTAL HEALTH AND AGING

Edited by
Helen Lavretsky, MD, MS
UNIVERSITY OF CALIFORNIA, LOS ANGELES

Martha Sajatovic, MD
CASE WESTERN UNIVERSITY SCHOOL OF MEDICINE,
AND UNIVERSITY HOSPITALS OF CLEVELAND

Charles Reynolds III, MD
WESTERN PSYCHIATRIC INSTITUTE AND CLINIC,
AND UNIVERSITY OF PITTSBURGH SCHOOL OF MEDICINE

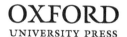

OXFORD
UNIVERSITY PRESS

OXFORD
UNIVERSITY PRESS

Oxford University Press is a department of the University of Oxford. It furthers
the University's objective of excellence in research, scholarship, and education
by publishing worldwide. Oxford is a registered trade mark of Oxford University
Press in the UK and certain other countries.

Published in the United States of America by Oxford University Press
198 Madison Avenue, New York, NY 10016, United States of America.

Library of Congress Cataloging-in-Publication Data
Complementary and integrative therapies for mental health and aging/edited by Helen Lavretsky,
Martha Sajatovic, Charles Reynolds III.
p. ; cm.
Includes bibliographical references.
ISBN 978–0–19–938086–2 (alk. paper)
I. Lavretsky, Helen, editor. II. Sajatovic, Martha, editor. III. Reynolds, Charles F., III, 1947– , editor.
[DNLM: 1. Aged. 2. Mental Disorders—therapy. 3. Complementary Therapies—methods.
4. Geriatric Psychiatry—methods. 5. Integrative Medicine—methods. WT 150]
RC451.4.A5
618.97′689—dc23
2015020578

To the healing of humanity: healing one person at a time.

CONTENTS

PREFACE

THE GLOBAL population is aging rapidly. Over the next four decades, the number of individuals aged 60 years and older *will nearly triple* to more than two billion in 2050 (UN, 2013). With the aging of the population, the burden and cost of chronic disease will escalate worldwide. In order to ensure healthy and successful aging and reduce the cost of care for this huge increase, building resilience and well-being among the aging becomes a top priority for individuals, families, and society at large. More and more, clinicians and family caregivers will need guidance in finding successful strategies to support resilience and effective coping with aging-related diseases. More researchers will face the issue of inadequate treatment response in the presence of neuropsychiatric and medical comorbid disorders, and psychosocial issues like bereavement and caregiver stress, or in the presence of the social isolation and loneliness that often perpetuate a course of chronic physical and mental illness, and determine poor treatment outcomes. Complementary, alternative, and integrative medicine (CAIM) is well positioned

to offer interventions leading to the prevention of major mental and physical diseases of aging and the improvement of the quality of life for aging individuals and their families. This volume provides a concise update on recent advances in our conceptual understanding of complementary, alternative, and integrative therapies in the context of physical and mental disorders of aging, as well asthe latest research on the mechanisms of response to CAIM interventions directed to prevent and treat major disease of aging.

According to the National Center for Complementary and Integrative Health, complementary and alternative medicine "is a group of diverse medical and health care systems, practices, and products that are not presently considered part of conventional medicine." Some of these therapies provide promise as novel and effective therapies for the treatment and prevention of late-life psychiatric disorders with generally more modest side-effect profiles. *Complementary* generally refers to using a non-mainstream approach together with conventional Western medicine. *Alternative* refers to using a non-mainstream approach in place of conventional

Western medicine. "*Integrative medicine*" is another term often used in this field; it aims to combine alternative and complementary medicine with evidence-based Western medicine. For the purpose of this book, we will refer to such therapies as complementary, alternative, and integrative medicine (CAIM).

CAIM interventions have varying levels of efficacy and evidence for the therapies that can include mind–body practices, conventional physical activity, dietary interventions, and natural products, as well as body-based practices and other medical system practices. Our book reflects such heterogeneity of the available evidence and its application to the clinical practice and research. Some chapters provide solid evidence with scientific data and careful analyses, and some only outline the potential for use. The search for effective CAIM interventions is especially timely because of the characteristics and needs of aging Baby Boomers, who are more inclined to be involved in preventive health care and more self-deterministic in directing their care compared to earlier generations. This rapid change in the population has created an urgent need for a book that would provide much-needed information about CAIM interventions for mental health and aging for geriatric practitioners, both clinicians and researchers, dealing with the diseases of aging, and laypersons interested in prevention and positive aging and the latest approaches in preventive care for older adults. A broad audience of clinical researchers and clinicians from several disciplines involves those who are practicing complementary, alternative, and integrative medicine techniques (e.g., nurses, psychologists, acupuncturists, chiropractors, and allopathic, osthopathic, and naturopathic physicians), those in medical specialties (geriatric medicine and psychiatry, neurology, pain medicine, palliative and hospice settings, sleep disorders medicine), and students interested in integrative and complementary interventions. The book provides an update on recent advances in clinical and neuroscience research on CAIM approaches to treatment and prevention applied to mental health and aging. Our hope is that the content of the book will educate and increase clinicians' familiarity with recent research findings in the field of CAIM, and will broaden their understanding of the nature of the interventions and how to use these interventions in their clinical populations of older adults.

This volume will increase clinicians' and researchers' literacy about recent research findings with respect to CAIM interventions, will broaden their therapeutic perspectives, and will better prepare them to deal with the challenges of finding appropriate, effective treatments to boost resilience and well-being in older adults. Another target audience is family caregivers who are looking for better solutions to reduce their own burden and improve the quality of life for their family members with chronic diseases of aging. Those who are dedicated to preventing the stress-related diseases of aging might consider this volume an essential part of their libraries. We are grateful to the international group of contributing authors, consisting of the experts and opinion leaders and researchers in their respective areas of expertise. In the Overview, we provide new information on relevant science in biological aging across different disciplines of medicine and psychosocial sciences. Part II and III of this book describe interventions are focused on wellness promotion and stress reduction; the last section describes interventions devoted to the treatment and prevention of specific mental and physical disorders in older adults and in end-of life care settings. Also included is a detailed summary of the practical implications of evidence-based interventions, with descriptions of emerging interventions designed to enhance resilience and positive aging. And, finally, the Conclusion and Epilogue will focus on the new developments in the neuroscience of interventions with the use of biomarkers in research and clinical practice, followed by suggestions for future directions.

A key difference between this volume and other publications is that it brings together (1) a wide variety of clinical issues, (2) the latest neuroscientific discoveries of the mechanisms of the diseases of aging and CAIM interventions, and (3) the issues most relevant for public policy-makers to understand in pursuing CAIM interventions for aging adults. Thirty-three chapters bridge science and clinical practices, identifying viable models of treatment and fruitful future directions for preventive interventions with direct relevance to reimbursement for quality and evidence-based interventions. In sum, it is our hope that this book will disseminate important knowledge, point to exciting research possibilities, and increase both professional and public awareness of the CAIM interventions, ultimately leading to widened options for personalized medicine, prevention of the major diseases of aging, and improved treatment outcomes, with reduced cost of chronic disease to the individuals, families, and society.

Helen Lavretsky, MD, MS
Martha Sajatovic, MD
Charles Reynolds III, MD

CONTRIBUTORS

Acharya Balkrishna
Acharya Chairman
Patanjali Research Foundation
Patanjali Yogpeeth,
Haridwar
Uttarakhand, India

Daniele Balzafiore, MS, MA
Stanford University School of Medicine
Center for Neuroscience in Women's Health
Stanford, CA, USA

Michael Bauer, PhD, RN, ND
Australian Centre for Evidence
 Based Aged Care
Faculty of Science, Health and Engineering
La Trobe University
Melbourne Victoria, Australia

Bernhard T. Baune, PhD, MD, MPH, FRANZCP
Head, Discipline of Psychiatry
University of Adelaide
Adelaide, South Australia

Julienne E. Bower, PhD
Department of Psychology
Cousins Center for Psychoneuroimmunology
Department of Psychiatry and Biobehavioral
 Sciences
University of California, Los Angeles
Los Angeles, CA, USA

Chloe C. Boyle, MS
Department of Psychology
University of California, Los Angeles
Los Angeles, CA, USA

Richard P. Brown, MD
Associate Clinical Professor in Psychiatry
Columbia University College of Medicine
New York, NY, USA

Alison C. Burggren, PhD
Associate Adjunct Professor
Department of Psychiatry and Biobehavioral Sciences
University of California, Los Angeles
Los Angeles, CA USA

Tricia L. da Silva, MA
Institute of Medical Sciences
University of Toronto
Division of Mood and Anxiety Disorders
Centre for Addiction and Mental Health
Toronto, Ontario, Canada

Ellen Gay Detlefsen, DLS
Associate Professor
School of Information Sciences—the iSchool
    at Pitt; and
Training Program Faculty Department
    of Biomedical Informatics
School of Medicine University of Pittsburgh
Pittsburgh, PA, USA

Bruce J. Diamond, M.Ed, PhD
Professor, Department of Psychology
William Paterson University
Director, Neuropsychology, Cognitive
    Neuroscience and Treatment Outcomes Lab
Wayne, NJ, USA

Michelle L. Dossett, MD, PhD, MPH
Assistant in Medicine
Benson-Henry Institute for Mind Body Medicine
Massachusetts General Hospital;
    and Instructor
Harvard Medical School
Boston, MA, USA

Richelin V. Dye, PhD
Health Sciences Clinical Instructor (Voluntary)
Department of Psychiatry and
    Biobehavioral Science
David Geffen School of Medicine at UCLA
Los Angeles, CA, USA

Linda M. Ercoli, PhD
Health Sciences Clinical Professor
Psychiatry and Biobehavioral Sciences
David Geffen School of Medicine at UCLA
Los Angeles, CA, USA

Harris Eyre, MBBS, PhD
University of Adelaide
Adelaide, South Australia
And Semel Institute of Neuroscience
    and Human Behavior
University of California, Los Angeles
Los Angeles, CA, USA;

Jarred V. Gallegos, BA
Department of Psychiatry
University of California, San Diego
San Diego, CA, USA

John Geirland, PhD
Health Sciences Clinical Instructor (Voluntary)
Department of Psychiatry and Biobehavioral Sciences
University of California, Los Angeles
Los Angeles, CA, USA

Megan E. Gomez, PhD
Post-doctoral Scholar
Department of Neurology
University of Southern California
Los Angeles, CA, USA

Patricia L. Gerbarg, MD
Assistant Clinical Professor in Psychiatry
New York Medical College
Valhalla, NY, USA

Natasha Ghani, BA
Department of Psychiatry
University of California, San Diego
San Diego, CA, USA

Ronald M. Glick, MD
Assistant Professor of Psychiatry and Physical
    Medicine and Rehabilitation
University of Pittsburgh School of Medicine
Pittsburgh, PA, USA

Brenda Golianu, MD
Associate Professor
Department of Anesthesiology
Stanford University
Stanford, CA, USA

Bart N. Green, DC, MSEd
Associate Editor, *Journal of Manipulative and*
    Physiological Therapeutics
Department of Publication and Editorial Review
National University of Health Sciences
Lombard, IL, USA

Aikisha Harley, MS
Palo Alto University
Palo Alto, CA, USA

Alexandrea L. Harmell, MS
Doctoral Student
San Diego State University/University of California
San Diego
Joint Doctoral Program in Clinical Psychology
San Diego, CA, USA

Ka-Kit Hui, MD
Professor and Director
UCLA Department of Medicine
Center for East-West Medicine
Los Angeles, CA, USA

Scott A. Irwin, MD, PhD
Moores Cancer Center
Psychiatry & Psychosocial Services
Patient & Family Support Services;
Department of Psychiatry
University of California, San Diego
San Diego, CA, USA

Najmeh Jafari, MD
George Washington Institute for Spirituality and Health
The George Washington University School
of Medicine & Health Sciences
Washington, DC, USA

Dilip V. Jeste, PhD
Professor of Psychiatry and Neurosciences
Department of Psychiatry
University of California, San Diego
San Diego, CA, USA

Claire D. Johnson, DC, MSEd
Editor, *Journal of Manipulative and
Physiological Therapeutics*
Department of Publication and Editorial Review
National University of Health Sciences
Lombard, IL, USA

Susan K. Johnson, PhD
Professor of Psychology
University of North Carolina at Charlotte
Charlotte, North Carolina, United States

Rujvi Kamat, PhD
Postdoctoral Research Fellow
Department of Psychiatry
University of California, San Diego
San Diego, CA, USA

Edward Kwok-ho Hui, MD
Associate Clinical Professor of Medicine
UCLA Department of Medicine
Center for East-West Medicine
Los Angeles, CA, USA

Sachin Kumar Sharma
Senior Research Fellow in the Department
of Yoga Research
Patanjali Research Foundation
Patanjali Yogpeeth
Uttarakhand, India

Helen Lavretsky, MD, MS
Professor of Psychiatry
Semel Scholar in Integrative Mental Health
Director, Late-Life Mood, Stress and Wellness
Research Program
Semel Institute for Neuroscience and
Human Behavior
University of California, Los Angeles
Los Angeles, CA, USA

S. Melanie Lee, MD, PhD
Resident physician at UCLA Semel Institute for
Neuroscience and Human Behavior
UCLA Department of Psychiatry
Los Angeles, CA, USA

Sermsak Lolak, MD
Department of Psychiatry and Behavioral Sciences
The George Washington University School of
Medicine & Health Sciences
Washington, DC, USA

Stephanie Magou, BA
Department of Psychology,
William Paterson University
Neuropsychology, Cognitive Neuroscience
and Treatment Outcomes Lab
Wayne, NJ, USA

Cathy A. Malchiodi, PhD
Trauma-Informed Practices and Expressive
Arts Therapy Institute
Louisville, KY, USA

Isadora Sande Mathias
Faculdade de Medicina da Bahia
Universidade Federal da Bahia (UFBA)
Salvador, Bahia, Brasil

Emily A. Meier, PhD
Moores Cancer Center
Psychiatry & Psychosocial Services;
Patient & Family Support Services
Department of Psychiatry
University of California, San Diego
San Diego, CA, USA

David A. Merrill, MD, PhD
Assistant Clinical Professor of Psychiatry &
    Biobehavioral Sciences
Division of Geriatric Psychiatry Associate Director
    of Ambulatory Care
Semel Institute for Neuroscience & Human
    Behavior
David Geffen School of Medicine at UCLA
Los Angeles, CA, USA

Karen J. Miller, PhD
Health Sciences Associate Clinical Professor
Division of Geriatric Psychiatry
UCLA Longevity Center
David Geffen School of Medicine at UCLA
Los Angeles, CA, USA

Darlinda K. Minor, MD
Department of Psychiatry
    and Behavioral Sciences
The George Washington University School
    of Medicine & Health Sciences
Washington, DC, USA

David Mischoulon, MD, PhD
Depression Clinical and Research Program
Department of Psychiatry
Massachusetts General Hospital
Boston, MA, USA

Lori P. Montross Thomas, PhD
Moores Cancer Center
Psychiatry & Psychosocial Services
Patient & Family Support Services;
Department of Psychiatry;
Department of Family & Preventive Medicine
University of California, San Diego
San Diego, CA, USA

Elizabeth P. Neale PhD, BND (Hons.) APD
Research Fellow
Smart Foods Centre
School of Medicine/Faculty of Science,
    Medicine and Health
Illawarra Health and Medical Research Institute
University of Wollongong
New South Wales, Australia

Shelley Ochs, PhD
Instructor
International Institute
Beijing University of Chinese Medicine
Beijing, China

Olivia I. Okereke, MD, SM
Departments of Psychiatry and Medicine
Brigham and Women's Hospital
Boston, MA, USA

Nancy A. Pachana, PhD
Professor of Clinical Psychology and
Director of Clinical Training Program
School of Psychology
The University of Queensland
Queensland, Australia

Barton W. Palmer, PhD
Professor of Psychiatry
University of California, San Diego
San Diego, CA, USA

Alexander Panossian, PhD, Dr. Chem. Sci.
Head of Research & Development,
    Swedish Herbal Institute
Editor-in-Chief, International Journal
    of Phytotherapy and Phytopharmacology
Sweden

Sonya E. Pritzker, PhD, Lac
Assistant Professor
Department of Anthropology
University of Alabama
Tuscaloosa, AL, USA;
UCLA Center for East-West Medicine
Los Angeles, CA, USA

James O. Prochaska, PhD
Director
Cancer Prevention Research Center
University of Rhode Island
Kingston, Rhode Island, USA

Janice M. Prochaska, PhD
President and CEO
Pro-Change Behavior Systems, Inc.
South Kingstown, Rhode Island, USA

Christina Puchalski, MD, FACP, FAAHPM
Professor, Medicine and Health Sciences
Director, George Washington Institute for
    Spirituality
    and Health
Co-Director, GWU-MFA Supportive and Palliative
    Care Clinic
The George Washington University School
    of Medicine & Health Sciences
Washington, DC, USA

Arun V. Ravindran, MBBS, MSc, PhD, FRCPC, FRCPsych
Department of Psychiatry
University of Toronto;
Division of Mood and Anxiety Disorders
Centre for Addiction and Mental Health
Toronto, Ontario, Canada

Jo-Anne Rayner, PhD
Australian Centre for Evidence Based Aged Care
Faculty of Science, Health and Engineering
La Trobe University
Melbourne Victoria, Australia

Charles Reynolds III, MD
Western Psychiatric Institute and Clinic; and
University of Pittsburgh School of Medicine
Pittsburgh, PA, USA

Martha Sajatovic, MD
Case Western University School of Medicine; and
University Hospitals of Cleveland
Cleveland, OH, USAS

Theresa L. Scott, PhD
School of Psychology

The University of Queensland
Queensland, Australia

Karen J. Sherman, PhD, MPH
Senior Scientific Investigator
Group Health Research Institute; and
Affiliate Professor
Department of Epidemiology
University of Washington
Seattle, WA, USA

Ankura Singh, MPH
Department of Medicine
Brigham and Women's Hospital
Boston, MA, USA

Nilkamal Singh, PhD
Patanjali Research Foundation
Patanjali Yogpeeth
Uttarakhand, India

David Spiegel, MD
Willson Professor and Associate Chair of
    Psychiatry & Behavioral Sciences
Director of the Center on Stress and Health
Medical Director of the Center for Integrative
    Medicine
Stanford University School of Medicine
Stanford, CA, USA

Briana Stanfield, BS
Behavioral & Neural Sciences Program
Rutgers University
Newark, NJ, USA

Linda C. Tapsell, AM FDAA PhD
 Discipline Leader, Nutrition and Dietetics
Smart Foods Centre
School of Medicine/Faculty of Science,
    Medicine and Health
Illawarra Health and Medical Research Institute
University of Wollongong
New South Wales, Australia

Shirley Telles, PhD
Director
Patanjali Research Foundation
Patanjali Yogpeeth
Haridwar
Uttarakhand, India

Michael Teut, MD
Institute for Social Medicine, Epidemiology
    and Health Economics
Charité Universitätsmedizin Berlin
Berlin, Germany
Esther G. Teverovsky, MD
Clinical Assistant Professor of Psychiatry
University of Pittsburgh School of Medicine
Pittsburgh, PA, USA

Esther Teverovsky, MD
Geriatric Psychiatrist
University of Pittsburgh
Pittsburgh, PA, USA

Katelyn Van Clef, MA
 Department of Psychology,
    William Paterson University
Neuropsychology, Cognitive Neuroscience
    and Treatment Outcomes Lab
Wayne, NJ, USA

Taya Varteresian, DO, MS
Psychiatrist
Los Angeles County Department of Mental
    Health; and
Health Science Assistant Clinical Professor
University of California Irvine
Irvine, CA, USA

Shu-Ming Wang, MD
Professor in Residence
Department of Anesthesiology and
    Perioperative Health
University of California Irvine
Orange, CA, USA; and
Clinical Professor
Department of Anesthesiology
University of Connecticut
Farmington, CT, USA

Tonita E. Wroolie, PhD, ABPP
Board Certified in Geropsychology
Associate Clinical Professor
Stanford University School of Medicine
Center for Neuroscience in Women's Health

Arti Yadav
Junior Research Fellow in the Department of Yoga
    Research
Patanjali Research Foundation
Patanjali Yogpeeth
Uttarakhand, India

PART I

OVERVIEW

SECTION A

BASIC BIOLOGY OF AGING
UNDERLYING DISORDERS
OF AGING

1

EXPLORING THE EFFECTS OF COMPLEMENTARY, ALTERNATIVE, AND INTEGRATIVE MEDICINE INTERVENTIONS ON LATE-LIFE MENTAL ILLNESS THROUGH THE BASIC MECHANISMS OF AGING

Harris Eyre, Bernhard T. Baune, and Helen Lavretsky

INTRODUCTION

The aging of the world population in the twenty-first century is unprecedented in human history, and will place substantial pressure on health systems across the world with concurrent rises in chronic diseases, particularly age-related cognitive disorders and late-life affective disorders. A recent United Nations World Population Ageing Report provides the most up-to-date, current and projected figures in relation to world aging (UN, 2013). The report suggests that the global share of older people (aged ≥ 60 years) increased from 9.2% in 1990 to 11.7% in 2013 and will continue to grow as a proportion of the world population, reaching 21.1% by 2050. Globally, the number of older persons (aged ≥ 60 years) is expected to more than double, from 841 million people in 2013 to more than 2 billion in 2050. Moreover, the share of older persons aged ≥ 80 years (the "oldest old") within the older population was 14% in 2013 and is projected to reach 19% in 2050. Maintaining health and

health-promoting behaviors is becoming the main objective of preventive medicine in aging adults and includes the use of complimentary, alternative, and integrative medicine (CAIM) interventions and therapies (Arcury et al., 2013; Oberg et al., 2014).

In correlation with global population aging, there are robust predictions suggesting that rates of cognitive impairment, specifically dementia, will rise dramatically in the twenty-first century with devastating consequences. The World Alzheimer Report 2013 (ADI, 2013), produced by the Alzheimer's Disease International Organization, provides concerning statistics. As of 2013, there were an estimated 44.4 million people worldwide with dementia. This number will increase to an estimated 75.6 million in 2030, and 135.5 million in 2050. There are 7.7 million new cases of dementia each year, inferring that there is a new case of dementia every four seconds.

Late-life depression is a significant mental illness in older aged populations, with a rising burden expected in this century (Ferrari et al., 2013). The most recent global data on late-life depression comes from a contemporary analysis of the World Health Organization's (WHO) Global Burden of Disease Study 2010. This study was conducted by Ferrari et al. (2013) and identified depressive disorders as a leading cause of burden internationally; it suggested that major depressive disorder (MDD) was also a contributor of burden allocated to suicide and ischemic heart disease. Depressive disorders were the second leading cause of years lived with disability (YLD) in 2010. MDD accounted for 8.2% (5.9%–10.8%) of global YLDs and dysthymia for 1.4% (0.9%–2.0%). The burden of depressive disorders was highest in adults of working age (15–64 years) with 60.4 million in 2010, versus adults aged ≥ 65 years with 6.1 million YLDs.

Anxiety disorders are chronic, disabling conditions, which are believed to have a substantial prevalence. Surprisingly, it was only recently that the global burden of anxiety disorders has been calculated comprehensively. A recent study by Baxter et al. (Baxter, Vos, Scott, Ferrari, & Whiteford, 2014) has analyzed the WHO's Global Burden of Disease Study 2010 to explore the estimated burden due to morbidity and mortality. These data suggest that anxiety disorders were the sixth leading cause of YLDs of all diseases, accounting for 390 disability-adjusted life years (DALYs) per 100,000 persons in 2010. The highest burden occurred between the ages of 15 and 34 years. The burden of anxiety disorders was still substantial for males and females aged ≥ 60 years, with males accounting for between 200 and 280 DALYs per 100,000 persons and females accounting for between 380 and 520 DALYs per 100,000 persons. This burden is logically expected to rise with population aging.

Conventional treatments of late-life mental illnesses are limited by modest efficacy, significant side-effect profiles, and a limited pipeline of new pharmacological agents; therefore, new and more efficacious therapies with a better side-effect profile are needed. In Alzheimer's disease, pharmacological agents temporarily treat symptoms without having an effect on the underlying pathophysiology of the disease. In late-life depression, a recent meta-analysis of clinical trials suggests a response rate of 48% and a remission rate of 33.7% (Kok, Nolen, & Heeren, 2012), both very similar to response and remission rates found in adult patients. In late-life anxiety disorders, few randomized clinical trials (RCTs) have been conducted with psychotropic agents, with further systematic research required in this area (Wolitzky-Taylor,

Castriotta, Lenze, Stanley, & Craske, 2010). The common and inappropriate use of benzodiazepines for anxiety symptoms in the elderly is associated with significant adverse effects (e.g., hip fracture, cognitive dysfunction, and impaired psychomotor functioning). A number of factors are associated with increased side-effect profiles in late-life mental illness treated with pharmacotherapy compared to adult populations. These factors include age-related pharmacokinetic changes, resulting in a wider range of drug concentrations in the elderly, and pharmacodynamic changes, which make elderly patients more sensitive to the side effects of antidepressants (Pollock, 2004); in addition, oversimplified modifications for elderly patients from general dosing guidelines can lead to over- and under-dosing of medications (Kok, 2013).

CAIM interventions include therapies that are used instead of, or in addition to, conventional therapies. These therapies provide promise as novel and effective therapies for the treatment and prevention of aging-related disorders with generally more modest side-effect profiles. "Complementary" generally refers to using a non-mainstream approach, together with conventional medicine. "Alternative" refers to using a non-mainstream approach in place of conventional medicine. Integrative medicine aims to combine alternative and complementary medicine with evidence-based Western medicine. CAIM interventions have varying levels of efficacy and evidence; they can include mind-body practices, physical activity, dietary interventions, natural products, and body-based and other practices. Mind-body practices refer to practices in which physical and mental activity may be combined during training and typically include yoga, tai chi, qi gong, and meditation. Physical activity refers to any bodily movement produced by skeletal muscles that requires energy expenditure and may include aerobic, resistance, or combination activities. Dietary interventions explore the effect of dietary patterns on health and illness and may include Western, traditional, and Mediterranean dietary patterns, as well as caloric restriction, among others. Natural products may include herbs, vitamins, minerals, natural supplements, and probiotics. Body-based practices may include acupuncture, relaxation therapy, and massage therapy. Other whole-systems therapies may include homeopathy, Ayurveda, or traditional Chinese medicine. There is a growing evidence that Baby Boomers (adults born from 1946 to 1964) report significantly higher rates of CAIM use than the Silent Generation (born from 1925 to 1945) for both chronic diseases of aging and painful conditions (Ho, Rowland-Seymour, Frankel, Li, & Mao, 2014). Therefore, research into the efficacy, mechanisms, and side effects of CAIM interventions is very important. These therapies may be able to prevent aging-related diseases, they may augment the efficacy of conventional therapies, and they may have fewer side effects than conventional therapies. Regardless of their efficacy, they are utilized widely in society, so there is an impetus to understand their biological effects on aging-related diseases.

Researchers have begun to explore the effect of CAIM therapies on established research biomarkers of late-life cognitive and affective disorders. These biomarkers for disease neuropathology include neuroimaging (e.g., functional, volumetric, and structural magnetic resonance imaging, and positron emission tomography), neuroplasticity (e.g., brain-derived neurotrophic factor, hippocampal volume) and Alzheimer's-related biomarkers (e.g., amyloid-β and tau testing in cerebrospinal fluid and serum). For example, the effects of aerobic exercise have been extensively researched in the context of late-life psychiatric disorders. For a thorough review of the effects of aerobic exercise on late-life cognitive dysfunction and associated biomarkers, see Brown et al. (Brown, Peiffer, & Martins, 2013). These biomarkers, however, are shown to have limitations with ongoing quality control challenges, high clinical costs, and, for some biomarkers, a lack of evidence for clinical utility; therefore effort is required to find novel biomarkers.

Age-related disease is arguably the greatest challenge for health and biomedicine in the twenty-first century. For some time, the growing awareness of population aging has focused researchers toward specific age-related diseases. Investigation into the development and treatment of age-related diseases such as Alzheimer's disease and cancer have proven effective; however, there is now a growing awareness of the need for new avenues of investigation. One such avenue is to understand aging, which is the largest risk factor for non-genetic, age-related conditions such as cancer, Parkinson's disease, and Alzheimer's disease. Understanding the core mechanisms of aging and slowing down the process of aging represent a novel approach to addressing the burden of chronic diseases affecting the elderly. The area of exploration of the mechanisms of aging has been termed *geroscience*, an interdisciplinary field that aims to understand the relationship between aging and age-related diseases (Burch et al., 2014). In geroscience, researchers in a variety of disciplines may work together, sharing data and ideas, with a common goal of explaining and intervening in age-related diseases. *Compression of morbidity* is a major focus of geroscience research. Compression of morbidity is a concept whereby scientists discover ways to decrease the period of an individual's life when there is poor health. With this aim, individuals hope to postpone and reduce disease onset, disability, dependency, and suffering. The exact mechanisms of aging are still under debate; however, there are a number of mechanisms that are generally agreed upon (see, for discussion, Lopez-Otin, Blasco, Partridge, Serrano, & Kroemer, 2013). The mechanisms we will explore in this chapter include genomic instability, telomere attrition, epigenetic alterations, loss of proteostasis, mitochondrial dysfunction, cellular senescence, and chronic inflammation.

The aim of this review is to explore the effect of clinically active CAIM therapies on the mechanisms of aging for the treatment and prevention of aging-related diseases. We will overview clinical evidence for the use of CAIM therapies and the mechanisms of aging, and then will explore the effect of these therapies on the mechanisms of aging. We will then outline recommendations for the future of this field.

CAIM INTERVENTIONS FOR THE TREATMENT AND PREVENTION OF LATE-LIFE MENTAL ILLNESS: EXPLORING CLINICAL EFFICACY

The Importance of Exploring Complimentary, Alternative, and Integrative Interventions

Research into the efficacy, mechanisms, and side effects of CAIM interventions is highly important given their widespread use. A recent systematic review of prevalence studies from 1998 onward explored the use of these therapies internationally and included 51 reports from 49 surveys in 15 countries (Harris, Cooper, Relton, & Thomas, 2012). Estimates of 12-month prevalence of any usage ranged from 9.8% to 76%, and from 1.8% to 48.7% for visits to relevant practitioners. Estimates of 12-month prevalence of any usage (excluding prayer) from surveys using consistent measurement methods showed remarkable stability in Australia (49%, 52%, 52%; 1993, 2000, 2004) and the United States (36%, 38%; 2002, 2007).

Clinical Evidence for CAIM Therapies in Late-Life Mental Health

There is promising evidence for the use of various CAIM therapies in late-life mental health; alternatively, there is mixed, contradictory, or no evidence for other therapies. In this section we will provide an overview of the salient findings for therapies that show promise for evidence-based use in clinical populations.

CLINICAL EVIDENCE FOR MIND-BODY PRACTICES

Mind-body practices are varied and may include yoga, tai chi, qi gong, and mindfulness meditation. When considering the effect of tai chi on age-related cognitive decline, a recent meta-analysis by Wu et al. (Wu, Wang, Burgess, & Wu, 2013) noted eight studies in older adults (aged 55 years and older, with varying degrees of cognitive decline), of which two were cross-sectional and six were interventional studies. In total, nine cognitive variables were included in the meta-analysis with four of the nine variables (representing global cognitive function and memory) being significantly improved after tai chi exercise with effect sizes ranging from 0.20 to 0.46 (small to medium). The positive variables included the mini mental status examination (MMSE), digit span test backward, visual span test backward, and verbal fluency test. An RCT (Lavretsky et al., 2011) of elderly subjects (> 60 years)—who were non-responders to escitalopram—found that a 10-week tai chi exercise intervention augmented antidepressant treatment versus control (health education). A recent study by Shahidi et al. (2011) compared the effectiveness of laughter yoga, group exercise therapy, and control in decreasing depression in older adult women (aged 60–80 years). In this study, 70 depressed women were chosen if their Geriatric Depression Score was > 10. This study went for 10 sessions and found a significant improvement in depression score with both yoga and group exercise therapy as compared with control. While the evidence supporting the use of these therapies in the treatment of late-life mental illnesses is not strong, there are

some interesting early results, which require further high-quality research (Abbott & Lavretsky, 2013).

CLINICAL EVIDENCE FOR PHYSICAL ACTIVITY

The effects of physical activity on depression and cognitive impairment are increasingly studied, and have shown some promising results to date. Importantly, there are a variety of subtypes of physical activity, from aerobic activity to resistance and mind-body; this section will focus on aerobic and resistance activity. A recent systematic review examining the role of physical exercise in the treatment of depression in older adults was conducted by Blake et al. (Blake, Mo, Malik, & Thomas, 2009). This study examined 11 RCTs with a total of 641 participants aged > 60 years. The study noted that short-term (0–3 months) positive outcomes were found in nine studies, although there was variation in the type, intensity, and duration of exercise. The efficacy of exercise in the medium and long term (3–12 months and > 12 months, respectively) was less clear. Issues were noted, with only five studies showing appropriate allocation of concealment, and five studies showing intention to treat analysis; blinding occurred in seven studies. A recent meta-analysis by Gates et al. (Gates, Fiatarone Singh, Sachdev, & Valenzuela, 2013) has examined the efficacy of exercise on cognition in older adults with MCI. Fourteen RCTs (1695 participants, aged 65–95 years) were utilized and, overall, 42% of effect sizes (ESs) were potentially clinically relevant (ES > 0.20) with only 8% of cognitive outcomes statistically significant. The meta-analysis revealed negligible but significant effects of exercise on verbal fluency (ES: 0.17 [0.04, 0.30]). No significant benefit was found for additional executive measures, memory, or information processing. Further intervention research is needed to better understand what type of exercise is effective, depending on illness and illness severity.

CLINICAL EVIDENCE FOR NUTRITIONAL INTERVENTIONS

Examining the effect of nutrition and nutritional interventions is a new area of research showing favorable results. A recent meta-analysis of epidemiological trials by Psaltopoulous et al. (2013) concluded that adherence to the Mediterranean dietary pattern (i.e., a diet high in olive oil, legumes, unrefined grains, fruits, vegetables, fish, and wine, and low in meat) was protective against both depression and cognitive decline. In this meta-analysis there were nine studies covering depression and eight covering cognitive impairment. High adherence to the Mediterranean diet was consistently associated with reduced risk of depression (relative risk (RR) = 0.68; 95% CI = 0.54–0.86), and cognitive impairment (RR = 0.60; 95% CI = 0.43–0.83). A recent RCT by Martinez-Lapiscina et al. (2013) has provided insights into the effect of nutritional trials in cognitive impairment. This study was a multicenter, randomized, primary prevention trial titled Prevención con Dieta Mediterránea (PREDIMED) and assessed the effects of a nutritional intervention using the Mediterranean diet (MeDi; supplemented with either extra-virgin olive oil [EVOO] or mixed nuts) in comparison with a low-fat control diet. This study assessed 522 participants at high vascular risk (age 74.6±5.7) and examined cognitive performance (MMSE and Clock Drawing Test [CDT]) after 6.5 years of nutritional intervention. After full adjustment, the MeDi EVOO group showed higher mean MMSE and CDT scores versus control (adjusted differences: +0.62 [95% CI +0.18 to +1.05], p = 0.005 for MMSE; and +0.51 [95% CI +0.20 to +0.82], p = 0.001 for CDT). Similarly, the MeDi+Nuts group showed higher mean MMSE and CDT scores (adjusted differences: +0.57 [95% CI +0.11 to +1.03], p = 0.015 for MMSE; and +0.33 [95% CI +0.003 to +0.67], p = 0.048 for CDT) versus control. In a prospective cohort study of older Australians by Hodge et al. (Hodge, Almeida, English, Giles, & Flicker, 2013), stronger adherence to not only the Mediterranean diet but also the traditional Australian-style eating pattern (i.e., some foods high in fat and sugar content along with whole foods) was associated with lower psychological distress (Kessler Psychological Distress Scale) after 12 years. The field of nutritional psychiatry is developing with regard to general adult populations and cognitive impairment; however, there is a paucity of research into late-life depression and anxiety.

CLINICAL EVIDENCE FOR NATURAL PRODUCTS

Natural products that have been examined in late-life affective and cognitive disorders—with mixed results—include omega-3 polyunsaturated fatty acids ($\Omega 3$ PUFAs), S-adenosyl-L-methionine (SAMe), St. John's wort, Ginkgo biloba, Huperzine

A, B vitamins, and curcumin (see, for review, Varteresian & Lavretsky, 2014; Varteresian, Merrill, & Lavretsky, 2013). Data from a recent review suggests that some studies support the role of omega-3 PUFAs in slowing cognitive impairment prior to the onset of dementia (Varteresian et al., 2013). However, a recent Cochrane Database systematic review by Syndenham et al. (Sydenham, Dangour, & Lim, 2012) explored the effects of $\Omega 3$ PUFAs on the prevention of dementia and cognitive decline in cognitively healthy older people. Information was available from 3 RCTs including 3536 participants in total. This meta-analysis found no evidence to support a preventative effect following 24 or 40 months of intervention. Studies evaluating an antidepressant effect of supplementation with B vitamins are mixed. An RCT in older adults showed no effect of folic acid and vitamin B_{12} with mild depressive symptoms (Walker et al., 2010). Another RCT in post-stroke older adults found that supplementation with vitamins B_6, B_9, and B_{12} prevented the development of depression (Almeida et al., 2010). Despite the growing use of natural supplements and vitamins by an aging population, there is an urgent need to establish the efficacy and safety in well-designed rigorous RCTs.

GEROSCIENCE OF AGING: A FIELD AIMED AT INVESTIGATING THE MECHANISMS OF AGING

Aging is the largest risk factor for non-genetic, age-related conditions. Understanding the core mechanisms of aging and slowing down the process of aging represent a novel approach to addressing the burden of chronic diseases affecting the elderly. The exact mechanisms of aging are still under debate; however, there are a number of mechanisms that are generally agreed upon (Lopez-Otin et al., 2013). The mechanisms include genomic instability, telomere attrition, epigenetic alterations, loss of proteostasis, mitochondrial dysfunction, cellular senescence, and chronic inflammation. These mechanisms are ideally classified according to a number of hallmarks: (1) the mechanism should manifest during normal aging; (2) aggravation of the mechanism should accelerate aging; and (3) attenuation of the mechanism should slow aging. Of course, not all mechanisms carry all three hallmarks; however, there is work underway to explore this issue further. A graphical representation of potential biomarkers

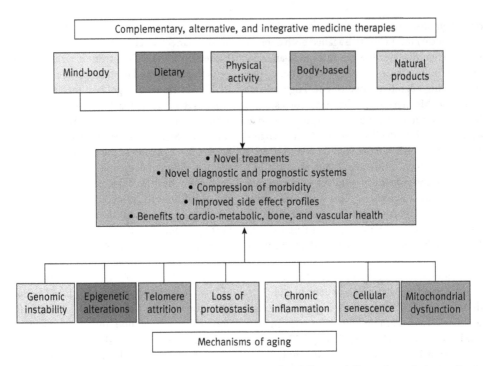

FIGURE 1.1   Exploring the effects of CAIM interventions on late-life mental illness through the mechanisms of aging.

Note: This figure outlines the types of complementary, alternative and integrative medicine (CAIM) interventions, as well as the mechanisms of aging. In the middle box, we provide benefits to exploring how CAIM therapies affect the mechanisms of aging.

relating to the mechanisms of aging are outlined in Figure 1.1.

Genomic Instability

Genomics is a branch of molecular biology concerned with the structure, function, evolution, and mapping of genomes (the complete set of nuclear deoxyribonucleic acid [DNA] within a single cell of an organism). Genomic instability encompasses mutations, deletions, and dysfunction of DNA, mitochondrial (mt)DNA, and processes associated with maintaining nuclear architecture (Lopez-Otin et al., 2013). Genomic instability and damage can occur from intrinsic or extrinsic stressors. Intrinsic stressors may include DNA replication errors, spontaneous hydrolytic reactions, and reactive oxygen species (ROS); extrinsic stressors may arise due to physical, chemical, and biological agents (Lopez-Otin et al., 2013). Genomic damage due to these stressors may include point mutations, translocations, chromosomal gains and losses, telomere shortening, and gene disruption caused by the integration of viruses or transposons. Numerous

premature aging diseases, such as Werner syndrome, Bloom syndrome, and progeria syndromes are the consequences of increased DNA damage accumulation (Lopez-Otin et al., 2013). DNA damage may affect gene functioning, possibly resulting in dysfunctional cells that—if not eliminated via apoptosis or senescence—may adversely affect organismal homeostasis and tissue functioning. Mice overexpressing BubR1, a mitotic/cell division checkpoint component that ensures the accurate segregation of chromosomes, exhibit an extended life span (Baker et al., 2013). Damage to mtDNA is associated with aging. Clinical evidence supporting the role of mtDNA damage in processes of aging come from multisystem disorders caused by mutations (Lopez-Otin et al., 2013). Preclinical evidence supporting this model comes from mice deficient in mtDNA polymerase γ, an enzyme critical for mtDNA maintenance (Vermulst et al., 2008). These mice exhibit premature aging in associated with elevated random point mutations and mtDNA deletions (Vermulst et al., 2008). Defects in the nuclear lamina, an important functional component within the nucleus helping to maintain genomic instability, are also associated with accelerated aging (see, for review, Lopez-Otin et al., 2013).

Telomere Attrition

Telomeres play an important role in cell fate and are particularly susceptible to age-related deterioration; telomere shortening is associated with aging in rodent and human populations (Aubert & Lansdorp, 2008). The telomere is a compound structure at the end of a chromosome. The telomere is a region of repetitive nucleotide sequences at each end of a chromatid with a function of protecting the end of the chromosome from deterioration or fusion with neighboring chromosomes. Telomerase, a specialized DNA reverse transcriptase, functions to replicate the terminal ends of the telomere, and has a critical role in cellular senescence. Genetically modified rodent models have found associations between telomere length, cellular senescence, and organismal aging—that is, mice with shortened or lengthened telomeres exhibit decreased or increased life span, respectively (Lopez-Otin et al., 2013). Telomerase deficiency in humans is associated with the premature development of diseases associated with a loss of regenerative capacity of various tissues, such as pulmonary fibrosis, dyskeratosis congenita, and aplastic anemia (Lopez-Otin et al., 2013). Premature aging in telomerase-deficient mice can be reversed when telomerase is genetically reactivated (Jaskelioff et al., 2011).

Epigenetic Alterations

Epigenetics refers to the study of changes in our genome that occur without altering DNA coding. In aging, epigenetic alterations may include histone modifications, DNA methylation, chromatin remodeling, and transcriptional alterations (Lopez-Otin et al., 2013). Histones are found in the nucleus and help condense DNA into a smaller volume, by forming molecular complexes around which the DNA winds. Histone methylation determines gene activity and is a hallmark of aging. Fly and nematode models suggest that deletion of histone methylation complexes extend life span (Lopez-Otin et al., 2013). Histone demethylases modulate life span by targeting important longevity-related pathways such as the insulin/insulin-like growth factor-1 signaling pathway (Jin et al., 2011). Sirtuin proteins, deacylase enzymes, have been shown to contribute to healthy aging in mammals. For example, SIRT6

extends life span likely via beneficial effects including improving genomic stability, NF-κB signaling, and glucose homeostasis via histone H3K9 deacetlyation (Kanfi et al., 2012). DNA methylation is found in cells from patients and mice with progeroid/early aging syndromes; however, at present there is no direct experimental evidence to demonstrate prolonged life span with altered patterns of DNA methylation (Lopez-Otin et al., 2013). Global heterochromatin loss and redistribution is a characteristic feature of aging that results from complex epigenetic processes. Heterochromatin has been associated with several functions, from gene regulation to the protection of the integrity of chromosomes. One possible process affecting chromatin modeling is a failure of heterochromatin assembly, causing genomic instability, due to failure of trimethylation of histones H3K0 and H4K20, as well as heterochromatin protein 1α binding (Schotta et al., 2004). A variety of transcriptional alterations occur in aging—these include aberrant production and maturation of mRNAs and non-coding RNAs as well as miRNAs (Lopez-Otin et al., 2013).

Loss of Proteostasis

Proteostasis is the portmanteau of "protein homeostasis." Proteostasis involves biological pathways and processes within cells that control the generation, folding, transport, and degradation of proteins both inside and outside the cells. Aging is associated with impaired proteostasis. Dysfunctional systems and proteins relevant to proteostasis include heat-shock proteins, chaperones, and proteolysis malfunction, and may result in misfolding, protein accumulation, and resultant toxicity (Lopez-Otin et al., 2013). Mice deficient in various co-chaperones of the heat-shock family exhibit accelerated-aging phenotypes (Swindell et al., 2009), whereas activation of the transcription factor heat shock protein-1, a regulator of the heat-shock response, increases longevity in nematodes (Chiang, Ching, Lee, Mousigian, & Hsu, 2012). The autophagy-lysosomal system and the ubiquitin-proteasome system are noted to decline with aging (Lopez-Otin et al., 2013). The induction of macroautophagy with rapamycin and spermidine, pharmacological compounds, are shown to promote longevity in yeast and flies (Lopez-Otin et al., 2013), with minimal evidence available for these effects in mammalian species. Experimental enhancement of proteasome activity by a number of compounds has been shown to increase clearance of toxic proteins in cell culture (Morimoto & Cuervo, 2014).

Mitochondrial Dysfunction

Mitochondria are membrane-bound organelles found in most cells of the body, and they are involved in adenosine triphosphate (ATP) generation (an integral component of intracellular energy transfer). With aging, the efficacy of the respiratory chain tends to diminish; thus there is increased electron leakage and reducing ATP production. Key factors involved in this age-related dysfunction include ROS, accumulation of mutations and deletions in mtDNA, destabilization of the respiratory chain, changes in the composition of mitochondrial membranes, and defective mitophagy (Lopez-Otin et al., 2013). ROS creation was initially believed to be associated with mitochondrial deterioration and global cellular damage, and hence associated with age-related cellular dysfunction. However, recent work has found that ROS actually does not affect life span in rodents and actually extends the life span of yeast and C. elegans (Hekimi, Lapointe, & Wen, 2011). These lines of evidence can be harmonized if ROS is seen as a stress-elicited survival signal aimed at compensating for the progressive deterioration associated with aging (Hekimi et al., 2011). As age advances, ROS levels increase in order to maintain survival until they negate their original purpose and eventually aggravate rather than alleviate age-associated damage (Hekimi et al., 2011). Sirtuins, mentioned previously, may act as metabolic sensors to control mitochondrial function and may protect against age-related dysfunction. For example, SIRT1 modulates mitochondrial biogenesis through a process involving peroxisome proliferator-activated receptor-gamma coactivator (PGC)-1α, a transcriptional co-activator, and the removal of damaged mitochondria by autophagy (Lee et al., 2008).

Chronic Inflammation

Inflammaging is a low-grade, chronic pro-inflammatory phenotype known to accompany aging in mammals. This inflammation may arise from the accumulation of tissue damage, dysfunctional immune cells, senescent cells secreting pro-inflammatory cytokines, the enhanced activation of NF-κB, or defective autophagy (Lopez-Otin et al., 2013). NF-κB inhibition via genetic or pharmacological approaches is shown to prevent age-associated features in aging-related mouse models. The mRNA decay factor AUF1, which mediates cytokine mRNA degradation, may be involved in aging-related pathology. AUF1-deficient mice demonstrated marked cellular senescence and a premature aging phenotype that can be pharmacologically rescued (Pont, Sadri, Hsiao, Smith, & Schneider, 2012). SIRT1 may prevent inflammatory responses in mice (Lopez-Otin et al., 2013), possibly via down-regulating inflammation-related genes by deacetylating histones and NF-κB (Xie, Zhang, & Zhang, 2013). Interestingly, the long-term administration of the anti-inflammatory agent aspirin may increase longevity in mice (Strong et al., 2008).

Cellular Senescence

Cellular senescence is the phenomenon by which normal cells cease to divide and the cell cycle stops. A common cause of senescence is telomere shortening with other non-telomeric mechanisms also involved. Cellular senescence does contribute to aging; however, there are also physiological purposes to senescence, such as preventing the development of damaged cells (e.g., oncogenic cells or toxic cells). In aging, damage may ensue when senescent cells are not replaced, and the senescent cells may then contribute to further damage and aging. The functional decline of stem cells is an obvious characteristic of aging. Stem cell populations decline in a variety of tissues during aging, including the brain (Lopez-Otin et al., 2013). The senescence-associated secretory phenotype may confer damage to surrounding tissues via the release of pro-inflammatory cytokines and matrix metalloproteinases (Rodier & Campisi, 2011). The mitogen-controlling locus, INK4a/ARF, is robustly correlated with chronological age across tissues and species, and is linked to the highest number of age-related pathologies of any genomic locus (Jeck, Siebold, & Sharpless, 2012). This locus encodes p16[INK4a] and p19[ARF], which are tumor-suppressor proteins associated with aging. Mice with a mild and systemic increase in p16[INK4a], p19[ARF], and p53 tumor suppressors exhibit extended longevity (Matheu et al., 2007).

CAIM THERAPIES INFLUENCING THE MECHANISMS OF AGING

To this point of the chapter, a number of points are clear. First, late-life psychiatric disorders create a sizable burden of disease at the present time, and this will only increase in the future. Second, some CAIM therapies provide promising evidence in the treatment and prevention of late-life psychiatric disorders. Finally, the mechanisms of aging are an important facet of research in the goal of addressing the risk factor of aging in disease. Therefore, given the promising clinical effect of some CAIM therapies in late-life psychiatric disorders, it is important to explore how they affect, or fail to affect, the mechanisms of aging. Benefits to exploring how CAIM therapies affect the mechanisms of aging include novel treatments and diagnostic and prognostic systems; compression of morbidity; improved side-effect profiles; and benefits for cardio-metabolic, bone, and vascular health. See Figure 1.2 for a graphical representation of this topic.

In the following sections, we will summarize studies examining the effects of CAIM therapies on the mechanisms of aging.

The Effect of Mind-Body Practices on the Mechanisms of Aging

Relatively few studies have explored the effects of mind-body practices on the mechanisms of aging; however, established research shows promising findings. A recent RCT study by Black et al. (2013) examined whether yogic meditation, Kirtan Kriya Meditation (KKM), might alter the activity of inflammatory and antiviral transcription control pathways that shape immune cell gene expression, as compared to relaxing music (RM). This study was conducted for a total of 8 weeks of active intervention, with 8 weeks of follow-up, and involved 39 family dementia caregivers, mean age 60.5 years ± 28.2 years. Genome-wide transcription profiles from peripheral blood mononuclear cells (PBMCs) were examined at 0 and 8 weeks; depression was measured by the Hamilton Depression Rating Scale (HDRS). In the KKM group, 65.2% of the participants showed 50% improvement on the HDRS. In RM group, 31.2% of the participants showed 50% improvement. After adjusting for sex, illness burden, and BMI, 68 genes were differentially expressed (19 up-regulated, 49 down-regulated). Up-regulated genes included immunoglobulin-related transcripts

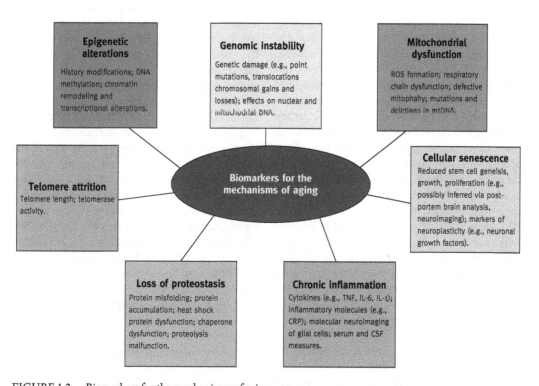

FIGURE 1.2   Biomarkers for the mechanisms of aging.

(e.g., *IGJ*, *IGLL3*). Down-regulated transcripts included pro-inflammatory cytokines (e.g., *IL8*) and activation-related immediate-early genes (e.g., *JUN*, *FOSB*). *IL-1β* and *IL-6* showed 0.94-fold reductions in KKM versus RM, whereas *TNF* showed a 1.07-fold increase. Transcript origin analyses identified plasmacytoid dendritic cells and B lymphocytes as the primary cellular context of these transcriptional alterations. Promoter-based bioinformatics analysis implicated reduced NF-κB signaling and increased IRF1 in structuring these effects. It was not possible to pinpoint the specific effects of KKM that are responsible for these biological effects (e.g., chanting, breathing, focused meditation, or mudras). Another recent study by Bhasin et al. (2013) explored the rapid genomic changes during one session of relaxation response (RR) practice among healthy practitioners with 4–20 years of RR practice versus novices with 8 weeks of RR training. RR practice is broad and may include yoga, tai chi, qi gong, meditation, and repetitive prayer. In this study, the transcriptome, RNA production, of PBMCs was measured prior to, immediately after, and 15 minutes after listening to an RR-eliciting or a health education CD. Greater gene expression changes were noted in experienced practitioners versus novices. RR practice enhanced the expression of genes associated with energy metabolism, mitochondrial function, insulin secretion, and telomere maintenance, and reduced the expression of genes linked to inflammatory response and stress-related pathways. Interactive network analyses of RR-affected pathways identified mitochondrial ATP synthase and insulin as the top up-regulated critical molecules (focus hubs) and NF-κB pathway genes as the top down-regulated focus hubs. A study by this research group (Lavretsky et al., 2013) examined the effects of brief daily yogic meditation on neuropsychological markers and immune cell telomerase activity in family dementia caregivers with mild depressive symptoms. In this study, 39 individuals (mean age 60.3 years; SD 10.2) were randomized to KKM or relaxation music for 12 minutes per day for 8 weeks. Two major genes were upregulated in PBMCs by yogic practice: *AVIL* and *Nuclear Factor Erythroid 2* (*NFE2*). AVIL may activate the directed secretion of lytic granule contents at the immunological synapse (IS), and thereby increase NK cell cytotoxicity. *NFE2* encodes a basic leucine zipper transcription factor that has an essential role in megakaryocyte maturation and platelet production; therefore yoga may have effects on megakaryocyte maturation and

platelet production. A study by Kaliman et al. (2014) compared the biological impact of 1 day of intensive mindfulness meditation on experienced subjects (min. 3 years experience; *n* = 19) versus controls with no meditation experience who engaged in leisure activities in the same environment (*n* = 21). Biological measures included PBMC expression of genes relating to circadian rhythms, chromatin modulation, and inflammation. After the intervention, meditators had reduced expression of histone deacetylase genes (*HDAC* 2, 3, and 9), alterations in global modification of histones (H4ac, H3K4me3), and decreased expression of pro-inflammatory genes (*RIPK2* and *COX2*).

The Effect of Physical Activity on the Mechanisms of Aging

Physical activity researchers have extensively explored the effects of physical activity on the mechanisms of aging; however, this is a relatively poor understanding of the unique effects of aerobic and resistance activities. A recent study by Rethorst et al. (2012) investigated the extent to which inflammatory markers can be used to predict response to exercise treatment after an incomplete response to a selective serotonin reuptake inhibitor (SSRI). This neuroimmune investigation was conducted with the cohort from the Treatment with Exercise Augmentation for Depression (TREAD) study, a randomized, parallel dose comparison trial. Incomplete response was qualified as having at least moderate residual depressive symptomatology, quantified by a 17-item HDRS score ≥ 14. This study randomized 73 participants (aged 18 to 70 years) to 12 weeks of either 4 or 16 kilocalories per kilogram of body weight per week (KWW), via aerobic PA. The study examined serum IFN-γ, IL-1β, IL-6, TNF-α and made a number of interesting findings. From a clinical perspective, both doses of exercise showed significant improvements over time ($F_{1,121} = 39.9$, $p < .0001$). Adjusted remission rates at week 12 were 28.3% versus 15.5% for the 16-KKW and 4-KKW groups, respectively. There was a trend for higher remission rates in the higher-dose exercise group ($p < 0.06$). High baseline TNF-α (> 5.493 pg/ml) was associated with a greater reduction in depressive symptoms (measured by Inventory for Depressive Symptomatology Clinical [IDS-C]). There was also a significant correlation between reductions of IL-1β and depressive symptoms in the 16-KWW group, but not the 4-KWW group. Otherwise, there was no significant change in cytokine levels following the 12-week PA intervention, and a non-significant association between PA dose and change in cytokine levels. A study by Savela et al. (2013) investigated the association between physical activity in midlife and leukocyte telomere length (LTL) in old age. The study cohort utilized was the Helsinki Businessmen Study and enrolled 782 men in 1974 (mean age 47), had them fill out a physical activity questionnaire at baseline, then followed them up after 29 years in 2003. Teleomeres were measured from the DNA of a random subcohort of survivors ($n = 204$, mean age 76 years). The moderate physical activity group had longer mean LTL (8.27 kB, SE 0.05) than the low (8.10 kB, SE 0.07), or high (8.10 kB, SE 0.05) physical activity groups ($p = 0.03$ between groups). Conversely, the proportion of short telomeres was lowest in the moderate physical activity group (11.35%, SE 0.25), and higher in the high (12.39%, SE 0.29), and the low (12.21%, SE 0.39) physical activity groups ($p = 0.02$ between groups). The difference between mean LTL of the moderate and low activity groups was 172 base pairs, corresponding to a difference of approximately 4 to 6 years in "biological age," assuming an annual mean LTL shortening of 30–40 base pairs. A study by Abubaker et al. (2013) explored the effect of 3 months of moderate intensity, aerobic and resistance exercise training on inflammatory and stress response, proteostasis markers in lean and obese adult subjects. Both PBMCs and subcutaneous adipose tissue were tested. The expression of DNAJB3, a co-chaperone member of the HSP-40, a factor important in proteostasis and the stress response, as well as JNK—and inflammatory response pathway—was reduced in obese subjects and physical activity restored the expression. DNAJB3 formed a complex with JNK, IKKβ, and HSP-72. This suggests that physical activity improved proteostasis and inflammation in obese subjects. A mouse study by Steiner et al. (Steiner, Murphy, McClellan, Carmichael, & Davis, 2011) examined the effects of exercise training on markers of both brain and muscle mitochondrial biogenesis in relation to endurance capacity. In this study, mice were assigned to an exercise group (treadmill running) or sedentary conditions for 8 weeks. Exercise training increased PGC-1α, Silent Information Regulator T 1 (SIRT1), and citrate synthase (CS) mRNA and mtDNA in most brain

regions in addition to the soleus muscle. These findings suggest that exercise increases mitochondrial biogenesis.

The Effect of Nutritional Interventions on the Mechanisms of Aging

To date, the Mediterranean and caloric restriction diets are the most thoroughly explored with respect to the mechanisms of aging, with encouraging results. A recent sub-analysis of the PREDIMED trial provides an example of a clinical trial utilizing a healthy dietary pattern and assessing inflammatory effects (Mena et al., 2009; Urpi-Sarda et al., 2012). To recap, PREDIMED was a large, parallel-group, multicenter, randomized, controlled, 5-year clinical trial that aimed to assess the effects of the Mediterranean diet on the primary prevention of cardiovascular disease for individuals aged 55–80 years. In this study, the authors analysed the effects at 3 months of two Mediterranean diet interventions supplemented with either virgin olive oil (VOO) or nuts compared with a control low-fat diet (LFD). Both Mediterranean diets showed an anti-inflammatory effect reducing serum C-reactive protein, interleukin-6 (IL6), and endothelial and monocyte adhesion molecules (i.e., E-selectin and P-selectin) and chemokines (i.e., ICAM-1 and VCAM-1), whereas these parameters increased after the LFD intervention. A study by Boccardi et al. (2013) explored the association between telomere length, telomerase activity, and different adherence to the Mediterranean diet. This cross-sectional cohort study occurred in 217 elderly subjects (mean age ~ 78 years). The high adherence group showed longer PBMC telomere length and higher telomerase activity compared to low- and medium-adherence groups. Telomerase was negatively modulated by inflammation and oxidative stress. A study by Dai et al. (2008) examined the association between the Mediterranean diet and oxidative stress in a well-controlled study of 159 twins aged 51.6 to 57 years. The oxidative stress marker used was the ratio of reduced to oxidized glutathione, a strong anti-oxidant (GSH/GSSG). A one-unit increment in the diet score was associated with a 7% higher GSH/GSSG ratio.

The best known "anti-aging" diet is the caloric restriction (CR) without malnutrition diet. This diet is the only non-genetic intervention that has consistently been found to extend both mean and maximal life span across a variety of species

(Anton & Leeuwenburgh, 2013). A recent review (Anton & Leeuwenburgh, 2013) summarizes evidence suggesting that moderate caloric restriction increases mean and maximal life span in rodents and non-human primates, as well as delaying the onset of age-associated conditions in these species such as cancer and diabetes. In overweight humans, there is evidence to suggest that caloric restriction reduces several cardiac risk factors, improves insulin sensitivity, and enhances mitochondrial function (Anton & Leeuwenburgh, 2013). Biological investigations suggest this diet may exert its effects by reducing oxidative damage to both DNA and RNA in PBMCs, as well as mitochondrial biogenesis, enhanced cellular quality control through autophagy, and improved functioning of the ubiquitin-proteosome system (Anton & Leeuwenburgh, 2013). There is currently no large-scale evidence supporting the use of caloric restriction on markers of aging in non-overweight human populations; however, the CALERIE phase 2 study is now underway to explore this issue (Rochon et al., 2011). This study is examining the long-term effects of a 25% reduction of ad libitum energy intake in non-obese, middle-aged men and women (21–50 years) on markers of aging, cardiovascular disease risk, insulin sensitivity and secretion, immune function, neuroendocrine function, quality of life, and cognitive function.

The Effect of Natural Products on the Mechanisms of Aging

A number of natural products stand out for their effects on the mechanisms of aging, including Ω3 PUFAs, zinc, curcumin, B vitamins, and vitamin D. In this section, we will focus on Ω3 PUFAs. A significant number of analyses of the biological effects of Ω3 PUFAs come from the OmegAD study (Freund-Levi et al., 2006). The OmegAD study was a randomized controlled trial of 174 patients with mild to moderate AD and compared 1.7g Docosahexaenoic acid (DHA) and 0.6g eicosapentaenoic acid (EPA) to a placebo for 6 months (Freund-Levi et al., 2006). In a subset of 23 subjects from the OmegAD study, Ω-3 PUFA supplementation was found to reduce the in vitro PBMC expression of IL-1β and IL-6, but not TNF-α, in response to lipopolysaccharide (LPS) stimulation (Vedin et al., 2008). In another subset involving 21 subjects of the OmegAD study, plasma Ω-3 PUFA concentration was inversely correlated with in vitro PBMC expression of prostaglandin (PG)-$F_{2\alpha}$ in response to LPS (Vedin et al., 2010). $PGF_{2\alpha}$ is a known metabolite and surrogate marker of PGE_2, which is thought to enhance immune and inflammatory reactivity through inducing pro-stimulatory molecules of the TNF cytokine/receptor family (Vedin et al., 2010). Furthermore, in yet another OmegAD subset study of 16 subjects, Ω-3 PUFA supplementation was demonstrated to up- and down-regulate the PBMC expression of a multitude of genes (Vedin et al., 2012). Up-regulated genes included MS4A3, NAIP, DRG1, CD63, HSD17B11, RAB27A, CASP4, SUPT4H1, UBE2V1. Down-regulated genes included RHOB, VCP, LOC399491, ZNF24, SORL1, MANA2A1, PARP1, SSRP1, ARIH1, and ANAPC5. Overall, these genes might influence a variety of processes including inflammation regulation, neurodegeneration, and ubiquitination. An in vitro study by Mizwicki et al. (2013) found that soluble Aβ administration increased the secretion of cytokines (e.g., IL-1 and IL-6) and chemokines (e.g., CCLs and CXCLs) from PBMCs extracted from five AD patients and three controls. The authors report that resolvin D1 (a derivative of DHA) administration improved the phagocytosis of Aβ and inhibited fibrillar Aβ-induced apoptosis, while reversing most of the pro-inflammatory cytokine secretion. A recent study by Farzaneh-Far et al. (Farzaneh-Far et al., 2010) investigated the association between Ω-3 PUFA bloods levels with telomere length in a 5-year prospective cohort study of 608 ambulatory outpatients with stable coronary heart disease, mean age ~ 65 years. Individuals in the lowest quartile of DHA+EPA experienced the fastest rate of telomere shortening (0.13 telomere-to-single-copy gene ratio [T/S] units over 5 years; 95% CI, 0.09–0.17), whereas those in the highest quartile experienced the slowest rate of telomere shortening shortening (0.05 T/S units over 5 years; 95% CI, 0.02–0.08; $p < .001$ for linear trend across quartiles). Each 1-SD increase in DHA+EPA levels was associated with a 32% reduction in the odds of telomere shortening (adjusted odds ratio, 0.68; 95% CI, 0.47–0.98).

RECOMMENDATIONS FOR THIS FIELD

The field exploring the effects of CAIM therapies on the mechanisms of aging is promising and requires further systematic, empirical research. At present, given the large number of treatment modalities and the novelty of the area, more quality data is needed. Important considerations in clinical studies include careful and expert design with high clinical trials standards, control groups, clear and robust endpoints, appropriate sample sizes, and so on. In this field, careful consideration must be given to manufacturing control of botanical and non-botanical natural products to ensure safety and consistency in products. Clearly, in the area of psychiatry, given the limitations of biological analyses in human populations, clinical neuroimaging modalities and rodent models must be effectively utilized to ensure a detailed understanding of neurobiology. Examples of neuroimaging modalities for chronic inflammation include microglia-related positron emission tomography (PET) ligands. Neuroimaging biomarkers for telomere health and cellular senescence include structural MRI imaging. In rodent models, in vivo studies with gain- or loss-of-function models are necessary. Moving forward, the field must be clear as to the veracity of the proposed mechanisms of aging. It is clear that there are some mechanisms absolutely core to aging, such as DNA damage; however, there are other mechanisms whose function depends on their level of intensity. For example, high-level acute inflammation may be neuroprotective, whereas chronic, low-grade inflammation is likely neurodegenerative.

SUMMARY

As the world's population ages and late-life psychiatric disorders become more prevalent, novel therapies are required to treat and prevent illness. It is hoped that understanding the impact of CAIM therapies on the fundamental mechanisms of aging will lead to therapeutic developments in the future. Robust and systematic empirical research is needed to develop this field.

REFERENCES

Abbott, R., & Lavretsky, H. (2013). Tai chi and gigong for the treatment and prevention of mental disorders. *Psychiatr Clin N Am*, 36(1), 109–119. doi: 10.1016/j.psc.2013.01.011

Abubaker, J., Tiss, A., Abu-Farha, M., Al-Ghimlas, F., Al-Khairi, I., Baturcam, E., . . . Dehbi, M. (2013). DNAJB3/HSP-40 cochaperone is downregulated in obese humans and is restored by physical exercise. *PLoS One*, 8(7), e69217. doi: 10.1371/journal.pone.0069217

ADI. (2013). *World Alzheimer Report: journal of caring: an analysis of long-term care for dementia.* London: Alzheimer's Disease International.

Almeida, O. P., Marsh, K., Alfonso, H., Flicker, L., Davis, T. M., & Hankey, G. J. (2010). B-vitamins reduce the long-term risk of depression after stroke: the VITATOPS-DEP trial. *Ann Neurol*, 68(4), 503–510. doi: 10.1002/ana.22189

Anton, S., & Leeuwenburgh, C. (2013). Fasting or caloric restriction for healthy aging. *Exp Gerontol*, 48(10), 1003–1005. doi: 10.1016/j.exger.2013.04.011

Arcury, T. A., Nguyen, H. T., Sandberg, J. C., Neiberg, R. H., Altizer, K. P., Bell, R. A., . . . Quandt, S. A. (2013). Use of complementary therapies for health promotion among older adults. *J Appl Gerontol*. 2015 August; 34(5): 552–572 doi: 10.1177/0733464813495109

Aubert, G., & Lansdorp, P. M. (2008). Telomeres and aging. *Physiol Rev*, 88(2), 557–579. doi: 10.1152/physrev.00026.2007

Baker, D. J., Dawlaty, M. M., Wijshake, T., Jeganathan, K. B., Malureanu, L., van Ree, J. H., . . . van Deursen, J. M. (2013). Increased expression of BubR1 protects against aneuploidy and cancer and extends healthy lifespan. *Nat Cell Biol*, 15(1), 96–102. doi: 10.1038/ncb2643

Baxter, A. J., Vos, T., Scott, K. M., Ferrari, A. J., & Whiteford, H. A. (2014). The global burden of anxiety disorders in 2010. *Psychol Med*, 44(11):2363–2374. doi: 10.1017/S0033291713003243

Bhasin, M. K., Dusek, J. A., Chang, B. H., Joseph, M. G., Denninger, J. W., Fricchione, G. L., . . . Libermann, T. A. (2013). Relaxation response induces temporal transcriptome changes in energy metabolism, insulin secretion and inflammatory pathways. *PLoS One*, 8(5), e62817. doi: 10.1371/journal.pone.0062817

Black, D. S., Cole, S. W., Irwin, M. R., Breen, E., St Cyr, N. M., Nazarian, N., . . . Lavretsky, H. (2013). Yogic meditation reverses NF-kappaB and IRF-related transcriptome dynamics in leukocytes of family dementia caregivers in a randomized controlled trial. *Psychoneuroendocrinology*, 38(3), 348–355. doi: 10.1016/j.psyneuen.2012.06.011

Blake, H., Mo, P., Malik, S., & Thomas, S. (2009). How effective are physical activity interventions for alleviating depressive symptoms in older people? A systematic review. *Clin Rehabil*, 23(10), 873–887. doi: 10.1177/0269215509337449

Boccardi, V., Esposito, A., Rizzo, M. R., Marfella, R., Barbieri, M., & Paolisso, G. (2013). Mediterranean diet, telomere maintenance and health status among elderly. *PLoS One, 8*(4), e62781. doi: 10.1371/journal.pone.0062781

Brown, B. M., Peiffer, J. J., & Martins, R. N. (2013). Multiple effects of physical activity on molecular and cognitive signs of brain aging: can exercise slow neurodegeneration and delay Alzheimer's disease? *Mol Psychiatry, 18*(8), 864–874. doi: 10.1038/mp.2012.162

Burch, J. B., Augustine, A. D., Frieden, L. A., Hadley, E., Howcroft, T. K., Johnson, R., . . . Wise, B. C. (2014). Advances in geroscience: impact on healthspan and chronic disease. *J Gerontol A Biol Sci Med Sci, 69*(Suppl 1), S1–3. doi: 10.1093/gerona/glu041

Chiang, W. C., Ching, T. T., Lee, H. C., Mousigian, C., & Hsu, A. L. (2012). HSF-1 regulators DDL-1/2 link insulin-like signaling to heat-shock responses and modulation of longevity. *Cell, 148*(1–2), 322–334. doi: 10.1016/j.cell.2011.12.019

Dai, J., Jones, D. P., Goldberg, J., Ziegler, T. R., Bostick, R. M., Wilson, P. W., . . . Vaccarino, V. (2008). Association between adherence to the Mediterranean diet and oxidative stress. *Am J Clin Nutr, 88*(5), 1364–1370.

Farzaneh-Far, R., Lin, J., Epel, E. S., Harris, W. S., Blackburn, E. H., & Whooley, M. A. (2010). Association of marine omega-3 fatty acid levels with telomeric aging in patients with coronary heart disease. *JAMA, 303*(3), 250–257. doi: 10.1001/jama.2009.2008

Ferrari, A. J., Charlson, F. J., Norman, R. E., Patten, S. B., Freedman, G., Murray, C. J., . . . Whiteford, H. A. (2013). Burden of depressive disorders by country, sex, age, and year: findings from the global burden of disease study 2010. *PLoS Med, 10*(11), e1001547. doi: 10.1371/journal.pmed.1001547

Freund-Levi, Y., Eriksdotter-Jonhagen, M., Cederholm, T., Basun, H., Faxen-Irving, G., Garlind, A., . . . Palmblad, J. (2006). Omega-3 fatty acid treatment in 174 patients with mild to moderate Alzheimer disease: OmegAD study: a randomized double-blind trial. *Arch Neurol, 63*(10), 1402–1408. doi: 10.1001/archneur.63.10.1402

Gates, N., Fiatarone Singh, M. A., Sachdev, P. S., & Valenzuela, M. (2013). The effect of exercise training on cognitive function in older adults with mild cognitive impairment: a meta-analysis of randomized controlled trials. *Am J Geriatr Psychiatry, 21*(11), 1086–1097. doi: 10.1016/j.jagp.2013.02.018

Harris, P. E., Cooper, K. L., Relton, C., & Thomas, K. J. (2012). Prevalence of complementary and alternative medicine (CAM) use by the general population: a systematic review and update. *Int J Clin Pract, 66*(10), 924–939. doi: 10.1111/j.1742-1241.2012.02945.x

Hekimi, S., Lapointe, J., & Wen, Y. (2011). Taking a "good" look at free radicals in the aging process. *Trends Cell Biol, 21*(10), 569–576. doi: 10.1016/j.tcb.2011.06.008

Ho, T. F., Rowland-Seymour, A., Frankel, E. S., Li, S. Q., & Mao, J. J. (2014). Generational differences in complementary and alternative medicine (CAM) use in the context of chronic diseases and pain: baby boomers versus the silent generation. *J Am Board Fam Med, 27*(4), 465–473. doi: 10.3122/jabfm.2014.04.130238

Hodge, A., Almeida, O. P., English, D. R., Giles, G. G., & Flicker, L. (2013). Patterns of dietary intake and psychological distress in older Australians: benefits not just from a Mediterranean diet. *Int Psychogeriatr, 25*(3), 456–466. doi: 10.1017/S1041610212001986

Jaskelioff, M., Muller, F. L., Paik, J. H., Thomas, E., Jiang, S., Adams, A. C., . . . Depinho, R. A. (2011). Telomerase reactivation reverses tissue degeneration in aged telomerase-deficient mice. *Nature, 469*(7328), 102–106. doi: 10.1038/nature09603

Jeck, W. R., Siebold, A. P., & Sharpless, N. E. (2012). Review: a meta-analysis of GWAS and age-associated diseases. *Aging Cell, 11*(5), 727–731. doi: 10.1111/j.1474-9726.2012.00871.x

Jin, C., Li, J., Green, C. D., Yu, X., Tang, X., Han, D., . . . Han, J. D. (2011). Histone demethylase UTX-1 regulates C. elegans life span by targeting the insulin/IGF-1 signaling pathway. *Cell Metab, 14*(2), 161–172. doi: 10.1016/j.cmet.2011.07.001

Kaliman, P., Alvarez-Lopez, M. J., Cosin-Tomas, M., Rosenkranz, M. A., Lutz, A., & Davidson, R. J. (2014). Rapid changes in histone deacetylases and inflammatory gene expression in expert meditators. *Psychoneuroendocrinology, 40*, 96–107. doi: 10.1016/j.psyneuen.2013.11.004

Kanfi, Y., Naiman, S., Amir, G., Peshti, V., Zinman, G., Nahum, L., . . . Cohen, H. Y. (2012). The sirtuin SIRT6 regulates lifespan in male mice. *Nature, 483*(7388), 218–221. doi: 10.1038/nature10815

Kok, R. M. (2013). What is the role of medications in late life depression? *Psychiatr Clin N Am, 36*(4), 597–605. doi: 10.1016/j.psc.2013.08.006

Kok, R. M., Nolen, W. A., & Heeren, T. J. (2012). Efficacy of treatment in older depressed patients: a systematic review and meta-analysis of double-blind randomized controlled trials with antidepressants. *J Affect Disord, 141*(2–3), 103–115. doi: 10.1016/j.jad.2012.02.036

Lavretsky, H., Alstein, L. L., Olmstead, R. E., Ercoli, L. M., Riparetti-Brown, M., Cyr, N. S., &

Irwin, M. R. (2011). Complementary use of tai chi chih augments escitalopram treatment of geriatric depression: a randomized controlled trial. *Am J Geriatr Psychiatry, 19*(10), 839–850. doi: 10.1097/JGP.0b013e31820ee9ef

Lavretsky, H., Epel, E. S., Siddarth, P., Nazarian, N., Cyr, N. S., Khalsa, D. S., . . . Irwin, M. R. (2013). A pilot study of yogic meditation for family dementia caregivers with depressive symptoms: effects on mental health, cognition, and telomerase activity. *Int J Geriatr Psychiatry, 28*(1), 57–65. doi: 10.1002/gps.3790

Lee, I. H., Cao, L., Mostoslavsky, R., Lombard, D. B., Liu, J., Bruns, N. E., . . . Finkel, T. (2008). A role for the NAD-dependent deacetylase Sirt1 in the regulation of autophagy. *Proc Natl Acad Sci U S A, 105*(9), 3374–3379. doi: 10.1073/pnas.0712145105

Lopez-Otin, C., Blasco, M. A., Partridge, L., Serrano, M., & Kroemer, G. (2013). The hallmarks of aging. *Cell, 153*(6), 1194–1217. doi: 10.1016/j.cell.2013.05.039

Martinez-Lapiscina, E. H., Clavero, P., Toledo, E., Estruch, R., Salas-Salvado, J., San Julian, B., . . . Martinez-Gonzalez, M. A. (2013). Mediterranean diet improves cognition: the PREDIMED-NAVARRA randomised trial. *J Neurol Neurosurg Psychiatry, 84*(12):1318–1325. doi: 10.1136/jnnp-2012-304792

Matheu, A., Maraver, A., Klatt, P., Flores, I., Garcia-Cao, I., Borras, C., . . . Serrano, M. (2007). Delayed ageing through damage protection by the Arf/p53 pathway. *Nature, 448*(7151), 375–379. doi: 10.1038/nature05949

Mena, M. P., Sacanella, E., Vazquez-Agell, M., Morales, M., Fito, M., Escoda, R., . . . Estruch, R. (2009). Inhibition of circulating immune cell activation: a molecular antiinflammatory effect of the Mediterranean diet. *Am J Clin Nutr, 89*(1), 248–256. doi: 10.3945/ajcn.2008.26094

Mizwicki, M. T., Liu, G., Fiala, M., Magpantay, L., Sayre, J., Siani, A., . . . Teplow, D. B. (2013). 1alpha,25-dihydroxyvitamin D3 and resolvin D1 retune the balance between amyloid-beta phagocytosis and inflammation in Alzheimer's disease patients. *J Alzheimers Dis, 34*(1), 155–170. doi: 10.3233/JAD-121735

Morimoto, R. I., & Cuervo, A. M. (2014). Proteostasis and the aging proteome in health and disease. *J Gerontol A Biol Sci Med Sci, 69 Suppl 1,* S33–38. doi: 10.1093/gerona/glu049

Oberg, E. B., Thomas, M. S., McCarty, M., Berg, J., Burlingham, B., & Bradley, R. (2014). Older adults' perspectives on naturopathic medicine's impact on healthy aging. *Explore (NY), 10*(1), 34–43. doi: 10.1016/j.explore.2013.10.003

Pollock, B. G. (2004). Pharmacokinetics and pharmacodynamics in late life. In H. A. Sackein (Ed.), *Late-life depression* (pp. 185–191). New York: Oxford University Press.

Pont, A. R., Sadri, N., Hsiao, S. J., Smith, S., & Schneider, R. J. (2012). mRNA decay factor AUF1 maintains normal aging, telomere maintenance, and suppression of senescence by activation of telomerase transcription. *Mol Cell, 47*(1), 5–15. doi: 10.1016/j.molcel.2012.04.019

Psaltopoulou, T., Sergentanis, T. N., Panagiotakos, D. B., Sergentanis, I. N., Kosti, R., & Scarmeas, N. (2013). Mediterranean diet, stroke, cognitive impairment, and depression: a meta-analysis. *Ann Neurol, 74*(4), 580–591. doi: 10.1002/ana.23944

Rethorst, C. D., Toups, M. S., Greer, T. L., Nakonezny, P. A., Carmody, T. J., Grannemann, B. D., . . . Trivedi, M. H. (2012). Pro-inflammatory cytokines as predictors of antidepressant effects of exercise in major depressive disorder. *Mol Psychiatry.* doi: 10.1038/mp.2012.125

Rochon, J., Bales, C. W., Ravussin, E., Redman, L. M., Holloszy, J. O., Racette, S. B., . . . Group, C. S. (2011). Design and conduct of the CALERIE study: comprehensive assessment of the long-term effects of reducing intake of energy. *J Gerontol A Biol Sci Med Sci, 66*(1), 97–108. doi: 10.1093/gerona/glq168

Rodier, F., & Campisi, J. (2011). Four faces of cellular senescence. *J Cell Biol, 192*(4), 547–556. doi: 10.1083/jcb.201009094

Savela, S., Saijonmaa, O., Strandberg, T. E., Koistinen, P., Strandberg, A. Y., Tilvis, R. S., . . . Fyhrquist, F. (2013). Physical activity in midlife and telomere length measured in old age. *Exp Gerontol, 48*(1), 81–84. doi: 10.1016/j.exger.2012.02.003

Schotta, G., Lachner, M., Sarma, K., Ebert, A., Sengupta, R., Reuter, G., . . . Jenuwein, T. (2004). A silencing pathway to induce H3-K9 and H4-K20 trimethylation at constitutive heterochromatin. *Genes Dev, 18*(11), 1251–1262. doi: 10.1101/gad.300704

Shahidi, M., Mojtahed, A., Modabbernia, A., Mojtahed, M., Shafiabady, A., Delavar, A., & Honari, H. (2011). Laughter yoga versus group exercise program in elderly depressed women: a randomized controlled trial. *Int J Geriatr Psychiatry, 26*(3), 322–327. doi: 10.1002/gps.2545

Steiner, J. L., Murphy, E. A., McClellan, J. L., Carmichael, M. D., & Davis, J. M. (2011). Exercise training increases mitochondrial biogenesis in the brain. *J Appl Physiol, 111*(4), 1066–1071. doi: 10.1152/japplphysiol.00343.2011

Strong, R., Miller, R. A., Astle, C. M., Floyd, R. A., Flurkey, K., Hensley, K. L., . . . Harrison, D. E. (2008). Nordihydroguaiaretic acid and aspirin increase lifespan of genetically heterogeneous male mice. *Aging Cell, 7*(5), 641–650. doi: 10.1111/j.1474-9726.2008.00414.x

Swindell, W. R., Masternak, M. M., Kopchick, J. J., Conover, C. A., Bartke, A., & Miller, R. A. (2009). Endocrine regulation of heat shock protein mRNA levels in long-lived dwarf mice. *Mech Ageing Dev, 130*(6), 393–400. doi: 10.1016/j.mad.2009.03.004

Sydenham, E., Dangour, A. D., & Lim, W. S. (2012). Omega 3 fatty acid for the prevention of cognitive decline and dementia. *Cochrane Database Syst Rev, 6*, CD005379. doi: 10.1002/14651858. CD005379.pub3

UN. (2013). World Population Ageing 2013. In Department of Economic and Social Affairs, Population Division (2013). World Population Ageing 2013. ST/ESA/SER.A/348.

Urpi-Sarda, M., Casas, R., Chiva-Blanch, G., Romero-Mamani, E. S., Valderas-Martinez, P., Arranz, S., . . . Estruch, R. (2012). Virgin olive oil and nuts as key foods of the Mediterranean diet effects on inflammatory biomakers related to atherosclerosis. *Pharmacol Res, 65*(6), 577–583. doi: 10.1016/j.phrs.2012.03.006

Varteresian, T., & Lavretsky, H. (2014). Natural products and supplements for geriatric depression and cognitive disorders: an evaluation of the research. *Curr Psychiatry Rep, 16*(8), 456. doi: 10.1007/s11920-014-0456-x

Varteresian, T., Merrill, D., & Lavretsky, H. (2013). The use of natural products and supplements in late-life mood and cognitive disorders. *Focus: Psychiatry, 11*(1), 15–21.

Vedin, I., Cederholm, T., Freund-Levi, Y., Basun, H., Garlind, A., Irving, G. F., . . . Palmblad, J. (2012). Effects of DHA-rich n-3 fatty acid supplementation on gene expression in blood mononuclear leukocytes: the OmegAD study. *PLoS One, 7*(4), e35425. doi: 10.1371/journal. pone.0035425

Vedin, I., Cederholm, T., Freund Levi, Y., Basun, H., Garlind, A., Faxen Irving, G., . . . Palmblad, J. (2008). Effects of docosahexaenoic acid-rich n-3 fatty acid supplementation on cytokine release from blood mononuclear leukocytes: the OmegAD study. *Am J Clin Nutr, 87*(6), 1616–1622.

Vedin, I., Cederholm, T., Freund-Levi, Y., Basun, H., Hjorth, E., Irving, G. F., . . . Palmblad, J. (2010). Reduced prostaglandin F2 alpha release from blood mononuclear leukocytes after oral supplementation of omega3 fatty acids: the OmegAD study. *J Lipid Res, 51*(5), 1179–1185. doi: 10.1194/jlr.M002667

Vermulst, M., Wanagat, J., Kujoth, G. C., Bielas, J. H., Rabinovitch, P. S., Prolla, T. A., & Loeb, L. A. (2008). DNA deletions and clonal mutations drive premature aging in mitochondrial mutator mice. *Nat Genet, 40*(4), 392–394. doi: 10.1038/ng.95

Walker, J. G., Mackinnon, A. J., Batterham, P., Jorm, A. F., Hickie, I., McCarthy, A., . . . Christensen, H. (2010). Mental health literacy, folic acid and vitamin B12, and physical activity for the prevention of depression in older adults: randomised controlled trial. *Br J Psychiatry, 197*(1), 45–54. doi: 10.1192/bjp.bp.109.075291

Wolitzky-Taylor, K. B., Castriotta, N., Lenze, E. J., Stanley, M. A., & Craske, M. G. (2010). Anxiety disorders in older adults: a comprehensive review. *Depress Anxiety, 27*(2), 190–211. doi: 10.1002/da.20653

Wu, Y., Wang, Y., Burgess, E. O., & Wu, J. (2013). The effects of Tai Chi exercise on cognitive function in older adults: a meta-analysis. *J Sport Health Sci, 2*(4), 193–203. doi: 10.1016/j.jshs.2013.09.001

Xie, J., Zhang, X., & Zhang, L. (2013). Negative regulation of inflammation by SIRT1. *Pharmacol Res, 67*(1), 60–67. doi: 10.1016/j.phrs.2012.10.010

SECTION B

RESEARCH METHODOLOGY AND THE RESEARCH AGENDA IN DEVELOPING INTEGRATIVE INTERVENTIONS FOR OLDER ADULTS

2

METHODOLOGICAL CHALLENGES IN DEVELOPING AND DELIVERING PREVENTIVE HEALTH INTERVENTIONS FOR MENTAL HEALTH AND AGING

James O. Prochaska and Janice M. Prochaska

THE CHALLENGE

A major challenge facing the field of prevention is how to most effectively change multiple health risk behaviors to prevent heart disease, diabetes, cancer, and other chronic diseases. Populations with co-occurring multiple health behavior risks suffer greater morbidity, disability, and premature mortality (Doll, Peto, Boreham & Sutherland, 2004; Khaw et al., 2008; Kvaavik Batty, Ursin, Huxley & Gale, 2010; Mokdad, Marks, Stroup, & Gerberding, 2004). The majority of the US population has co-occurring multiple behavioral risks (Fine, Philogene, Gramling, Coups, & Sinha, 2004; Poortinga, 2007). The challenge with aging populations and those with severe mental illness (SMI) is even greater, where most have multiple modifiable risks. The presence of multiple risk behaviors has a negative synergistic influence on health. For example, with tobacco and alcohol use, the risk of head and neck cancers is multiplied beyond the sum of the two risks individually (Allison et al., 1999; McElroy, 2002). A poor diet and being physically inactive greatly increases the likelihood of cancer, diabetes, and cardiovascular disease (Irwin & Mayne, 2008; USDHHS, 1996).

Excess risks also lead to excess costs. Modifiable health risks such as tobacco use and overweight status are associated with short-term increases in both the likelihood and magnitude of incurring health expenditures (Goetzel et al., 1998). Effectively treating two behaviors in an individual reduces medical costs by about $2,000 per year (Edington, 2001). Consequently, multiple health behavior change (MHBC) offers the potential for increased health benefits, maximized disease prevention, and reduced healthcare costs. Of special significance is that the development of multiple health-risk behaviors begins at younger ages in populations with SMI, who have dramatic decreases in longevity with adults dying an average of 11 years earlier than adults with no mental disorders (Druss, Zhao, Von Esenwein, Morrato, & Marcus, 2011). Also of special significance is that besides the number of risk behaviors, age is the other major driver of poorer health and increased healthcare costs, so changing multiple risks in older adults can have an even greater impact on health and healthcare costs.

In recent years, there has been a dramatic increase in MHBC research as a result of the funding initiatives of the National Institutes of Health (NIH) and foundations (Prochaska & Prochaska, 2011). For example, our innovative research applying computer-tailored interventions (CTIs) based on the Transtheoretical Model of Behavior Change (TTM) to simultaneously treat multiple behaviors has produced unprecedented impacts with adolescents and adults (Johnson et al., 2008; Prochaska et al., 2004; Prochaska et al., 2005; Prochaska et al., 2008). Our CTIs have had clinically significant impacts across a broad range of populations. These include populations that are often perceived as not having the same ability to change risk behaviors. Older adults, for example, are often stereotyped as "old dogs who cannot be taught new tricks." Across our population-based randomized controlled trials, smokers over 65 whom we treated had the highest abstinence rates at long-term follow-ups (Velicer, Redding, Sun & Prochaska, 2007). The Surgeon General's Report on adolescent smokers concluded in one page that such populations would not participate in cessation programs and if they did, they would not quit. Collaborating with partners at Kaiser Permanente, we found that 65% of teens in primary care practices would participate, and their abstinence rates of 25% were comparable to ordinary adult smokers (Hollis et al., 2005). With African-American smokers and with Hispanic smokers, we produced abstinence rates that were higher than non-Hispanic Caucasians (Velicer et al., 2007). These results suggest that the issue may not be the ability to change, but rather access to quality change programs.

Of particular importance are the results produced with smokers with mental disorders. Smokers attending clinics for depression were proactively recruited to cessation treatments that integrated our CTIs plus counseling, delivered first in the clinic and then via telephone. The long-term abstinence rates of 26.7% were surprisingly comparable to our average population outcomes (Hall et al., 2006). Also, of importance was that people treated for smoking had comparable outcomes on depression as did control groups (Prochaska et al., 2008). These results challenged the belief that even a history of depression would lead to failure in quitting smoking and that quitting smoking could lead to poorer outcomes with depression (Lasser et al., 2000).

In a population with SMI, hospitalized for acute episodes of their disorders, smokers were proactively recruited to a cessation program applying our CTIs, with research assistants providing cognitive and social support when needed. With our standard practice of three CTI sessions, pre- and post-discharge delivered digitally over 6 months, the treatment group had 2.5 times greater abstinence rates (20% vs. 8%) than controls (Prochaska, Hall, Delucchi, & Hall, 2013). Of special significance here was the finding that compared to controls, people treated for smoking had significantly fewer re-hospitalizations over the next 12 months after discharge. These results support the hypothesis that the smoking cessation intervention may have had significant effects on people's well-being and functioning outside the hospital.

Those results also support the guiding principles of the Substance Abuse and Mental Health Services Administration (SAMHSA, 2011) for recovery from substance abuse and mental health disorders. Recovery from mental and substance abuse disorders is defined as "[a] voluntary and individually determined process of change through which individuals work to improve their own health and well-being, live a productive life and welcome opportunities for growth. Recovery is holistic and exists on a continuum of improved health and well-being. Recovery involves addressing and transcending, discrimination, shame and stigma."

When those results of the study with smokers with SMI were reported in the *New York Times*, there were positive letters from readers, but there were also very upsetting letters (Prochaska et al., 2013). Stigmatizing letters included questions as to why special efforts should be made to extend the lives of such populations, and why pleasures like smoking should be removed from people who have so few pleasures in life. As the SAMHSA guiding principles indicate, helping to increase health and well-being in these understudied and underserved populations involves transcending discrimination, shame, and stigma.

A key question is why our Transtheoretical Model of Behavior Change CTIs produce comparable outcomes across populations that differ in age, race, ethnicity, and mental health status, even when experts and stereotypes would predict otherwise. Our TTM interventions are developed for and evaluated on entire at-risk populations, including those in the *preparation* stage who are ready to take action, those in *contemplation* who are getting ready, and those in *precontemplation* who are not yet ready. Contrast that to the vast number of smoking cessation studies included in the Clinical Guidelines for the Treatment of Tobacco (Fiore et al., 2000; Fiore et al., 2008). With more than 6,000 studies available, there were plenty of evidence-based treatments for "motivated" smokers, defined as people in the preparation stage who were ready to quit in the next month. There were no evidence-based treatments for the more than 80% of smokers in the United States who are not "motivated" and are in the precontemplation stage (about 40%) and contemplation stage (about 40%). Of special significance is that there were no evidence-based treatments for smokers with mental illness, even though today, such smokers consume about 40% of all cigarettes in the United States (Lasser et al., 2000). In two cessation studies with SMI, only 15% were "motivated" and about 44% were in precontemplation, and 41% in contemplation (Prochaska et al., 2013; DiClemente et al., 2011). These stage distributions indicate the importance of applying interventions for participants at each stage, if population treatments are to be effective.

THE TRANSTHEORETICAL MODEL OF BEHAVIOR CHANGE

The Transtheoretical Model of Behavior Change (TTM) uses stages to integrate principles and processes of change derived from major theories of intervention—hence, the name *Transtheoretical*. This model emerged from a comparative analysis of leading theories grounded in psychotherapy and behavior change. Because more than 300 psychotherapy theories were found, the TTM developers determined that there was a need for systematic integration (Prochaska, 1979). Ten processes of change emerged, including consciousness raising from the Freudian tradition, reinforcement management from the Skinnerian tradition, and helping relationships from the Rogerian tradition.

Stages of change lie at the heart of the TTM. Studies of change have found that people move through a series of stages when modifying behavior. While the time a person can stay in each stage is variable, the tasks required to move to the next stage are not. Certain principles and processes of change work best at each stage to reduce resistance, to facilitate progress, and to prevent relapse. Those include decisional balance, self-efficacy, and processes of change. Only a minority (usually less than 20%) of a population at risk is prepared to take action at any given time. Thus, action-oriented advice mis-serves individuals in the early stages. Guidance based on the TTM results in increased participation in the change process because it appeals to the entire population, rather than the minority ready to take action.

Stages of Change

The stage construct represents a temporal dimension. Change implies phenomena occurring over time. Surprisingly, none of the leading theories of therapy contained a core construct representing time. Traditionally, behavior change was often construed as an event, such as quitting

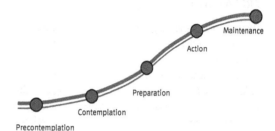

FIGURE 2.1   Stages of change.

smoking, drinking, or overeating, but the TTM recognizes change as a process that unfolds over time, involving progress through a series of stages (Figure 2.1).

PRECONTEMPLATION

People in the precontemplation stage do not intend to take action in the foreseeable future, usually measured as the next 6 months. Being uninformed or underinformed about the consequences of one's behavior may cause a person to be in the precontemplation stage. Multiple unsuccessful attempts at change can lead to demoralization about the ability to change. Both the uninformed and underinformed tend to avoid reading, talking, or thinking about their high-risk behaviors. They are often characterized in other theories as resistant, unmotivated, or unready for health promotion programs. In fact, traditional population health promotion programs were not ready for such individuals and were not designed to meet their needs.

CONTEMPLATION

Contemplation is the stage in which people intend to change in the next 6 months. They are more aware of the pros of changing, but are also acutely aware of the cons. In a meta-analysis across 48 health-risk behaviors, the pros and cons of changing were equal (Hall & Rossi, 2008). This weighting between the costs and benefits of changing can produce profound ambivalence, which can cause people to remain in this stage for long periods of time. This phenomenon is often characterized as chronic contemplation or behavioral procrastination. Individuals in the contemplation stage are not ready for traditional action-oriented programs that expect participants to act immediately.

PREPARATION

Preparation is the stage in which people intend to take action in the immediate future, usually measured as the next month. Typically, they have already taken some significant action in the past year. These individuals have a plan of action, such as joining a health education class, consulting a counselor, talking to their physician, buying a self-help book, or relying on a self-change approach. These are the people who should be recruited for action-oriented programs.

ACTION

Action is the stage in which people have made specific overt modifications in their lifestyles within the past 6 months. Because action is observable, the overall process of behavior change often has been equated with action. But in the TTM, action is only one of six stages. Typically, not all modifications of behavior count as action in this model. In most applications, people have to attain a criterion that scientists and professionals agree is sufficient to reduce risk of disease. For example, reduction in the number of cigarettes and switching to low-tar and low-nicotine cigarettes were formerly considered acceptable actions. Now the consensus is clear—only total abstinence counts.

MAINTENANCE

Maintenance is the stage in which people have made specific overt modifications in their lifestyles and are working to prevent relapse; however, they do not apply change processes as frequently as do people in action. While in the maintenance stage, people are less tempted to relapse and grow increasingly more confident that they can continue their changes. Based on self-efficacy data, researchers have estimated that maintenance lasts from 6 months to about 5 years. While this estimate may seem somewhat pessimistic, longitudinal data in the 1990 Surgeon General's report support this temporal estimate. After 12 months of continuous abstinence, 43% of individuals returned to regular smoking. It was not until 5 years of continuous abstinence that the risk for relapse dropped to 7% (USDHHS, 1990).

TERMINATION

Termination is the stage in which individuals are not tempted; they have 100% self-efficacy. Whether depressed, anxious, bored, lonely, angry, or stressed, individuals in this stage are sure they will not return to unhealthy habits as a way of coping. It is as if their new behavior has become an automatic habit. Examples include adults who have developed automatic seatbelt use or who automatically take their anti-hypertensive medication at the same time and place each day. In a study of former smokers and alcoholics, researchers found that less than 20% of each group had reached the criteria of zero temptation and total self-efficacy (Snow, Prochaska & Rossi, 1992). The criterion of 100% self-efficacy may be too strict, or it may be that this stage is an ideal goal for population health efforts. In other areas, like exercise, consistent condom use, and weight control, the realistic goal may be a lifetime of maintenance.

Decisional Balance

The process of reflecting and weighing the pros and cons of changing is termed *decisional balance*. According to Janis and Mann (1977), sound decision-making requires the consideration of the potential gains (pros) and losses (cons) associated with a behavior's consequences. Figure 2.2 illustrates the systematic relationship between the pros and cons of changing and the stages of change for 48 health risk behaviors. Practical implications are clear: to help people progress from precontemplation to action, the pros of changing need to be increased. To progress from contemplation, the cons need to decrease. To be prepared to take action, the pros need to outweigh the cons. TTM programs tell people, for example, that there are more than 65 scientific benefits of regular physical activity, and they encourage people to make a list to see how many they can identify. They can also list the cons and think about how they can decrease key cons. Time is the number one con for people in Taiwan, Mexico, and even any retired Americans. But, if we are aware of gaining 65 benefits rather than 6, then time can decrease dramatically as a con. The more the list of pros outweighs the cons, the better prepared people will be to take effective action (Figure 2.2).

Self-Efficacy

Self-efficacy is the situation-specific confidence that people have while coping with high-risk situations without relapsing to their unhealthy habit (Bandura, 1982). Temptation reflects the intensity of urges to

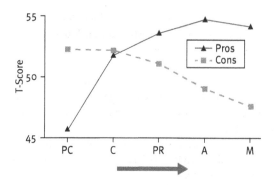

FIGURE 2.2   Pros and cons by stage of change.

engage in a specific risky habit while in the midst of difficult situations. Typically, three factors reflect the most common types of tempting situations: negative affect or emotional distress, social situations, and craving. Asking people how they will cope with emotional distress without relying on a cigarette or comfort foods can help them cope more effectively and thereby build their confidence or self-efficacy.

Processes of Change

Processes of change are the 10 experiential and behavioral activities that people use to progress through the stages. It is important for practitioners of population health to understand these progressions. They provide important guides for intervention programs, serving as independent variables that are applied to move from stage to stage.

CONSCIOUSNESS-RAISING

Consciousness-raising involves increased awareness about the causes, consequences, and cures for a particular problem behavior. Interventions that can increase awareness include feedback, interpretations, and bibliotherapy. Sedentary people, for example, may not be aware that their inactivity can have the same risk as smoking a pack of cigarettes a day.

DRAMATIC RELIEF

Dramatic relief initially produces increased emotional experiences, followed by reduced affect or anticipated relief if appropriate action is taken. Health promotion programs can provide fear-arousing feedback on health risks or success stories in order to move people emotionally.

ENVIRONMENTAL REEVALUATION

Environmental reevaluation combines both affective and cognitive assessments of how the presence or absence of a personal habit affects one's social environment, such as the effect of smoking on others. It can also include the awareness that one can serve as a positive or negative role model for others.

SELF-REEVALUATION

Self-reevaluation combines both cognitive and affective assessments of one's self-image with and without a particular unhealthy habit, such as one's image as a couch potato versus an active person. Values clarification, identifying healthy role models, and imagery are techniques that health promotion programs can use to move people toward self-reevaluation. During interaction with a TTM computerized tailored intervention, the program might ask, "Imagine you were free from smoking. How would you feel about yourself?"

SELF LIBERATION

Self liberation is both the belief that one can change and the commitment, as well as the recommitment, to act on that belief. Encouraging people to make New Year's resolutions, public testimonies, or a contract are ways of enhancing willpower. The TTM program might say, "Telling others about your commitment to take action can strengthen your willpower. Whom are you going to tell?"

SOCIAL LIBERATION

Social liberation requires an increase in social opportunities or alternatives, especially for people who are relatively deprived or oppressed. For example, advocacy, empowerment procedures, and appropriate policies can produce increased opportunities for mental health promotion, gay health promotion, and health promotion for impoverished segments of the population. These same procedures can also be used to help populations change; examples include smoke-free zones, healthy food at day centers, and easy access to condoms and other contraceptives.

COUNTER CONDITIONING

Counter conditioning requires learning healthy behaviors as substitutes for problem behaviors. Examples of counter conditioning include recommendations for use of nicotine replacement as a safe substitute for smoking, and walking as a healthier alternative than "comfort foods" as a way to cope with stress.

HELPING RELATIONSHIPS

Helping relationships combine caring, trust, openness, and acceptance, as well as support for healthy behavior change. Rapport building, a therapeutic alliance, supportive calls, and buddy systems can be sources of social support. Silver Sneakers, an exercise program often covered by Medicare, is an example of a program that could be suggested to older adults.

REINFORCEMENT MANAGEMENT

Reinforcement management provides consequences for taking steps in a positive direction. While contingency management can include the use of punishment, we found that self-changers rely on reward much more than punishment. So, we recommend an emphasis on reinforcement in order to work in harmony with how people change naturally. People expect to be reinforced by others more frequently than reinforcement occurs, so they should be encouraged to reinforce themselves through self-statements like "Nice going—you handled that temptation." They also need to treat themselves at milestones as a way to provide reinforcement and to increase the probability that healthy responses will be repeated.

STIMULUS CONTROL

Stimulus control removes cues for unhealthy habits and adds prompts for healthier alternatives. In this process, TTM programs can recommend removing all the ashtrays from the house and car or removing high-fat foods that are tempting cues for unhealthy eating.

Critical Assumptions

The Transtheoretical Model is also based on critical assumptions about the nature of behavior change and population health interventions that can best facilitate such change. The following set of assumptions drives Transtheoretical Model theory, research, and practice:

1. Behavior change is a process that unfolds over time through a sequence of stages, and health population programs need to assist people as they progress over time.
2. Stages are both stable and open to change, just as chronic behavioral risk factors are both stable and open to change.
3. Population health initiatives can motivate change by enhancing the understanding of the pros and diminishing the value of the cons.
4. The majority of at-risk populations are not prepared for action and will not be served by traditional action-oriented prevention programs. Helping people set realistic goals, like progressing to the next stage, will facilitate the change process.
5. Specific principles and processes of change need to be emphasized at specific stages in order for progress through the stages to occur. Figure 2.3 outlines which principles and processes to apply at each stage.
6. Interventions can also be tailored to the special needs of older adults (Greene et al., 2008; Jones et al., 2003) and populations with mental health problems (Hall et al., 2006; Prochaska et al., 2013).

These critical assumptions need to be taken into consideration when developing a population-based approach to behavior change and facilitating progress through the stages (see Figure 2.3).

COMPUTERIZED TAILORED INTERVENTIONS

TTM-based computer-tailored interventions (CTIs) rely on a computer to create tailored feedback for individuals from a feedback library using algorithms and pre-programmed decision rules. The TTM and the interrelationships among the core constructs provide the theoretical and empirical basis for creating CTIs. In addition, CTIs require advanced statistical analyses to determine decision rules for tailoring interventions to individuals—rules that link responses to particular feedback. At the outset of a CTI, participants are assessed on all TTM variables relevant for them (stage of change, decisional balance, self-efficacy, and processes of change). In the first (baseline) session, participants receive individualized feedback on how their responses

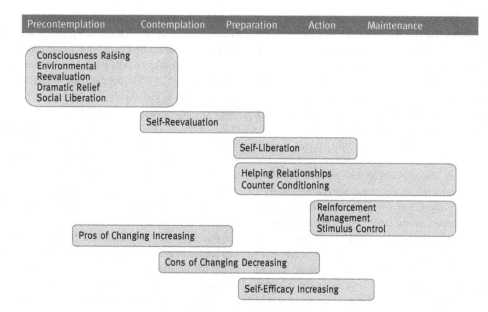

FIGURE 2.3   Stages by Principles and Processes of Change.

compare to the responses of other individuals in the same stage of change who successfully progressed on the same behavior change (normative comparisons).

At follow-up, users receive updated normative feedback based on their most recent responses, as well as "ipsative feedback" that compares their most recent scores to their previous scores. Interventions that offer multiple contacts where messages are dynamically tailored over time are more effective (Noar, Benac, & Harris, 2007). Though the tailoring is done via computer, CTI feedback can be delivered in multiple channels, including mail, telephonic coach, onscreen, interactive voice response (IVR), or short message service (SMS) text messages.

Computer-based programs combine the advantages of a clinic approach, which emphasizes individualized interaction between the client and provider, with the goals of the public health approach, which targets entire populations. On-screen assessments and programming allow for extensively tailored and immediate feedback. Fidelity to treatment is enhanced with consistent and reliable feedback delivered to participants. In addition, the embedded interactivity gives the user an active role with more control over his or her participation. Rich media such as audio, animated graphics, and video can be incorporated. Users enjoy these features as well as the flexibility

of engaging in the program at their convenience. With improved program retention, wider reach, and less reliance on staff for delivery, interactive technologies offer a cost effective means of delivering behavior change interventions.

CTIs often include stage-matched personal activity centers that are populated with a variety of tools, tips, and resources specifically chosen for participants based on their stage of change. The personal activity center provides more content and specifics on how to apply each of the principles and processes of change that users were encouraged to use in the CTI. Activities are presented in a variety of media, including video, interactive quizzes and activities, tips and worksheets, and links to external websites. Users may visit the portal and choose any activity at any time to facilitate progress between CTI sessions (for a video of a CTI see www.prochange.com/exercisedemo).

ADAPTING THE TTM CTI FOR POPULATIONS WITH SMI

We recommended that a participatory design approach be employed in which qualitative research and usability testing is conducted on existing intervention components with participants, healthcare providers, and other key stakeholders to ensure that the needs of stakeholders are met. The qualitative phase should involve an iterative process. We further recommend that the modification and enhancement of the existing interventions begin with a comprehensive review by a patient advisory panel and mental health clinicians. Their feedback on necessary modifications can be incorporated, along with health literacy testing. Focus groups with participants and mental health staff should be conducted. The sessions would employ moderator guides that include open-ended questions and discussion probes. Participants would provide input on (1) the sequentially delivered program flow, user interface, images, and tone; (2) recruitment messages intended to motivate participants to complete the intervention; and (3) how they would like a mental health staff person to work with them. Additional participants could be invited to share their stories about working to eat healthy, exercise, or quit smoking. These interviews would be used to enhance program content. A series of usability tests and cognitive interviews should then be conducted. In rounds of cognitive testing, clients would be shown sections of content to determine whether they understand instructions, language, worksheets, and graphics as intended. Experienced staff trained in cognitive testing can then use "think aloud" and intensive probing methodologies.

ADAPTING THE TTM CTI FOR AGING POPULATIONS

Our programs have worked successfully with aging populations and have not needed the previously noted kinds of adaptations. In a diabetes self-management multiple behavior change TTM trial, older adults were able to move to self-monitoring blood glucose, healthy eating, and smoking cessation. For those receiving the TTM intervention, 43% of those receiving the program plus testing strips moved to the action stage as well as 30.5% of those receiving the program alone, 27% of those receiving usual care plus strips, compared to 18.4% of those receiving usual treatment alone. For the healthy eating intervention, more participants who received the TTM program than usual care (32.5% vs. 25.8%) moved to action or maintenance. For the smoking intervention, more participants receiving the TTM program (24.3%) than usual care (13.4%) moved to an action stage. This study demonstrated that the TTM has the potential of

positively impacting the health of broad populations of individuals with diabetes, not just the minority who were ready for change (Jones et al., 2003).

Recently, the American Psychological Association (2014) outlined "Guidelines for Psychological Practice with Older Adults." Rather than a strong focus on advocating for changes in programs for older adults, it assisted psychologists in evaluating their own readiness for working with older adults and in seeking and using appropriate education and training to increase their knowledge, skills, and experience in their area of practice. Twenty-one guidelines were given, including one urging practitioners to strive to recognize and address issues related to the provision of prevention and health promotion services with older adults. The guidelines stated, "It might be useful to advocate for more health promotion activities to facilitate older adult participation in exercise, good nutrition, and healthy lifestyle." (p. 51) Because depression and suicide prevention are of particular concern for preventive efforts with older adults, improved recognition of depressive symptoms and other risk factors and referral to appropriate treatment were recommended.

INNOVATION

The process of applying our TTM CTI programs to populations with SMI involves a series of innovations. While we and collaborators have been successful in applying our smoking cessation programs to populations with mental disorders, targeting MHBC is new. Based on how readily our programs for the single behavior of smoking generalized to such populations, we might assume that programs for MHBC might require little innovation. But MHBC is considerably more complicated, especially in the context of populations with complicated conditions.

A major concern is that asking a population with SMI to receive simultaneous treatment on three risk behaviors could be overwhelming for some important percentage of the people. One major adaptation is to treat smoking separately, in part because our evidence is that smoking cessation is the most difficult behavior change, as reflected in the lowest rates of success across different behaviors. This adaptation is also supported by recent discoveries that in a combined population of nearly 10,000 people, smokers who put their most efforts into just quitting smoking were about four times more successful than those who changed two behaviors (e.g., smoking and diet) (Yin et al., 2013). With energy balance behaviors (like exercise and diet), individuals who made their best efforts on changing both behaviors were about 50% more successful than those who changed just diet. We can use the strategy of one primary behavior and one secondary, and simultaneously treat both exercise and diet, reducing treatment demands. But the impact can be at least 50% greater.

Our adaptation or best practice of three CTI sessions over 6 months for smoking, and three sessions for exercise and diet during a separate 6 months, is recommended. Clients with all three risks should be treated first for the behavior that they are most ready to change.

Integrating an MHBC program should begin with close collaboration with mental health workers, whose experience with their population with SMI is a major determining factor in such choices as (1) providing our best practice of CTIs alone to reduce demands on case managers; (2) limiting treatment to a maximum of two energy balance behaviors to limit demands on participants; (3) type of incentives that would be most effective for recruitment and retention; (4) how to build the MHBC program into the service procedures at therapy clinics, including scheduling the CTI sessions concurrently with other service opportunities, utilizing regularly scheduled tests for biometric measures, and utilizing their pharmacy services for nicotine replacement therapy (NRT) paid for by Medicaid; and (5) how to best train case managers in TTM and the TTM CTIs so they can assist participants in a time-effective manner.

We have learned from a study with 3391 high-risk and high-cost older adults how to lessen the burden of separate modules with full TTM tailoring for each separate MHBC, and we innovated with more user-friendly alternatives. The participants were 3391 from 39 states who had an average age of 4.2 chronic health conditions and nearly four health risk behaviors (Prochaska et al., 2012). About 80% reported some depression, 45% were obese, and 30% were overweight, the majority were suffering or struggling with impaired functioning. They were randomly assigned to (1) three sessions of telephonic TTM tailored coaching with exercise as primary target and only stage targeting on stress management; (2) three sessions of an online TTM-tailored program with stress management as primary and exercise as secondary; or (3) controls.

At 6 months the effects of coaching compared to controls on exercise (57.3%) was about two-thirds higher, was about 50% higher on stress management (74.9%) and diet (30.7%) and 20% higher on effective depression management (67.3%), even though diet and depression were not treated. The online program produced results midway between coaching and controls with significant effects on exercise (46.6%) and stress (64.7%) and total risk reduction. Of special relevance is that the coaching and online programs had even higher differences than controls in improvements on multiple domains of well-being: (1) 90% to 50% higher on emotional health (reduced depression, anxiety, and stress, and increased happiness and enjoyment); and (2) 2.5 times and 80% higher on physical health, and 3 times and 2.5 times greater increases in the percentage that progressed from suffering or struggling to thriving.

One should not conclude that telephonic coaching was superior to online programs, because coaching had a different primary behavior (exercise) than did online (stress management). In a recent population trial on MHBC with energy balance behaviors in middle schools, the CTI alone treatment had exercise as the primary behavior and diet and TV watching as secondary (Velicer et al., 2013). The outcomes were clear, with significant impacts on each risk behavior. The significance of this body of evidence for dissemination is that simultaneous treatments for energy balance behaviors can apply an approach that can reduce the demands on participants, compared to applying a separate fully tailored module for each behavior.

SUMMARY

The evidence is clear that populations with multiple health risks who also are older or have SMI are at greater risk for chronic diseases, premature death, impaired functioning, and increased healthcare costs. In spite of stereotypes that such populations do not have the same abilities to change, the evidence to date suggests that the problem is not the ability to change, but accessibility to quality change programs.

The methodological challenge for the future is how to deliver high-impact prevention programs to older populations with and without mental health problems. TTM tailored interventions could be delivered by counselors serving such populations, by providers in patient-centered medical homes designed to deliver more integrative and holistic health care, or in health homes designed to provide best practices for populations with SMI.

We have been asked by the director of Rhode Island's Behavior Health and Disabilities Division to participate in an initiative to transform statewide services for populations with mental health and substance abuse disorders. Our proposal is to provide the prevention training and tools for counselors and their clients that can impact on risk behaviors that account for the majority of chronic diseases, disability, lost productivity, and premature death. The initial focus would be on the four behaviors that account for about 70% of chronic diseases: smoking, alcohol abuse, unhealthy diet, and inadequate exercise. These behaviors are so critical to health and health care, in part, because they represent fundamental processes of life: breathing, drinking, eating, and moving. Changing these behaviors from high risk to low risk can enhance physical well-being, and emotional, social, financial, and work well-being. Perhaps even more important, they can help segments of older populations with mental health problems to progress from suffering or struggling to thriving. In the future, we need to deliver services that not only prevent disease but also enhance life.

DISCLOSURE STATEMENTS

Dr. James O. Prochaska is the founder of Pro-Change Behavior Systems, Inc., and serves as a consultant to the company.

Dr. Janice M. Prochaska is the President and CEO of Pro-Change Behavior Systems, Inc.

REFERENCES

Allison, D. B., Fontaine, K. R., Heo, M. et al. (1999). The distribution of body mass index among individuals with and without schizophrenia. *J Clin Psychiatry, 60*(4), 215–220.

American Psychological Association. (2014). Guidelines for psychological practice with older adults. *Am Psychol, 69,* 34–65.

Bandura, A. (1982). Self-efficacy mechanism in human agency. *Am Psychol, 37,* 122–147.

DiClemente, C. C., Delahanty, J. C., Kofeldt, M. G., Dixon, L., Goldberg, R., & Lucksted, A. (2011). Stage movement following a 5A's intervention in tobacco dependent individuals with serious mental illness (SMI). *Addict Behav, 36*(3), 261–264. PMID: 21146317.

Doll, R., Peto, R., Boreham, J., & Sutherland, I. (2004). Mortality in relation to smoking: 50 years' observations on male British doctors. *Brit Med J, 328,* 1519.

Druss B. G., Zhao, L., Von Esenwein, S., Morrato, E. H., & Marcus, S. C. (2011). Understanding excess mortality in persons with mental illness: 17-year follow up of a nationally representative US survey. *Med Care, 49*(6), 599–604. doi: 10.1097/MLR.0b013e31820bf86e. PMID: 21577183.

Edington, D. W. (2001). Emerging research: a view from one research center. *Am J Health Promot, 15,* 341–349.

Fine, L. J., Philogene, G. S., Gramling, R., Coups, E. J., & Sinha, S. (2004). Prevalence of multiple chronic disease risk factors; 2001 National Health Interview Survey. *Am J Prev Med, 27,* 18–24.

Fiore, M. C., Bailey, W. C., Cohen, S. J., Dorfman, S. F., Goldstein, M. G., & Gritz, E. R. (2000). *Treating tobacco use and dependence: clinical practice guideline.* Rockville, MD: US DHHS, Public Health Service.

Fiore, M. C., Jaen, C. R., Baker, T. B. et al. (2008). *Treating tobacco use and dependence: 2008 update, clinical practice guideline.* Rockville, MD: USDHHS. PHS.

Goetzel, R. Z., Anderson, D. R., Whitmer, R. W., Ozminkowski, R. J., Dunn, R. L., & Wasserman J. (1998). The relationship between modifiable health risks and health care expenditures: an analysis of the multi-employer HERO health risk and cost database. *J Occup Environ Med, 40,* 843–854.

Greene, G. W., Fey-Yensan, N., Padula, C., Rossi, S. R., Rossi, J. S., & Clark, P. G. (2008). Change in fruit and vegetable intake over 24-months in older adults: results of the SENIOR project intervention. *Gerontologist, 48,* 378–387.

Hall, K. L. and Rossi, J. S. (2008). Meta-analytic examination of the strong and weak principles across 48 health behaviors. *Prev Med, 46*(3), 266–274.

Hall, S. M., Tsoh, J., Prochaska, J. J., Eisendrath, S., Rossi, J. S., Redding, C. A., et al. (2006). Treatment of depressed mental health outpatients for cigarette smoking: a randomized clinical trial. *Am J Public Health, 96*(10), 1808–1814. (PMCID: PMC1586139)

Hollis, J. F., Polen, M. R., Whitlock, E. P., Lichtenstein, E., Mulloly, J., Velicer, W. F., & Redding, C. A. (2005). Teen REACH: outcomes from a randomized controlled trial of a tobacco reduction program for teens seen in primary medical care. *Pediatrics, 115*(4), 981–989. PMID: 15805374.

Irwin, M. L., & Mayne, S. T. (2008). Impact of nutrition and exercise on cancer survival. *Cancer J, 14*, 435–441.

Janis, I. L., & Mann L. (1977). *Decision making: a psychological analysis of conflict, choice, and commitment.* London: Cassel & Collier Macmillan.

Johnson, S. S., Paiva, A. L., Cummins, C., Johnson, J. L., Dyment, S., Wright, J. A., Prochaska, J. O., Prochaska, J. M., & Sherman, K. (2008). Evidence-based multiple behavior intervention for weight management: effectiveness on a population basis. *Prev Med, 46*, 238–246. PMCID: PMC2327253.

Jones, H., Edwards, L., Vallis, T. M., Ruggiero, L. et al. (2003). Changes in diabetes self-care behaviors make a difference in glycemic control: The Diabetes Stages of Change (DISC) Study. *Diabetes Care, 26*, 732–737.

Khaw, K. T., Wareham, N., Bingham, S., Welch, A., Luben, R., & Day, N. (2008) Combined impact of health behaviors and mortality in men and women: The EPIC-Norfolk Prospective Population Study. *PLoS Med, 5*(1), e12. doi:10.1371/journal.pmed.0050012

Kvaavik, E., Batty, G. D., Ursin, G., Huxley, R., & Gale, C. R. (2010). Influence of individual and combined health behaviors on total and cause-specific mortality in men and women. *Arch Intern Med, 170*(8), 711–718. PMID: 20421558.

Lasser, K., Boyd, J. W., Woolhandler, S., Himmelstein, D. U., McCormick, D., & Bor, D. H. (2000). Smoking and mental illness: a population-based prevalence study. *JAMA, 284*(20), 2606–2610.

McElroy, S. L. (2002). Correlates of overweight and obesity in 644 patients with bipolar disorder. *J Clin Psychiatry, 63*, 207–213.

Mokdad, A. H., Marks, J. S., Stroup, D. F., & Gerberding, J. L. (2004). Actual causes of death in the United States, 2000. *JAMA, 291*(10), 1238–1245.

Noar, S. M., Benac, C. M., & Harris, M. S. (2007). Does tailoring matter? Meta-analytic review of tailored print health behavior change interventions. *Psychol Bull, 133*(4), 673–693.

Poortinga, W. (2007). The prevalence and clustering of four major lifestyle risk factors in an English adult population. *Prev Med, 44*, 124–128.

Prochaska, J. J., Hall, S. E., Delucchi, K., & Hall, S. M. (2013). Efficacy of initiating tobacco dependence treatment in inpatient psychiatry: a randomized controlled trial. *Am J Public Health,*

e1–e9. doi:10.2105/AJPH.2013.301403. PMID: 23948001.

Prochaska, J. J., Hall, S. M., Tsoh, J. Y., Eisendrath, S., Rossi, J. S., Redding, C. A. et al. (2008). Treating tobacco dependence in smokers with clinical depression: impact on mental health functioning. *Am J Public Health, 98*(3), 446–448. PMCID: PMC2253568.

Prochaska, J. J., & Prochaska, J. O. (2011). A review of multiple health behavior change interventions for primary prevention. *Am J Lifestyle Med, 5*(3), 208–221. PMID: 11162323.

Prochaska, J. O., Butterworth, S. Redding, C., Burden, V., Perrin, N., Leo, M. (2008). Initial efficacy of MI, TTM tailoring and HRI's with multiple behaviors for employee health promotion. *Preven Med, 45*, 226–231. PMCID: PMC3384542.

Prochaska, J. O., Evers, K. E., Castle, P. H., Johnson, J. L., Prochaska, J. M., Rula, E. Y., Coberley, C., & Pope, J. E. (2012). Enhancing multiple domains of wellbeing by decreasing multiple risk behaviors: a randomized clinical trial. *Popul Health Manage, 15*(5), 276–286. PMID: 22352379.

Prochaska, J. O., Velicer, W. F, Redding, C. A., Rossi, J. S., Goldstein, M., et al. (2005). Stage-based expert systems to guide a population of primary care patients to quit smoking, eat healthier, prevent skin cancer and receive regular mammograms. *Prev Med, 41*, 406–416. PMID: 15896835.

Prochaska, J. O., Velicer, W. F., Rossi, J. S., Redding, C., et al. (2004). Multiple risk expert systems interventions: impact of simultaneous stage-matched expert system interventions for smoking, high-fat diet and sun exposure on a population of parents. *Health Psychol, 23*(5), 503–516. PMID: 15367070.

SAMHSA. (2011). Working definition of recovery from mental health. www.samhsa.gov.

Snow, M. G., Prochaska, J. O., & Rossi, J. S. (1992). Stages of change for smoking cessation among former problem drinkers: a cross-sectional analysis. *J Subst Abuse, 4*(2), 107–116.

US Department of Health and Human Services (USDHHS). (1990). *The health benefits of smoking cessation: a report of the Surgeon General.* Washington, DC: US Department of Health and Human Services. DHHS Publication No. (CDC) 90–8416.

US Department of Health and Human Services (USDHHS). (1996). *Physical activity and health: a report of the Surgeon General.* Atlanta, GA: USDHHS.

Velicer, W. F., Redding, C. A., Paiva, A. L., Blissmer, B., Mauriello, L. M., Oatley, K., et al. (2013). Multiple risk factor intervention to prevent substance abuse and increase energy balance behaviors in middle school students. *Transl Behav Med, 3*(1), 82–93. PMID: 23585821.

Velicer, W. F., Redding, C. A., Sun, X., & Prochaska, J. O. (2007). Demographic variables, smoking variables, and outcome across five studies. *Health Psychol, 26*(3), 278–287. PMID: 17500614.

Yin, H-Q, Prochaska, J. O., Rossi, J. S., Redding, C. A., Paiva, A. L., Blissmer, B., et al. (2013). Treatment enhanced paired action contributes substantially to change across multiple health behaviors: secondary analyses of five randomized controlled trials. *Transl Behav Med, 3*(1), 62–71. (PMID: 23630546)

PART II

PROMOTING WELL-BEING THROUGH HOLISTIC INTERVENTIONS

SECTION A

NUTRITIONAL AND HERBAL MEDICINE

3

HEALTH BENEFITS OF HERBS AND SPICES IN AGING ADULTS

Linda C. Tapsell and Elizabeth P. Neale

DRAWING THE LINKS BETWEEN HEALTHY AGING AND CONSUMPTION OF HERBS AND SPICES

Lifetime dietary patterns are known to play a substantial role in promoting healthy aging (Anderson et al., 2011; Samieri et al., 2013), a concept that relates to both longevity and cognitive function. Positive effects on these two attributes have been shown in the Mediterranean diet and the Okinawan diet (Samieri et al., 2013; Tangney et al., 2011; Willcox, Willcox, Todoriki, & Suzuki, 2009), both of which use culinary herbs and spices, such as garlic, turmeric, and chili, extensively. In comparison, herbs and spices are less commonly used in Western-style dietary patterns, which are associated with increased risk of diseases such as cardiovascular disease and cancer (Heidemann et al., 2008). It is not fully known how herbs and spices contribute protective effects, but they do possess compounds with strong antioxidant properties (Srinivasan, 2012).

The prevention of oxidative damage and inflammation is a key component in healthy aging. Over the life span, accumulation of oxidative damage from free radicals and reactive oxygen species results in the development of oxidative stress (De la Fuente & Miquel, 2009). This oxidative stress is likely to have an effect on the immune system, resulting in the release of pro-inflammatory compounds and a state of chronic inflammation (De la Fuente & Miquel, 2009). The combined effects of oxidation and inflammation underpin a number of diseases associated with aging, including dementia, atherosclerosis, and type II diabetes mellitus (De la Fuente & Miquel, 2009; De Martinis, Franceschi, Monti, & Ginaldi, 2005; Ferencík, Stvrtinová, Hulín, & Novák, 2007).

From a clinical perspective, the emergence of these diseases usually occurs after earlier presentations of chronic disease risk factors, such as overweight and obesity, high blood glucose levels, hypertension, and dyslipidemia (AIHW, 2012). Thus research that exposes links between healthy aging and the consumption of herbs and spices might reasonably address these disease risk factors, in addition to other markers of healthy aging such as cognitive function. For example, both fasting glucose levels and glycated hemoglobin A1c (HbA1c) provide an indication of glucose control and predict diabetes progression and associated complications (Ai-Lawati & Al-Lawati, 2007; Edelman, Olsen, Dudley, Harris, & Oddone, 2004; Inoue, Matsumoto, & Kobayashi, 2007; Pradhan, Rifai, Buring, & Ridker, 2007). Similarly, increased levels of low-density lipoprotein cholesterol (LDL-C) and triglycerides, and decreased levels of high-density lipoprotein cholesterol (HDL-C) are associated with an increased risk of cardiovascular disease (Assmann, 2006; Musunuru, 2010).

The consumption of herbs and spices might also have indirect effects on healthy aging by promoting a protective dietary pattern. In this sense, other research parameters may be considered, such as overall food intake and liking of specific foods. Research indicating a positive influence of herbs and spices on food choices would add to the evidence of how they may contribute to positive effects on health aging.

Finally, there are many classes of herbs and spices, they occur in many forms (for example, fresh and dried), and they appear in the diet in many ways, in conjunction with many different types of foods. Healthy aging is the result of the total diet, so isolating the effects of herbs and spices in a culinary sense presents a great challenge. Nevertheless, searching the literature in a transparent fashion and systematically reporting outcomes shows there is a mounting body of research indicating that including herbs and spices in a healthy diet is advantageous.

LITERATURE SEARCH METHODS

To conduct this review, the Web of Science and Scopus databases were searched from 2000–June 2014 using the search terms: "herb" OR "spice" OR "functional food" AND "aging" AND ("health" OR "cardiovascular disease" OR "dementia" OR "stroke" OR "obesity*" OR "hypertension" OR "diabete*" OR "cognition"). The search was limited to studies published in the English language that examined the effects of consumption of herbs and/or spices on health or behavioral outcomes. Additional relevant

articles were also sourced from the reference lists of original articles. The literature search methods were based on the PRISMA (preferred reporting items for systematic reviews and meta-analyses) framework, and followed the guidelines for determining and reporting eligibility criteria, information sources, and study selection (Moher, Liberati, Tetzlaff, Altman, & The Prisma Group, 2009) (Figure 3.1). Culinary herbs and spices were considered in the first instance, while those examining traditional herbal medicines were then included in the discussion for comparison.

RESEARCH ASSESSING THE EFFECTS OF HERBS AND SPICES ON HEALTH OUTCOMES

The search conducted produced 27 articles on culinary herbs and spices for inclusion in this review. Within these articles, a range of clinical and behavioral outcomes were assessed (Table 3.1), including blood glucose levels ($n = 9$), lipid levels ($n = 8$), cognitive function ($n = 3$), energy intake or satiety ($n = 7$), and liking of meals with added herbs and spices ($n = 2$). This demonstrates the breadth of investigation addressing the impact of herbs and spices on health outcomes. A summary of the research pathways examining clinical and behavioral effects of culinary herbs and spices is shown in Figure 3.2.

Effects on Blood Glucose Control

Blood glucose levels are a well-utilized indicator of metabolic profile, particularly in relation to diabetes. Most of the research on the effects of herbs and spices on blood glucose has focused on cinnamon.

Studies have shown that the consumption of cinnamon can lead to improvements in blood glucose levels and measures of blood glucose control. One study in people with type II diabetes compared the effects of consuming 1, 3, or 6 g of cinnamon daily over a 40-day period. There were significant reductions in fasting serum glucose levels, but no evidence of a dose-dependent response, suggesting that small amounts are effective (Khan, Safdar, Mohammad Muzaffar Ali, Khan Nawaz, & Anderson, 2003). This was confirmed in another randomized controlled trial (RCT) that showed the effect of cinnamon on blood glucose was not dose-dependent in type II diabetes (Lu et al., 2012). In this trial, consumption

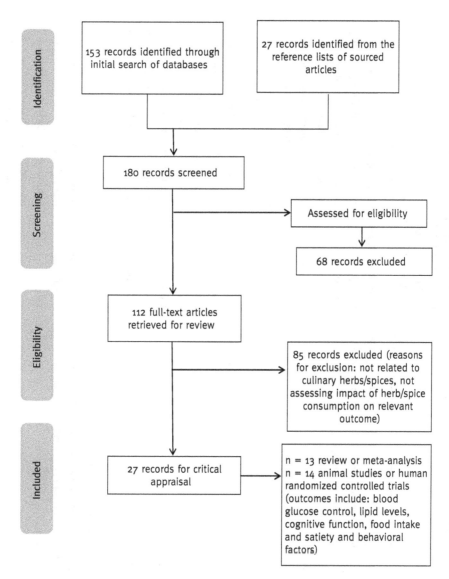

FIGURE 3.1 Flowchart of the search strategy used in this review.

of cinnamon extract at levels of 120 mg/day and 360 mg/day, taken with gliclazide (an anti-diabetic agent which acts by increasing insulin release by binding to sulfonylurea receptors [SUR-1] on beta cells in the pancreas), resulted in significant reductions in HbA1c and fasting glucose levels over 3 months. No significant changes were seen in the group on gliclazide alone.

Effects have also been seen in participants without type II diabetes. In a sample of normal weight and obese individuals without type II diabetes, a dose of 6 g of cinnamon added to cereal was found to significantly reduce blood glucose responses up to 1 hour after consumption (Magistrelli & Chezem, 2012). Blood glucose levels were found to be higher at 120 minutes, but the authors indicated that this could have reflected a decrease in variability of blood glucose levels. Similarly, when individuals with pre-diabetes were provided with 500 mg/day of Cinnulin PF (a water soluble cinnamon extract) for a 12-week period, significant decreases in fasting blood glucose (> 8%) were found in the experimental group compared to controls (Ziegenfuss, Hofheins, Mendel, Landis, & Anderson, 2006).

While these studies are informative, systematic reviews of the literature provide more consolidated

Table 3.1. Summary of Clinical and Behavioral Effects of Herb and Spice Consumption

AUTHOR	DESIGN	N	SOURCE	DOSE	MEASUREMENT (RELEVANT TO OUTCOMES OF INTEREST)	OUTCOME
Janssens et al. (2014)	RCT	15	Capsaicin (red pepper chili)—served in either 100% or 75% of energy balance	7.68 mg (divided over 3 meals)	Appetite profile, perception of taste of food, amount of ad libitum food consumed	Consumption of capsaicin in an isocaloric diet resulted in significantly higher satiety and fullness than isocaloric control meals ($p < 0.05$). Desire to eat, fullness, and satiety did not differ between the energy deficit meals with capsaicin and the isocaloric control meals.
Ahuja and Ball (2006)	RCT	27	Capsaicin (chili)	30 g chili/day	Lipids, lipoproteins, total antioxidant status, Cu-induced lipoprotein oxidation	Consumption of chili resulted in a significantly lower rate of oxidation in all participants ($p = 0.04$) and significantly increased lag time before commencement of oxidation in women ($p < 0.001$). No differences in lipids, lipoproteins, or antioxidant status were found.
Westerterp-Plantenga et al. (2005)	RCT	24	Capsaicin: red pepper in tomato juice or capsules, to be taken 30 min before set meals	0.9 g red pepper (0.25% capsaicin)	Daily food intake, self-reported hunger and satiety	Energy intake was significantly reduced following consumption of capsaicin in either capsules ($p < 0.01$) or juice ($p < 0.001$), compared to placebo. Capsaicin also resulted in a significant increase in self-reported satiety ($p < 0.01$), and resulted in a reduction in the percentage energy from fat ($p < 0.01$).

Reference	Study type	N	Supplement	Dose	Outcomes	Results
Whiting et al. (2012)	SLR	20 RCTs	Capsaicinoids—capsaicin, dihydrocapsaicin, nordihydrocapsaicin, capsiate, dihydrocapsiate, nordihydrocapaiate	1 mg–135 mg/day	Weight loss, satiety, thermogenesis, energy expenditure	Increases in energy expenditure were found in 13 of 15 trials (included increased metabolic rate, body temperature, oxygen consumption). Beneficial effects on lipid thermogenesis found in 7 of 11 studies (included increased lipid oxidation and decrease in fat stores). Five of seven studies found reductions in energy intake and reductions in hunger/increases in satiety.
Whiting et al. (2014)	SLR and meta-analysis	10 RCTs	Capsaicinoids (in the form of chili)	0.2 mg–30 mg	Energy intake	Consuming capsaicinoids resulted in statistically significant reductions in ad libitum energy intake of 74.0 kcal per meal ($p < 0.001$). A minimum of 2 mg of capsaicinoids was required to yield the effect.
Ziegenfuss et al. (2006)	RCT	22	Cinnulin PF (water-soluble cinnamon extract)	500 mg/day	Fasting blood glucose, systolic blood pressure, body composition	Consumption of cinnulin resulted in significant decreases in fasting blood glucose (-8.4%, $p < 0.01$), systolic blood pressure (-3.8%, $p < 0.001$), and increased in lean mass (1.1%, $p < 0.002$) compared to controls.

(continued)

Table 3.1. Continued

AUTHOR	DESIGN	N	SOURCE	DOSE	MEASUREMENT (RELEVANT TO OUTCOMES OF INTEREST)	OUTCOME
Markey et al. (2011)	RCT	9	Cinnamon	3 g cinnamon served with high-fat meal, followed by ad libitum buffet meal	Plasma glucose, blood lipids, subjective appetite ratings	Cinnamon consumption did not result in significant changes in any outcome.
Magistrelli and Chezem (2012)	RCT	30	Cinnamon	6 g served with cereal	Blood glucose at a range of time points until 120 min post-meal	Addition of cinnamon to cereal significantly reduced 120-min glucose area under the curve (AUC) ($p = 0.008$) and blood glucose at 15, 30, 45, 60 (all $p = 0.001$) minutes. However, at 120 minutes, blood glucose levels were significantly higher following cinnamon intake ($p = 0.001$)
Khan et al. (2003)	RCT	60	Cinnamon	1, 3 or 6 g daily	Fasting serum glucose, blood lipids	All three levels of cinnamon intake reduced mean fasting glucose (18%–29%), triglycerides (23%–30%), LDL-C (7%–27%), total cholesterol (12%–26%). No evidence of dose-dependent response

Study	Study type	N	Intervention	Dose	Outcomes	Results
Lu et al. (2012)	RCT	66	Cinnamon extract	360 mg/day (high dose) or 120 mg/day (low dose)	HbA1c, fasting glucose levels, blood lipids	Consumption of cinnamon significantly reduced HbA1c and fasting glucose levels in both the low ($p < 0.01$) and high ($p < 0.01$) cinnamon groups. Triglyceride levels were significantly reduced in the low-dose group only ($p < 0.01$). No significant changes were found in other outcomes.
Leach and Kumar (2012)	SLR	10 RCTs	Cinnamon	Mean dose 2 g/day	Fasting blood glucose, postprandial glucose levels, HbA1c, serum insulin, insulin sensitivity	The impact of cinnamon on fasting blood glucose levels was inconclusive. There was no significant difference between cinnamon and control groups for HbA1c, serum insulin, or postprandial glucose.
Akilen et al. (2012)	SLR and meta-analysis	6 RCTs	Cinnamon	1–6 g/day	HbA1c, fasting glucose	Cinnamon significantly improved HbA1c compared to placebo, and significantly reduced fasting plasma glucose compared to placebo.
Allen et al. (2013)	SLR and meta-analysis	10 RCTs	Cinnamon	120 mg/day–6 g/day	HbA1c, fasting glucose, blood lipids	Following cinnamon supplementation, significant reductions were found in fasting glucose, total cholesterol, LDL-C, and triglycerides. Cinnamon supplementation also resulted in increased HDL-C levels. No significant effect on HbA1c was found.

(continued)

Table 3.1. Continued

AUTHOR	DESIGN	N	SOURCE	DOSE	MEASUREMENT (RELEVANT TO OUTCOMES OF INTEREST)	OUTCOME
Davis and Yokoyama (2011)	SLR and meta-analysis	8 RCTs	Cinnamon (as whole cinnamon or as extract)	Whole cinnamon (1–6 g), cinnamon extract (250 mg–3 g equivalent)	Fasting plasma glucose	Cinnamon intake as whole or extract significantly lowered fasting plasma glucose ($p = 0.025$), and intake of cinnamon extract alone also lowered fasting glucose ($p = 0.008$).
Sahebkar (2014)	SLR and meta-analysis	5 RCTs	Curcumin	45 mg–6 g curcuminoids/day	Blood lipids	No significant effect of curcumin on any outcomes (small increases in total cholesterol, LDL-C, and small decreases in HDL-C and TG).
Dong et al. (2012)	Animal study	Aged rats	Curcumin	12 mg per day	Non-spatial and spatial memory, neurogenesis	Consumption of curcumin for 6 and 12 weeks significantly increased non-spatial memory ($p < 0.01$), while spatial memory improved after 12 weeks only ($p < 0.05$). 12-week curcumin intake also resulted in the development of new neural cells and the up-regulation of genes associated with brain development.
Prior et al. (2013)	Animal study	Aged mice with Alzheimer's disease	J147 (curcumin derivative)	200 ppm (10 mg/kg/day)	Memory, neuroprotective pathways, amyloid metabolism	J147 attenuated the cognitive decline found in aged mice with Alzheimer's disease. It also resulted in reduced levels of soluble β-amyloid.

Author	Study type	N	Spice/intervention	Dose	Outcomes	Findings
Brondino et al. (2014)	SLR	2 RCTs, 1 case-study	Curcumin	100 mg–4 g/day	Cognitive impairment and neuropsychiatric symptoms in individuals with dementia	RCTs found no difference in cognitive impairment following curcumin consumption, while a case study found improvements in neuropsychiatric symptoms.
Li et al. (2013)	SLR	9 SLRs	Garlic		Blood lipids	Evidence for the effect of garlic consumption on lipid levels was contentious, and the study authors were unable to draw a conclusion.
Ried et al. (2013)	SLR and meta-analysis	39 RCTs	Garlic (garlic powder, garlic oil, aged garlic extract, raw garlic)	Garlic powder (600–5600 mg/day), garlic oil (9–19 mg/day), aged garlic extract (1000–7200 mg/day), raw garlic (4–10 g/day)	Blood lipids	Consumption of garlic resulted in significant reductions in serum total cholesterol and LDL-C levels. Garlic was particularly effective in individuals with elevated total cholesterol levels, if garlic was used for more than 2 months. Small significant increases were also found in HDL-C levels.
Nakayama et al. (2014)	RCT	14	Mixed herbs and spices: curry containing cloves, coriander, cumin, garlic, ginger, onion, red pepper, turmeric	Cloves (0.9 g), coriander (1.8 g), cumin (0.9 g), garlic (3.6 g), ginger (2.7 g), onion (9 g), red pepper (0.09 g), turmeric (4.5 g)	Flow-mediated dilation, glucose, blood lipids, insulin, hsCRP, urine creatinine	Consumption of curry containing mixed herbs and spices resulted in a significant increase in postprandial flow-mediated dilation, compared to control meal ($p = 0.002$). No significant effect of curry on other outcomes.

(continued)

Table 3.1.   Continued

AUTHOR	DESIGN	N	SOURCE	DOSE	MEASUREMENT OUTCOME (RELEVANT TO OUTCOMES OF INTEREST)	
Peters et al. (2014)	RCT	148	Mixed herbs and spices: garlic and herb seasoning, basil, oregano, garlic powder, onion powder, dill weed, Italian seasoning, chervil, chives—added to reduced fat meatloaf, vegetables, and pasta sauce	Garlic and herb seasoning (0.27 g/serve), basil (0.03 g/serve), oregano (0.03 g/serve), garlic powder (30.76 g/serve), onion powder (17 g/serve), dill weed (4.06 g/serve), Italian seasoning (3 g/serve), chervil (1.5 g/serve), chives (1.5 g/serve)	Liking of the dish (amount consumed and self-reported liking)	Reducing fat by 60% caused a significant drop in liking, but adding herbs and spices attenuated drop in liking (so no significant difference was found between full- and low-fat meals).

Study	Design	N	Intervention	Outcomes measured	Key findings
Gregersen et al. (2013)	RCT	22	Mixed herbs and spices: ginger, horseradish, Dijon mustard, black pepper—each added to a separate test brunch	Ginger (20 g), horseradish (8.3 g), Dijon mustard (21 g), black pepper (1.3 g)	Subjective appetite sensations, taste, diet induced thermogenesis (DIT), blood lipids, glucose, insulin	Mustard increased DIT compared to ginger, horseradish and black pepper (all $p < 0.05$). No significant effect on ad libitium consumption was found, and there were no treatment effects on measures of subjective appetite. Black pepper decreased HDL-C significantly compared to placebo and horseradish ($p < 0.05$).
Ghawi et al. (2014)	RCT	148	Mixed herbs/spices: basil, cumin, and coriander or oregano added to low-salt soups	Urine sodium analysis, liking of soups	Liking of salt-reduced soup (57% lower salt content) was significantly lower than regular soup. While including herbs and spices did not result in an immediate improvement in liking, it enhanced the perception of salty taste of the low-salt soup to the same level as the standard soup. Repeated exposure to the soups with added herbs and spices also resulted in significant improvements in the liking of the soups.

SLR = systematic literature review; RCT = randomized controlled trial.

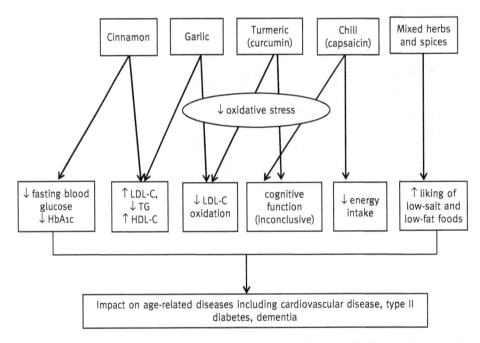

FIGURE 3.2   Summary of research pathways examining clinical and behavioral effects of culinary herbs and spices.

evidence than individual studies. For example, Davis and Yokoyama (2011) analyzed the results of eight RCTs investigating the effect of cinnamon intake on fasting plasma glucose in participants with type II diabetes. They found that adding cinnamon, taken as whole cinnamon or as cinnamon extract, significantly reduced fasting plasma glucose compared to controls. Similar results were published a year later (Akilen, Tsiami, Devendra, & Robinson, 2012) in a meta-analysis of six RCTs involving people with type II diabetes. This analysis found significant reductions in fasting plasma glucose and HbA1c following cinnamon consumption of 1–6 g/day. A more recent meta-analysis (Allen, Schwartzman, Baker, Coleman, & Phung, 2013) also found significant reductions in fasting glucose levels following consumption of 120 mg–6 g cinnamon per day, but not for HbA1c.

The lack of complete agreement in the literature is indicative of most studies on diet and health outcomes. In the case of cinnamon, differences may relate to the background diet in which the study of cinnamon consumption is conducted. For example, in one study where cinnamon (3 g) was served with a high-fat meal, no significant effects on postprandial glucose levels were observed (Markey et al., 2011). The choice of study populations may

also influence results. For example, one systematic review that included participants with both type I and type II diabetes found inconclusive evidence of effects on fasting blood glucose levels and no significant effects of cinnamon consumption on HbA1c (Leach & Kumar, 2012). These findings add layers to the understanding of how cinnamon may exert effects on blood glucose levels, suggesting that both dietary conditions and existing states of metabolic health need to be considered before making general statements.

Overall, however, the results of the studies taken as a whole suggest that cinnamon consumption may help to ameliorate high fasting blood glucose levels in individuals with and without type II diabetes. The mechanisms behind these effects are the subject of further research, with current findings suggesting an influence on the expression of peroxisome proliferator-activated receptors (Sheng, Zhang, Gong, Huang, & Zang, 2008) as well as the expression of genes such as protein-tyrosine phosphatase 1β (Eijaz, Salim, & Waqar, 2014). As these mechanisms result in improved insulin and glucose metabolism (Eijaz et al., 2014; Sheng et al., 2008), the observations made in clinical trials appear plausible.

While cinnamon is a single spice, very few studies have also been conducted using mixed herbs and spices. In one small study involving males only ($n = 14$), Nakayama et al. (2014) found the 1-hour postprandial glucose response to a curry containing mixed herbs and spices (cloves, coriander, cumin, garlic, ginger, onion, red pepper, turmeric) was no different from that to a herb- and spice-free control meal. Similarly, meals containing either ginger, horseradish, Dijon mustard, or black pepper had no impact on postprandial glucose levels, even when collected 4 hours post-meal. Thus short-term effects could not be demonstrated, although this says nothing of long-term effects in a dietary pattern. Either way, substantially more research is required.

Effects on Blood Lipids

Dyslipidemia, a clinical condition characterized by elevated LDL-C and triglyceride levels, and decreased HDL-C levels, is associated with an increased risk of cardiovascular disease (Musunuru, 2010). In addition, susceptibility of LDL-C to oxidation is a key component in the development of atherosclerosis, causing a buildup of fatty plaques in the arteries (Ahuja & Ball, 2006; Musunuru, 2010). The consumption of herbs and spices that may influence these parameters is now of great interest in promoting healthy aging.

As for blood glucose levels, many of the studies found for this review also focused on the effects of cinnamon on blood lipid levels. In addition to blood glucose, Khan et al. (2003) also examined the effect of varying levels of cinnamon intake on blood lipids after 40 days in people with type II diabetes ($n = 60$). They found significant reductions in total cholesterol, LDL-C, and triglyceride levels. There was no evidence of a dose-dependent effect and no significant effects on HDL-C levels. In another study where intakes of high (360 mg/day) and low (120 mg/day) cinnamon extract were compared, no significant changes in total cholesterol, LDL-C, or HDL-C were found (Lu et al., 2012). Triglyceride levels reduced significantly, but only in the low-dose group. These mixed results suggest that more research is required on the pharmacodynamics of cinnamon in relation to blood lipids, with careful attention to other dietary influencers on lipids, in particular dietary fat.

Once again, systematic reviews of the literature provide more consolidated evidence than individual studies. A recent meta-analysis (Allen et al., 2013) examining RCTs (including those referred to earlier: Khan et al., 2003; Lu et al., 2012) found

significant reductions in total cholesterol, LDL-C, and triglycerides with cinnamon consumption, along with significant increases in HDL-C levels. There appear to be some inconsistencies in lipid responses to cinnamon intake reported between studies, but significant effects are found when results are combined.

Unlike for blood glucose levels, there were more reports in the literature on the effects of other spices on blood lipids. For example, the effect of consumption of capsaicin from chili on lipids was investigated in a 4-week RCT (Ahuja & Ball, 2006). Participants were provided with 30 g of chili per day to be added to a prescribed diet, and outcomes were compared to those following consumption of a "bland" diet with minimal herbs or spices. At the conclusion of the study, no differences were found between diets in lipid levels or antioxidant status, although the rate of lipoprotein oxidation was significantly lower following the chili diet compared to the "bland" diet. The results of this study suggest that while the consumption of capsaicin may not lead to reductions in lipid levels, it may be associated with the attenuation of oxidation, which is linked with atherosclerosis. This association has been supported by the overview of the health benefits of capsaicin explored by Srinivasan (2012).

Turmeric appears as another spice of interest in lipids research. Here the compound of interest is curcumin. A recent meta-analysis examined the effect of consumption of curcumin on lipid levels (2014) in five RCTs with curcuminoid intake ranging from 45 mg to 6 g per day. No significant effect for curcumin consumption on total cholesterol, LDL-C, HDL-C or triglycerides was found when study results were pooled. As for capsaicin, however, curcumin may also play a role in decreasing the susceptibility of LDL-C to oxidation (Srinivasan, 2012).

While not strictly a spice, the potential for garlic to exert favorable effects on lipid levels and on the susceptibility of LDL-C to oxidation has been previously raised (Srinivasan, 2012; Tapsell et al., 2006). However, contention has arisen around the inconsistent use of inclusion and exclusion criteria in evaluating the research (Li et al., 2013), such that sound conclusions on the effect of garlic consumption on lipid levels remain problematic. Nevertheless, a meta-analysis involving more recent RCTs ($n = 39$) did examine the effect of a range of sources of garlic on total cholesterol, LDL-C, HDL-C, and triglyceride levels (Ried, Toben, & Fakler, 2013). Consumption of garlic for more than 2 months was found to result in significantly reduced levels of total cholesterol and LDL-C in individuals with elevated total cholesterol levels. Small improvements in HDL-C levels were found with garlic consumption, and no significant changes in triglycerides were found. Furthermore, the source of the garlic appeared to influence the effect, with aged garlic extract having the greatest impact on total cholesterol levels. The authors of that review suggested that the health outcomes of garlic consumption may be mediated by a number of factors, including study duration, cholesterol level, and garlic source. This may explain the inconsistent results found by others (for example, Li et al., 2013).

As with blood glucose, there are few studies examining the effects of mixed herbs and spices, even though this is how they are often consumed. One study examined the short-term effects of a dish rich in a number of herbs and spices on lipid levels (Nakayama et al., 2014). Consumption of a curry dish with mixed herbs and spices including garlic, turmeric, and red pepper did not affect total cholesterol, LDL-C, HDL-C, or triglyceride levels when measured 1 hour later. In another investigation, the short-term impact of ginger, horseradish, Dijon mustard, or black pepper on a number of lipid measures was studied 4 hours after a meal. Black pepper was found to significantly reduce HDL-C compared to placebo and horseradish (Gregersen et al., 2013). Clearly more research is needed in this area and in cuisine patterns that characteristically utilize these spices.

Effects on Cognitive Function

A number of herbs and spices have been used as complementary therapy for mental health therapy (Chiappedi, de Vincenzi, & Bejor, 2012). Dementia is an age-related condition associated with oxidative stress and inflammation, and maintaining cognitive function in individuals suffering from dementia is a key part of retaining quality of life in aging.

Research conducted in animals suggests that consumption of curcumin may improve cognitive function during aging. Dong et al. (2012) found improvements in non-spatial memory in aged rats fed curcumin for 6 weeks, and in spatial memory when curcumin was consumed over 12 weeks, suggesting that prolonged intake may be required for beneficial effects. Consumption of curcumin also resulted in the up-regulation of a number of genes, including those linked with brain development, and also led to the generation of new neural cells, which

has been linked to improvements in memory function.

While evidence exists for the effect of curcumin on cognitive function in animals, a recent systematic review found limited evidence for these effects in humans with dementia (Brondino et al., 2014). Two RCTs met the criteria for inclusion, and both found that curcumin consumption produced no difference in cognitive impairment, although the reviewers included a case study of three patients showing improvements in neuropsychiatric symptoms. The review did identify a number of clinical trials currently underway, which may shed further light on the potential relationship between curcumin and cognitive function. Even so, the bioavailability characteristics of naturally occurring curcumin may prove a challenge for studies aiming to show significant effects at clinically relevant doses (Brondino et al., 2014). Recent animal research using the curcumin derivative J147 found that it attenuated cognitive decline in aged mice with Alzheimer's disease (Prior, Dargusch, Ehren, Chiruta, & Schubert, 2013). J147 may provide an alternative vehicle for curcumin delivery in human studies.

Impact on Food Intake and Satiety

In addition to clinical outcomes, the inclusion of herbs and spices may influence behavioral outcomes such as food intake and perceived satiety. Of all the spices, the effect of capsaicin from chili on dietary intake has received the most attention. In one study, Westerterp-Plantenga et al. (2005) assessed the effect of 0.9 g red pepper (0.25% capsaicin) on subsequent food intake, hunger, and satiety. Twenty-four participants were provided with red pepper, either added to tomato juice or taken in capsule form (or a corresponding control), prior to consuming prescribed meals over a 2-day period. Consumption of capsaicin in tomato juice or as capsules resulted in significantly lower energy intakes compared to placebo, with the presentation of capsaicin in tomato juice found to be most effective (resulting in a 16% reduction in energy intake). Capsaicin consumption was also found to result in significant increases in self-reported satiety and significant decreases in hunger compared to placebo. The spiciness of capsaicin appeared to be central to its influence, with perceived spiciness found to be associated with the changes in energy intake and satiety for the tomato juice preparation, but not when capsaicin was consumed in capsule form. This result suggests that the method of providing capsaicin, as well as its sensory components, plays an important role in mediating its effect.

The inclusion of dietary capsaicin has also been found to attenuate the effects of negative energy balance in a recent RCT (Janssens, Hursel, & Westerterp-Plantenga, 2014). Participants were given food providing 100% or 75% of their energy requirements, both including a total of 7.68 mg of capsaicin, or corresponding control meals. The inclusion of capsaicin in an energy-deficient diet resulted in similar outcome measures for desire to eat, satiety, and fullness compared to the isocaloric control (without capsaicin). This suggests that capsaicin attenuates the effect on appetite that might result from a 25% reduction in energy intake. Similarly, when the results were compared for those given 100% energy with and without capsaicin, the meals containing capsaicin were found to result in significantly higher perceptions of satiety and fullness, suggesting that capsaicin mediates appetite in both negative and neutral energy balance models.

The mechanisms by which capsaicin may exert its effect have also been studied. It is suggested that capsaicin may influence appetite and energy intake through the activation of the transient receptor potential vanilloid 1 receptor, resulting in stimulation of the sympathetic nervous system and the corresponding release of catecholamines, which act to suppress appetite (Sharma, Vij, & Sharma, 2013; Whiting, Derbyshire, & Tiwari, 2014). In addition, the body of research has grown to the extent where consolidated analyses can be conducted. For example, a systematic review of 20 RCTs found evidence of the beneficial effects of capsaicinoids on energy expenditure and lipid thermogenesis, as well as on reductions in energy intake and hunger (Whiting, Derbyshire, & Tiwari, 2012). In a more recent meta-analysis (Whiting et al., 2014), the effect of chili containing capsaicinoids on energy intake was quantified. This study found that consuming a minimum of 2 mg of capsaicinoids prior to a meal resulted in reductions in ad libitum energy intake of 74 calories per meal. Though this may not appear to be a large decrease at a single point in time, the effects may be cumulative if the food pattern is maintained for extended periods.

Impact on Food Choice

The ability of herbs and spices to influence the choice of other foods and thereby the total diet is an indirect way in which herbs and spices may contribute to better health. In a recent study, the addition of mixed herbs and spices improved the perceived liking of reduced-fat and reduced-salt foods. Peters et al. (2014) assessed the impact of adding mixed herbs and spices, including garlic, basil, and oregano, to a reduced-fat meal of meatloaf, vegetables, and pasta sauce. The inclusion of herbs and spices to this 60% reduced fat meal was found to attenuate the drop in liking seen with reducing the fat content, with no difference in liking found between the control meal and the reduced-fat meal for most components. Similarly, Ghawi et al. (2014) found that adding basil, cumin, and coriander or oregano to low-salt soups enhanced the perception of salty taste, and significantly improved the liking of the low-salt soups following repeated exposure. The results of these studies suggest that adding herbs and spices may improve the acceptability of meals with reduced fat and salt contents, and thus may be supportive of consumption of a diet that better protects health.

Traditional Herbal Preparations

While this review has focused on culinary herbs and spices and their effect on health and behavioral outcomes, traditional herbal preparations such as those included in traditional Chinese medicine form another consideration in examining the contribution of herbs and spices to health.

As with most plant foods, traditional Chinese herbal medicines have been shown to demonstrate antioxidant capacity in in vitro studies (Shen, Truong, Helliwell, Govindaraghavan, & Sucher, 2013; Zhao, Dou, Wu, & Aisa, 2013). As stated earlier, antioxidant mechanisms may be considered in addressing possible effects on cognitive function. There have been reports of traditional Chinese medicines linked to improvements in cognitive function in both healthy individuals (Park et al., 2005) and those suffering from Alzheimer's disease and dementia (Wang, Huang, Tang, & Zhang, 2010; Wang & Tang, 2005).

Specific attention has also been paid to the individual components of traditional Chinese herbal medicine, including ginseng and ginkgo biloba. Research suggests that the consumption of ginseng may improve cognitive function both in individuals with dementia (Wang et al., 2010) and in healthy individuals, including those with some age-related memory loss (Geng et al., 2010; Kim et al., 2008).

These effects may be due to an increase in acetylcholine levels due to an improvement in cholinergic function, and the inhibition of the inflammation cascade (Wang et al., 2010). Evidence for the impact of ginkgo biloba on cognitive function is currently inconsistent, with mixed results found both for healthy individuals and those experiencing cognitive decline (Canter & Ernst, 2007; Holtzman, 2013; Meletis & Bramwell, 2001; Snitz et al., 2009; Wesnes, 2006). These results suggest that while some evidence exists for specific components of traditional Chinese medicine, additional research is required to fully elucidate the effects of these herbs on clinical outcomes.

SUMMARY

Evidence from the literature suggests that herbs and spices and their components, such as cinnamon, garlic, curcumin, and capsaicin, may have beneficial effects on health and behavioral outcomes. These outcomes characterize age-related chronic diseases, and the effects reported here may be mediated by the antioxidant actions of herbs and spices. The inclusion of herbs and spices in protective dietary patterns, such as the Mediterranean and Okinawan diets, may play a role in contributing to their effects. Conversely, a paucity of herbs and spices may be linked to the detrimental health outcomes associated with the Western diet. The food or meal vehicle providing the herb or spice should also be considered when translating to dietary advice to preserve the beneficial role within a specific dietary pattern. Encouragement of a diet rich in herbs and spices may also improve acceptability of protective dietary patterns, suggesting that the impact of herbs and spices on healthy aging may be multifaceted.

DISCLOSURE STATEMENTS

Financial Disclosure information from Linda Tapsell:

Research grants: from the Australian Research Council, Illawarra Health and Medical Research Institute, California Walnut Commission. Advisory Committees: Australian Government, Department of Health and Aging, Nutrient Reference Values Advisory Committee and Expert Working Group, California Walnut Commission, McCormick's Science Institute. Editorial Committees: *Nutrition and Dietetics* (Dietitians Association of Australia), *Nutrition Today, Perspective Newsletter* (Unilever).

Dr. Neale is a Research Fellow at the University of Wollongong. Dr. Neale is also a director of Landmark Nutrition, and in this role has received funding from the Pork Cooperative Research Centre, Nuts for Life, Safcol Australia, Oxford University Press, and the Australian Government Department of Health.

REFERENCES

Ahuja, K. D. K., & Ball, M. J. (2006). Effects of daily ingestion of chilli on serum lipoprotein oxidation in adult men and women. *Brit J Nutrition, 96*(2), 239–242. doi: 10.1079/bjn20061788

Ai-Lawati, J. A., & Al-Lawati, A. M. (2007). The utility of fasting plasma glucose in predicting glycosylated hemoglobin in type 2 diabetes. *Ann Saudi Med, 27*(5), 347–351.

AIHW. (2012). *Risk factors contributing to chronic disease.* (Cat. no. PHE 157). Canberra: Retrieved from http://www.aihw.gov.au/publication-detail/?id=10737421466.

Akilen, R., Tsiami, A., Devendra, D., & Robinson, N. (2012). Cinnamon in glycaemic control: systematic review and meta analysis. *Clin Nutr, 31*(5), 609–615. doi: http://dx.doi.org/10.1016/j.clnu.2012.04.003

Allen, R. W., Schwartzman, E., Baker, W. L., Coleman, C. I., & Phung, O. J. (2013). Cinnamon use in type 2 diabetes: an updated systematic review and meta-analysis. *Ann Family Med, 11*(5), 452–459. doi: 10.1370/afm.1517

Anderson, A. L., Harris, T. B., Tylavsky, F. A., Perry, S. E., Houston, D. K., Hue, T. F., . . . Sahyoun, N. R. (2011). Dietary patterns and survival of older adults. *J Am Dietetic Assoc, 111*(1), 84–91. doi: http://dx.doi.org/10.1016/j.jada.2010.10.012

Assmann, G. (2006). Dyslipidaemia and global cardiovascular risk: clinical issues. *Eur Heart J Suppl, 8*(suppl F), F40–F46. doi: 10.1093/eurheartj/sul040

Brondino, N., Re, S., Boldrini, A., Cuccomarino, A., Lanati, N., Barale, F., & Politi, P. (2014). Curcumin as a therapeutic agent in dementia: a mini systematic review of human studies. *Scientific World J, 2014*, 174282. doi: 17428210.1155/2014/174282

Canter, P. H., & Ernst, E. (2007). Ginkgo biloba is not a smart drug: an updated systematic review of randomised clinical trials testing the nootropic effects of G-biloba extracts in healthy people.

Human Psychopharm Clin Exper, 22(5), 265–278. doi: 10.1002/hup.843

Chiappedi, M., de Vincenzi, S., & Bejor, M. (2012). Nutraceuticals in psychiatric practice. *Recent Pat CNS Drug Discov, 7*(2), 163-72. doi: 10.2174/157488912800673119

Davis, P. A., & Yokoyama, W. (2011). Cinnamon intake lowers fasting blood glucose: meta-analysis. *J Med Food, 14*(9), 884–889. doi: 10.1089/jmf.2010.0180

De la Fuente, M., & Miquel, J. (2009). An update of the oxidation-inflammation theory of aging: the involvement of the immune system in oxi-inflamm-aging. *Curr Pharmaceut Design, 15*(26), 3003–3026.

De Martinis, M., Franceschi, C., Monti, D., & Ginaldi, L. (2005). Inflamm-ageing and lifelong antigenic load as major determinants of ageing rate and longevity. *FEBS Letters, 579*(10), 2035–2039. doi: http://dx.doi.org/10.1016/j.febslet.2005.02.055

Dong, S. Z., Zeng, Q. W., Mitchell, E. S., Xiu, J., Duan, Y., Li, C. X., . . . Zhao, Z. (2012). Curcumin enhances neurogenesis and cognition in aged rats: implications for transcriptional interactions related to growth and synaptic plasticity. *Plos One, 7*(2), e31211 doi: e3121110.1371/journal.pone.0031211

Edelman, D., Olsen, M. K., Dudley, T. K., Harris, A. C., & Oddone, E. Z. (2004). Utility of hemoglobin A1c in predicting diabetes risk. *J Gen Intern Med, 19*(12), 1175–1180. doi: 10.1111/j.1525-1497.2004.40178.x

Eijaz, S., Salim, A., & Waqar, M. A. (2014). Possible molecular targets of cinnamon in the insulin signaling pathway. *J Biochem Technol, 5*(2), 708–717.

Ferencík, M., Stvrtinová, V., Hulín, I., & Novák, M. (2007). Inflammation—a lifelong companion: attempt at a non-analytical holistic view. *Folia microbiologica, 52*(2), 159–173. doi: 10.1007/bf02932155

Geng, J. S., Dong, J. C., Ni, H. J., Lee, M. S., Wu, T. X., Jiang, K., . . . Malouf, R. (2010). Ginseng for cognition. *Cochrane Database Syst Rev, 12*, CD007769. doi: 10.1002/14651858.CD007769.pub2

Ghawi, S. K., Rowland, I., & Methven, L. (2014). Enhancing consumer liking of low salt tomato soup over repeated exposure by herb and spice seasonings. *Appetite, 81*(0), 20–29. doi: http://dx.doi.org/10.1016/j.appet.2014.05.029

Gregersen, N. T., Belza, A., Jensen, M. G., Ritz, C., Bitz, C., Hels, O., . . . Astrup, A. (2013). Acute effects of mustard, horseradish, black pepper and ginger on energy expenditure, appetite, ad libitum energy intake and energy balance in human subjects. *Brit J Nutrition, 109*(3), 556–563. doi: http://dx.doi.org/10.1017/S0007114512001201

Heidemann, C., Schulze, M. B., Franco, O. H., van Dam, R. M., Mantzoros, C. S., & Hu, F. B. (2008). Dietary patterns and risk of mortality from cardiovascular disease, cancer, and all causes in a prospective cohort of women. *Circulation, 118*(3), 230–237. doi: 10.1161/circulationaha.108.771881

Holtzman, J. L. (2013). Cellular and animal models for high-throughput screening of therapeutic agents for the treatment of the diseases of the elderly in general and alzheimer's disease in particular. *Front Pharmacology, 4*, article 59. doi: 10.3389/fphar.2013.00059.

Inoue, K., Matsumoto, M., & Kobayashi, Y. (2007). The combination of fasting plasma glucose and glycosylated hemoglobin predicts type 2 diabetes in Japanese workers. *Diabetes Res Clin Pr, 77*(3), 451–458. doi: 10.1016/j.diabres.2007.01.024

Janssens, P. L. H. R., Hursel, R., & Westerterp-Plantenga, M. S. (2014). Capsaicin increases sensation of fullness in energy balance, and decreases desire to eat after dinner in negative energy balance. *Appetite, 77*(0), 46–51. doi: http://dx.doi.org/10.1016/j.appet.2014.02.018

Khan, A., Safdar, M., Mohammad Muzaffar Ali, K., Khan Nawaz, K., & Anderson, R. A. (2003). Cinnamon improves glucose and lipids of people with type 2 diabetes. *Diabetes Care, 26*(12), 3215–3218.

Kim, J., Chung, S. Y., Park, S., Park, J. H., Byun, S., Hwang, M., . . . Kim, H. (2008). Enhancing effect of HT008-1 on cognitive function and quality of life in cognitively declined healthy adults: a randomized, double-blind, placebo-controlled, trial. *Pharmacol Biochem Behav, 90*(4), 517–524. doi: 10.1016/j.pbb.2008.03.033

Leach, M. J., & Kumar, S. (2012). Cinnamon for diabetes mellitus. *Cochrane Database Syst Rev, 9*, CD007170. doi: Cd00717010.1002/14651858.CD007170.pub2

Li, L., Sun, T., Tian, J., Yang, K., Yi, K., & Zhang, P. (2013). Garlic in clinical practice: an evidence-based overview. *Crit Rev Food Sci Nutr, 53*(7), 670–681. doi: 10.1080/10408398.2010.537000

Lu, T., Sheng, H., Wu, J., Cheng, Y., Zhu, J., & Chen, Y. (2012). Cinnamon extract improves fasting blood glucose and glycosylated hemoglobin level in Chinese patients with type 2 diabetes. *Nutr Res, 32*(6), 408–412. doi: http://dx.doi.org/10.1016/j.nutres.2012.05.003

Magistrelli, A., & Chezem, J. C. (2012). Effect of ground cinnamon on postprandial blood glucose concentration in normal-weight and obese adults. *J Acad Nutr Diet, 112*(11), 1806–1809. doi: 10.1016/j.jand.2012.07.037

Markey, O., McClean, C., Medlow, P., Davison, G., Trinick, T., Duly, E., & Shafat, A. (2011). Effect of cinnamon on gastric emptying, arterial stiffness, postprandial lipemia, glycemia, and appetite responses to high-fat breakfast. *Cardiovasc Diabetol, 10*(1), 78.

Meletis, C. D., & Bramwell, B. (2001). Natural therapies to preserve and enhance cognition and memory. *Altern Complem Ther, 7*(5), 273–276.

Moher, D., Liberati, A., Tetzlaff, J., Altman, D. G., & The Prisma Group. (2009). Preferred reporting items for systematic reviews and meta-analyses: the PRISMA statement. *PLoS Med, 6*(7), e1000097. doi: 10.1371/journal. pmed.1000097

Musunuru, K. (2010). Atherogenic dyslipidemia: cardiovascular risk and dietary intervention. *Lipids, 45*(10), 907–914. doi: 10.1007/s11745-010-3408-1

Nakayama, H., Tsuge, N., Sawada, H., Masamura, N., Yamada, S., Satomi, S., & Higashi, Y. (2014). A single consumption of curry improved postprandial endothelial function in healthy male subjects: a randomized, controlled crossover trial. *Nutrition J, 13*(1), 67.

Park, E., Kang, M., Oh, J. W., Jung, M., Park, C., Cho, C., . . . Bae, H. (2005). Yukmijihwang-tang derivatives enhance cognitive processing in normal young adults: a double-blinded, placebo-controlled trial. *Am J Chinese Med, 33*(1), 107–115.

Peters, J. C., Polsky, S., Stark, R., Zhaoxing, P., & Hill, J. O. (2014). The influence of herbs and spices on overall liking of reduced fat food. *Appetite, 79*(0), 183–188. doi: http://dx.doi.org/10.1016/j. appet.2014.04.019

Pradhan, A. D., Rifai, N., Buring, J. E., & Ridker, P. M. (2007). Hemoglobin A1c predicts diabetes but not cardiovascular disease in nondiabetic women. *Am J Med, 120*(8), 720–727. doi: http://dx.doi. org/10.1016/j.amjmed.2007.03.022

Prior, M., Dargusch, R., Ehren, J., Chiruta, C., & Schubert, D. (2013). The neurotrophic compound J147 reverses cognitive impairment in aged Alzheimer's disease mice. *Alzheimer's Res Ther, 5*(3), 25.

Ried, K., Toben, C., & Fakler, P. (2013). Effect of garlic on serum lipids: an updated meta-analysis. *Nutr Rev, 71*(5), 282–299. doi: 10.1111/ nure.12012

Sahebkar, A. (2014). A systematic review and meta-analysis of randomized controlled trials investigating the effects of curcumin on blood lipid levels. *Clin Nutr, 33*(3), 406–414. doi: http:// dx.doi.org/10.1016/j.clnu.2013.09.012

Samieri, C., Sun, Q., Townsend, M. K., Chiuve, S. E., Okereke, O. I., Willett, W. C., . . . Grodstein, F. (2013). The association between dietary patterns at midlife and health in aging: an observational study. *Ann Intern Med, 159*(9), 584–591. doi: 10.7326/0003-4819-159-9-201311050-00004

Sharma, S. K., Vij, A. S., & Sharma, M. (2013). Mechanisms and clinical uses of capsaicin. *Eur J Pharmacol, 720*(1–3), 55–62. doi: http://dx.doi. org/10.1016/j.ejphar.2013.10.053

Shen, B. J., Truong, J., Helliwell, R., Govindaraghavan, S., & Sucher, N. J. (2013). An in vitro study of neuroprotective properties of traditional Chinese herbal medicines thought to promote healthy ageing and longevity. *BMC Complem Altern Med, 13.* doi: 10.1186/1472-6882-13-373

Sheng, X. Y., Zhang, Y. B., Gong, Z. W., Huang, C., & Zang, Y. Q. (2008). Improved insulin resistance and lipid metabolism by cinnamon extract through activation of peroxisome proliferator-activated receptors. *PPAR Res, 2008*, 581348. doi: 58134810.1155/2008/581348

Snitz, B. E., O'Meara, E. S., Carlson, M. C., Arnold, A. M., Ives, D. G., Rapp, S. R., . . . DeKosky, S. T. (2009). Ginkgo biloba for preventing cognitive decline in older adults a randomized trial. *JAMA, 302*(24), 2663–2670.

Srinivasan, K. (2012). Antioxidant potential of spices and their active constituents. *Crit Rev Food Sci Nutr, 54*(3), 352–372. doi: 10.1080/10408398.2011.585525

Tangney, C. C., Kwasny, M. J., Li, H., Wilson, R. S., Evans, D. A., & Morris, M. C. (2011). Adherence to a Mediterranean-type dietary pattern and cognitive decline in a community population. *Am J Clin Nutr, 93*(3), 601–607. doi: 10.3945/ ajcn.110.007369

Tapsell, L. C., Hemphill, I., Cobiac, L., Patch, C. S., Sullivan, D. R., Fenech, M., . . . Inge, K. E. (2006). Health benefits of herbs and spices: the past, the present, the future. *Med J Australia, 185*(4 Suppl), S4–24.

Wang, R., & Tang, X. C. (2005). Neuroprotective effects of huperzine A—A natural cholinesterase inhibitor for the treatment of Alzheimer's disease. *Neurosignals, 14*(1–2), 71–82. doi: 10.1159/000085387

Wang, Y., Huang, L. Q., Tang, X. C., & Zhang, H. Y. (2010). Retrospect and prospect of active principles from Chinese herbs in the treatment of dementia. *Acta Pharm Sinic, 31*(6), 649–664.

Wesnes, K. A. (2006). Cognitive function testing: the case for standardization and automation. *J Brit Menopause Soc, 12*(4), 158–163.

Westerterp-Plantenga, M. S., Smeets, A., & Lejeune, M. P. G. (2005). Sensory and gastrointestinal satiety effects of capsaicin on food intake. *Int J Obes Relat Metab Disord, 29*(6), 682–688.

Whiting, S., Derbyshire, E., & Tiwari, B. K. (2012). Capsaicinoids and capsinoids: a potential role for weight management? A systematic review of the evidence. *Appetite, 59*(2), 341–348. doi: http://dx.doi.org/10.1016/j.appet.2012.05.015

Whiting, S., Derbyshire, E. J., & Tiwari, B. (2014). Could capsaicinoids help to support weight management? A systematic review and meta-analysis of energy intake data. *Appetite,* 73(0), 183–188. doi: http://dx.doi.org/10.1016/j.appet.2013.11.005

Willcox, D. C., Willcox, B. J., Todoriki, H., & Suzuki, M. (2009). The Okinawan diet: health implications of a low-calorie, nutrient-dense, antioxidant-rich dietary pattern low in glycemic load. *J Am College Nutr, 28*(4), 500S–516S.

Zhao, Y. X., Dou, J., Wu, T., & Aisa, H. A. (2013). Investigating the antioxidant and acetylcholinesterase inhibition activities of Gossypium herbaceam. *Molecules, 18*(1), 951–962. doi: 10.3390/molecules18010951

Ziegenfuss, T., Hofheins, J., Mendel, R., Landis, J., & Anderson, R. (2006). Effects of a water-soluble cinnamon extract on body composition and features of the metabolic syndrome in pre-diabetic men and women. *J Int Soc Sports Nutr, 3*(2), 45–53.

4

NATURAL REMEDIES FOR MENTAL HEALTH AND AGING

Isadora Sande Mathias and David Mischoulon

INTRODUCTION

The application of alternative medicine in the elderly, especially for mood disorders and dementia, is a developing area of psychiatry. Because of their relative ease of access and good tolerability, natural supplements are very attractive for elderly individuals seeking health balance and quality of life. However, clinicians need to be aware of their degree of efficacy, mechanisms of action, and possible side effects, in order to advise their patients and obtain positive outcomes. In this chapter, we will synthesize the most recent data on the utilization of some popular natural remedies, such as Ginkgo biloba (EGb 761), folate (particularly in Cerefolin/Deplin preparations), Rhodiola, omega-3 fatty acids, and Vayacog, St John's Wort (SJW), and S-adenosyl methionine (SAMe) in psychiatric disorders in the elderly, focusing on dementia and depression with emphasis on recommended dosage and safety considerations.

GINKGO BILOBA FOR DEMENTIA

Extracts from the leaves of the maidenhair tree, Ginkgo biloba (Gb), have been used in China for health-related purposes for centuries. In the Western community, standardized extracts from the leaves are administered as oral tablets or liquid, or intravenously. EGb 761 is the extract standardized with 24% of ginkgo-flavone glycosides, and it is the most administered version. EGb 761 has demonstrated antioxidant and vasoactive properties, as well as the potential to act as a cognitive enhancer in people with dementia. The effects of Ginkgo biloba may be due to single or combined actions from their active components, most importantly flavonoids and terpenoids (1,2,3). Many clinical trials and meta-analyses have been performed to examine the effectiveness of EGb 761 for dementia and cognitive impairment. However, data remain unclear, and more evidence is needed to recommend ginkgo's use.

Clinical Evidence

A Cochrane review and meta-analysis from 2009 (2) stated that, although safe and with no excessive unwanted effects, there was no consistent evidence of Ginkgo biloba's efficacy for dementia and cognitive impairment to date. However, several more recent trials have been performed, yielding different and often positive outcomes. These trials are outlined in the following paragraphs.

Ihl et al. (4), tested the efficacy of a once-daily formulation of EGb 761 (240 mg) for dementia in a randomized controlled trial. Their results showed improvement in cognitive performance, neuropsychiatric symptoms, functional abilities, and overall well-being when compared to placebo. A study with middle-aged healthy individuals (5) reported that a daily dose of 240 mg of EGb 761 produced benefits on free recall of appointments.

Herrschaft et al. (6) performed a clinical trial with outpatients older than 50 years, diagnosed with mild to moderate Alzheimer's disease (AD) or vascular dementia, receiving a daily dose of 240 mg of EGb 761. Their results showed significant efficacy of EGb 761 when compared to placebo.

Nasab et al. (7) compared the effectiveness of Ginkgo biloba (120 mg) to rivastagmine, a cholinesterase inhibitor, in patients with Alzheimer's disease. They found that rivastagmine is superior to EGb 761 and recommended that it not be replaced by ginkgo.

Dong et al. (8) found significant improvement in mild cognitive impairment after 1 year of a regimen of Ginkgo biloba tablets, 3 times a day. They also observed a reduction in the rate of conversion to dementia. On the other hand, a GuidAge clinical trial (9) showed that 120 mg/day of EGb 761 did not reduce the risk of progression to AD in 5 years in patients with memory complaints compared to placebo. Brondino et al. (3) also concluded that Ginkgo biloba is better than placebo, providing benefits in cognition and daily activities.

More recent studies, such as Canavelli et al. (10), suggested that EGb 761 in a daily dose of 120 mg led to positive cognitive effects in patients undergoing cholinesterase inhibitors. Finally, a meta-analysis from 2014 (11) showed that EGb 761 (240 mg) is able to stabilize or slow decline in cognition and functioning in dementia.

Dosage

The majority of significant recent trials and meta-analyses favoring Ginkgo biloba (4–6,11) have supported a daily dose of 240 mg as effective and safe. Some clinical trials have used a daily dose of 120 mg leading to negative outcomes (7,9). Indeed, the majority of studies reviewed by the Cochrane meta-analysis (2), in 2009, administered daily doses of 120 mg. They did not conclude significant benefits of EGb 761. A recent study showed efficacy of 120 mg when added to a cholinesterase inhibitor (10). The mode of administration of Ginkgo biloba may be oral or intravenous (infusion or injection) (2).

The Ginkgo One Tablet a Day (GOTADAY) study (4) was designed to assess the clinical efficacy and tolerability of a once-daily formulation containing 240 mg of Ginkgo biloba extract in demented individuals. The study found no issues with safety and tolerability of daily 240 mg of EGb 761. The dose was safe and effective for dementia, especially in cases with neuropsychiatric features.

Mechanisms

Mechanisms of action for Ginkgo biloba include an enhancement of cerebral blood flow by dilation of blood vessels, reduction of blood viscosity, antioxidant anti-inflammatory effects, and modification of neurotransmitters. Anti-platelet effects have been attributed to flavone and terpene lactone components. Ginkgo seems to act through anti–platelet activating factor (PAF) activity, exerting antioxidant effects as well. Additionally, it may protect mitochondria, damage to which has been implicated in the pathophysiology of dementia (2,12,13).

The components of EGb 761 may act in different stages of cognitive decline by several pathways (1). In dementia, it has been shown that a disturbed supply of oxygen and glucose can cause neurodegeneration and hence loss of intellectual function. Furthermore, EGb 761's properties may include the protection of neuronal cells against ischemia and reperfusion injury (2).

Side Effects and Precautions

Cases of bleeding have been reported when Ginkgo biloba was used with concurrent anti-platelet or anticoagulant drugs. EGb 761 is generally safe, but patients should be aware of possible risks of bleeding, particularly when used with anticoagulants (12). A classic review from *The Lancet* (1) found neither side effects nor drug interactions. Indeed, Tan et al. (2014) (11) support a good safety profile and tolerability of EGb 761 for dementia and cognitive impairment.

Conclusion

The most recent clinical trials and meta-analyses have supported the potential benefits of Ginkgo biloba extract (EGb 761) in the treatment of dementia, especially at a daily dose of 240 mg. Considering its reported safety and ease of access, this natural supplement seems to be attaining a significant niche in dementia care, benefiting both patients and caregivers.

RHODIOLA ROSEA L. FOR DEPRESSION AND DEMENTIA

Rhodiola rosea L., the most investigated species of Rhodiola, is traditionally used in Eastern Europe and Asia to stimulate the nervous system, treating various disorders, including depression. *Rhodiola rosea L.*'s influence on psychiatric disorders may be related to its effect on changes in neurotransmitter levels and in the activity of the central nervous system (14). Despite its potential benefits in the nervous system, there are relatively few clinical trials with Rhodiola for depression and dementia.

Clinical Evidence

A randomized, double-blind clinical trial (15) compared two different doses of a standardized extract from *Rhodiola rosea L.* (SHR-5) to a placebo during 6 weeks in 89 mild to moderately depressed patients. The Rhodiola group showed improvement in overall depression and symptoms such as insomnia, emotional stability, and also self-esteem for the higher dose group. Indeed, important positive outcomes were mood stabilization and energy restoration.

Dosage

Darbinyan et al. (15) showed positive effects in depression with either 340 mg/day (2 tablets of 170 mg, daily) or 680 mg (2 tablets of 170 mg, twice a day)

of *Rhodiola rosea L.* extract (SHR-5) monotherapy. The difference between doses yielded a positive effect on self-esteem reported in the higher dose group, in addition to the above-mentioned improvement in depression symptoms.

Mechanisms

A study from 2009 (14) tested three extracts of *Rhodiola rosea L.* roots against the enzymes monoamine oxidase (MAOs) A and B. Interestingly, they found a potent inhibitory effect of *Rhodiola* on MAO-A, suggesting a potential antidepressant mechanism. The inhibition of MAO-A and B may affect serotonin and norepinephrine levels in the nerve terminals. *Rhodiola rosea L.* extracts' inhibition of MAO-A and B may also shed light onto the treatment of senile dementia and Alzheimer's disease.

Side Effects and Precautions

No side effects were reported in Darbinyan et al.'s trial (15). However, more clinical trials have to be performed under different conditions to better address safety and efficacy issues for *Rhodiola rosea L.*

Conclusion

Although there is not much evidence, especially for treatment of dementia, *Rhodiola* has been shown to have a positive effect in the treatment of depression (15). *Rhodiola's* reported MAO-B inhibitory activity (14) remains a key issue to be addressed in future clinical trials for a novel and beneficial treatment for senile dementia and Alzheimer's disease.

FOLATE (CEREFOLIN NAC/DEPLIN) FOR DEPRESSION AND DEMENTIA

Folate is a water-soluble B vitamin, naturally available in foods such as yeast, spinach, lentils, and orange juice. Adequate levels of folate are fundamental for brain function (16). In 1996, the US Federal Drug Administration (FDA) mandated the fortification of grains with folate, which successfully improved folate levels in the population. Studies have associated folate deficiencies with a higher risk of cognitive impairment and dementia, as well as an increased risk of depression and a dampened response to antidepressant treatment (16).

There has been a growing interest in the active form of folate, 5-methyltetrahydrofolate (5-MTHF), which has the capacity of crossing the blood–brain barrier (BBB) and reaching the cerebral spinal fluid without the need for interconversions that folic acid and other folate forms require (16–18). Two different 5-MTHF based supplements have been a focus of the treatment and prevention of depression and dementia: Deplin (L-methylfolate or 5-MTHF) and Cerefolin. The latter contains, besides L-methylfolate, methylcobalamin and N-acetyl-cysteine, and may confer a potential anti-oxidant effect in addition to antidepressant effect (18,19).

Clinical Evidence

Some studies (20–22) have found an inverse relationship between folate intake and levels and dementia. The Baltimore Longitudinal Study of Aging (20) related daily folate intake at or higher than recommended to a decreased risk of Alzheimer's disease. Indeed, another study found an association between low levels of serum folate and worse cognitive function and higher risk of cognitive decline (22). Meanwhile, according to Mischoulon and Raab (16), some clinical trials have found a relationship between low folate and a lower likelihood of response to antidepressant treatment, also slowing clinical improvement in these patients.

Two trials (18) were performed comparing different doses of L-methylfolate to placebo as adjuncts to selective serotonin reuptake inhibitors (SSRIs). These studies suggested that the higher daily dose administered (15 mg/day) was effective, safe, and relatively well tolerated when given to patients with poor or no response to SSRIs.

As for Cerefolin NAC, clinical evidence still remains unclear and lacks specific clinical trials to assess efficacy (19). Nevertheless, there is a considerable argument for its effectiveness, given the role of folate and B vitamins in dementia and the growing data relating oxidative disorders to psychiatric illnesses (19).

Dosage

The two different trials for Deplin administered either 7.5 mg/day or 15.0 mg/day of L-methylfolate (18). In the first trial, 7.5 mg/day of adjunctive L-methylfolate did not show efficacy compared to placebo. However, in the same trial, response rates increased when L-methylfolate was increased to 15.0 mg/day, although with low statistical significance. The second trial of 15.0 mg/day supported a potential role for L-methylfolate as an adjunctive treatment for patients with poor response to SSRIs.

Cerefolin NAC's marketed dosage is 5.6 mg of L-methylfolate, 2 mg methylcobalamin, and 600 mg of N-acetylcysteine. Whether this dosage is optimal for mood disorders remains to be determined.

Mechanisms

The role of folate in depression and dementia care relies on its potential impact on the 1-carbon cycle. In this pathway, folate is converted into methylfolate, which contributes to the methylation of homocysteine, synthesizing S-adenosyl-L-methionine (SAMe). Impairments in the 1-carbon cycle can lead to the accumulation of homocysteine and also can affect the synthesis of neurotransmitters, such as dopamine, norepinephrine, and serotonin. Indeed, Deplin can work as one of the regulators of monoamine levels (16,18).

Additionally, the impairment of the 1-carbon cycle leads to suppression of the neuroprogenitor cell proliferation. That may contribute to neurodegeneration and hence to cognitive decline and dementia. Nevertheless, lower levels of folate may result in higher levels of homocysteine, which can act as a neurotoxin with a DNA-damaging potential that may promote cell death. The promise of Cerefolin NAC is related to the relationship between oxidative stress, vitamin B deficiency, and dementia. B vitamin supplements added to NAC might also have a potential to lower homocysteine levels. (16,19).

Side Effects and Precautions

Both recent trials from Papakostas et al. (18) have showed safety and good tolerability for the highest dose administered of L-methylfolate. Although there is not much evidence for the combination of L-methylfolate with methylcobalamin and N-acetylcysteine, the rationale for its use suggests a potentially safe and tolerable supplement (19).

There have been some concerns about folate supplementation as potentially masking B$_{12}$ deficiency anemia and possibly being associated with cancer, particularly colorectal cancer. Certain forms, such as L-methylfolate, are less likely to mask B$_{12}$ deficiency, and should be used in cases where such masking is a concern. The association with cancer is not clear, and studies have in fact shown mixed results. There is, as of this time, no definitive human study evidence conclusively showing any pro or anti-cancer effects of folate supplementation. Caution should always be exercised with patients considered at high risk for colon cancer or B$_{12}$ deficiency, prior to initiating folate therapy (23).

Conclusion

Considering that adequate folate levels may play a key role in the treatment of depression and dementia, preparations such as L-methylfolate that can cross the blood–brain barrier, seem to be a viable strategy in the prevention and treatment of these disorders. According to McCaddon and Hudson (19), there is not much clinical evidence proving the efficacy of Cerefolin NAC. However, considering the role of oxidative and inflammatory pathways in dementia and the known benefits of folate, it seems a reasonable option for the prevention of and adjunctive treatment for psychiatric illnesses. Novel clinical trials have yet to be performed to analyze its potential effects in dementia and depression.

Despite the FDA's initiative to increase dietary folate levels, deficiencies of this vitamin still exist, due not always to lack of intake but to problems with its absorption in the gastrointestinal tract or its utilization. It is therefore important to target these deficiencies so as to optimize the treatment of psychiatric disorders.

OMEGA-3 FATTY ACIDS FOR MOOD DISORDERS

Omega-3 polyunsaturated fatty acids (PUFAs) are found mainly in oily fish and seafood (24). Omega-3s are thought to act by altering cell membrane structure and function, particularly membrane fluidity,

cellular communication, and inflammatory pathways (24). Also, omega-3s support neural development and prevent nervous system disorders (25). We will review the specific effects of omega-3s in the elderly, particularly concerning dementia, depression, and bipolar disorder.

Clinical Evidence

DEPRESSION

Omega-3 has been reported as a supplement with good adherence and minimum side effects (26). Yet, according to a Cochrane review from 2014 (27), not all studies reported beneficial effects of omega-3 in major depressive disorder.

Gertsik and colleagues (28) showed that the combination of omega-3 with selective serotonin reuptake inhibitors (SSRIs) decreases the signs and symptoms of major depressive disorder.

A study (29) with 46 depressed elderly women (66–95 years old) administered a daily dose of 2.5 g omega-3 (1.67 EPA and 0.83 DHA) and evaluated improvements in depressive symptoms (Geriatric Depression Scale) and quality of life related to health. The results showed that omega-3 led to a significant reduction in depressive symptoms and amelioration of quality of life as well, with improved physical and mental function.

Another study with 66 depressed patients (26), older than 65 years, compared a daily low dose of omega-3 (1 g/day) to placebo over 6 months. The authors found that low dose omega-3 supplementation was associated with some efficacy in the treatment of mild to moderate depression in that group. However, more studies are needed to assess the efficacy in severe depression.

BIPOLAR DISORDER

A Cochrane meta-analysis from 2009 found that omega-3 fatty acids appear to ameliorate at least some features of bipolar disorder, especially depressive symptoms measured by the Hamilton Depression Rating Scale, although they report some limitations from the studies reviewed (24). A systematic review from (30) did not report improvement related to manic symptoms in patients supplemented with omega-3. However, some data suggest efficacy without definitive results.

DEMENTIA

A randomized, double-blind trial ($n=174$) (31) with 1.7 g DHA and 0.6 g EPA or placebo for 6 months in patients with Alzheimer's disease was performed by Freund-Levi et al. (31). The Mini-Mental State Examination (MMSE) and Alzheimer's Disease Assessment Scale with a modified cognitive portion (ADAS-COG) were used to evaluate the outcomes. Their results showed that omega-3 did not improve cognitive decline in patients with mild to moderate AD, but positive effects were observed in patients with mild AD.

Indeed, the supplementation with omega-3 did not produce effects on neuropsychiatric symptoms, although there were some possible beneficial effects on depressive symptoms (32). A prospective study (33) measured erythrocyte membrane total omega-3, DHA, and EPA and the incidence of dementia in 663 non-demented individuals. Their analyses did not find evidence of a reduced risk of dementia among individuals with higher omega-3, DHA, or EPA concentrations. However, they state that a protective effect of those fatty acids could be related to long-term dietary intake, which cannot be accurately measured by erythrocyte levels.

Dosage

In the Cochrane meta-analysis of omega-3 in bipolar disorder, the doses ranged between 1 g and 9.6 g per day (24). It is generally accepted that optimal doses for depression are in the range of 1–2 g per day. Some studies in bipolar disorder have used higher doses. Recent evidence suggests that preparations that contain at least 60% EPA (as opposed to DHA) are more effective (34).

Mechanisms

In all likelihood, the psychotropic mechanism of the omega-3s is multifactorial. Omega-3s can influence many neurotransmitters within the brain, such as dopamine, serotonin, and norepinephrine. This occurs by direct influence or by changes in the neuronal membranes (24). Omega-3s have also been shown to lower inflammation in overweight and sedentary older adults (35). Other mechanisms of action may include the regulation of the phosphatidyl inositol cascade, and calcium flux inhibition (36).

Side Effects and Precautions

Side effects tend to be mild (29). While omega-3s are well tolerated and safe, care should be observed with patients who are taking anticoagulants, due to risk of bleeding if omega-3s are combined with anticoagulants. There are cases of cycling to mania in bipolar patients, and such individuals should take omega-3s in conjunction with a mood stabilizer (37).

Conclusion

Omega-3 fatty acids are a promising intervention for mood disorders, given their easy accessibility, tolerability, and safety. Considering the likely relationship between inflammatory processes and mood disorders (36), omega-3s still have to be thoroughly evaluated as a therapeutic tool for bipolar disorder, dementia, and depression.

PHOSPHATIDYLSERINE OMEGA-3 (PS-DHA; VAYACOG) FOR DEMENTIA

Phosphatidylserine enriched with docosahexaenoic acid (PS-DHA; Vayacog) is a novel natural supplement combination that may be indicated for dementia and the prevention and treatment of cognitive decline. To date, there are only a few studies addressing the efficacy and safety of PS combined with omega-3 among individuals with memory complaints. These include a double-blind clinical trial (38), which was extended as an open-label trial (39), and a pilot open-label study (40). Though few, these studies showed impressive results for this supplement in memory improvement. We will review the details of Vakhapova et al. (38), to examine the potential promise of PS-DHA as a new treatment for dementia and cognitive decline.

Clinical Evidence

Vakhapova et al. (38) performed the first double-blind, placebo-controlled clinical trial ($n = 131$) to analyze the effect of phosphatidylserine with attached omega-3 fatty acids (mainly DHA) for 15 weeks in patients without dementia but with memory complaints. The supplement's efficacy was measured by several cognitive and memory assessment tools, with objective and subjective evaluations. Results showed a better recall of immediate verbal memories in the intervention group. Indeed, there was also better treatment responsiveness among patients receiving PS-DHA when compared to the placebo group.

This clinical trial was extended as an open-label trial ($n = 122$), in which the researchers administered a lower dose of PS-DHA in prior completing patients for another 15 weeks. Similarly to their previous findings, they observed memory benefits in prior placebo subjects and the maintenance of improvements in prior treated subjects (39).

Finally, Richter et al. (40) published a pilot open-label study in which PS with omega-3 (EPA+DHA) was administered daily for 6 weeks in eight elderly volunteers with memory complaints. Despite not being a placebo-controlled and double-blind trial, the results were significant and impressive, showing a 42% increase in patients' ability of verbal recall of memory.

Mechanisms

Considering the key role of phospholipids in brain mechanisms, the reasoning proposed by Vakhapova et al. (38) is related to the function of phosphatidylserine in neural physiology through several different mechanisms. Nevertheless, Vakhapova et al. state that the exact mechanisms by which PS-DHA acts are still not clear (38), although they are potentially related to influence in neuronal membrane physiology and thus are implicated in many neurotransmitting pathways (40).

Dosage

In the study by Richter et al. (40), doses of PS-DHA were PS 300 mg/day + DHA/EPA 37.5 mg/day. The two Vakhapova et al. (38,39) studies used preparations consisting of PS 300 mg/day + DHA/EPA 79 mg/day (3:1 ratio) and PS 100 mg/day + EPA/DHA 26 mg/day (3:1 ratio), respectively.

Side Effects and Precautions

Vakhapova and colleagues measured laboratory values and clinical examination features to address safety, tolerability, and adverse effects of PS-DHA. No significant complaints were reported, showing good toleranbility for the administered dose. Some cases of gastrointestinal symptoms were reported in the treatment group, but were alleviated by simultaneous food intake. Interestingly, the authors have also published a single paper describing the safety issues of this trial (41). Neither the extension study nor the open label pilot study reported adverse episodes or significant side effects administering the above-mentioned doses.

Conclusion

The results of these three studies on phosphatidylserine combined with omega-3 fatty acids were interesting and promising, supporting this natural supplement as a potential member of the armamentarium for dementia care, especially regarding the prevention of cognitive worsening. Indeed, the significant effects in elderly patients with memory loss complaints should pave the way for future studies aiming to unveil the mechanisms of PS-DHA. These findings will be crucial for further establishment of a novel and potential option for patients dealing with degenerative memory loss disorders.

ST. JOHN'S WORT FOR DEPRESSION

St. John's wort (SJW) is the popular name for the extract of *Hypericum perforatum L.*, from the *Hypericaceae* family (42,43). SJW can be found over the counter in preparations containing active ingredients such as hyperforin, hypericin, and flavonoids (44). Due to its potential antidepressant effect, SJW has been widely prescribed for the treatment of depression (43). In this section, we will discuss some evidence and mechanistic reasoning for its use in depression, and its potential use in dementia.

Clinical Evidence

A Cochrane review (43) for the potential effects of St. John's wort in depression compared its effectiveness to standard antidepressants and placebo. The authors concluded that SJW was superior to placebo, with effects similar to antidepressants and a lower rate of adverse effects. Nevertheless, a trial from Rapaport et al. (45) compared SJW, an SSRI (citalopram), and a matching placebo for minor depression and found no advantage for either of the active treatments over placebo. According to Sarris (46),

SJW is most effective for mild to moderate depression, although its benefits in some other psychiatric disorders are yet to be determined.

Dosage

The dosage of St. John's wort typically varies between 900 mg/day and 1800 mg/day (47). On the other hand, in the studies analyzed by the Cochrane review (43), dosages went as low as 240 mg/day and usually were in the range of 500–1200 mg/day in different preparations. Rapaport et al. (45) administered 810 mg/day in three daily tablets. Because of different manufacturing standards, it is fundamental to pay close attention to specific preparations of SJW that may have different amounts of active components such as hypericin or hyperforin (hence different strengths) when prescribing this herbal supplement (42,47).

Mechanisms

The exact pathway by which St. John's wort acts is still unclear. Hyperforin, one of its active components, has been reported to exert an inhibiting effect in serotonin reuptake, and as well for norepinephrine and acetylcholine (42,44). Also, there seems to be a monoamine oxidase inhibiting (MAOI) effect in some components of SJW (flavonoids), but their small concentrations are probably not effective for depression treatment (42). A review by Russo et al. (44) also reported MAOI effects for hypericin. Moreover, there is some evidence reporting that hyperforin acts by diminishing beta-amyloid accumulation within the brain, potentially preventing the progression of dementia and cognitive decline (44, 46–48).

Side Effects and Precautions

Overall, SJW has shown good tolerability and a low rate of adverse effects (43,47). However, physicians must keep in mind its potential herbal–drug interactions when prescribing SJW. Mischoulon (42) cautioned about SJW's induction of the cytochrome p450 enzyme 3A4, which in turn can decrease the activity of various drugs, including protease inhibitors, cancer chemotherapies, and immunosuppressive drugs, among others. Moreover, the combination of SJW and SSRIs can cause serotonin syndrome, a severe and potentially life-threatening condition (42,44). Some phototoxicity effects have been reported, but can be addressed with general UV light protection such as sunscreen (42). When using preparations with more than 1 mg of hyperforin, physicians should keep in mind possible interactions (46).

Conclusion

Given its well-studied antidepressant features and potential effects in lowering the progression of cognitive decline, St. John's wort seems to be a reasonable herbal option for the elderly with depression, though additional investigation is needed with regard to dementia. However, due to SJW's large spectrum of adverse interactions, its utilization must be closely monitored by a physician, carefully administering the optimal dose as appropriate for each patient.

S-ADENOSYLMETHIONINE (SAME)

S-adenosylmethionine (SAMe) is a nutritional supplement with potential effects in depression, both as monotherapy and in combination with other antidepressants (42,47,49). SAMe serves as a methyl donor in metabolic reactions, and the reasoning for its use is based on its role in several chemical reactions in the brain (47,50). However, the existing body of trials of this supplement has not yet provided definitive conclusions (51).

Clinical Evidence

According to a review and update in natural remedies (42), more than 40 studies have shown efficacy for SAMe in depression and in dementia-like cognitive decline. In a recent clinical trial, Mischoulon et al. (52) reported no advantage for SAMe or SSRI monotherapy compared to placebo for depression. Papakostas et al. found efficacy of SAMe augmentation in SSRI- and SNRI-resistant patients, however (49). Preliminary data from Levkovitz et al. (50) showed that adjunctive SAMe is able to ameliorate memory issues in patients with depression, suggesting a potential role in dementia.

Table 4.1. Summary of Guidelines for the Clinician

MEDICATION	INDICATIONS	DAILY DOSES REPORTED	TREATMENT DURATIONS REPORTED	EFFECT SIZES REPORTED*	MAIN ADVERSE EFFECTS REPORTED
Ginkgo biloba	Dementia	120 mg–240 mg	Up to 1 year	Cognition: $d = 0.413$ [95% CI 0.22 to 0.61] (ref. 53); SMD: −0.89 [95% CI −1.82 to 0.04] (ref. 54); SMD = −0.65 [95% CI −1.22 to −0.09] (refs. 2,54). ADAS-cog: Bivariate random effect estimate of difference: −2.65 [95% CI −4.53 to −0.76] (ref 55); SMD = −0.05 [95% CI −0.41 to 0.30] (ref. 3); WMD = −2.86 [95% CI −3.18 to −2.54] (ref. 11). SKT: SMD = −0.72 [95% CI −1.28 to −0.017] (ref. 3). ADL: (< 200 mg): SMD = −0.16 [95% CI −0.31 to −0.01] (refs. 2,54); SMD = −0.598 [95% CI −0.954 to −0.251] (ref. 3); SMD = −0.36 [95% CI −0.44 to −0.28] (ref. 11). CGI: OR = 1.66 [95% CI 1.12 to 2.46] (> 200 mg) (refs. 2,54); OR = 1.88 [95% CI 1.54 to 2.29] (ref. 11).	Gastrointestinal disturbance, headaches, irritability, dizziness. Bleeding when combined with anticoagulants or when undergoing surgery.
Rhodiola rosea	Dementia Depression	340 mg–680 mg	Up to 12 weeks	Depression monotherapy: $d \approx 1.6$–2.0 (ref. 15).	Irritability, insomnia, fatigue (at higher doses).
Folic Acid/5-MTHF (Deplin)	Depression, Dementia	7.5 mg–15.0 mg	Up to 60 days	Depression augmentation (15.0 mg): $d \approx 0.4$ (ref. 18); RR $\approx$ 2.2 (ref. 18).	Gastrointestinal disturbance. Possibility of masking B$_{12}$ deficiency anemia.
Cerefolin NAC		5.6 mg L-methylfolate, 2 mg methylcobalamin, 600 mg NAC	No trials	Dementia (2 mg): No significant advantage (ref. 56).	Unclear association with colorectal cancer.

(continued)

Table 4.1.   Continued

MEDICATION	INDICATIONS	DAILY DOSES REPORTED	TREATMENT DURATIONS REPORTED	EFFECT SIZES REPORTED*	MAIN ADVERSE EFFECTS REPORTED
Omega-3	Depression Dementia Bipolar disorder	1.0 g–2.5 g 2.3 g 1.0–9.6 g	Up to 6 months Up to 6 months Up to 4 months	Depression: g = 0.532 [95% CI 0.277 to 0.733 (EPA ≥ 60%) (ref. 34); SMD = 0.69 [95% CI: 0.24 to 1.13] (ref. 57). Bipolar depression: g = 0.34 [95% CI: 0.035 to 0.641] (ref. 58).SMD = 0.69 [95% CI: 0.28 to 1.10] (ref. 57). Mania: g = 0.2 [95% CI: −0.037 to 0.433] (ref. 58). Dementia: g = −0.455 [95% CI −0.727 to −0.184] (ref. 59)	Gastrointestinal disturbance, "fishy taste." Risk of bleeding when taken with anticoagulants. Cycling to mania in bipolar disorder.
Vayacog	Dementia	300 mg PS + 79 mg O3, 100 mg PS + 26 mg O3, 300 mg PS + 37.5 mg O3	Up to 15 weeks (+15 weeks follow up)	Dementia: d ≈ 2.3–2.5; OR ≈ 2.8 (refs. 38,39)	Gastrointestinal disturbance (alleviated by food intake).
St. John's wort (SJW)	Depression	500–1800 mg	Up to 12 weeks	SJW vs. Placebo: RR = 1.48 [95% CI 1.23 to 1.77] (ref. 43); RR = 1.22 [95% CI 1.03 to 1.45], WMD = 1.33 [95% CI = 1.15 to 1.51] (ref. 60). SJW vs. older antidepressants: RR = 1.02 [95% CI 0.90 to 1.15] (ref. 43). SJW vs SSRI: RR = 1.00 [95% CI 0.90 to 1.12] (ref. 43); RR = 0.99 [95% CI = 1.15 to 1.51], WMD = 0.32 [95% CI −1.28 to 0.64] (ref. 60).	Drug–drug interactions (via Cytochrome p450 3A4 induction) with Warfarin, Cyclosporin, oral contraceptives, Theophylline, Fenprocoumon, Digoxin, Indinavir, Camptosar, Zolpidem, Irinotecam, Olanzapine. Serotonin syndrome when combined with SSRIs or other serotonergic agents. Phototoxicity. Cycling to mania in bipolar disorder.

SAMe	Depression	200–3200 mg	Up to 12 weeks	Augmentation: RR ≈ 2.62 (ref. 49). Monotherapy: SAMe vs. Placebo: $d = -0.65$ [95% CI −1.05 to −0.25] (ref. 61). Monotherapy: SAMe vs. TCA: $d = 0.08$ (95% CI −0.17 to 0.32] (ref. 61).	Gastrointestinal discomfort, diarrhea. Cycling to mania in bipolar disorder.

*Estimates of effect sizes (ES) are difficult to ascertain due to heterogeneity of studies, methodologies employed, selection criteria used for meta-analyses, and patient samples. For this table, most effect sizes were obtained from selected meta-analyses and systematic reviews, as noted. Due to small numbers of available studies, and the absence of adequate meta-analyses, we calculated our own effect sizes for Rhodiola, Vayacog, Deplin, and SAMe augmentation, based on articles referenced. *These data should be regarded only as estimates to help guide the practitioner's clinical decisions, and may not be representative of the body of evidence as a whole.* Reported ES are against placebo unless otherwise specified.

For continuous measures (e.g., improvement in HAM-D score), effect sizes reported here include Cohen's $d = (\text{mean}_1 - \text{mean}_2)/\text{SQR}[(SD_1{}^2 + SD_2{}^2)/2]$, where mean refers to improvement in HAM-D for treatment 1 (drug) vs. treatment 2 (placebo or standard comparator), and SD refers to the standard deviation for each respective mean (62,63). Cohen's effect sizes are generally categorized as small (0.0–0.3), moderate (0.3–0.6) and large (> 0.6). Hedges' g (64) is similar to Cohen's d, but includes a correction for biases due to smaller samples, and effect sizes may be interpreted as for Cohen's.

For categorical measures (e.g., response rates), we report the odds ratio for response, OR $_{[R_x/PBO]} = (R_1/N_1)/(R_2/N_2)$, where R_1 = number of responders to treatment 1 (drug), R_2 = number of responders to treatment 2 (placebo), and N_1 and N_2 refer to the number of respective nonresponders. Alternatively we report Risk Ratio for response, RR = P_1/P_2 is where P_1 = the probability of response to treatment 1 (drug) and P_2 = the probability of response to treatment 2 (placebo). These measures give an estimate of how much more likely a patient is to respond to treatment compared to placebo (or to a comparator treatment).

In meta-analysis, the standardized mean difference (SMD) is used when the studies assess the same outcome in different ways (65). Results are standardized to a uniform scale expressing the size of the intervention effect in each study relative to the variability observed in that study. SMD = difference in mean outcomes between groups/SD of outcome among subjects. Alternatively, weighted means are similarly calculated by combining measures and weighting each study based on the precision of its estimate of effect. The weighted mean is calculated for groups pre- and post-treatment (e.g., decrease in HAM-D score), and the weighted mean difference (WMD) represents the difference between baseline and final values. The difference is calculated as the sum of the differences in the individual studies, weighted by the individual variances for each study. Weighting can also be done based on sample size, to give greater weight to larger studies.

Where 95% confidence intervals (CI) are reported, results are considered *nonsignificant* if the interval range crosses 1.0.

Abbreviations:

ADAS-Cog: Alzheimer's Disease Assessment Scale, cognitive subscale

ADL: Activities of daily living

CGI: Clinical Global Improvement Scale

HAM-D: Hamilton Depression Rating Scale

SKT: Syndrom-Kurz test, a short cognitive performance test for assessing deficits of memory and attention

SSRI: Selective serotonin reuptake inhibitor

TCA: Tricyclic antidepressant

Dosing

Reported SAMe doses in published clinical trials have typically ranged from 200 to 1600 mg/day (42,47). The recent study by Mischoulon et al. (52) used doses up to 3200 mg/day with good tolerability. In clinical practice, we have found that many patients require doses as high as 2000–3000 mg/day.

Mechanisms

SAMe acts in different chemical reactions in the brain, serving as a methyl donor and impacting hormone and neurotransmitters synthesis, particularly norepinephrine, serotonin, and dopamine (42). Folate deficiencies can lead to SAMe deficiencies, the latter of which have a key role in the 1-carbon cycle (42). Thus, the reasoning for SAMe's prescription for depression is similar to the one for L-methylfolate.

Side Effects and Precautions

According to recent reviews and trials, SAMe seems to be a safe drug in general, without significant adverse effects and unwanted interactions (42,51,52). Most notably, SAMe can cause mild gastrointestinal discomfort and sometimes diarrhea, but has a generally good tolerability profile (51,52).

Conclusions

Considering its apparent safety and easy accessibility, studies elucidating SAMe's potential benefits for depression and in the elderly seem to be a path for another novel and safe natural option in psychiatry.

CONCLUSIONS AND RECOMMENDATIONS

Natural remedies continue to grow in popularity, and in the past two decades there has been increasing evidence of efficacy. Nonetheless, these remedies do not yet have as much data to support their efficacy compared to FDA-registered medications. Likewise, there are lingering questions about their safety. While many of these treatments may eventually find a place in the psychopharmacologist's armamentarium, more research needs to be carried out to determine the optimal use for these agents,

both in elderly patients as well as in the general population.

In the absence of more data, we generally recommend that patients approach these remedies with caution, and preferably under the supervision of a physician. Patients with milder forms of illness may be the better candidates for these therapies. Elderly patients may seem like especially good candidates, in view of the relatively mild side-effect profiles of these natural products. However, this population often may be receiving polypharmacy for various indications, and therefore caution with potential adverse interactions needs to be upmost on the mind of the prescribing physician.

Finally, caution should be undertaken with bipolar patients, who may be at risk of cycling to mania or hypomania when treated with some of these natural products; they should preferably use these agents in combination with a mood stabilizer.

A summary of indications, doses, safety concerns, range of treatment duration in studies, and estimated effect sizes is provided in Table 4.1 as a quick reference for the reader.

DISCLOSURE STATEMENT

Dr. Mischoulon has received research support from the Bowman Family Foundation, FisherWallace, Nordic Naturals, Methylation Sciences, Inc. (MSI), and PharmoRx Therapeutics. He has received honoraria for consulting, speaking, and writing from Pamlab, and the Massachusetts General Hospital Psychiatry Academy. He has received royalties from Lippincott Williams & Wilkins for the published book *Natural Medications for Psychiatric Disorders: Considering the Alternatives.*

Ms. Mathias has no conflicts of interest to report.

REFERENCES

1. Kleijnen J, Knipschild P. Ginkgo biloba. *Lancet.* 1992 Nov 7;340(8828):1136–1139.
2. Birks J, Grimley Evans J. Ginkgo biloba for cognitive impairment and dementia. *Cochrane Database Syst Rev.* 2009, Issue 1. Art. No. CD003120. doi: 10.1002/14651858.CD003120. pub3.
3. Brondino N, De Silvestri A, Re S, Lanati N, Thiemann P, Verna A, et al. a systematic review and meta-analysis of ginkgo biloba in neuropsychiatric disorders: from

ancient tradition to modern-day medicine. *Evid Based Complement Alternat Med.* 2013;2013:915691.

4. Ihl R, Bachinskaya N, Korczyn AD, Vakhapova V, Tribanek M, Hoerr R, Napryeyenko O; GOTADAY Study Group. Efficacy and safety of a once-daily formulation of Ginkgo biloba extract EGb 761 in dementia with neuropsychiatric features: a randomized controlled trial. *Int J Geriatr Psychiatry.* 2011 Nov;26(11):1186–1194.

5. Kaschel R. Specific memory effects of Ginkgo biloba extract EGb 761 in middle-aged healthy volunteers. *Phytomedicine.* 2011 Nov 15;18(14):1202–1207.

6. Herrschaft H, Nacu A, Likhachev S, Sholomov I, Hoerr R, Schlaefke S. Ginkgo biloba extract EGb 761® in dementia with neuropsychiatric features: a randomized, placebo-controlled trial to confirm the efficacy and safety of a daily dose of 240 mg. *J Psychiatr Res.* 2012 Jun;46(6):716–723.

7. Nasab NM, Bahrammi MA, Nikpour MR, Rahim F, Naghibis SN. Efficacy of rivastigmine in comparison to ginkgo for treating Alzheimer's dementia. *J Pak Med Assoc.* 2012 Jul;62(7):677–680.

8. Dong ZH, Zhang CY, Pu BH. Effects of ginkgo biloba tablet in treating mild cognitive impairment. *Zhongguo Zhong Xi Yi Jie He Za Zhi.* 2012 Sep;32(9):1208–1211.

9. Vellas B, Coley N, Ousset PJ, Berrut G, Dartigues JF, Dubois B, et al. Long-term use of standardised Ginkgo biloba extract for the prevention of Alzheimer's disease (GuidAge): a randomised placebo-controlled trial. *Lancet Neurol.* 2012 Oct;11(10):851–859.

10. Canevelli M, Adali N, Kelaiditi E, Cantet C, Ousset PJ, Cesari M; ICTUS/DSA Group. Effects of Gingko biloba supplementation in Alzheimer's disease patients receiving cholinesterase inhibitors: data from the ICTUS study. *Phytomedicine.* 2014 May 15;21(6):888–892.

11. Tan MS, Yu JT, Tan CC, Wang HF, Meng XF, Wang C, Jiang T, Zhu XC, Tan L. Efficacy and adverse effects of ginkgo biloba for cognitive impairment and dementia: a systematic review and meta-analysis. *J Alzheimers Dis.* 2015;43(2):589–603.

12. Diamond BJ, Bailey MR. Ginkgo biloba: indications, mechanisms, and safety. *Psychiatr Clin North Am.* 2013 Mar;36(1):73–83.

13. Diamond BJ, Shiflett SC, Feiwel N, et al. Ginkgo biloba extract: mechanisms and clinical indications. *Arch Phys Med Rehabil.* 2000;81:668–678.

14. van Diermen D, Marston A, Bravo J, Reist M, Carrupt PA, Hostettmann K. Monoamine oxidase inhibition by Rhodiola rosea L. roots. *J Ethnopharmacol.* 2009 Mar 18;122(2):397–401. doi: 10.1016/j.jep.2009.01.007. Epub 2009 Jan 9.

15. Darbinyan V, Aslanyan G, Amroyan E, Gabrielyan E, Malmström C, Panossian A. Clinical trial of Rhodiola rosea L. extract SHR-5 in the treatment of mild to moderate depression. *Nord J Psychiatry.* 2007;61(5):343–348. Erratum in: *Nord J Psychiatry.* 2007;61(6):503.

16. Mischoulon D, Raab MF. The role of folate in depression and dementia. *J Clin Psychiatry.* 2007;68 Suppl 10:28–33.

17. Wu D, Pardridge WM. Blood-brain barrier transport of reduced folic acid. *Pharm Res.* 1999;16:415–419

18. Papakostas GI, Shelton RC, Zajecka JM, Etemad B, Rickels K, Clain A, et al. Am J Psychiatry. L-methylfolate as adjunctive therapy for SSRI-resistant major depression: results of two randomized, double-blind, parallel-sequential trials. 2012 Dec 1;169(12):1267–1274.

19. McCaddon A, Hudson PR. L-methylfolate, methylcobalamin, and N-acetylcysteine in the treatment of Alzheimer's disease-related cognitive decline. *CNS Spectr.* 2010 Jan;15 (1 Suppl 1):2–5; discussion 6.

20. Corrada MM, Kawas CH, Hallfrisch J, et al. Reduced risk of Alzheimer's disease with high folate intake: the Baltimore Longitudinal Study of Aging. *Alzheimers Dement.* 2005;1:11–18

21. Kado DM, Karlamangla AS, Huang MH, et al. Homocysteine versus the vitamins folate, B6, and B12 as predictors of cognitive function and decline in older high-functioning adults: MacArthur Studies of Successful Aging. *Am J Med.* 2005;118:161–167

22. Ramos MI, Allen LH, Mungas DM, et al. Low folate status is associated with impaired cognitive function and dementia in the Sacramento Area Latino Study on Aging. *Am J Clin Nutr.* 2005;82:1346–1352

23. Mischoulon D, Fava M, Stahl S. Folate supplementation. [Response to letter] *J Clin Psychiatry.* 2009;70:767–769

24. Montgomery P, Richardson AJ. Omega-3 fatty acids for bipolar disorder. Cochrane Database Syst Rev. 2008 Apr 16;(2):CD005169. doi: 10.1002/14651858.CD005169.pub2.

25. Janssen CIF, Kiliaan A. Long-chain polyunsaturated fatty acids (LCPUFA) from genesis to senescence: the influence of LCPUFA on neural development, aging, and neurodegeneration. *Prog Lipid Res.* 2014 Jan;53:1–17.

26. Tajalizadekhoob Y, Sharifi F, Fakhrzadeh H, Mirarefin M, Ghaderpanahi M, Badamchizade Z, Azimipour S. The effect of low-dose omega 3 fatty acids on the treatment of mild to moderate depression in the elderly: a double-blind, randomized, placebo-controlled study. *Eur Arch Psychiatry Clin Neurosci*. 2011 Dec;261(8):539–549.

27. Appleton KM, Perry R, Sallis HM, Ness AR, Churchill R. *Omega-3 fatty acids for depression in adults (Protocol).* . The Cochrane Library 2014; DOI: 10.1002/14651858.CD004692.pub3; http://onlinelibrary.wiley.com/doi/10.1002/14651858.CD004692.pub3/full

28. Gertsik L, Poland RE, Bresee C, Rapaport MH. Omega-3 fatty acid augmentation of citalopram treatment for patients with major depressive disorder. *J Clin Psychopharmacol*. 2012 Feb;32(1):61–64.

29. Rondanelli M, Giacosa A, Opizzi A, Pelucchi C, La Vecchia C, Montorfano G, Negroni M, Berra B, Politi P, Rizzo AM. Effect of omega-3 fatty acids supplementation on depressive symptoms and on health-related quality of life in the treatment of elderly women with depression: a double-blind, placebo-controlled, randomized clinical trial. *J Am Coll Nutr*. 2010 Feb;29(1):55–64.

30. Sylvia LG, Peters AT, Deckersbach T, Nierenberg AA. Nutrient-based therapies for bipolar disorder: a systematic review. *Psychother Psychosom*. 2013;82(1):10–19.

31. Freund-Levi Y, Eriksdotter-Jönhagen M, Cederholm T, Basun H, Faxén-Irving G, Garlind A, Vedin I, Vessby B, Wahlund LO, Palmblad J. Omega-3 fatty acid treatment in 174 patients with mild to moderate Alzheimer disease: OmegAD study: a randomized double-blind trial. *Arch Neurol*. 2006 Oct;63(10):1402–1408.

32. Freund-Levi Y, Basun H, Cederholm T, Faxén-Irving G, Garlind A, Grut M, Vedin I, Palmblad J, Wahlund LO, Eriksdotter-Jönhagen M. Omega-3 supplementation in mild to moderate Alzheimer's disease: effects on neuropsychiatric symptoms. *Int J Geriatr Psychiatry*. 2008 Feb;23(2):161–169.

33. Kröger E, Verreault R, Carmichael PH, Lindsay J, Julien P, Dewailly E, Ayotte P, Laurin D. Omega-3 fatty acids and risk of dementia: the Canadian Study of Health and Aging. *Am J Clin Nutr*. 2009 Jul;90(1):184–192. doi: 10.3945/ajcn.2008.26987.

34. Sublette ME, Ellis SP, Geant AL, Mann JJ. Meta-analysis of the effects of eicosapentaenoic acid (EPA) in clinical trials in depression. *J Clin Psychiatry*. 2011 Dec;72(12):1577–1584.

35. Kiecolt-Glaser JK, Belury MA, Andridge R, Malarkey WB, Hwang BS, Glaser R. *Brain Behav Immun*. 2012 Aug;26(6):988–995. doi: 10.1016/j.bbi.2012.05.011. Epub 2012 May 26.

36. Stoll AL. Omega-3 fatty acids in mood disorders: a review of neurobiological and clinical actions. In: Mischoulon D, Rosenbaum J (Eds.). *Natural medications for psychiatric disorders: considering the alternatives*. Philadelphia: Lippincott Williams & Wilkins, 2008, pp. 39–67.

37. Mischoulon D, Freeman MP. Omega-3 fatty acids in psychiatry. *Psychiatr Clin North Am*. 2013 Mar;36(1):15–23.

38. Vakhapova V, Cohen T, Richter Y, Herzog Y, Korczyn AD. Phosphatidylserine containing omega-3 fatty acids may improve memory abilities in non-demented elderly with memory complaints: a double-blind placebo-controlled trial. *Dement Geriatr Cogn Disord*. 2010;29(5):467–474. doi: 10.1159/000310330. Epub 2010 Jun 3.

39. Vakhapova V, Cohen T, Richter Y, Herzog Y, Kam Y, Korczyn AD. Phosphatidylserine containing omega-3 fatty acids may improve memory abilities in nondemented elderly individuals with memory complaints: results from an open-label extension study. *Dement Geriatr Cogn Disord*. 2014;38(1–2):39–45. doi: 10.1159/000357793. Epub 2014 Feb 20.

40. Richter Y, Herzog Y, Cohen T, Steinhart Y. The effect of phosphatidylserine-containing omega-3 fatty acids on memory abilities in subjects with subjective memory complaints: a pilot study. *Clin Interv Aging*. 2010 Nov 2;5:313–316. doi: 10.2147/CIA.S13432.

41. Vakhapova V, Richter Y, Cohen T, Herzog Y, Korczyn AD. Safety of phosphatidylserine containing omega-3 fatty acids in non-demented elderly: a double-blind placebo-controlled trial followed by an open-label extension. *BMC Neurol*. 2011 Jun 28;11:79. doi: 10.1186/1471-2377-11-79.

42. Mischoulon D. Update and critique of natural remedies as antidepressant treatments. *Obstet Gynecol Clin North Am*. 2009 Dec;36(4):789–807, x. doi: 10.1016/j.ogc.2009.10.005.

43. Linde K, Berner MM, Kriston L. St John's wort for major depression. *Cochrane Database Syst Rev*. 2008; (4): CD000448.

44. Russo E, Scicchitano F, Whalley BJ, Mazzitello C, Ciriaco M, Esposito S, Patanè M, Upton R, Pugliese M, Chimirri S, Mammì M, Palleria C, De Sarro G. Hypericum

perforatum: pharmacokinetic, mechanism of action, tolerability, and clinical drug-drug interactions. *Phytother Res.* 2014 May;28(5):643–655.

45. Rapaport MH, Nierenberg AA, Howland R, Dording C, Schettler PJ, Mischoulon D. The treatment of minor depression with St. John's wort or citalopram: failure to show benefit over placebo. *J Psychiatr Res.* 2011 Jul;45(7):931–941.

46. Sarris J. St. John's wort for the treatment of psychiatric disorders. *Psychiatr Clin North Am.* 2013 Mar;36(1):65–72.

47. Nyer M, Doorley J, Durham K, Yeung AS, Freeman MP, Mischoulon D. What is the role of alternative treatments in late-life depression? *Psychiatr Clin North Am.* 2013 Dec;36(4):577–596. doi: 10.1016/j.psc.2013.08.012. Epub 2013 Oct 6.

48. Dinamarca MC, Cerpa W, Garrido J, Hancke JL, Inestrosa NC. Hyperforin prevents beta-amyloid neurotoxicity and spatial memory impairments by disaggregation of Alzheimer's amyloid-beta-deposits. *Mol Psychiatry.* 2006 Nov;11(11):1032–1048.

49. Papakostas GI, Mischoulon D, Shyu I, Alpert, JE, Fava M. S-adenosyl methionine (SAMe) augmentation of serotonin reuptake inhibitors (sris) for sri- non-responders with major depressive disorder: a double-blind, randomized clinical trial. *Am J Psychiatry.* 2010; 167:942–948.

50. Levkovitz Y, Alpert JE, Brintz CE, Mischoulon D, Papakostas GI. Effects of S-adenosylmethionine augmentation of serotonin-reuptake inhibitor antidepressants on cognitive symptoms of major depressive disorder. *J Affect Disord.* 2012 Feb;136(3):1174–1178.

51. Luberto CM, White C, Sears RW, Cotton S. Integrative medicine for treating depression: an update on the latest evidence. *Curr Psychiatry Rep.* 2013 Sep;15(9):391.

52. Mischoulon D, Price LH, Carpenter LL, Tyrka AR, Papakostas GI, Baer L, Dording CM, Clain AJ, Durham K, Walker R, Ludington E, Fava M. A double-blind, randomized, placebo-controlled clinical trial of S-adenosyl-L-methionine (SAMe) versus escitalopram in major depressive disorder. *J Clin Psychiatry.* 2014 Apr;75(4):370–376.

53. Oken BS, Storzbach DM, Kaye JA.The efficacy of Ginkgo biloba on cognitive function in Alzheimer disease. *Arch Neurol.* 1998 Nov;55(11):1409–1415.

54. Birks J, Grimley Evans J. Ginkgo biloba for cognitive impairment and dementia. *Cochrane Database Syst Rev.* 2007 Apr 18;(2):CD003120.

55. Wang BS, Wang H, Song YY, Qi H, Rong ZX, Wang BS, Zhang L, Chen HZ. Effectiveness of standardized ginkgo biloba extract on cognitive symptoms of dementia with a six-month treatment: a bivariate random effect meta-analysis. *Pharmacopsychiatry.* 2010 May;43(3):86–91

56. Malouf M, Grimley EJ, Areosa SA. Folic acid with or without vitamin B12 for cognition and dementia. *Cochrane Database Syst Rev.* 2003;(4):CD004514.

57. Lin PY, Su KP. A meta-analytic review of double-blind, placebo-controlled trials of antidepressant efficacy of omega-3 fatty acids. *J Clin Psychiatry.* 2007 Jul;68(7):1056–1061

58. Sarris J, Mischoulon D, Schweitzer I. Omega-3 for bipolar disorder: meta-analyses of use in mania and bipolar depression. *J Clin Psychiatry.* 2012 Jan;73(1):81–86.

59. Lin PY, Chiu CC, Huang SY, Su KP. A meta-analytic review of polyunsaturated fatty acid compositions in dementia. *J Clin Psychiatry.* 2012 Sep;73(9):1245–1254.

60. Rahimi R, Nikfar S, Abdollahi M. Efficacy and tolerability of Hypericum perforatum in major depressive disorder in comparison with selective serotonin reuptake inhibitors: a meta-analysis. *Prog Neuropsychopharmacol Biol Psychiatry.* 2009 Feb 1;33(1):118–127.

61. US Departments of Health and Human Services Agency for Healthcare Research and Quality (AHRQ). S-adenosyl-L-methionine for treatment of depression, osteoarthritis, and liver disease. Summary, Evidence Report/Technology Assessment: Number 64. AHRQ Publication No. 02-E033. August 2002. Accessed October 8, 2007, from http://www.ahrq.gov/clinic/epcsums/samesum.htm.

62. Cohen J. *Statistical power analysis for the behavioral sciences* (2nd ed.). New York: Academic Press, 1988.

63. Cohen J. A power primer. *Psychol Bull.* 1992:112; 155–159.

64. Hedges LV, Olkin I. *Statistical methods for meta-analysis.* Orlando, FL: Academic Press, 1985.

65. Weighted mean or weighted mean difference. Accessed November 8, 2014, from http://www.medicine.ox.ac.uk/bandolier/booth/glossary/wmd.html.

5

HUMAN INTESTINAL MICROBIOTA AND HEALTHY AGING

S. Melanie Lee and Helen Lavretsky

INTRODUCTION

Advancements in science and medicine, as well as improved living standards, have led to a steady increase in life expectancy in affluent countries. Unfortunately, the elderly population often suffers from increased susceptibility to degenerative or infectious diseases and overall degradation of health beyond the normal expected regression of physiological function due to the aging process. Developing preventive strategies to promote healthy aging and maintain quality of life is critical for preserving the period of independence and dignity of the elderly.

Over a century ago, Elie Metchnikoff, the father of cellular immunology, best known for his discovery of the phagocytes, theorized that health could be enhanced and senility could be delayed by ingesting health-promoting live micro-organisms found in fermented milk. Today, probiotics are not only the subject of intense medical research but also the source of a multibillion-dollar global industry (1). The gut

microbiota is intimately tied to the host health and disease and plays a major role in the development and modulation of the host metabolism, immunity, and the nervous system (2).

In this chapter, we review the physiological changes in bowel function and immune function with aging and how the gut microbiota of the elderly may reflect these changes. We also explore a possible link between the gut microbiome changes and various aging-related disorders such as Alzheimer's disease, cardiovascular diseases, and cancer. Finally, we review the literature on how manipulating the gut flora with diet and probiotics may have beneficial outcomes.

AGING-RELATED CHANGES IN THE GASTROINTESTINAL TRACT

The effects of aging itself as well as other concomitant changes can have adverse effects on the gastrointestinal (GI) function. The elderly are especially at risk for poor nutritional status for several reasons. Delayed gastric emptying and changes in satiety peptide expression may cause loss of appetite and unbalanced energy intake in the elderly (3). Increased thresholds for taste and smell, coupled with mastication dysfunction caused by loss of teeth and muscle bulk and swallowing difficulties, can lead to the consumption of a narrow, nutritionally imbalanced diet (4–6). In the stomach, hypochlorhydria is highly prevalent in the elderly, which can subsequently result in decreased absorption of calcium, ferric iron, and vitamin B_{12}, as well as microbial overgrowth in the small intestine (7,8).

Decreased intestinal motility and impaired thirst mechanism, leading to frequent dehydration, often result in fecal impaction and constipation in the older adults (9). Age-related neurodegeneration in the enteric nervous system may partly explain the decline in peristaltic motor function (10). Increased transit time of the colonic content results in increased bacterial protein fermentation, which releases toxic products, including ammonia and phenol from the putrefactive process (11).

The use of medications increases with age, with more than 75% of people aged 65 or older taking at least one prescription medication (12). Many commonly prescribed medications cause dry mouth and hyposalivation, affecting approximately 30% of those aged 65 years and older. It can produce serious negative effects on the patient's quality of life by limiting dietary habits, speech, and mucosal defense, and by increasing risk of oral infection (13). Frequent use of broad-spectrum antibiotics among the elderly, especially in hospitals or long-term care facilities, increases the risk of *Clostridium difficile*–associated diarrhea and poses a serious threat to their well-being (14). Proton pump inhibitors (PPIs) are widely used to treat peptic ulcers. The suppression of gastric acid has been shown to alter the bacterial flora of the upper GI tract, raising concern for bacterial overgrowth in the small intestine and malabsorption of nutrients (15). Although PPI therapy rarely causes overt complications, it is important to only use it if the benefits will outweigh the small risks. Yet another commonly used medication in the elderly is opioid therapy, which is well known to cause constipation, compounding the already decreased gut motility of the elderly and in turn resulting in the increased use of laxatives with aging (16).

Taken together, it is important to be alerted to the dangers of polypharmacy in the elderly population, and to the importance of health maintenance using non-pharmacological methods including diet, exercise, and complementary, alternative, and integrative medicine (CAIM).

AGING-RELATED CHANGES IN IMMUNE FUNCTION

Immunosenescence is a process of gradual deterioration of the immune function brought on by the advancement of age. It is a major contributory factor to the increased morbidity and mortality among the elderly (17). Several mechanisms contribute to the age-related decline of immune function. The thymus gland, a central lymphoid organ responsible for the production of naïve T cells, undergoes chronic involution and atrophy starting in year 1 of life and shrinks down to less than 10% of the total thymic tissue by age 70, critically impacting the peripheral T cell pool with a in naïve T cells and a shift toward memory CD4+ T cells (18). Peripheral lymphoid organs also undergo architectural and cellular changes that reflect the cumulative effect of lifelong stimulation with more and more antigens with age, including a decrease in CD8+ T cells, naïve T cells, IgM-expressing B cells and smaller germinal centers (19). Humoral immune response is defective in old age due to the decreased ability of B cells to produce immunoglobulins and a shift toward memory B cells (20). Natural killer (NK) cells are a critical component of the innate immunity against viral pathogens, and aging is associated with a significant impairment in cytotoxic ability of NK cells (21). Chronic, low-grade inflammation is another hallmark of immunosenescence and is linked to most age-related health problems that share an inflammatory pathogenesis, such as Alzheimer's disease and atherosclerosis (22).

The gut mucosa is the largest immunological environment of the body and it is constantly exposed to a vast array of foreign antigens from foods and the commensal bacteria of the gut, as well as the pathogenic microorganisms and parasites. As such, the gut microbiota has a critical role in instructing the host immune system, and age-related changes in the gut community may have a role in mediating immunosenescence and chronic low-grade inflammation in an elderly host.

AGING-RELATED CHANGES IN THE GUT MICROBIOTA

Humans and other mammals are born sterile until the first major colonization event occurs at contact with the vaginal flora during birth (23). For the first two years of life, many abrupt changes in the fecal bacterial community occur due to the combination of breast milk effects, the introduction of solid food, the developing immune system, and weaning. By approximately 2 years of age, the gut community will stabilize and become adult-like (24). During adult life, the gut microbiota is remarkably stable over time, as one longitudinal experiment found that 60% of bacterial strains in an individual's gut persisted over the length of the 5-year study (25). Even after major perturbation events such as antibiotic therapy, after a week-long recovery, membership and relative abundance will largely be restored to pre-treatment state (26). However, this relative stability is reduced in old age. Age-related physiological changes in the GI tract and the immune system, compounded by the poor nutritional status and the use of medications, will inevitably change the intestinal community in several different ways.

Fecal microbiota enumeration studies to define which species are found in the human GI tract and to quantify the relative abundance of each species are notorious for generating inconsistent or even contradicting results. Many studies are limited by the small cohort size and the use of culture-dependent enumeration methods which will miss majority of the species found in the gut as we do not have the technology to culture them. Other confounding factors in interpreting fecal microbiota data include cultural, geographical and dietary effects on the gut microbiome which contribute to the inevitable noise (24). Nevertheless, there are a few changes in the community composition with aging that are worth noting.

One of the signature changes in the bacterial community of the aging gut is the marked reduction in number and diversity of Bifidobacteria (27–32). It appears that aging leads to poor adhesion between the bacteria and the host mucus layer. Ouwehand et al. (1999) tested the adhesion of four Bifidobacterium strains to intestinal mucus isolated from subjects of different age and found that all strains bound significantly less to the mucus preparation of the elderly subjects. Furthermore, Bifidobacterium strains isolated from elderly subjects were functionally distinct from those isolated from younger adults in their adhesive abilities as shown by in vitro mucus-binding experiments (28).

Some studies have shown a decline in Bacteroides in number and diversity with increased age (31–33). In another study, a reduction in Bacteroides was only observed in elderly hospitalized patients, especially following antibiotic treatments, but not in healthy elderly subjects (30). The mechanism of decrease in Bacteroides as a function of aging is unclear. However, Bacteroides plays a major role in the metabolism of dietary polysaccharide (34), as well as in the maintenance of intestinal immune homeostasis (35,36) and thus represents an important member of the gut flora to promote healthy aging.

Several studies have noted a rise in proteolytic bacteria such as Fusobacteria, Propionibacteria, and Clostridia in antibiotic-treated elderly subjects (29–31). These bacteria ferment amino acids, which then result in the production of several detrimental end products such as ammonia and indoles. Short-chain fatty acids (SCFA) are the main saccharolytic fermentation products of colonic microbes with known beneficial roles, including the promotion of barrier function against pathogens and of colonic motility (37). Aging leads to decreased Bifidobacteria and Bacteroides, both important saccharolytic bacteria, with concomitant increase in proteolytic bacteria and changes in the colonic microbial activity from saccharolytic metabolism toward unfavorable putrefactive metabolism (31,38).

THE ROLE OF GUT MICROBIOME IN AGING-RELATED DISORDERS

Alteration from the normal gut microbiota, also known as dysbiosis, has a broad implication across various organ systems and disease types including inflammatory bowel disease (39–42), obesity (43–45), diabetes (46), asthma (47,48), and even autism (49). Moreover, changes in gut microbiome have been linked with diseases that are seen with increasing frequency with aging such as atherosclerosis and cardiovascular disease (CVD), cancer, and Alzheimer's disease.

In a seminal study by Wang et al. (2011), a large clinical cohort of patients ($n = 1876$) was screened for their plasma level of metabolites, which showed choline, trimethylamine N-oxide (TMAO), and betaine, all metabolites of dietary lipid phosphatidylcholine that were predictive of CVD risk. They went on to show that TMAO production from dietary choline was gut microbiota dependent as the mice treated with broad-spectrum antibiotics showed significant suppression of plasma TMAO levels compared to the control group while on a choline-supplemented diet (50). Koeth et al. (2013) demonstrated that dietary L-carnitine, a trimethylamine abundant in red meat, is also metabolized by intestinal microbiota to produce TMAO and to accelerate atherosclerosis in both mice and humans. To identify which members of the gut microbiota may be responsible for TMAO production, they profiled the fecal microbial composition and found enrichment of the genus *Prevotella* and depletion of the genus *Bacteroides* were significantly associated with increased plasma TMAO concentrations. These studies show that in addition to reducing dietary choline, phosphatidylcholine, and L-carnitine intake, gut microbiota modification may provide a novel preventive and therapeutic strategy for CVD.

Cancer susceptibility and progression is an outcome of a complex interplay between genetic and environmental factors. The microbial community that inhabits our gastrointestinal tract is emerging as a formidable environmental factor that can modulate the risk of carcinogenesis. Here, we briefly discuss recent findings in colorectal cancer (CRC)–associated dysbiosis in the gut. One of the dysbiotic features of the fecal microbiota in CRC patients compared to healthy controls is the enrichment of pro-inflammatory opportunistic pathogens such as *Fusobacterium*, *Enterococcaceae*, and *Campylobacter* (51). Unsurprisingly, severity of inflammation is highly associated with risk of CRC in ulcerative colitis patients (52). In the same comparative study, *Faecalibacterium prausnitzii* and *Roseburia*, both members of the *Clostridium* cluster IV and well-known butyrate producers, were found to be depleted in the CRC patients (51). Butyrate is one of the short-chain fatty acids, microbial carbohydrate fermentation products, with a known role in the regulation of inflammation and protection from colon and liver cancer (53,54). In addition to the inflammatory and metabolic effects of the dysbiotic microbiome, a novel oncogenic bacterial species was found when cancerous tissue samples were compared to adjacent healthy tissues and an enrichment of *Fusobacterium nucleatum* was found in tumors (55,56). *F. nucleatum* expresses a unique FadA adhesin molecule that binds to E-cadherin and activates β-catenin signaling in the CRC cells, thereby promoting inflammation and tumor cell growth (57). There is a wealth of both clinical and preclinical evidence linking dysbiotic microbiota and various cancer types through inflammatory, metabolic, and direct toxic effects (58,59). Therefore, the gut microbiome is beginning to be recognized as a promising marker of cancer prediction as well as a target of intervention.

Alzheimer's disease (AD) is a progressive neurodegenerative disorder and the leading cause of cognitive and behavioral impairment in later life. About 5% of all AD cases have a genetic or familial cause, but the vast majority of AD cases are of sporadic origin (60). As of yet, no direct evidence of the human microbiome being linked to the pathophysiology of AD is available. However, there is an increasing appreciation for the gut microbiota as an active participant of the brain-gut communication via the enteric nervous system, the hypothalamic-pituitary-adrenal axis, and the immune system (61). Germ-free (GF) animal studies have allowed us to directly assess the role of microbiome on all aspects of host physiology (62). As for cognition, GF mice demonstrate a deficit in nonspatial memory and impaired working memory, with concomitant reduction in two proteins that play important roles in the hippocampal-dependent memory formation, namely brain-derived neurotropic factor (BDNF) and c-fos (63). BDNF is also found to be decreased in brains and serum from patients with schizophrenia, anxiety, and AD (64,65). Therefore, identifying the bacterial species responsible for modulation of host BDNF expression may shed light on how the brain-gut-microbiota axis may be involved in AD pathophysiology. From a metabolic and inflammatory standpoint, there is a clear link between gut dysbiosis with obesity and metabolic disorders including type 2 diabetes (66). Given the presence of an undeniable link between type 2 diabetes and AD on an epidemiological and biological level (67), comparative analysis of gut microbiota between healthy subjects and patients with AD may provide further insight into the complex pathophysiology of AD and a target of preventive and/or therapeutic intervention, with the goal of restoring cognitive health-promoting gut microbiota.

BENEFICIAL EFFECTS OF PREBIOTICS, PROBIOTICS, AND SYNBIOTICS IN THE ELDERLY

Changes in gastrointestinal function in advanced age appear to be at least partly responsible for the dysbiotic changes in the gut microbial community of the elderly, which is functionally more putrefactive, less efficient at harvesting energy and nutrients, more inflammatory, and less protective against invading organisms. To break this vicious cycle and start a healthy aging process, it appears necessary to restore the composition and/or activity of the intestinal microbiota back to health. Probiotics are defined as "live microorganisms which when administered in adequate amounts confer a health benefit on the host" (68). Prebiotics are "selectively fermented ingredients that allow specific changes, both in the composition and/or activity in the gastrointestinal microflora that confer benefits upon host well being and health," whereas synergistic combinations of pro- and prebiotics are called synbiotics (69). We summarize here clinical trials involving probiotics and prebiotics in the elderly which were generally targeting the following beneficial effects: (1) improved gut microbiota composition; (2) improved bowel function; and (3) improved immune function. We also include other probiotics/prebiotics trials not limited to the elderly population but still demonstrating beneficial outcomes that will impact the well-being of the aging population, such as cholesterol-lowering effects and improvements in depression and anxiety scale. Primary literature papers and relevant review articles were searched in PubMed using various search keywords including "elderly," "probiotic," "prebiotic," "gut microbiota," "constipation," "aging," "cholesterol," "CVD," and "immune function."

Several feeding trials with known probiotics, prebiotics, or synbiotics interventions in elderly healthy volunteers have demonstrated increase in proportion of *Bifidobacteria* in the fecal community (70–77). Some studies also report concomitant increase in *Lactobacilli* (72,77) or decrease in *Proteobacteria* (74). Although the direct benefit of having an increased proportion of *Bifidobacteria* in the gut microbiota is unknown, these studies show successful correction of aging-related dysbiotic patterns. The immunomodulatory effects of probiotic/prebiotic feeding trials have been most pronounced in the increased phagocytic activity of the PMNs (polymorphonuclear cells) and tumor-killing activity of the NK (natural killer) cells isolated from the peripheral blood samples (78–84). It has also been shown to reduce pro-inflammatory cytokine production from the leukocytes (85). These findings may be translated to beneficial clinical outcomes in the elderly, as probiotic ingestions were associated with significantly reduced duration of illness caused by infectious agents (86–89). Interestingly, no difference has been appreciated with regard to the incidence of infections. Constipation and defecation difficulty is a common complaint of the elderly. Probiotics and prebiotics have been shown to have a normalizing effect on defecation frequency. In subjects with existing constipation, feeding trials have significantly increased the frequency of bowel movement as well as ease of defecation (75,76,90–94). Interestingly, in subjects with loose stools and diarrhea at baseline, probiotic/prebiotic feeding trials have demonstrated the opposite effect by decreasing the defecation frequency (77,90,94).

As aberrant gut microbiota composition is associated with metabolic risk factors such as obesity, diabetes, and CVD, probiotic and prebiotic feeding trials have been shown to improve blood lipid profile, especially in hypercholesterolemic and/or obese adults (95–104) as well as in the elderly (105,106). Most studies targeting healthy, normolipidemic volunteers show no significant change in the lipid profile (107–110). Interestingly, in a study of Italian young healthy male volunteers, consumption of 11% inulin-enriched pasta for 5 weeks resulted in significantly decreased serum triglycerides and lipoproteins and increase in HDL cholesterol levels (111), which highlights the impact of culturally significant dietary contribution to the effects of probiotics and prebiotics supplementation. It is also important to understand that different probiotic strains can have different degrees of lipid-modulating effects, as 10-week-long *Lactobacillus fermentum* ingestion in hypercholesterolemic individuals did not produce any detectable changes in the serum lipid levels (112).

BENEFICIAL EFFECTS OF PROBIOTICS IN PSYCHIATRIC DYSFUNCTION

Clinical studies demonstrating the beneficial effects of probiotics on anxiety, depression, or stress response are few and far between, and no studies targeting an elderly population exist thus far. One of the

Table 5.1. Beneficial Effects of Probiotics and Prebiotics on Elderly Health

TARGET	STUDY DESIGN	PROBIOTIC/PREBIOTIC	TREATMENT DOSE AND DURATION	SUBJECTS	OUTCOME	REFERENCE
Microbiota composition	Randomized, placebo-controlled trial	B. longum 46+ B. longum 2C	Daily ingestion of fermented oat drink containing 10^9 CFU/ml probiotics (quantity undocumented) 6 months	$n = 66$ 84 ± 8 yrs Nursing home residents	Significant increase in fecal bifidobacteria*	Lahtinen et al. (2009)
Microbiota composition	No placebo-controlled, pre-post intervention trial	Short-chain FOS (Actilight)	8 g/day 4 weeks	$n = 12$ 69 ± 2 yrs Healthy volunteers	Increase in fecal bifidobacteria* Increase in fecal cholesterol excretion*	Bouhnik et al. (2007)
Microbiota composition	Randomized, double-blind, placebo-controlled trial	B. bifidum BB-02 + B. lactis BL-01 + Raftilose Synergy1	Raftilose Synergy1 6g/day B. bifidum 3.5×10^{10} CFU/day B. lactis 3.5×10^{10} CFU/day 4 weeks	$n = 18$ $63–90$ yrs Healthy female volunteers	Increase in fecal bifidobacteria* and lactobacilli* compared to placebo group and pre-intervention levels	Bartosch et al. (2005)
Microbiota composition	Randomized, double-blind, placebo-controlled trial	B. lactis HN019	5×10^9 CFU/day (high) 1×10^9 CFU/day (medium) 6.5×10^7 CFU/day (low) 4 weeks	$n = 80$ $60–87$ yrs Healthy volunteers	Significant increase in fecal bifidobacteria compared to placebo and pre-intervention levels** Decrease in enterobacteria No significant difference between dose groups	Ahmed et al. (2007)

Focus	Study design	Intervention	Dose/duration	Sample	Results	Reference
Microbiota composition and immune function	Randomized, double-blind, placebo-controlled crossover study	B. longum + Synergy1 (inulin-based prebiotic)	Synergy1 12 g/day B. longum 4×10^{11} CFU/day 4 weeks	n = 43 65–90 yrs Healthy volunteers	Significant increase in fecal bifidobacteria***, Actinobacteria***, and Firmicutes**** and decrease in proteobacteria**** Increased butyrate production* Significant reduction in pro-inflammatory cytokine TNF-α*	Macfarlane et al. (2013)
Immune function	Randomized, pre-post intervention trial	L. rhamnosus HN001 (Group A) or B. lactis HN019 (Group B)	HN001: 5×10^{10} CFU/day HN019: 5×10^{9} CFU/day 3 weeks	n = 27 60–84 yrs Healthy volunteers	Increased tumoricidal activity of PBMCs following both probiotic supplementations**	Gill et al. (2001a)
Immune function	Randomized, pre-post intervention trial	B. lactis HN019	5×10^{10} CFU/day (typical dose) 5×10^{9} CFU/day (low dose) 3 weeks	n = 30 63–84 yrs Healthy volunteers	Increased phagocytic activity of PMNs** and mononuclear cells** and tumoricidal activity of NK cells* No significant difference between typical and low dose groups	Gill et al. (2001b)

(continued)

Table 5.1. Continued

TARGET	STUDY DESIGN	PROBIOTIC/PREBIOTIC	TREATMENT DOSE AND DURATION	SUBJECTS	OUTCOME	REFERENCE
Immune function	Randomized, double-blind, placebo-controlled trial	*B. lactis* HN019	3×10^{11} CFU/day 6 weeks	$n = 25$ 60–83 yrs Healthy volunteers	Increased IFNα production from PBMCs* and phagocytic capacity of PMNs*	Arunachalam et al. (2000)
Immune function	Double-blind, pre-post intervention trial	*B. lactis* HN019 (group A) vs. *B. lactis* HN019 + GOS (group B)	5×10^{10} CFU/day 3 weeks	$n = 50$ 41–81 yrs (median 60) Healthy volunteers	Increased phagocytic activity of PMNs* and tumor-killing activity of NK cells* compared to pre-intervention Relative increase in PMN cell activity ($p = 0.09$) and NK cell activity ($p = 0.043$) in group B compared to group A	Chiang et al. (2000)
Immune function	Randomized, double-blind, placebo-controlled, crossover study	*B. lactis* Bi-07 vs GOS vs Bi-07 + GOS vs maltodextrin (control)	Bi-07: 10^9 CFU/d GOS: 8 g/d Maltodextrin: 8 g/d 3 weeks	$n = 37$ > 60 yrs Healthy volunteers	Bi-07 (probiotic) consumption improves the phagocytic activity of monocytes*** and granulocytes* No significant effect observed with prebiotic and synbiotic intervention compared to control	Maneerat et al. (2013)

Immune function	Randomized, placebo-controlled, single-blind crossover study	L. casei Shirota (LcS)	1.3×10^{10} CFU/day 4 weeks	$n = 30$ 55–74 yrs Healthy volunteers	Increased tumor lysis activity of NK cells compared to pre-intervention** Decreased CD25 expression (marker of activation) of resting T cells compared to placebo**	Dong et al. (2013)
Immune function	Pre-post intervention trial	L. rhamnosus HN001	2.5×10^{10} CFU/day 3 weeks	$n = 52$ 44–80 yrs (median 63.5) Healthy volunteers	Increased phagocytic activity of PMNs* and tumor killing activity of NK cells* compared to pre-intervention.	Sheih et al. (2013)
Immune function	Randomized, double-blind, placebo-controlled trial	Oligosaccharides (OS)	1.3 g/day 12 weeks	$n = 74$ 84 ± 7 yrs Elderly individuals, undernourished or at risk of malnutrition	Diminished leukocyte pro-inflammatory cytokines TNF-α ($p = 0.05$) and IL-6* compared to control No significant differences in the fecal gut flora or in the nutritional parameters	Schiffrin et al. (2007)

(continued)

Table 5.1. Continued

TARGET	STUDY DESIGN	PROBIOTIC/ PREBIOTIC	TREATMENT DOSE AND DURATION	SUBJECTS	OUTCOME	REFERENCE
Effects on acute upper respiratory tract infection (URTI)	Randomized, double-blind, placebo-controlled, multicenter comparative study	L. casei Shirota (LcS)	4×10^{10} CFU/day 130.1 ± 31.3 days	$n = 154$ 83.2 ± 9.1 yrs Volunteers from day care facilities for the elderly population	No significant difference in total number of acute URTI events between probiotic and placebo groups Shorter mean duration of infection per infection event in the probiotic group compared to placebo*	Fujita et al. (2013)
Prevention of antibiotic-associated diarrhea (AAD)	Randomized, double-blind, placebo-controlled multicenter trial	L. acidophilus CUL60 + L. acidophilus CUL21 + B. bifidum CUL20 +B. lactis CUL 34	A multistrain preparation: 6×10^{10} CFU/day 3 weeks	$n = 2941$ ≥ 65 yrs Inpatients exposed to antibiotics	No significant difference in AAD occurrence between probiotics and placebo groups	Allen et al. (2013)
Effects on norovirus gastroenteritis	Placebo-controlled parallel study	L. casei Shirota (LcS)	4×10^{10} CFU/day 3 months	$n = 77$ Mean age: 84 yrs Long term care facility residents	No significant difference in the incidence of norovirus gastroenteritis Significantly reduced mean duration of fever after the onset of gastroenteritis* (1.5d vs 2.9d)	Nagata et al. (2011)

Effects on winter infections	Randomized, placebo-controlled study	L. casei DN-114001	Daily supplementation with fermented milk 3 weeks	n = 360 Elderly individuals, volunteers from the community (Italy)	No difference in the incidence of winter infections (GI and respiratory) 20% reduction in duration of all pathologies* acompared to control group	Turchet et al. (2003)
Bowel function and microbiota composition	Placebo-controlled, double-blind, parallel-group comparative study	L. casei Shirota (LcS)	4×10^{10} CFU/day 4 weeks	n = 30 Volunteers with loose stool, otherwise healthy	Defecation frequency significantly decreased compared to pre-intervention* Improved stool quality (hardened) compared to placebo** Significantly increased fecal bifidobacteria** and lactobacilli** compared to pre-intervention	Matsumoto et al. (2010)
Bowel function and microbiota composition	Randomized, double-blind, pre-post intervention trial	Inulin vs. lactose	20 g/day x 8 d stepwise increase to 40g/day x 3 d 40g/day x 8 d 19 days	n = 25 68–89 yrs Inpatients with constipation, No abx in 4 wks	Increased stool frequency (from 2x/wk to 8-9x/wk) on inulin. Increase in bifidobacteria* and decrease in enterobacteria** on inulin	Kleessen et al. (1997)

(continued)

Table 5.1. Continued

TARGET	STUDY DESIGN	PROBIOTIC/ PREBIOTIC	TREATMENT DOSE AND DURATION	SUBJECTS	OUTCOME	REFERENCE
Bowel function and microbiota composition	Randomized, double-blind, placebo-controlled trial	Lactitiol + L. acidophilus NCFM vs. Sucrose (placebo)	Lactitol 5 g/day L.acidophilus 1×10^{10} CFU/day 2 weeks	$n = 47$ ≥ 65 yrs Healthy volunteers	Increased defecation frequency in synbiotic group compared to placebo** Significantly increased fecal bifidobacteria compared to placebo*	Ouwehand et al. (2009)
Bowel function	Placebo-controlled, open parallel study	L. reuteri vs L. rhamnosus + P. freudenreichii vs placebo	L. reuteri 7.2×10^8 CFU/day L. rhamnosus 3×10^{10} CFU/day P. freudenreichii 6×10^{10} CFU/day 4 weeks	$n = 28$ 70–96 yrs Nursing home residents with self-reported constipation	24% increase in defecation frequency* after L. rhamnosus+ P. freudenreichii consumption	Ouwehand et al. (2008)

Bowel function	Randomize, double-blind, placebo-controlled trials	*B. longum* BB536	Trial 1: 5×10^{10} CFU/d (high) Trial 2: 2.5×10^{10} CFU/d (low) 5×10^{10} CFU/d (high) 16 weeks	Trial 1: $n = 83$ 67–101 yrs Trial 2: $n = 123$ 65–102 yrs Long-term inpatients receiving enteral feeding	Trial 1 and 2 combined results: Significantly increased defecation frequency in the low frequency group (< 4 x/wk at baseline) compared to pre-intervention and placebo** Significantly decreased defecation frequency in the high frequency group (> 10 x/wk at baseline) compared to pre-intervention**	Kondo et al. (2013)
Bowel function	Randomized, double-blind, placebo-controlled trial	*B. longum* strains vs. *B.lactis* vs. placebo	*B. longum* 10^9 CFU/day *B. lactis* 10^9 CFU/day 7 months	$n = 209$ Elderly nursing home residents	Increased defecation frequency in *B. longum* group** and *B. lactis* group** compared to placebo	Pitkala et al. (2007)
Bowel function	Randomized, double-blind, cross-over study	GOS + prunes + linseed in yogurt	GOS 12 g/day Prunes 12 g/day Linseed 6 g/day 3 weeks	$n = 43$ 61–92 yrs Volunteers with self-reported constipation	Significantly increased defecation frequency* and ease of defecation* compared to control period.	Sairanen et al. (2007)

(continued)

Table 5.1. Continued

TARGET	STUDY DESIGN	PROBIOTIC/ PREBIOTIC	TREATMENT DOSE AND DURATION	SUBJECTS	OUTCOME	REFERENCE
Bowel function	Randomized, double-blind, placebo-controlled trial	VSL#3 (*L.plantarum* + *L. paracasei* + *L.bulgaricus* + *L.acidophilus* + *B.breve* + *B.longum* + *B.infantis* + *S.thermophilus*)	4.5×10^{11} CFU/ day 45 days	$n = 243$ ≥ 65 yrs Inpatients in Geriatric Orthopedic Rehab Dept	Significantly lower incidence of diarrhea* and laxative use* Significantly increased serum albumin* and protein* in age [3] 80 yrs	Zaharoni et al. (2011)

CFU = (colony-forming units)
PBMCs = (peripheral blood mononuclear cells)
PMNs = (polymorphonuclear cells)
NK = (natural killer)
FOS = (fructo-oligosaccharides)
GOS = (galacto-oligosaccharides)
*$p < 0.05$, ** $p < 0.01$, ***$p < 0.001$, ****$p < 0.0001$

Table 5.2   Beneficial Effects of Probiotics and Prebiotics on Cardiovascular Health

REFERENCE	STUDY DESIGN	PROBIOTIC/PREBIOTIC	TREATMENT DOSE AND DURATION	SUBJECTS	OUTCOME
Anderson & Gilliland (1999)	Randomized, double-blind, placebo controlled, cross-over trial	L. acidophilus L1 fermented milk	200 ml/day 4 weeks	n = 29 Hypercholesterolemic adults	2.9% reduction in total cholesterol concentration**
Bertolami et al. (1999)	Randomized, double-blind, placebo-controlled, cross-over trial	E. faecium + S. thermophilus fermented milk product (Giao)	Gaio: 200 g/day 8 weeks	n = 32 36–65 yrs Mild-to-moderate primary hypercholesterolemia	5.3% reduction in total cholesterol** and 6.15% reduction in LDL-cholesterol*
Simons et al. (2006)	Randomized, double-blind, placebo-controlled, parallel trial	L. fermentum capsules	8 × 10⁹ CFU/day 10 weeks	n = 44 Volunteers with TC ≥ 4 mmol/L	No significant changes in TC, LDL-C, HDL-C or TG.
Ataie-Jafari et al. (2009)	Randomized, placebo-controlled, cross-over trial	L. acidophilus + B. lactis fermented yogurt	300 g/day 6 weeks	n = 14 Mild-to-moderate primary hypercholesterolemia	Significant decrease in serum total cholesterol* compared to control. No significant change in LDL-C, HDL-C, TG
Ejtahed et al. (2011)	Randomized, double-blind, placebo-controlled trial	L. acidophilus La5 + B. lactis Bb12 containing yogurt	300 g/day 6 weeks	n = 60 Type 2 diabetes and LDL-C > 2.6 mmol/L	4.54% decrease in TC and 7.45% decrease in LDL-C compared to control
Fuentes et al. (2013)	Randomized, double-blind, placebo-controlled trial	L. plantarum (CECT 7527, CECT 7528 and CECT 7529) capsule	1.2 × 10⁹ CFU/day 12 weeks	n = 60 18–65 yrs Hypercholesterolemic patients	13.6% decrease in TC compared to control

(continued)

Table 5.2. Continued

REFERENCE	STUDY DESIGN	PROBIOTIC/ PREBIOTIC	TREATMENT DOSE AND DURATION	SUBJECTS	OUTCOME
Jones et al. (2012a)	Randomized, double-blind, placebo-controlled, multicenter trial	*L. reuteri* NCIMB 30242 microencapsulated, in yogurt	250 g 6 weeks	n = 114	4.81% decrease in TC* and 8.92% decrease in LDL-C* compared to control
Jones et al. (2012b)	Randomized, double-blind, placebo-controlled, multicenter trial	*L. reuteri* NCIMB 30242 capsule	2×10^9 CFU/day 9 weeks	n = 127 Hypercholesterolemic patients	9.14% decrease in TC*** and 11.64% decrease in LDL-C***
Hlivak et al. (2005)	Randomized, double-blind, placebo-controlled trial	*E. faecium* M-74 capsule	2×10^9 CFU/day 1 year	n = 43 Mean age: 75.4 ± 1.5 yrs	Significant reduction in TC *** and LDL-C*** after 56 weeks of probiotic ingestion
Pedersen et al. (1997)	Randomized, double-blind, crossover	Inulin	14 g/d 4 weeks	n = 66 Young, healthy females	No significant differences between TC, HDL-C, LDL-C, and TG Significant higher degree of discomfort from flatulence and other GI symptoms during inulin period*
van Dokkum et al (1999)	Randomized, double-blind, diet-controlled, crossover study	Inulin vs. FOS vs. GOS vs. control	15 g/d 3 weeks	n = 12 Mean age: 23 yrs Healthy male volunteers	No significant change in blood lipid concentration and glucose absorption

Reference	Study design	Prebiotic	Dose/duration	Subjects	Results
Jackson et al. (1999)	Randomized, double-blind, placebo-controlled, parallel study	Inulin	10 g/d 8 weeks	n = 54 Mean age: 52 ± 9 Healthy men and women with moderately raised fasting plasma TC and TAG	Significantly lower insulin level at 4 weeks compared to pre-intervention** Significantly lower TAG levels at 8 weeks on inulin compared to control*
Russo et al. (2008)	Randomized, double-blind, placebo-controlled crossover study	11% inulin-enriched pasta	11 g/d 5 weeks	n = 22 Young healthy male volunteers	35.9% increase in HDL-C** 22.2% decrease in TC/HDL-C ratio** 23.4% decrease in TG* 16.5% decrease in LPa*
Vulevic et al. (2008)	Randomized, double-blind, placebo-controlled crossover study	B-GOS	5.5 g/d 10 weeks	n = 44 64–79 yrs Healthy elderly	No significant effect on TC or HDL-C levels.
Yen et al. (2011)	Randomized, double-blind, placebo-controlled, diet-controlled parallel study	FOS	10 g/d 3 weeks	n = 10 Normolipidemic, constipated nursing-home residents	7% decrease in TC compared to placebo*
Giacco et al. (2004)	Randomized, double-blind, placebo-controlled crossover study	scFOS (Actilight) with tea and/or coffee	10.6 g/d 8 weeks	n = 30 45.5 ± 9.9 yrs Mildly hyperlipidemic, otherwise healthy adults	No significant difference in fasting TC, TG, vLDL, LDL, HDL levels

(continued)

Table 5.2. Continued

REFERENCE	STUDY DESIGN	PROBIOTIC/ PREBIOTIC	TREATMENT DOSE AND DURATION	SUBJECTS	OUTCOME
Balcazar-Munoz et al. (2003)	Randomized, double-blind, placebo-controlled parallel study	Inulin	7 g/d 4 weeks	$n = 12$ 19–32 yrs Dyslipidemic obese subjects	Significant reduction in TC*, LDL*, vLDL* and TG* No effect on insulin sensitivity
Vulevic et al. (2013)	Randomized, double-blind, placebo-controlled crossover study	B-GOS	5.5 g/d 12 weeks	$n = 45$ 44.6 ± 11.2 yrs Overweight adults with metabolic syndrome	Significantly decreased TC***, TG*** and serum TC:HDL-C ratio**** compared to placebo (male > female)

TC (total cholesterol)
LDL-C (low-density lipoprotein cholesterol)
vLDL (very low density lipoprotein)
HDL-C (high-density lipoprotein cholesterol)
TG (triglycerides)
TAG (triacylglycerol)
CFU (colony-forming units)
FOS (fructo-oligosaccharides)
scFOS (short-chain FOS)
OFS (oligofructose)
GOS (galacto-oligosaccharides)
B-GOS (trans-galactooligosaccharide mixture)
LPa (lipoprotein)
*$p < 0.05$, **$p < 0.01$, ***$p < 0.001$, ****$p < 0.0001$

first studies was a double-blind, placebo-controlled study on healthy volunteers, which showed consumption of *Lactobacillus casei* strain Shirota (LcS) containing milk drink for 3 weeks improved mood (113). More recently, Messaoudi and colleagues demonstrated in a double-blind, randomized parallel group study that ingestion of probiotics, *L. helveticus* and *B. longum*, for 30 days resulted in beneficial effects on general signs of anxiety and depression (especially evident in the global severity index of the HSCL-90 and global scores of Hospital Anxiety and Depression Scale) and decreased serum cortisol levels in healthy human volunteers (114).

Other human studies were conducted in the setting of physiological disorders with comorbid psychiatric symptoms such as chronic fatigue syndrome and irritable bowel syndrome (IBS). In a randomized, double-blind, placebo-controlled pilot study of patients with chronic fatigue syndrome, 8-week-long treatment with LcS consumption led to significant improvement in anxiety levels (115). According to the most recent meta-analysis of the effects of probiotics on IBS symptoms, five of the 12 studies that evaluated IBS quality of life (QOL) showed significant improvement (116). Typically, most IBS studies do not formally assess the psychiatric symptoms beyond QOL. However, a recent randomized, placebo-controlled pilot study measured the effect of a newer probiotic *L. casei rhamnosus* LCR35 on the IBS severity score as well as the hospital anxiety and depression scale (HADS) (117). Although no clinically relevant changes were noted in the HADS, future clinical studies with an adequate sample size, different probiotic strains, and possibly longer treatment duration are warranted to properly assess the changes in mood and anxiety symptoms.

SUMMARY

Many physiological changes found with normal aging process have direct and indirect association with the changes in the composition of the gut microbiota. Restoring a healthy gut microbial community with probiotics or prebiotic supplementation may be key to promoting the health and well-being of our elderly population by modulating the risk of cardiovascular disease, malignancy, and neuropsychiatric decline. It is important to expect a range in the types and degrees of beneficial outcomes with different probiotics and prebiotics.

Individual differences in the gut microbiota composition, diet, immune status, and genetic background can contribute to the heterogeneity of outcomes. Therefore, evidence-based practice and adequate trials of a few different probiotics/prebiotics preparations may be necessary for maximal beneficial outcome. In conclusion, probiotics and prebiotics comprise an important CAIM intervention for various aspects of the health of the elderly population.

REFERENCES

1. Podolsky SH. Metchnikoff and the microbiome. *Lancet.* Nov 24 2012;380(9856):1810–1811.
2. Sekirov I, Russell SL, Antunes LC, Finlay BB. Gut microbiota in health and disease. *Physiol Rev.* Jul 2010;90(3):859–904.
3. Hays NP, Roberts SB. The anorexia of aging in humans. *Physiol Behav.* Jun 30 2006;88(3):257–266.
4. Weiffenbach JM, Baum BJ, Burghauser R. Taste thresholds: quality specific variation with human aging. *J Gerontol.* May 1982;37(3):372–377.
5. Laurin D, Brodeur JM, Bourdages J, Vallee R, Lachapelle D. Fibre intake in elderly individuals with poor masticatory performance. *J Can Dent Assoc.* May 1994;60(5):443–446, 449.
6. Doty RL, Shaman P, Applebaum SL, Giberson R, Siksorski L, Rosenberg L. Smell identification ability: changes with age. *Science.* Dec 21 1984;226(4681):1441–1443.
7. Husebye E, Skar V, Hoverstad T, Melby K. Fasting hypochlorhydria with gram positive gastric flora is highly prevalent in healthy old people. *Gut.* Oct 1992;33(10):1331–1337.
8. Russell RM. Changes in gastrointestinal function attributed to aging. *Am J Clin Nutr.* Jun 1992;55(6 Suppl):1203S–1207S.
9. McCrea GL, Miaskowski C, Stotts NA, Macera L, Varma MG. Pathophysiology of constipation in the older adult. *World J Gastroenterol.* May 7 2008;14(17):2631–2638.
10. Camilleri M, Lee JS, Viramontes B, Bharucha AE, Tangalos EG. Insights into the pathophysiology and mechanisms of constipation, irritable bowel syndrome, and diverticulosis in older people. *J Am Geriatr Soc.* Sep 2000;48(9):1142–1150.
11. Macfarlane GT, Cummings JH, Macfarlane S, Gibson GR. Influence of retention time on degradation of pancreatic enzymes by human colonic bacteria grown in a 3-stage continuous culture system. *J Appl Bacteriol.* Nov 1989;67(5):520–527.

12. Chrischilles EA, Foley DJ, Wallace RB, et al. Use of medications by persons 65 and over: data from the established populations for epidemiologic studies of the elderly. *J Gerontol.* Sep 1992;47(5):M137–144.

13. Gupta A, Epstein JB, Sroussi H. Hyposalivation in elderly patients. *J Can Dent Assoc.* Nov 2006;72(9):841–846.

14. Simor AE, Bradley SF, Strausbaugh LJ, Crossley K, Nicolle LE. Clostridium difficile in long-term-care facilities for the elderly. *Infect Control Hosp Epidemiol.* Nov 2002;23(11):696–703.

15. Williams C, McColl KE. Review article: proton pump inhibitors and bacterial overgrowth. *Aliment Pharmacol Ther.* Jan 1 2006;23(1):3–10.

16. Pappagallo M. Incidence, prevalence, and management of opioid bowel dysfunction. *Am J Surg.* Nov 2001;182(5A Suppl):11S–18S.

17. Gruver AL, Hudson LL, Sempowski GD. Immunosenescence of ageing. *J Pathol.* Jan 2007;211(2):144–156.

18. George AJ, Ritter MA. Thymic involution with ageing: obsolescence or good housekeeping? *Immunol Today.* Jun 1996;17(6):267–272.

19. Lazuardi L, Jenewein B, Wolf AM, Pfister G, Tzankov A, Grubeck-Loebenstein B. Age-related loss of naive T cells and dysregulation of T-cell/B-cell interactions in human lymph nodes. *Immunology.* Jan 2005;114(1):37–43.

20. Weksler ME, Szabo P. The effect of age on the B-cell repertoire. *J Clin Immunol.* Jul 2000;20(4):240–249.

21. Solana R, Tarazona R, Gayoso I, Lesur O, Dupuis G, Fulop T. Innate immunosenescence: effect of aging on cells and receptors of the innate immune system in humans. *Semin Immunol.* Oct 2012;24(5):331–341.

22. Giunta S. Exploring the complex relations between inflammation and aging (inflamm-aging): anti-inflamm-aging remodelling of inflamm- aging, from robustness to frailty. *Inflamm Res.* Dec 2008;57(12):558–563.

23. Dominguez-Bello MG, Costello EK, Contreras M, et al. Delivery mode shapes the acquisition and structure of the initial microbiota across multiple body habitats in newborns. *Proc Natl Acad Sci U S A.* Jun 29 2010;107(26):11971–11975.

24. Yatsunenko T, Rey FE, Manary MJ, et al. Human gut microbiome viewed across age and geography. *Nature.* Jun 14 2012;486(7402):222–227.

25. Faith JJ, Guruge JL, Charbonneau M, et al. The long-term stability of the human gut microbiota. *Science.* Jul 5 2013;341(6141):1237439.

26. Dethlefsen L, Relman DA. Incomplete recovery and individualized responses of the human distal gut microbiota to repeated antibiotic perturbation. *Proc Natl Acad Sci U S A.* Mar 15 2011;108 Suppl 1:4554–4561.

27. Mitsuoka T. Intestinal flora and aging. *Nutr Rev.* Dec 1992;50(12):438–446.

28. He F, Ouwehand AC, Isolauri E, Hosoda M, Benno Y, Salminen S. Differences in composition and mucosal adhesion of bifidobacteria isolated from healthy adults and healthy seniors. *Curr Microbiol.* Nov 2001;43(5):351–354.

29. Hopkins MJ, Sharp R, Macfarlane GT. Age and disease related changes in intestinal bacterial populations assessed by cell culture, 16S rRNA abundance, and community cellular fatty acid profiles. *Gut.* Feb 2001;48(2):198–205.

30. Hopkins MJ, Macfarlane GT. Changes in predominant bacterial populations in human faeces with age and with Clostridium difficile infection. *J Med Microbiol.* May 2002;51(5):448–454.

31. Woodmansey EJ, McMurdo ME, Macfarlane GT, Macfarlane S. Comparison of compositions and metabolic activities of fecal microbiotas in young adults and in antibiotic-treated and non-antibiotic-treated elderly subjects. *Appl Environ Microbiol.* Oct 2004;70(10):6113–6122.

32. Mueller S, Saunier K, Hanisch C, et al. Differences in fecal microbiota in different European study populations in relation to age, gender, and country: a cross-sectional study. *Appl Environ Microbiol.* Feb 2006;72(2):1027–1033.

33. Enck P, Zimmermann K, Rusch K, Schwiertz A, Klosterhalfen S, Frick JS. The effects of ageing on the colonic bacterial microflora in adults. *Z Gastroenterol.* Jul 2009;47(7):653–658.

34. Xu J, Bjursell MK, Himrod J, et al. A genomic view of the human-Bacteroides thetaiotaomicron symbiosis. *Science.* Mar 28 2003;299(5615):2074–2076.

35. Round JL, Mazmanian SK. Inducible Foxp3+ regulatory T-cell development by a commensal bacterium of the intestinal microbiota. *Proc Natl Acad Sci U S A.* Jul 6 2010;107(27):12204–12209.

36. Shen Y, Giardino Torchia ML, Lawson GW, Karp CL, Ashwell JD, Mazmanian SK. Outer membrane vesicles of a human commensal mediate immune regulation and disease protection. *Cell Host Microbe.* Oct 18 2012;12(4):509–520.

37. Macfarlane S, Macfarlane GT. Regulation of short-chain fatty acid production. *Proc Nutr Soc.* Feb 2003;62(1):67–72.

38. Tiihonen K, Tynkkynen S, Ouwehand A, Ahlroos T, Rautonen N. The effect of ageing with and without non-steroidal anti-inflammatory drugs on gastrointestinal microbiology and immunology. *Br J Nutr*. Jul 2008;100(1):130–137.

39. Frank DN, St Amand AL, Feldman RA, Boedeker EC, Harpaz N, Pace NR. Molecular-phylogenetic characterization of microbial community imbalances in human inflammatory bowel diseases. *Proc Natl Acad Sci U S A*. Aug 21 2007;104(34):13780–13785.

40. Sokol H, Seksik P, Furet JP, et al. Low counts of Faecalibacterium prausnitzii in colitis microbiota. *Inflamm Bowel Dis*. Aug 2009;15(8):1183–1189.

41. Walker AW, Sanderson JD, Churcher C, et al. High-throughput clone library analysis of the mucosa-associated microbiota reveals dysbiosis and differences between inflamed and non-inflamed regions of the intestine in inflammatory bowel disease. *BMC Microbiol*. 2011;11:7.

42. Ott SJ, Musfeldt M, Wenderoth DF, et al. Reduction in diversity of the colonic mucosa associated bacterial microflora in patients with active inflammatory bowel disease. *Gut*. May 2004;53(5):685–693.

43. Ley RE, Turnbaugh PJ, Klein S, Gordon JI. Microbial ecology: human gut microbes associated with obesity. *Nature*. Dec 21 2006;444(7122):1022–1023.

44. Turnbaugh PJ, Hamady M, Yatsunenko T, et al. A core gut microbiome in obese and lean twins. *Nature*. Jan 22 2009;457(7228):480–484.

45. Zuo HJ, Xie ZM, Zhang WW, et al. Gut bacteria alteration in obese people and its relationship with gene polymorphism. *World J Gastroenterol*. Feb 28 2011;17(8):1076–1081.

46. Karlsson FH, Tremaroli V, Nookaew I, et al. Gut metagenome in European women with normal, impaired and diabetic glucose control. *Nature*. Jun 6 2013;498(7452):99–103.

47. Thavagnanam S, Fleming J, Bromley A, Shields MD, Cardwell CR. A meta-analysis of the association between Caesarean section and childhood asthma. *Clin Exp Allergy*. Apr 2008;38(4):629–633.

48. Abrahamsson TR, Jakobsson HE, Andersson AF, Bjorksten B, Engstrand L, Jenmalm MC. Low gut microbiota diversity in early infancy precedes asthma at school age. *Clin Exp Allergy*. Jun 2014;44(6):842–850.

49. Finegold SM, Dowd SE, Gontcharova V, et al. Pyrosequencing study of fecal microflora of autistic and control children. *Anaerobe*. Aug 2010;16(4):444–453.

50. Wang Z, Klipfell E, Bennett BJ, et al. Gut flora metabolism of phosphatidylcholine promotes cardiovascular disease. *Nature*. Apr 7 2011;472(7341):57–63.

51. Wu N, Yang X, Zhang R, et al. Dysbiosis signature of fecal microbiota in colorectal cancer patients. *Microb Ecol*. Aug 2013;66(2):462–470.

52. Rutter M, Saunders B, Wilkinson K, et al. Severity of inflammation is a risk factor for colorectal neoplasia in ulcerative colitis. *Gastroenterology*. Feb 2004;126(2):451–459.

53. Maslowski KM, Vieira AT, Ng A, et al. Regulation of inflammatory responses by gut microbiota and chemoattractant receptor GPR43. *Nature*. Oct 29 2009;461(7268):1282–1286.

54. Hu S, Dong TS, Dalal SR, et al. The microbe-derived short chain fatty acid butyrate targets miRNA-dependent p21 gene expression in human colon cancer. *PLoS One*. 2011;6(1):e16221.

55. Kostic AD, Gevers D, Pedamallu CS, et al. Genomic analysis identifies association of Fusobacterium with colorectal carcinoma. *Genome Res*. Feb 2012;22(2):292–298.

56. Castellarin M, Warren RL, Freeman JD, et al. Fusobacterium nucleatum infection is prevalent in human colorectal carcinoma. *Genome Res*. Feb 2012;22(2):299–306.

57. Rubinstein MR, Wang X, Liu W, Hao Y, Cai G, Han YW. Fusobacterium nucleatum promotes colorectal carcinogenesis by modulating E-cadherin/beta-catenin signaling via its FadA adhesin. *Cell Host Microbe*. Aug 14 2013;14(2):195–206.

58. Schwabe RF, Jobin C. The microbiome and cancer. *Nat Rev Cancer*. Nov 2013;13(11):800–812.

59. Bultman SJ. Emerging roles of the microbiome in cancer. *Carcinogenesis*. Feb 2014;35(2):249–255.

60. Hill JM, Clement C, Pogue AI, Bhattacharjee S, Zhao Y, Lukiw WJ. Pathogenic microbes, the microbiome, and Alzheimer's disease (AD). *Front Aging Neurosci*. 2014;6:127.

61. Rhee SH, Pothoulakis C, Mayer EA. Principles and clinical implications of the brain-gut-enteric microbiota axis. *Nat Rev Gastroenterol Hepatol*. May 2009;6(5):306–314.

62. Smith K, McCoy KD, Macpherson AJ. Use of axenic animals in studying the adaptation of mammals to their commensal intestinal microbiota. *Semin Immunol*. Apr 2007;19(2):59–69.

63. Gareau MG, Wine E, Rodrigues DM, et al. Bacterial infection causes stress-induced

memory dysfunction in mice. *Gut.* Mar 2011;60(3):307–317.

64. Carlino D, De Vanna M, Tongiorgi E. Is altered BDNF biosynthesis a general feature in patients with cognitive dysfunctions? *Neuroscientist.* Aug 2013;19(4):345–353.

65. Lu B, Nagappan G, Guan X, Nathan PJ, Wren P. BDNF-based synaptic repair as a disease-modifying strategy for neurodegenerative diseases. *Nat Rev Neurosci.* Jun 2013;14(6):401–416.

66. Sommer F, Backhed F. The gut microbiota: masters of host development and physiology. *Nat Rev Microbiol.* Apr 2013;11(4):227–238.

67. Barbagallo M, Dominguez LJ. Type 2 diabetes mellitus and Alzheimer's disease. *World J Diabetes.* Dec 15 2014;5(6):889–893.

68. Gareau MG, Sherman PM, Walker WA. Probiotics and the gut microbiota in intestinal health and disease. *Nat Rev Gastroenterol Hepatol.* Sep 2010;7(9):503–514.

69. de Vrese M, Schrezenmeir J. Probiotics, prebiotics, and synbiotics. *Adv Biochem Eng Biotechnol.* 2008;111:1–66.

70. Lahtinen SJ, Tammela L, Korpela J, et al. Probiotics modulate the Bifidobacterium microbiota of elderly nursing home residents. *Age (Dordr).* Mar 2009;31(1):59–66.

71. Ahmed M, Prasad J, Gill H, Stevenson L, Gopal P. Impact of consumption of different levels of Bifidobacterium lactis HN019 on the intestinal microflora of elderly human subjects. *J Nutr Health Aging.* Jan-Feb 2007;11(1):26–31.

72. Bartosch S, Woodmansey EJ, Paterson JC, McMurdo ME, Macfarlane GT. Microbiological effects of consuming a synbiotic containing Bifidobacterium bifidum, Bifidobacterium lactis, and oligofructose in elderly persons, determined by real-time polymerase chain reaction and counting of viable bacteria. *Clin Infect Dis.* Jan 1 2005;40(1):28–37.

73. Bouhnik Y, Achour L, Paineau D, Riottot M, Attar A, Bornet F. Four-week short chain fructo-oligosaccharides ingestion leads to increasing fecal bifidobacteria and cholesterol excretion in healthy elderly volunteers. *Nutr J.* 2007;6:42.

74. Macfarlane S, Cleary S, Bahrami B, Reynolds N, Macfarlane GT. Synbiotic consumption changes the metabolism and composition of the gut microbiota in older people and modifies inflammatory processes: a randomised, double-blind, placebo-controlled crossover study. *Aliment Pharmacol Ther.* Oct 2013;38(7):804–816.

75. Ouwehand AC, Tiihonen K, Saarinen M, Putaala H, Rautonen N. Influence of a combination of Lactobacillus acidophilus NCFM and lactitol on healthy elderly: intestinal and immune parameters. *Br J Nutr.* Feb 2009;101(3):367–375.

76. Kleessen B, Sykura B, Zunft HJ, Blaut M. Effects of inulin and lactose on fecal microflora, microbial activity, and bowel habit in elderly constipated persons. *Am J Clin Nutr.* May 1997;65(5):1397–1402.

77. Matsumoto K, Takada T, Shimizu K, et al. Effects of a probiotic fermented milk beverage containing Lactobacillus casei strain Shirota on defecation frequency, intestinal microbiota, and the intestinal environment of healthy individuals with soft stools. *J Biosci Bioeng.* Nov 2010;110(5):547–552.

78. Gill HS, Rutherfurd KJ, Cross ML. Dietary probiotic supplementation enhances natural killer cell activity in the elderly: an investigation of age-related immunological changes. *J Clin Immunol.* Jul 2001;21(4):264–271.

79. Gill HS, Rutherfurd KJ, Cross ML, Gopal PK. Enhancement of immunity in the elderly by dietary supplementation with the probiotic Bifidobacterium lactis HN019. *Am J Clin Nutr.* Dec 2001;74(6):833–839.

80. Arunachalam K, Gill HS, Chandra RK. Enhancement of natural immune function by dietary consumption of Bifidobacterium lactis (HN019). *Eur J Clin Nutr.* Mar 2000;54(3):263–267.

81. Chiang BL, Sheih YH, Wang LH, Liao CK, Gill HS. Enhancing immunity by dietary consumption of a probiotic lactic acid bacterium (Bifidobacterium lactis HN019): optimization and definition of cellular immune responses. *Eur J Clin Nutr.* Nov 2000;54(11):849–855.

82. Dong H, Rowland I, Thomas LV, Yaqoob P. Immunomodulatory effects of a probiotic drink containing Lactobacillus casei Shirota in healthy older volunteers. *Eur J Nutr.* Dec 2013;52(8):1853–1863.

83. Maneerat S, Lehtinen MJ, Childs CE, et al. Consumption of Bifidobacterium lactis Bi-07 by healthy elderly adults enhances phagocytic activity of monocytes and granulocytes. *J Nutr Sci.* 2013;2:e44.

84. Sheih YH, Chiang BL, Wang LH, Liao CK, Gill HS. Systemic immunity-enhancing effects in healthy subjects following dietary consumption of the lactic acid bacterium Lactobacillus rhamnosus HN001. *J Am Coll Nutr.* Apr 2001;20(2 Suppl):149–156.

85. Schiffrin EJ, Thomas DR, Kumar VB, et al. Systemic inflammatory markers in older persons: the effect of oral nutritional supplementation with prebiotics. *J Nutr Health Aging*. Nov-Dec 2007;11(6):475–479.

86. Fujita R, Iimuro S, Shinozaki T, et al. Decreased duration of acute upper respiratory tract infections with daily intake of fermented milk: a multicenter, double-blinded, randomized comparative study in users of day care facilities for the elderly population. *Am J Infect Control*. Dec 2013;41(12):1231–1235.

87. Nagata S, Asahara T, Ohta T, et al. Effect of the continuous intake of probiotic-fermented milk containing Lactobacillus casei strain Shirota on fever in a mass outbreak of norovirus gastroenteritis and the faecal microflora in a health service facility for the aged. *Br J Nutr*. Aug 2011;106(4):549–556.

88. Allen SJ, Wareham K, Wang D, et al. Lactobacilli and bifidobacteria in the prevention of antibiotic-associated diarrhoea and Clostridium difficile diarrhoea in older inpatients (PLACIDE): a randomised, double-blind, placebo-controlled, multicentre trial. *Lancet*. Oct 12 2013;382(9900):1249–1257.

89. Turchet P, Laurenzano M, Auboiron S, Antoine JM. Effect of fermented milk containing the probiotic Lactobacillus casei DN-114001 on winter infections in free-living elderly subjects: a randomised, controlled pilot study. *J Nutr Health Aging*. 2003;7(2):75–77.

90. Kondo J, Xiao JZ, Shirahata A, et al. Modulatory effects of Bifidobacterium longum BB536 on defecation in elderly patients receiving enteral feeding. *World J Gastroenterol*. 2013;19(14):2162–2170.

91. Ouwehand AC, Bergsma N, Parhiala R, et al. Bifidobacterium microbiota and parameters of immune function in elderly subjects. *FEMS Immunol Med Microbiol*. Jun 2008;53(1):18–25.

92. Pitkala KH, Strandberg TE, Finne Soveri UH, Ouwehand AC, Poussa T, Salminen S. Fermented cereal with specific bifidobacteria normalizes bowel movements in elderly nursing home residents: a randomized, controlled trial. *J Nutr Health Aging*. Jul-Aug 2007;11(4):305–311.

93. Sairanen U, Piirainen L, Nevala R, Korpela R. Yoghurt containing galacto-oligosaccharides, prunes and linseed reduces the severity of mild constipation in elderly subjects. *Eur J Clin Nutr*. Dec 2007;61(12):1423–1428.

94. Zaharoni H, Rimon E, Vardi H, Friger M, Bolotin A, Shahar DR. Probiotics improve bowel movements in hospitalized elderly patients: the PROAGE study. *J Nutr Health Aging*. Mar 2011;15(3):215–220.

95. Anderson JW, Gilliland SE. Effect of fermented milk (yogurt) containing Lactobacillus acidophilus L1 on serum cholesterol in hypercholesterolemic humans. *J Am Coll Nutr*. Feb 1999;18(1):43–50.

96. Ataie-Jafari A, Larijani B, Alavi Majd H, Tahbaz F. Cholesterol-lowering effect of probiotic yogurt in comparison with ordinary yogurt in mildly to moderately hypercholesterolemic subjects. *Ann Nutr Metab*. 2009;54(1):22–27.

97. Bertolami MC, Faludi AA, Batlouni M. Evaluation of the effects of a new fermented milk product (Gaio) on primary hypercholesterolemia. *Eur J Clin Nutr*. Feb 1999;53(2):97–101.

98. Ejtahed HS, Mohtadi-Nia J, Homayouni-Rad A, et al. Effect of probiotic yogurt containing Lactobacillus acidophilus and Bifidobacterium lactis on lipid profile in individuals with type 2 diabetes mellitus. *J Dairy Sci*. Jul 2011;94(7):3288–3294.

99. Fuentes MC, Lajo T, Carrion JM, Cune J. Cholesterol-lowering efficacy of Lactobacillus plantarum CECT 7527, 7528 and 7529 in hypercholesterolaemic adults. *Br J Nutr*. May 28 2013;109(10):1866–1872.

100. Balcazar-Munoz BR, Martinez-Abundis E, Gonzalez-Ortiz M. [Effect of oral inulin administration on lipid profile and insulin sensitivity in subjects with obesity and dyslipidemia]. *Rev Med Chil*. Jun 2003;131(6):597–604.

101. Jackson KG, Taylor GR, Clohessy AM, Williams CM. The effect of the daily intake of inulin on fasting lipid, insulin and glucose concentrations in middle-aged men and women. *Br J Nutr*. Jul 1999;82(1):23–30.

102. Vulevic J, Juric A, Tzortzis G, Gibson GR. A mixture of trans-galactooligosaccharides reduces markers of metabolic syndrome and modulates the fecal microbiota and immune function of overweight adults. *J Nutr*. Mar 2013;143(3):324–331.

103. Jones ML, Martoni CJ, Parent M, Prakash S. Cholesterol-lowering efficacy of a microencapsulated bile salt hydrolase-active Lactobacillus reuteri NCIMB 30242 yoghurt formulation in hypercholesterolaemic adults. *Br J Nutr*. May 2012;107(10):1505–1513.

104. Jones ML, Martoni CJ, Prakash S. Cholesterol lowering and inhibition of sterol absorption by Lactobacillus reuteri NCIMB 30242: a randomized controlled trial. *Eur J Clin Nutr*. Nov 2012;66(11):1234–1241.

105. Hlivak P, Odraska J, Ferencik M, Ebringer L, Jahnova E, Mikes Z. One-year application of probiotic strain Enterococcus faecium M-74 decreases serum cholesterol levels. *Bratisl Lek Listy.* 2005;106(2):67–72.

106. Yen CH, Kuo YW, Tseng YH, Lee MC, Chen HL. Beneficial effects of fructo-oligosaccharides supplementation on fecal bifidobacteria and index of peroxidation status in constipated nursing-home residents: a placebo-controlled, diet-controlled trial. *Nutrition.* Mar 2011;27(3):323–328.

107. Giacco R, Clemente G, Luongo D, et al. Effects of short-chain fructo-oligosaccharides on glucose and lipid metabolism in mild hypercholesterolaemic individuals. *Clin Nutr.* Jun 2004;23(3):331–340.

108. Pedersen A, Sandstrom B, Van Amelsvoort JM. The effect of ingestion of inulin on blood lipids and gastrointestinal symptoms in healthy females. *Br J Nutr.* Aug 1997;78(2):215–222.

109. van Dokkum W, Wezendonk B, Srikumar TS, van den Heuvel EG. Effect of nondigestible oligosaccharides on large-bowel functions, blood lipid concentrations and glucose absorption in young healthy male subjects. *Eur J Clin Nutr.* Jan 1999;53(1):1–7.

110. Vulevic J, Drakoularakou A, Yaqoob P, Tzortzis G, Gibson GR. Modulation of the fecal microflora profile and immune function by a novel trans-galactooligosaccharide mixture (B-GOS) in healthy elderly volunteers. *Am J Clin Nutr.* Nov 2008;88(5):1438–1446.

111. Russo F, Chimienti G, Riezzo G, et al. Inulin-enriched pasta affects lipid profile and Lp(a) concentrations in Italian young healthy male volunteers. *Eur J Nutr.* Dec 2008;47(8):453–459.

112. Simons LA, Amansec SG, Conway P. Effect of Lactobacillus fermentum on serum lipids in subjects with elevated serum cholesterol. *Nutr Metab Cardiovasc Dis.* Dec 2006;16(8):531–535.

113. Benton D, Williams C, Brown A. Impact of consuming a milk drink containing a probiotic on mood and cognition. *Eur J Clin Nutr.* Mar 2007;61(3):355–361.

114. Messaoudi M, Lalonde R, Violle N, et al. Assessment of psychotropic-like properties of a probiotic formulation (Lactobacillus helveticus R0052 and Bifidobacterium longum R0175) in rats and human subjects. *Br J Nutr.* Mar 2011;105(5):755–764.

115. Rao AV, Bested AC, Beaulne TM, et al. A randomized, double-blind, placebo-controlled pilot study of a probiotic in emotional symptoms of chronic fatigue syndrome. *Gut Pathog.* 2009;1(1):6.

116. Ortiz-Lucas M, Tobias A, Saz P, Sebastian JJ. Effect of probiotic species on irritable bowel syndrome symptoms: a bring up to date meta-analysis. *Rev Esp Enferm Dig.* Jan 2013;105(1):19–36.

117. Dapoigny M, Piche T, Ducrotte P, Lunaud B, Cardot JM, Bernalier-Donadille A. Efficacy and safety profile of LCR35 complete freeze-dried culture in irritable bowel syndrome: a randomized, double-blind study. *World J Gastroenterol.* May 7 2012;18(17):2067–2075.

6

HORMONE THERAPY, MOOD, AND COGNITION

Aikisha Harley, Danielle Balzafiore, and Tonita E. Wroolie

INTRODUCTION

There are five major classes of human steroid hormones: estrogens, progestogens, androgens, mineral corticoids, and glucocorticoids. These hormones play an important role in the central nervous system by regulating bodily functions, and some hormones are believed to be able to penetrate the blood–brain barrier (Genazzani, Pluchino, Luisi, & Luisi, 2007). In addition, steroid hormones may impact how the body regulates stress as well as have neuropathic affects (Genazzani et al., 2007; Keller et al., 2006; G. E. Miller, Chen, & Zhou, 2007). When prescribed, hormone therapy (HT) most often includes an estrogen with or without a progestogen.

Estrogen, one of the sex steroid hormones, affects a number of biological systems, helping to regulate autonomic, affective, and cognitive functioning (for a review, see Fischer, Gleason, & Asthana, 2014). There are three different classes of estrogens: estrone (E1), 17-β estradiol (E2), and estriol (E3).

During a woman's reproductive years, E2 is the most prevalent of the estrogens, except during pregnancy when E3 is predominant (Coelingh Bennink, 2014). However, after menopause, E2 decreases and E1 becomes the predominant circulating estrogen (Asthana & Middleton, 2004; Rannevik et al., 1995). HT preparations most often contain E2 or conjugated equine estrogen (CEE), the latter being an estrogen derived from equine sources that is predominately composed of E1.

The term *progestogens* can be used to refer to both naturally occurring progestogens as well as synthetic compounds that have progestogenic activity similar to those that occur naturally (Rott, 2014). Progesterone is the naturally occurring progestogen and is secreted by the ovaries and adrenal glands in non-pregnant women (Rott, 2014). The synthetic progestogen is typically referred to as progestin (Conaway, 2011). In HT, progestogens are typically combined with estrogens to prevent endometrial hyperplasia (Rott, 2014) in women who have an intact uterus.

The majority of HT studies in postmenopause have focused on either synthetic or natural E2 with progestogen because women are vulnerable to the effects of decreases in these hormones across the life span due to menopause (Sood, Faubion, Kuhle, Thielen, & Shuster, 2014). Because the level of estrogens and progestogens have been found to impact higher order functions, including mood and cognition, several studies have looked at the use of HT to regulate hormone levels for the management of menopausal, psychiatric, and cognitive symptoms (Luine, 2014; Sood et al., 2014).

Prior to the Women's Health Initiative (WHI) study, the largest clinical trial of HT, the most widely prescribed estrogen in the United States was CEE (Carr, 1996). The use of HT became controversial following the WHI study, which showed an increased risk of cardiovascular disease, ischemic stroke, venous thromboembolism, and breast cancer (for a review, see Sood et al., 2014). The Women's Health Initiative Memory Study (WHIMS) also found increased probable dementia and/or cognitive decline in women who initiated CEE after the age of 65 years (Espeland et al., 2004; Rapp et al., 2003; Shumaker et al., 2003, 2004). Immediately following publication of the WHI results, HT use guidelines were developed and HT use dropped dramatically (Kelly et al., 2005; Silverman & Kokia, 2009; Stefanick, 2005).

In the years to follow, evidence has emerged that suggests that the type of HT compound and the timing of initiation may play a significant role in the risk versus benefit profile of use. Commonly referred to as the "window of opportunity," the timing of HT initiation and the age at which hormone therapies are prescribed are critical in determining whether benefits could be obtained from HT use (Sood et al., 2014). Some studies have found that the benefits of hormone therapy outweigh the risks when prescribed to menopausal women younger than 60 years old or within 10 years of the start of menopause, but they are less beneficial or unfavorable when prescribed to women beyond this time frame (Sood et al., 2014). Finally, with regard to duration, the current standard is to prescribe hormone therapies at the lowest dose and shortest duration needed to manage symptoms, which for the average woman is between 3 to 5 years (North American Menopause Society, 2012).

This chapter reviews the effectiveness of HT use for mood and risk of cognitive decline or dementia in women. The use of HT for major depressive disorder and bipolar disorder will be discussed, following an overview of the effects of HT on cognitive functions during the menopause transition. Finally, a brief overview of the effects of HT on men will be provided, an area that is of growing interest and warrants further attention.

HORMONE THERAPY AND MOOD

Treatment of Major Depressive Disorder

Females have been found to have 1.5- to 3-fold higher rates of major depressive disorder compared to males (Kessler et al., 2003), with the prevalence disparity typically beginning during early adolescence through postmenopause. The higher rate of depressive symptoms among females is often associated with marked fluctuations in estrogen levels during reproductive cycle events, such as puberty, pregnancy, and menopause (Joinson et al., 2012; Wharton, Gleason, Olson, Carlsson, & Asthana, 2012). Although most women transitioning through menopause do not become depressed, it is a time of increased vulnerability for depression and the recurrence of depressive symptoms in women with a history of a mood disorder (North American Menopause Society, 2012; Wharton et al., 2012).

Although menopause transition is linked to significant fluctuations in estrogen, which may be associated with higher depression risk, the use of HT to treat depressive symptoms has not been clearly established (Wharton et al., 2012). Studies that examine the utility of antidepressant and adjunctive HT treatment of depression are limited, and many of these studies have yielded conflicting results (Amsterdam et al., 1999; Klaiber, Broverman, Vogel, & Kobayashi, 1979; Shapira et al., 1985). The variability in findings is due to a number of factors, including differences in study design (i.e., retrospective versus prospective study) and in HT preparations (i.e., type of estrogen, with or without a progestogen). There is also heterogeneity of study populations regarding depression severity, phase of menopause, and type of antidepressant prescribed (tricyclic antidepressants versus selective serotonin reuptake inhibitors [SSRIs]) (Amsterdam et al., 1999; Klaiber, Broverman, Vogel, & Kobayashi, 1979; Shapira et al., 1985).

In a retrospective study, Amsterdam et al. (1999) investigated the efficacy of HT in women over 45 years old diagnosed with major depressive disorder who were taking 20 mg of fluoxetine daily. The findings did not suggest any difference in outcome between women who were or were not using HT. Similarly, Shapira et al. (1985) found that adding CEE to a regimen of antidepressants did not significantly improve depressive symptoms in women aged 24 to 76 years with treatment-resistant depression.

Overall, placebo-controlled clinical trials have demonstrated significant group differences between placebo, HT use only, and antidepressant with adjunctive HT (Klaiber et al., 1979; Schneider et al., 1997). In an earlier study, Klaiber et al. (1979) found that a sample of women inpatients with severe, treatment-resistant depression who were given large doses (5–25 mg) of CEE had significant declines in Hamilton Depression Rating Scale (HDRS) scores when they were compared to a similar sample of women who received a placebo.

Schneider et al. (1997) investigated the efficacy of HT in women users or non-users combined with fluoxetine in women age 60 years and older with depression compared to an age-matched placebo control group. The results indicated a significant interaction between HT status and treatment effect. The women taking fluoxetine with HT had a greater improvement in depressive symptoms compared to women on placebo and HT. Additionally, the women who were not using HT did not have a significant improvement with fluoxetine treatment compared to the placebo group. The authors concluded that HT appeared to augment the response to fluoxetine in these depressed older adult women (Schneider et al., 1997).

More recent evidence suggests that transdermal E2 may accelerate the response to antidepressants (Rasgon et al., 2007). In a randomized placebo-controlled trial (Rasgon et al., 2007), postmenopausal women with major depressive disorder taking sertraline received either transdermal E2 with a release rate of 0.1 mg E2/day or a placebo patch. Overall, the results indicated similar improvements in depression for both groups by the end of the study. However, women receiving E2 showed a greater decline from baseline to weeks 2, 3, and 4 when compared to the placebo group, suggesting an accelerated response to antidepressant treatment.

Further evidence suggests that menopause status may affect the response of antidepressants to HT. More specifically, estrogen therapy (ET) has been found to be as effective as an antidepressant in perimenopausal women but not in women 5 to 10 years postmenopause (Schmidt, 2005). A possible explanation for this is that in older women, there are age-related decreases in serotonergic activity (Halbreich et al., 1995), which could delay antidepressant response. However, discontinuation of ET may also increase risk of depression. Evidence suggests that in women of reproductive age, treatment with estrogen may enhance serotonin synthesis or decrease serotonin reuptake (Shors & Leuner, 2003), augment serotonergin activity (Halbreich, Asnis, Shindledecker, Zumoff, & Nathan, 1985), inhibit monoaminoxidase (MAO; Luine, Khylchevskaya, & McEwen, 1975), and/or increase the number of sites available for active transport of serotonin into the brain cell (Sherwin & Suranyi-Cadotte, 1990). Additionally, regardless of age, ET may not be efficacious for the treatment of severe depression (Morrison et al., 2004; Schneider et al., 1997).

Moreover, it has been purported that the antidepressant effects of HT may be mitigated by preparations that contain progesterone (Soares, Poitras, & Prouty, 2003). Progesterone may increase monoamine oxidase activity and gamma-aminobutyric acid (GABA)–inhibitory action, resulting in mood-destabilization (Sherwin & Suranyi-Cadotte, 1990).

Overall, animal models have shown that estrogen may regulate serotonin pathways at various levels as well as increase serotonin availability (Kiss et al., 2012; Récamier-Carballo, Estrada-Camarena, Reyes, & Fernández-Guasti, 2012). Animal studies further elucidate the effectiveness of HT in the treatment of depression. Récamier-Carballo et al. (2012) studied the effects of antidepressants in young (2–4-month-old) and middle-aged (12–14-month-old) ovariectomized rats given suboptimal doses of E2 and fluoxetine. It was concluded that the combination of these suboptimal doses caused an antidepressant-like effect in both groups; specifically, both groups presented with increased mobility and swimming. Additionally, when the groups were exposed to chronic mild stress, the E2 and fluoxetine combination improved sucrose intake in both groups, but the middle-aged groups improved earlier than the young group. Kiss et al. (2012) found that E2 improved performance in the Morris water maze in both younger adult (7-month-old) and middle-aged adult (12-month-old) rats; however, the younger adult rats benefited from treatment more than the middle-aged rats.

Similar findings have been noted in human trials. Research has found that in human models, estrogen may alter mRNA and protein levels of various serotonin markers. In addition, estrogen may cause a decrease in serotonin breakdown (Lokuge, Frey, Foster, Soares, & Steiner, 2011).

In conclusion, many studies indicate that HT may be beneficial in the treatment of depression. However, there is conflicting evidence, likely due to factors such as study design, differences in HT preparations and route of administration, and heterogeneity of the study populations (Amsterdam et al., 1999; Klaiber, Broverman, Vogel, & Kobayashi, 1979; Shapira et al., 1985). Animal studies have helped to clarify some conflicts due to confounds frequently encountered in human investigations.

TREATMENT OF BIPOLAR DISORDER

Similar to epidemiological research on major depressive disorder, previous studies suggest that intense hormonal fluctuations during reproductive events can trigger mood episodes in women with bipolar disorder (for a review, see Frey & Dias, 2014). Overall, studies have indicated that approximately 20%–50% of women with bipolar disorder report intense mood symptoms during the menopause transition (Blehar et al., 1998; Freeman et al., 2002), specifically, increases in depressive symptoms and frequency of depressive episodes (Marsh, Ketter, & Rasgon, 2009; Marsh, Templeton, Ketter, & Rasgon, 2008). Menopausal transition may also precipitate new onset or worsening of bipolar disorder, increased irritability, increased hypomania/mania, more rapid cycling, and severe emotional distress (Blehar et al., 1998; Freeman et al., 2002; Kukopulos et al., 1980). Further, recent evidence shows a gradient of worsening mood state in women with bipolar disorder from the premenopausal to perimenopausal to postmenopausal periods (Marsh, Ketter, Crawford, Johnson, Kroll-Desrosiers, & Rothschild, 2012).

Few studies have examined the use of HT in bipolar disorder, and resultant findings are mixed. There is evidence to suggest that women using HT are less likely to report intensifying mood symptoms during perimenopause compared to non-users (Freeman et al., 2002). In contrast, Marsh et al. (2009) found no differences in the number of psychiatric clinic visits for depressed mood in perimenopausal and postmenopausal women HT users and non-users. Additional research on the effectiveness of HT in women with bipolar disorder is warranted.

HORMONE THERAPY AND COGNITION

Relationship Between Estrogen and Cognition

Research indicates that estrogens, specifically E2, mediate higher order cognitive functions in the cerebral cortex, basal forebrain, hippocampus, and striatum (Luine, 2014). There is evidence suggesting that E2, which is synthesized in these brain regions, may be involved in the consolidation of memory (Luine & Frankfurt, 2012). Animal models suggest that E2 influences synaptic plasticity in the hippocampus and prefrontal cortex and that HT containing E2 may improve cognitive functions that are implicated in these brain regions (for a review, see Luine, 2014) and that decreases in estrogen levels are associated with age-related declines in learning and memory (Luine, 2014). E2, along with other gonadal hormones, is indirectly involved in the maintenance of cognitive abilities because of neurotrophic interactions within the brain. Thus, decreases in E2 may be responsible for age-related cognitive declines. Such an implication would explain the cognitive complaints typically reported by women during menopause transition.

Hormone Therapy and Cognition

Results from the Seattle Midlife Women's Health Study and the Study of Women's Health Across the Nation suggest that timing, age, and menopause status play an important role in the presence of subjective cognitive complaints. More specifically, these studies showed that women who were in the early and middle menopause transition stage reported more subjective memory complaints compared to women in late transition or postmenopause (Woods, Mitchell, & Adams, 2000). Similarly, Elsabagh et al. (2007) found that women in the late postmenopausal stage (greater than 5 years since last menstrual period) performed worse on executive functioning tasks (i.e., cognitive flexibility and planning) compared to women early in the postmenopausal stage (5 years since last menstrual period). However, no significant differences in verbal memory or verbal fluency tasks were noted.

Drogos et al. (2013) showed a relationship between subjective memory complaints and objective cognitive test performance in middle-aged women who were transitioning into menopause. They found that objective measures of attention and memory were significantly correlated with forgetfulness ratings, and negative affect was associated with increased frequency of forgetting. Finally, lower positive affect and greater severity of vasomotor symptoms were related to higher reported retrospective memory functioning difficulties.

Moreover, E2 has been found to improve memory abilities in animal studies (Luine, 2014); however, findings regarding the effectiveness of HT as a treatment for cognitive deficits are limited. There is limited evidence indicating that estrogen levels are typically lower in women diagnosed with Alzheimer's disease when compared to age-matched healthy controls (Hideo et al., 1989), but in general HT use for patients with Alzheimer's disease does not appear to be beneficial (see Henderson, 2014 for a review). There is a growing body of evidence, however, suggesting a decreased risk of developing dementia in postmenopausal women who use or have ever used HT (Henderson, Paganini-Hill, Emanuel, Dunn, & Buckwalter, 1994; Kawas et al., 1997; Tang et al., 1996). Additional studies (Rasgon et al., 2005) suggest that unopposed E2 may be beneficial in preserving glucose metabolism in the posterior cingulate, an area known to decline early in Alzheimer's disease.

Numerous studies also show that healthy postmenopausal women using HT with E2, but not CEE, performed significantly better on verbal memory tasks (for a review, see Yaffe et al., 1998). Other studies show better performances on tasks of simple attention, working memory, abstract reasoning, and verbal fluency in E2 users compared to either non-users or CEE users (LeBlanc, Janowsky, Chan, & Nelson, 2001; K. Miller, Conney, Rasgon, Fairbanks, & Small, 2002; Wroolie et al., 2011). HT with E2 has also been found to be associated with better visuospatial abilities when prescribed during the early stages or soon after the onset of menopause (Luine, 2014). Use of E2 may also improve executive functioning when initiated earlier, rather than later, in postmenopausal women (Dunkin et al., 2005).

Although studies show that HT may be a protective factor against cognitive decline, with evidence that HT use may reduce the risk of Alzheimer's disease by approximately 50% (Hogervorst, Williams, Budge, Riedel, & Jolles, 2000; Simpkins et al., 2009), it appears that timing of initiation, duration of use, and type of HT are important considerations. Findings from WHIMS and from the Heart and Estrogen/Progestin Replacement Study (HERS) indicated that prolonged or later initiation (age > 65 years) of HT treatment with CEE was associated with increased risk of cognitive decline and poorer cognitive performance (Espeland et al., 2004; Grady et al., 2002; Rapp et al., 2003; Shumaker et al., 2003, 2004).

Currently, there is evidence to support the premise that HT use may be efficacious in managing both subjective and objective cognitive issues. Specifically, studies have found that HT, particularly with E2, is associated with improvements in verbal memory, executive functions, and visuospatial abilities (Luine, 2014; K. Miller et al., 2002). Studies also suggest that HT may act as a protective factor against cognitive decline and Alzheimer's disease (Yaffe et al., 1998). However, the literature is limited, and more studies need to be conducted investigating the potential benefits to cognition.

HORMONE THERAPY FOR MEN

Male testosterone levels are said to decrease by 40% from age 40 to age 70, and for some men, this can contribute to a number of mood or cognitive symptoms. The most common HT for men is testosterone therapy for the treatment of hypogonadism. Hypogonadism is a condition in which testosterone deficiency is associated with abnormal physical, mood, and cognitive symptoms. When present in elderly men, the condition is known as andropause, androgen deficiency, or late onset hypogonadism (LOH). Both hypogonadism and LOH can greatly impact men's quality of life. Common symptoms include decreased muscle mass, decreased strength, osteoporosis, cardiovascular disease, erectile dysfunction, and abdominal obesity (for a review, see Bassil, Alkaade, & Morley, 2009). Mood and cognitive symptoms are also common. These include decrease libido, insomnia, memory deficits, difficulties concentrating, depressed mood, and other cognitive impairments (Lunenfeld, Nieschlag, Lunenfeld, & Nieschlag, 2007). HT has been used to address some of the physical symptoms associated with hypogonadism. However, research regarding the efficacy of testosterone supplementation for mood and cognitive disorders is limited.

When compared to age-matched infertile and non-hypogonadal men, those with hypogonadism report higher levels of depression, anger, and confusion (Burris, Banks, Carter, Davidson, & Sherins, 1992). Given that studies have found that the prevalence of depression increases with age, the risk of developing depressive symptoms associated with LOH is even more concerning (Barrett-Connor, von Mühlen, & Kritz-Silverstein, 1999).

Current research investigating the efficacy of testosterone therapy in managing mood symptoms related to hypogonadism is conflicting. Some studies have suggested that hypogonadal men given testosterone supplementation saw an improvement in mood (Barrett-Connor et al., 1999; Burris et al., 1992; Wang et al., 1996). Similarly, one study (Wang et al., 1996) that included hypogonadal men prescribed testosterone therapy suggested significant positive correlations between testosterone supplementation and positive moods (i.e., energy, friendliness, increased sense of well-being). The authors also found significant negative correlations between testosterone therapy and negative moods (i.e., nervousness, irritability, anger, depression) when testosterone was given for a short course (3 weeks). However, prolonged (6 months) testosterone therapy did not lead to further improvements in mood.

Furthermore, when used as an augmentation to antidepressants or SSRIs, evidence suggests that testosterone therapy may be effective in improving depressive symptoms (Ehrenreich et al., 1999; Pope, Cohane, Kanayama, Siegel, & Hudson, 2003; Seidman & Rabkin, 1998). However, research suggests that the efficacy of testosterone supplementation is only effective in certain populations (e.g., some hypogonadal and antidepressant-resistant men). In addition, clinical studies investigating the relationship between testosterone therapy and mood in healthy males did not yield significant results (for review, see Amiaz & Seidman, 2008).

In elderly men, the findings are also variable and dependent upon the sample characteristics and duration of treatment. Some studies suggest a decrease in depression severity and improvements in mood and well-being, while others have found no differences (for a review, see Gruenewald & Matsumoto, 2003). In one 9-month double-blind study, Mårin et al. (1993) found testosterone therapy to be effective in improving feelings of overall well-being and energy in obese elderly men. In contrast, results from a 12-month randomized controlled trial of older hypogonadal men (Sih et al., 1997) and a double blind placebo-controlled study (Janowsky et al., 2000) did not indicate any significant improvement in mood.

There is also variability in the literature investigating the efficacy of testosterone therapy for the improvement of cognitive deficits. According to a population-based study that included 547 men between the ages of 59 and 89, bioavailable testosterone levels were better predictors of verbal memory and mental control (Barrett-Connor et al., 1999). Other studies have found that declines in age-related bioavailable testosterone were related to verbal memory and visuospatial deficits (for a review, see Bassil et al., 2009). The Baltimore Longitudinal Study of Aging investigated the relationship between testosterone levels, Alzheimer's disease, and age. The results indicated that the risk of Alzheimer's disease was reduced by approximately 26% for each 10-unit (nmol/nmol) increase of testosterone prescribed 2, 5, and 10 years prior to a diagnosis of Alzheimer's disease (Moffat et al., 2004). These findings suggest that testosterone levels are related to cognitive functioning and risk for Alzheimer's disease in men.

Further research regarding testosterone therapy and cognition suggests that in mildly hypogonadal men, testosterone supplementation may lead to improvements in verbal memory (Cherrier, Craft, & Matsumoto, 2003). Similarly, a study by Janowsky et al. (2000) indicated that testosterone supplementation may improve working memory performance in elderly men. In addition, the authors reported that in younger men, there was a positive relationship between working memory performance and testosterone therapy. Cherrier et al. (2005) found that testosterone therapy, when prescribed to elderly men diagnosed with Alzheimer's disease and mild cognitive impairment for 6 weeks, improved visual memory and visuospatial constructional abilities. Improvements were also seen during the peak hormone period of 24–48 hours post-injection. In contrast, Kenny et al.'s (2002) study did not yield significant improvements in cognition when testosterone was prescribed to older men (average age 76 years) with low levels of bioavailable testosterone. Given these inconsistencies, further research is necessary to determine the benefits of testosterone supplementation on cognition.

SUMMARY

Although the research regarding the efficacy of HT for the treatment of depression may be conflicting, there is a growing body of literature indicating that HT use may augment and/or accelerate antidepressant treatment response in women. Similarly, HT may help manage mood episodes in women with bipolar disorder. HT therapy, specifically preparations with E2, when initiated early in menopause are associated with improvements in verbal memory, attention, working memory, visuospatial abilities, executive functions, and preservation of metabolism in the posterior cingulate, suggesting that HT may protect against risk for Alzheimer's disease. In order for benefits to be realized, it is important to consider the age of HT initiation, duration, time since menopause, and HT preparation.

Regarding men, there is evidence suggesting that low testosterone levels may be associated with mood and cognitive deficits. The most common form of HT prescribed to men is testosterone therapy. However, the research regarding the efficacy of testosterone therapy for such issues is limited and conflicting. More research is necessary to determine the potential benefits of testosterone therapy for men.

REFERENCES

Amiaz, R., & Seidman, S. N. (2008). Testosterone and depression in men. *Curr Opin Endocrinol, Diabetes Obesity, 15*(3), 278–283.

Amsterdam, J., Garcia-España, F., Fawcett, J., Quitkin, F., Reimherr, F., Rosenbaum, J., & Beasley, C. (1999). Fluoxetine efficacy in menopausal women with and without estrogen replacement. *J Affect Disorders, 55*(1), 11–17.

Asthana, S., & Middleton, W. S. (2004). Estrogen and cognition: a true relationship? *J Am Geriatr Soc, 52*(2), 316–318.

Barrett-Connor, E., von Mühlen, D. G., & Kritz-Silverstein, D. (1999). Bioavailable testosterone and depressed mood in older men: The Rancho Bernardo Study. *The J Clin Endocrinol Metab, 84*(2), 573–577.

Bassil, N., Alkaade, S., & Morley, J. E. (2009). The benefits and risks of testosterone replacement therapy: a review. *Therapeut Clin Risk Manage, 5*, 427.

Blehar, M. C., DePaulo, J. R., Jr., Gershon, E. S., Reich, T., Simpson, S. G., & Nurnberger, J. I., Jr. (1998). Women with bipolar disorder: findings from the NIMH genetics initiative sample. *Psychopharmacol Bull. 34*(3) 239–243.

Burris, A. S., Banks, S. M., Carter, C., S. U. E., Davidson, J. M., & Sherins, R. J. (1992). A long-term, prospective study of the physiologic and behavioral effects of hormone replacement in untreated hypogonadal men. *J Androl, 13*(4), 297–304.

Cherrier, M. M., Craft, S., & Matsumoto, A. H. (2003). Cognitive changes associated with supplementation of testosterone or dihydrotestosterone in mildly hypogonadal men: A preliminary report. *J Androl, 24*(4), 568–576.

Carr, B.R. (1996). HRT management: the American experience. *Eur J Obstet Gynecol Reprod Biol 64* (S), 17-20.

Cherrier, M. M., Matsumoto, A. M., Amory, J. K., Asthana, S., Bremner, W., Peskind, E. R., . . . Craft, S. (2005). Testosterone improves spatial memory in men with Alzheimer disease and mild cognitive impairment. *Neurology, 64*(12), 2063–2068.

Coelingh Bennink, H. J. T. (2014). Are all estrogens the same? *Maturitas, 47*(4), 269–275.

Conaway, E. (2011). Bioidentical hormones: an evidence-based review for primary care providers. *J Am Osteopath Assoc, 111*(3), 153–164.

Drogos, L. L., Rubin, L. H., Geller, S. E., Banuvar, S., Shulman, L. P., & Maki, P. M. (2013). Objective cognitive performance is related to subjective memory complaints in midlife women with moderate to severe vasomotor symptoms. *Menopause, 20*(12), 1236–1242.

Dunkin, J., Rasgon, N., Wagner-Steh, K., David, S., Altshuler, L., & Rapkin, A. (2005). Reproductive events modify the effects of estrogen replacement therapy on cognition in healthy postmenopausal women. *Psychoneuroendocrinology, 30*, 284–296.

Ehrenreich, H., Halaris, A., Ruether, E., Hüfner, M., Funke, M., & Kunert, H. J. (1999). Psychoendocrine sequelae of chronic testosterone deficiency. *J Psychiatr Res, 33*(5), 379–387.

Elsabagh, S., Hartley, D. E., & File, S. E. (2007). Cognitive function in late versus early postmenopausal stage. *Maturitas, 56*(1), 84–93.

Espeland, M. A., Rapp, S. R., Shumaker, S. A., Brunner, R., Manson, J. E., Sherwin, B. B., . . . Hays, J. (2004). Conjugated equine estrogens and global cognitive function in postmenopausal women: Women's Health Initiative Memory Study. *JAMA, 291*(24), 2959–2968.

Fischer, B., Gleason, C., & Asthana, S. (2014). Effects of hormone therapy on cognition and mood. *Fertil Steril, 101*(4), 898–904.

Freeman, M. P., Smith, K. W., Freeman, S. A., McElroy, S. L., Kmetz, G. E., Wright, R., & Keck, P. E., Jr. (2002). The impact of reproductive events on the course of bipolar disorder in women. *J Clin Psychiatry, 63*(4), 284–287.

Frey, B. N., & Dias, R. D. (2014). Sex hormones and biomarkers of neuroprotection and neurodegeneration: implications for female reproductive events in bipolar disorder. *Bipolar Disord, 16*(1), 48–57.

Genazzani, A. R., Pluchino, N., Luisi, S., & Luisi, M. (2007). Estrogen, cognition and female ageing. *Human Reprod Update, 13*(2), 175–187.

Grady, D., Yaffe, K., Kristof, M., Lin, F., Richards, C., & Barrett-Connor, E. (2002). Effect of postmenopausal hormone therapy on cognitive function: The Heart and Estrogen/Progestin Replacement Study. *Am J Med, 113*, 543–548.

Gruenewald, D. A., & Matsumoto, A. M. (2003). Testosterone supplementation therapy for older men: potential benefits and risks. *J Am Geriatr Soc, 51*(1), 101–115.

Halbreich, U., Asnis, G. M., Shindledecker, R., Zumoff, B., & Nathan, R. S. (1985). Cortisol secretion in endogenous depression: time-related functions. *Arch Gen Psychiatry, 42*(9), 909.

Halbreich, U., Rojansky, N., Palter, S., Tworek, H., Hissin, P., & Wang, K. (1995). Estrogen augments serotonergic activity in postmenopausal women. *Biol Psychiatry, 37*(7), 434–441.

Henderson V. W. (2014). Alzheimer's disease: review of hormone therapy trials and implications for treatment and prevention after menopause. *J Steroid Biochem Mol Biol.* 142, 99-106.

Henderson, V. W., Paganini-Hill, A., Emanuel, C. K., Dunn, M. E., & Buckwalter, J. G. (1994). Estrogen replacement therapy in older women: comparisons between Alzheimer's disease cases and nondemented control subjects. *Arch Neurol, 51*(9), 896–900.

Hideo, H., Yoshio, O., Kazuo, N., Mamoru, U., Jo, K., Jinsuke, Y., . . . Toshio, N. (1989). In vivo effects by estrone sulfate on the central nervous system-senile dementia (Alzheimer's type). *J Steroid Biochem, 34*(1–6), 521–525.

Hogervorst, E., Williams, J., Budge, M., Riedel, W., & Jolles, J. (2000). The nature of the effect of female gonadal hormone replacement therapy on cognitive function in post-menopausal women: a meta-analysis. *Neuroscience, 101*(3), 485–512.

Janowsky, J. S., Chavez, B., & Orwoll, E. (2000). Sex steroids modify working memory. *J Cognitive Neurosci, 12*(3), 407–414.

Joinson, C., Heron, J., Araya, R., Paus, T., Croudace, T., Rubin, C., . . . Lewis, G. (2012). Association between pubertal development and depressive symptoms in girls from a UK cohort. *Psychol Med, 42*(12), 2579–2589.

Kawas, C., Resnick, S., Morrison, A., Brookmeyer, R., Corrada, M., Zonderman, A., . . . Metter, E. (1997). A prospective study of estrogen replacement therapy and the risk of developing Alzheimer's disease: The Baltimore Longitudinal Study of Aging. *Neurology, 48*(6), 1517–1521.

Keller, J., Flores, B., Gomez, R. G., Solvason, H. B., Kenna, H., Williams, G. H., & Schatzberg, A. F. (2006). Cortisol circadian rhythm alterations in psychotic major depression. *Biol Psychiatry, 60*(3), 275–281.

Kelly, J. P., Kaufman, D. W., Rosenberg, L., Kelley, K., Cooper, S. G., & Mitchell, A. A. (2005). Use of postmenopausal hormone therapy since the Women's Health Initiative findings. *Pharmacoepidem Drug Safety, 14*(12), 837–842.

Kenny, A. M., Bellantonio, S., Gruman, C. A., Acosta, R. D., & Prestwood, K. M. (2002). Effects of transdermal testosterone on cognitive function and health perception in older men with low bioavailable testosterone levels. *J Gerontol A, 57*(5), 321–325.

Kessler, R., Berglund, P., Demler, O., Jin, R., Merikangas, K., & Walters, E. (2003). The epidemiology of major depressive disorder: results from the National Comorbidity Survey Replication (NCS-R). *JAMA, 289*(23), 3095–3105.

Kiss, Á., Delattre, A. M., Pereira, S. I. R., Carolino, R. G., Szawka, R. E., Anselmo-Franci, J. A., . . . Ferraz, A. C. (2012). 17β-Estradiol replacement in young, adult and middle-aged female ovariectomized rats promotes improvement of spatial reference memory and an antidepressant effect and alters monoamines and BDNF levels in memory- and depression-related brain areas. *Behav Brain Res, 227*(1), 100–108.

Klaiber, E., Broverman, D., Vogel, W., & Kobayashi, Y. (1979). Estrogen therapy for severe persistent depressions in women. *Arch Gen Psychiatry, 36*(5), 550–554.

Kukopulos, A., Reginaldi, D., Laddomada, P., Floris, G., Serra, G., & Tondo, L. (1980). Course of the manic-depressive cycle and changes caused by treatments. *Pharmacopsychiatry, 13*(04), 156–167.

LeBlanc, E. S., Janowsky, J., Chan, B. K. S., & Nelson, H. D. (2001). Hormone replacement therapy and cognition: systematic review and meta-analysis. *JAMA, 285*(11), 1489–1499.

Lokuge, S., Frey, B. N., Foster, J. A., Soares, C. N., & Steiner, M. (2011). Depression in women: windows of vulnerability and new insights into the link between estrogen and serotonin. *J Clin Psychiatry, 72*(11), 1563–1569.

Luine, V. (2014). Estradiol and cognitive function: past, present and future. *Hormones Behav, 66*(4), 602–618.

Luine, V., & Frankfurt, M. (2012). Estrogens facilitate memory processing through membrane mediated mechanisms and alterations in spine density. *Front Neuroendocrinol, 33*(4), 388–402.

Luine, V., Khylchevskaya, R. I., & McEwen, B. (1975). Effect of gonadal steroids on activities of monoaminooxidase and choline acetylase in rat brain. *Brain Res, 86*, 293–306.

Lunenfeld, B., Nieschlag, E., Lunenfeld, B., & Nieschlag, E. (2007). Testosterone therapy in the aging male. *Aging Male, 10*(3), 139–153. doi: 10.1080/13685530701485998

Mårin, P., Holmtäng, S., Gustafsson, C., Elander, A., Eldh, J., Sjöström, L., . . . Björntorp, P. (1993). Androgen treatment of abdominally obese men. *Obesity Res, 1*(4), 245–251.

Marsh, W. K., Ketter, T. A., Crawford, S. L., Johnson, J. V., Kroll-Desrosiers, A., & Rothschild, A. (2012). Progression of reproductive stages associated with bipolar illness excerbation. *Bipolar Disord, 14*(5), 515–526.

Marsh, W. K., Ketter, T. A., & Rasgon, N. L. (2009). Increased depressive symptoms in menopausal age women with bipolar disorder: age and gender comparison. *J Psychiatric Res, 43*(8), 798–802.

Marsh, W. K., Templeton, A., Ketter, T. A., & Rasgon, N. L. (2008). Increased frequency of depressive episodes during the menopausal transition in women with bipolar disorder: preliminary report. *J Psychiatric Res, 42*(3), 247–251.

Miller, G. E., Chen, E., & Zhou, E. S. (2007). If it goes up, must it come down? Chronic stress and the hypothalamic-pituitary-adrenocortical axis in humans. *Psychol Bull, 133*(1), 24–45.

Miller, K., Conney, J., Rasgon, N., Fairbanks, L., & Small, G. (2002). Mood symptoms and cogntive performance in women estrogen users and nonusers and men. *J Am Geriatr, 50*, 1826–1830.

Moffat, S. D., Zonderman, A. B., Metter, E. J., Kawas, C., Blackman, M. R., Harman, S. M., & Resnick, S. M. (2004). Free testosterone and risk for Alzheimer disease in older men. *Neurology, 62*(2), 188–193.

Morrison, M. F., Kallan, M. J., Have, T. T., Katz, I., Tweedy, K., & Battistini, M. (2004). Lack of efficacy of estradiol for depression in postmenopausal women: a randomized, controlled trial. *Biol Psychiatry, 55*, 406–412.

North American Menopause Society. (2012). The 2012 hormone therapy position statement of the North American Menopause Society. *Menopause, 19*(3), 257–71.

Pope, H. G., Jr., Cohane, G. H., Kanayama, G., Siegel, A. J., & Hudson, J. I. (2003). Testosterone gel supplementation for men with refractory depression: a randomized, placebo-controlled trial. *Am J Psychiatry, 160*(1), 105–111.

Rannevik, G., Jeppsson, S., Johnell, O., Bjerre, B., Laurell-Borulf, Y., & Svanberg, L. (1995). A longitudinal study of the perimenopausal transition: altered profiles of steroid and pituitary hormones, SHBG and bone mineral density. *Maturitas, 21*(2), 103–113.

Rapp, S. R., Espeland, M. A., Shumaker, S. A., Henderson, V. W., Brunner, R. L., Manson, J. E., . . . Bowen, D. (2003). Effect of estrogen plus progestin on global cognitive function in postmenopausal women: The Women's Health Initiative Memory Study: a randomized controlled trial. *JAMA, 289*(20), 2663–2672.

Rasgon, N., Dunkin, J., Fairbanks, L., Altshuler, L. L., Troung, C., Elman, S., . . . Rapkin, A. (2007). Estrogen and response to sertraline in postmenopausal women with major depressive disorder: a pilot study. *J Psychiatr Res, 41*(3–4), 338–343.

Rasgon, N., Silverman, D., Siddarth, P., Miller, K., Ercoli, L., Elman, S., . . . Small, G. (2005). Estrogen use and brain metabolic change in postmenopausal women. *Neurobiol Aging, 26*, 229–235.

Récamier-Carballo, S., Estrada-Camarena, E., Reyes, R., & Fernández-Guasti, A. (2012). Synergistic effect of estradiol and fluoxetine in young adult and middle-aged female rats in two models of experimental depression. *Behav Brain Res, 233*(2), 351–358.

Rott, H. (2014). Prevention and treatment of venous thromboembolism during HRT: current perspectives. *Int J Gen Med, 7*, 433–40.

Schmidt, P. J. (2005). Mood, depression, and reproductive hormones in the menopausal transition. *Am J Med, 118*(12, Suppl 2), 54–58.

Schneider, L. S., Small, G. W., Hamilton, S. H., Bystritsky, A., Nemeroff, C. B., & Meyers, B. S. (1997). Estrogen replacement and response to fluoxetine in a multicenter geriatric depression trial. *Am J Geriatr Psychiatry, 5*(2), 97–106.

Seidman, S. N., & Rabkin, J. G. (1998). Testosterone replacement therapy for hypogonadal men with

SSRI-refractory depression. *J Affective Disord,* *48*(2), 157–161.

Shapira, B., Oppenheim, G., Zohar, J., Segal, M., Malach, D., & Belmaker, R. H. (1985). Lack of efficacy of estrogen supplementation to imipramine in resistant female depressives. *Biol Psychiatry, 20*(5), 576–579.

Sherwin, B. B., & Suranyi-Cadotte, B. E. (1990). Up-regulatroy effect of estrogen on platelet 3H-imipramine binding sites in sugically postmenopausal women. *Biol Psychiatry, 38,* 339–348.

Shors, T. J., & Leuner, B. (2003). Estrogen-mediated effects on depression and memory formation in females. *J Affective Disord, 74*(1), 85–96.

Shumaker, S. A., Legault, C., Kuller, L., Rapp, S. R., Thal, L., Lane, D. S., . . . Coker, L. H. (2004). Conjugated equine estrogens and incidence of probable dementia and mild cognitive impairment in postmenopausal women: Women's Health Initiative Memory Study. *JAMA, 291*(24), 2947–2958.

Shumaker, S. A., Legault, C., Rapp, S. R., Thal, L., Wallace, R. B., Ockene, J. K., . . . Wactawski-Wende, J. (2003). Estrogen plus progestin and the incidence of dementia and mild cognitive impairment in postmenopausal women: The Women's Health Initiative Memory Study: a randomized controlled trial. *JAMA, 289*(20), 2651–2662.

Sih, R., Morley, J. E., Kaiser, F. E., Perry III, H. M., Patrick, P., & Ross, C. (1997). Testosterone replacement in older hypogonadal men: a 12-month randomized controlled trial. *J Clin Endocrinol Metab, 82*(6), 1661–1667.

Silverman, B. G., & Kokia, E. S. (2009). Use of hormone replacement therapy, 1998–2007: sustained impact of the Women's Health Initiative findings. *Ann Pharmacother, 43*(2), 251–258.

Simpkins, J. W., Perez, E., Xiaofei Wang, ShaoHua Yang, Yi Wen, & Singh, M. (2009). Review: the potential for estrogens in preventing Alzheimer's disease and vascular dementia. *Ther Adv Neurol Disord, 2*(1), 31–49.

Soares, C. N., Poitras, J. R., & Prouty, J. (2003). Effect of reproductive hormones and selective estrogen receptor modulators on mood during menopause. *Drugs Aging, 20*(2), 85–100.

Sood, R., Faubion, S. S., Kuhle, C. L., Thielen, J. M., & Shuster, L. T. (2014). Prescribing menopausal hormone therapy: an evidence-based approach. *Int J Women's Health, 6,* 47–57.

Stefanick, M. L. (2005). Estrogens and progestins: background and history, trends in use, and guidelines and regimens approved by the US Food and Drug Administration. *Am J Med, 118*(12), 64–73.

Tang, M.-X., Jacobs, D., Stern, Y., Marder, K., Schofield, P., Gurland, B., . . . Mayeux, R. (1996). Effect of oestrogen during menopause on risk and age at onset of Alzheimer's disease. *Lancet, 348*(9025), 429–432.

Wang, C., Alexander, G., Berman, N., Salehian, B., Davidson, T., McDonald, V., . . . Swerdloff, R. S. (1996). Testosterone replacement therapy improves mood in hypogonadal men: a clinical research center study. *J Clin Endocrinol Metab, 81*(10), 3578–3583.

Wharton, W., Gleason, C. E., Olson, S. R., Carlsson, C. M., & Asthana, S. (2012). Neurobiological underpinnings of the estrogen-mood relationship. *Curr Psychiatry Rev, 8*(3), 247–256.

Woods, N. F., Mitchell, E. S., & Adams, C. (2000). Memory functioning among midlife women: observations from the Seattle Midlife Women's Health Study. *Menopause, 7*(4), 257–265.

Wroolie, T. E., Kenna, H. A., Williams, K. E., Powers, B. N., Holcomb, M., Khaylis, A., & Rasgon, N. L. (2011). Differences in verbal memory performance in postmenopausal women receiving hormone therapy: 17β-estradiol versus conjugated equine estrogens. *Am J Geriatr Psychiatry, 19*(9), 792.

Yaffe, K., Sawaya, G., Lieberburg, I., & Grady, D. (1998). Estrogen therapy in postmenopausal women: effects on cognitive function and dementia. *JAMA, 279*(9), 688–695.

7

THE EFFECTS OF CANNABIS USE AMONG OLDER ADULTS

Alison C. Burggren

INTRODUCTION

The use of marijuana, for both medicinal and non-medicinal purposes, among older adults is increasing, though the exact prevalence is not known. Recent results from a lively debate on medicinal marijuana published in the *New England Journal of Medicine* (*NEJM*) clearly demonstrate a dramatic shift in public perception of medical marijuana use and underscore an advancing divide between medical experts and the public about marijuana use, especially as it pertains to older adults, who are more likely to deal with pain management issues than younger people. In an interactive feature of controversial topics, readers were asked whether a 68-year-old woman with metastatic breast cancer should be prescribed medical marijuana (Bostwick, Reisfield, & DuPont, 2013). The first medical expert invited to comment on the issue provided a lukewarm argument regarding the issue, advocating use of marijuana "only when conservative options have failed for fully informed patients treated in

ongoing therapeutic relationships." The second expert concluded that "there is little scientific basis" for physicians to endorse smoked marijuana as medical therapy. However, the truly surprising outcome of the *NEJM* online poll of journal readers was that 76% voted in favor of the use of marijuana for medicinal purposes (Adler & Colbert, 2013). Additionally, responses were quite varied across state lines within the United States, with only 1% of respondents in Utah supporting medical marijuana, while 96% of Pennsylvania respondents were in support of the use of medicinal marijuana. Across both sides of the argument, reported the authors of the poll, "individual comments were as polarized as the experts' opinions." With the topic generating such heated discussions among medical experts as well as the general public, undoubtedly there is a pressing need for more research to move the discussion toward a stronger basis of evidence.

Marijuana (*Cannabis sativa*) has been used medically for centuries. Medical records dating as far back as 2727 B.C. by Pen-ts'ao Ching, the oldest known pharmacopoeia, describe the medicinal properties of cannabis as well as the psychiatric side effects (Murray, Morrison, Henquet, & Di Forti, 2007). For centuries, cannabis was perceived to possess both toxic as well as beneficial properties. However, over the course of the twentieth century, cannabis gradually lost its status as a useful remedy, and by the 1990s many believed that cannabis did not cause long-term harm to health ([Editorial], 1995). For many people, the use of cannabis became as normalized as the use of alcohol, nicotine, or tobacco, and to this day, some support the pro-legalization argument with this mantra: "If alcohol is legal, marijuana should be too."

However, the past 20 years have seen a rapid growth of research in this area, and many findings point to cannabis as having potential as both a potent medicine and a dangerous drug. Earlier this year, the first report of two adolescent deaths attributed to marijuana was published (Hartung, Kauferstein, Ritz-Timme, & Daldrup, 2014). While the majority of research in this area focuses on adolescent or young adult usage, cannabis use among older adults is increasing at a similar rate to use in other age groups, though it still falls far below usage levels of young adults (SAMHSA, US Department of Health and Human Services, 2012).

For the purposes of this chapter, an older adult is defined as a person aged 60 or older, though any age cutoff is simply arbitrary because age-related changes vary widely across individuals and even within a single person from body system to body system. It is possible, for example, for an 80-year-old to have better cardiovascular health than a 50-year-old, but in an individual 70-year-old, one might have "the spine of an 80-year-old, a heart typical of a 60-year-old, and a central nervous system equal in functioning to an average 60-year-old" (Altpeter, Schmall, Rakowski, Swift, & Campbell, 1994).

With respect to cannabis use, this makes it nearly impossible to extrapolate from clinical trials in younger subjects what the body's reactions might be to cannabis use in older subjects. Because of the age-related physiological changes that are found in this vulnerable population, as well as the high prevalence of polypharmacy use to manage these changes, results from investigations of young adults cannot be extrapolated to frail older adults. Unfortunately, none of the clinical trials that have investigated the therapeutic benefits of cannabis, or research studies of the effects of cannabis use, has aimed its recruitment at older adults. Additionally,

if clinical trials enrolled any subject from this age group (over 60 years old), they did not perform separate analysis that investigated age-related effects in such individuals.

The lack of evidenced-based medicine regarding the safety and efficacy of cannabis and cannabinoids in older adults warrants further research, especially adequately powered randomized controlled studies in order to assess the risk–benefit ratio in older individuals. There is a pressing need for current research to isolate the benefits of cannabinoids for medicinal purposes as well as establish dosage levels, formulations, and appropriate delivery mechanisms, and to determine whether the rapidly mounting reported health risks from continued cannabis use warrant its medicinal use. Until these studies are performed, individual evaluation of the benefits and risks must be weighed for each individual patient, and caution must be used in prescribing something for medicinal purposes that has not been fully investigated in older adults. Here, evidence is reviewed that focuses on known rationales for medical use among older persons, how age-related physiological changes *might* alter the effect of cannabis, and the future of cannabis use, for medicinal and non-medicinal purposes, in our growing population of older adults.

USE AMONG THE ELDERLY

Although cannabis use for recreational purposes is increasing among all demographics, including older adults, cannabis use among elderly patients remains mainly for therapeutic purposes, especially pain management (see Table 7.1). Recreational usage is primarily for the purposes of experiencing the euphoria that cannabis produces. As an analgesic, however, cannabinoids have been documented to have powerful analgesic purposes. Unfortunately, the distinction between medical and recreational cannabis use has become blurred over the past decade as legislative changes have advanced in various states within the United States. However, because cannabis use can have numerous adverse psychological effects (acute psychosis and paranoia, psychomotor and cognitive impairments, anxiety and panic attacks), widespread therapeutic usage may be limited. In a review article that detailed findings from nine randomized, controlled trials of cannabis use of pain management, all studies reported adverse effects while using cannabis for pain management, and the authors concluded that

Table 7.1.   Aggregation of the Various Hypotheses That Need to Be Tested with Well-Designed Studies of How Cannabis Use May Affect Older People

	HYPOTHESIS	TIME FRAME FOR RESULTS
1	The effects of adolescent cannabis use in the brain may interact with aging-related factors and result in a different endophenotype late in life compared to persons who have never used cannabis.	Retrospective method: A few years to gather and analyze neuroimaging and congitive assessments Prospective method: 40–50 years (possible alternative is to gain access to cognitive measures or any other metrics relevant to neurological integrity acquired before onset of use)
2	The effects of cannabis on brain morphology and/or cognition depend on age of onset.	A few years to a few decades. (Studies investigating this hypothesis are already yielding the initial results from age-related studies of the effects of cannabis use.)
3	Initiating recreational use of cannabis late in life similarly affects hippocampal mophology and cognitive performance compared to elderly subejcts who have been abstinent for decades, but did use cannabis as adolescents.	Unlikely to be investigated in the near future, but this design should be investigated once more longitudinal data are available from prospective studies.
4	Late-life recreational cannabis use does not affect brain morphology or impair cognitive performance after the acute effects of the drug have washed out.	A few years to recruit a population of older, current cannabis users
5	Cannabis used solely for medicinal purposes has greater beneficial effects compared to recreational use, especially in older persons, who have higher rates of cancer, pain management problems, nausea, and sleep disturbance.	A few years to recruit patient populations who have been prescribed marijuana
6	THC use actively inhibits the enzyme acetylcholinesterase and prevents aggregation of the amyloid beta peptide.	At least 5 years to recruit a prodromal population of cannabis users and follow these subjects longitudinally

Note that the majority of these hypotheses are not currently being tested, but rapidly advancing data available from the limited number of cannabis studies that are being conducted, as well as the growing number of cannabis users in every age demographic, strongly suggest that these hypotheses need to be tested in the near future.

cannabinoids were no more effective than codeine for controlling pain (Campbell et al., 2001).

Aging is, regrettably, known to be associated with increased prevalence of multiple chronic diseases, many of which result in the patient taking multiple drugs; according to one survey of 2590 participants in the contiguous United States, 50% took at least one prescription drug, and 57% of female Medicare recipients over 65 reported taking at least five medications (Kaufman, Kelly, Rosenberg, Anderson, & Mitchell, 2002). Because various definitions, models, and classifications of drug use do not account for age-related physiological and social changes, most simply do not apply to older adults. Optimizing recommendations and treatment in the face of multiple medications and comorbid conditions is a challenging task, especially given that the typical guidelines are not usually based on guidelines and practices specific to elderly subjects.

Additionally, elderly patients may frequently be excluded from clinical trials because of comorbid conditions (Van Spall, Toren, Kiss, & Fowler, 2007) and, therefore, evidence used to guide practice may not be generalizable to this unique population. Although there is some evidence that cannabinoids may be safe and modestly effective in neuropathic pain such as fibromyalgia and rheumatoid arthritis (Lynch & Campbell, 2011), there remains no reported randomized, clinical trial studies that have investigated the use of cannabinoids specifically in elderly subjects for pain management, thus making it difficult to generalize findings to this unique population. Any application of guidelines drawn from a dissimilar population would be problematic because the guidelines do not take into account the presence of comorbid conditions that are more frequent in older adults. Let us first consider the evidence gleaned from studies of younger cannabis users before considering the potential differential effect of cannabis in older adults.

THE ENDOCANNABINOID SYSTEM

For over a century, numerous attempts were made to isolate the active constituent in marijuana, unsuccessfully (Mechoulam & Hanus, 2000) There are more than 60 cannabis constituents, with closely related structures and physical properties, making the process of separating them difficult. In the mid-1960s, the major psychoactive component in cannabis Delta-9-tetrahydrocannabinol (THC), was finally isolated and subsequently synthesized by Raphael Mechoulam and colleagues (Gaoni & Mechoulam, 1964). The euphoric effects experienced by the cannabis user are primarily the results of stimulation of the cannabinoid (CB1) receptor (Huestis et al., 2001), first identified in 1988 (Devane, Dysarz, Johnson, Melvin, & Howlett, 1988) and cloned in 1990 (Matsuda, Lolait, Brownstein, Young, & Bonner, 1990). This receptor is the most common G-protein coupled receptor in the brain (Di Marzo, Bifulco, & De Petrocellis, 2004) with particularly high expression levels in several brain areas, including the hippocampus, cerebellum, basal ganglia, and neocortex (Egertová & Elphick, 2000). These areas are consistent with the regions involved in the typical cognitive and motor effects of THC administration (Bhattacharyya, Crippa, Martin-Santos, Winton-Brown, & Fusar-Poli, 2009). CB1 expression in peripheral nerve fibers, the dorsal root ganglion, the spinal dorsal horn, and the periaqueductal gray matter is most likely the source of the analgesic properties of THC (Ahluwalia, Urban, Capogna, Bevan, & Nagy, 2000; Calignano, La Rana, Giuffrida, & Piomelli, 1998; Hohmann et al., 2005). Typically, cannabis is ingested by smoking, as this method is the most efficient way to achieve the desired psychoactive effect (Iversen, 2007).

The discovery of the CB1 receptors responsible for the effects of THC prompted a search for the endogenous agonists that bind to them. These endocannabinoids act as retrograde messengers to presynaptically inhibit the release of neurotransmitters (Elphick & Egertová, 2001). Endocannabinoids are synthesized primarily in dendrites, and the CB1 receptors that respond to them have been found on the terminals of neighboring GABA-releasing and glutamatergic neurons (Eggan & Lewis, 2007; Yoshida et al., 2006). It is primarily output neurons, such as pyramidal neurons in the hippocampus and dopaminergic neurons in the midbrain, that are responsible for releasing the endocannabinoids and modulating the excitatory inputs of these CNS neurons (Freund, Katona, & Piomelli, 2003). These endogenous transmitters, therefore, play a crucial role in mediating and modulating synaptic activity. The endocannabinoid-mediated plasticity is expressed as reducing the possibility of neurotransmitter release. Naturally occurring endocannabinoids mediate synaptic plasticity, including cerebellar-dependent motor learning (Kishimoto & Kano, 2006), the extension of aversive memories in the amygdala (Marsicano et al., 2002), memory encoding via synapses in hippocampal cornu ammonis (CA) fields, reducing the threshold necessary to achieve long-term potentiation (LTP) in excitatory synapses adjacent to pyramidal neurons (Carlson, Wang, & Alger, 2002; Chevaleyre & Castillo, 2003, 2004; Zhu & Lovinger, 2007). These endocannabinoids, therefore, add another later of modulation of glutamate synapses to that which is provided by conventional transmitters such as serotonin or dopamine or serotonin (Bailey, Giustetto, Huang, Hawkins, & Kandel, 2000).

NEUROPROTECTIVE ACTIVITY OF CB1 RECEPTORS

The endogenous counterpart of cannabinoids, endocannabionoids, has long been reported to promote neuroprotection, but the mechanism is only beginning to be fully investigated. Findings from Chiarlone et al. (2014) reported on a unique and well-defined population of CA1 receptors on glutamatergic terminals. The authors use pharmacological and pharmacogenic tools to show that the CB1 receptors play an indispensable role in the neuroprotective activity of endocannabinoids and protect against excitotoxic damage in the mouse brain (Chiarlone et al., 2014), suggesting a target for future neuroprotective therapeutic strategies and reconceptualizing how the CB1 receptor evokes neuroprotection.

However, the use of cannabis-based medicines has existed for centuries. More recent uses include the licensing of THC in the 1980s as Dronabinol for the treatment of appetite stimulation and suppression of nausea in chemotherapy and AIDS patients. In addition to the value of cannabis in treating these patients, it has also been used to provide symptomatic relief of spasticity, pain, and sleep disturbance in patients with multiple sclerosis (Collin, Davies, Mutiboko, & Ratcliffe, 2007; Rog, Nurmikko, Friede, & Young, 2005; Zajicek et al., 2003) and has been approved in Canada for pain management in cancer patients. Other promising areas of research for the use of cannabis-based medicines include the management of Tourette's syndrome and glaucoma, as well as in the treatment of head injuries or inflammatory disorders (Mackie, 2006; Pacher, Bátkai, & Kunos, 2006).

It is likely that as we continue with advancing our understanding of the endocannabinoid system, future cannabis-based medicines will be developed. While one would hope that attitudes toward cannabis-based medicines would not be influenced by recreational cannabis use, especially when so many of the ailments mentioned earlier (cancer, pain, and sleep disturbance, to name a few) are more common among older adults who are less likely to use cannabis recreationally (US Department of Health and Human Services, 2012). It remains to be seen, however, how effective future efforts will be at distinguishing between useful cannabis-based medicines that should be developed and licensed for particular ailments and confusing their utility with recreational use.

ACUTE EFFECTS OF CANNABIS

In contrast to the subtle effects of endocannabinoids in mediating synaptic plasticity and neurotransmission, the acute administration of exogenous cannabinoids markedly disrupts neuronal signaling and circuit dynamics (Murray et al., 2007). The intoxicant effects of the active ingredient in cannabis, Δ9-tetrahydrocannabinol (THC), inhibits the long-term potentiation of CA3–CA1 synapses by activating CB1 receptors on glutamatergic terminals, inhibiting Ca2+ influx and suppressing glutamate release (Chevaleyre, Takahashi, & Castillo, 2006; Hampson & Deadwyler, 1999). By these findings, this mechanism appears to underlie the detrimental effect of THC on hippocampus-dependent learning and memory.

With respect to the cognitive effects of cannabis use, results show that the CB1 receptors located within the hippocampus play a necessary role in the memory-disruptive effects of cannabis (Wise, Thorpe, & Lichtman, 2009). These intoxicant effects of THC are mediated by CB1 cannabinoid receptors (Huestis et al., 2001), which are found primarily in the hippocampus, prefrontal cortex, anterior cingulate cortex, striatum, amygdala, and cerebellum (Burns et al., 2007). There is considerable evidence that cannabinoids impair hippocampal-dependent learning and memory processes, including spatial learning and context-dependent memory tasks (Ashtari et al., 2011; Yücel et al., 2010). In vitro experiments suggest that activation of CB1 receptors in the hippocampus reduces neurotransmitter release below the levels required to trigger long-term changes in synaptic strength in the hippocampus (Sullivan, 2000). These animal experiments support the connection between cannabinoid-mediated memory deficits and functional impairment within the hippocampus. In humans, cannabis use has been documented to acutely affect neuropsychological performance in the following domains: short-term memory, attention, and executive function (Lundqvist, 2010; O'Leary et al., 2002; Pope, Gruber, & Yurgelun-Todd, 1995; Schwartz, Gruenewald, Klitzner, & Fedio, 1989). However, findings also indicate that sustained cannabis use may alter brain structure and cognition, especially in regions such as the prefrontal cortex and medial temporal lobe, which are important for executive function and memory processes (Lyketsos, Garrett, Liang, & Anthony, 1999; van Holst & Schilt, 2011).

LONG-TERM EFFECTS OF EARLY LIFE USE

While some studies report little evidence for long-term impairments in cognitive function after a period of abstinence (Cousijn et al., 2011; Leslie Iversen, 2003), others have documented effects on learning (Gonzalez, Carey, & Grant, 2002; Pope, Gruber, Hudson, Huestis, & Yurgelun-Todd, 2001; Solowij, Stephens, Roffman, & Babor, 2002), intelligence (Fried, Watkinson, James, & Gray, 2002), memory (Riedel & Davies, 2005; Rubino et al., 2009; Yücel et al., 2010), attention (Ehrenreich et al., 1999; Schmetzer, 2000; Solowij, Michie, & Fox, 1995), motor function (Pillay et al., 2008), and executive function (Crean, Crane, & Mason, 2011; Pope & Yurgelun-Todd, 1996; Whitlow et al., 2004). In addition, psychopathological symptoms, including anxiety and anhedonia (Dorard, Berthoz, Phan, Corcos, & Bungener, 2008), psychotic symptoms (Moore et al., 2007; Semple, McIntosh, & Lawrie, 2005; Yücel et al., 2008), and depression (Moore et al., 2007) have also been linked to long-term cannabis use. Differences in dose, frequency, and duration (Gonzalez et al., 2002; Miller & Branconnier, 1983; Rubino et al., 2009; Sullivan, 2000; Yücel et al., 2010), as well as age of initiation of regular cannabis use (Ashtari et al., 2011; Jager & Ramsey, 2008; Pope et al., 2001), also affect the severity of these impairments.

Several more recent studies have been published documenting morphological brain change and alterations to IQ after sustained periods of heavy cannabis use in younger subjects. Lorenzetti et al. (2014) published results from a very small population (*n* = 15 heavy cannabis users and 16 control subjects) documenting reduced hippocampal and amygdalar volumes in subjects approximately 40 years old with 20 years of cannabis use in their past. Similarly, in 2012, Meier and colleagues published a report using retrospective data analysis in the Dunedin cohort of over 1000 subject; IQ decline was significant and persistent in those subjects who were tested before the onset of cannabis use and again at age 38 (Meier et al., 2012). These effects were more concentrated for adolescent-onset users and, perhaps most important, did *not* reverse upon cessation of use. Several other recent MRI studies (Yücel & Lubman, 2007) have also suggested an adverse effect of heavy cannabis use on adolescent brain development, particularly within the hippocampus

(Ashtari et al., 2011). One study by Yucel and colleagues of heavy cannabis users found bilaterally reduced hippocampal and amygdala volumes and provide some of the earliest imaging evidence that heavy cannabis use across protracted periods exerts harmful effects on brain tissue (Yücel et al., 2008).

LATE-LIFE EFFECTS: PERSISTENT EFFECTS AND DIFFERENCES IN OLDER ADULTS

The dense concentration of CB1 receptors in the hippocampus (Burns et al., 2007), the main structure for the encoding of new memories as well as the primary site of age-related changes in memory impairment and dementia (Hultsch, Hertzog, Small, McDonald-Miszczak, & Dixon, 1992; Johansson, Zarit, & Berg, 1992), suggests a potential interaction between heavy cannabis use and age-related changes in hippocampal morphology and cognition. The pattern of memory deficits seen following cannabis use is similar to that seen in patients with hippocampal dysfunction from disorders such as herpes simplex encephalitis, Korsakoff's syndrome, and Alzheimer's disease (Braak & Braak, 1991; Riedel & Davies, 2005; Yücel et al., 2010).

Advancing age is one of the primary risk factors for cognitive decline, especially in memory performance (Gély-Nargeot, Mure, Guérin-Langlois, Martin, & Descours, 1983; Luszcz & Bryan, 1999). As discussed earlier, because CB1 receptors are densely located within the hippocampus and mediate the effect of THC in this region (Cousijn et al., 2011), the resultant morphological effects of cannabis may interact with, and synergistically exacerbate, changes within the hippocampus during aging (Braak & Braak, 1996). The hippocampus is the first and, typically, most severely affected structure in age-related changes to brain morphology (Donix et al., 2010; Pruessner, Collins, Pruessner, & Evans, 2001), as well as Alzheimer's disease, whose primary risk factor is advancing age (Troncoso, Sukhov, Kawas, & Koliatsos, 1996; West, 1993). It is conceivable, therefore, that heavy cannabis use over time will have a compounding effect on age-related hippocampal and cognitive changes, particularly with respect to the formation of new memories.

Recent studies suggest that THC actively and competitively inhibits the enzyme acetylcholinesterase

(AChE) and prevents aggregation of the amyloid beta-peptide (Eubanks et al., 2006), a key pathological marker for Alzheimer's disease. However, whether or how this pathological marker is linked to the onset of Alzheimer's disease remains one of the most contested issues in the field to this day (Pimplikar, 2009). Additionally, the long-term effects of heavy cannabis use in the aging brain have, to our knowledge, never been studied. Also, because the still-developing adolescent brain differs anatomically and neurochemically from the adult brain (Chan, Hinds, Impey, & Storm, 1998; Pisanu, Acquas, Fenu, & Di Chiara, 2006) we anticipate the effects of cannabis on the brain to be greater in people who initiated use younger in life, when the brain is more susceptible to drug-mediated neuronal plasticity (Kreitzer, 2005; Pertwee, 2008). Overall, because declining cognition and subsequent dementia are best understood as the cumulative effects on the brain from diseases (e.g., cerebrovascular disease or Alzheimer's disease) and environmental factors such as drug use, against the background of age-related cognitive decline (DeCarlo, Tuokko, Williams, Dixon, & MacDonald, 2014), it is crucial to understand the long-term effects of cannabis use given the high usage rates among adolescents as well as the rapidly growing aging population.

Unfortunately, at this time, there are no available data on the relationship between cannabis use and advancing age on hippocampal morphology or cognitive decline in late life. People who used cannabis in the 1960s and 1970s are now entering a period of great risk for age-related cognitive decline and brain changes. Therefore, it is crucial to examine these questions now, in the early stages of late-life decline, with the goal of identifying whether age-related brain changes are greater in persons who report heavy cannabis use. Those people who were adolescents through the turbulent decades of the 1960s and 1970s, when cannabis use doubled (Robinson, 2002), are now entering late life, a period of high risk for memory and cognitive deficits related to aging (Grimby & Berg, 1995; Hultsch et al., 1992; Johansson et al., 1992; Schaie, 1994). However, there is little data with regard to the neurobiological and cognitive effects of cannabis use in older adults approaching late life. Such data might help to identify persons more likely to decline than their age-matched counterparts and may suggest early intervention in therapies aimed at slowing cognitive decline in late life.

DISCLOSURE STATEMENT

Dr. Burggren has no conflicts to disclose. She is funded by NIDA only. Grant Support: National Institute of Drug Abuse, NIH K01DA034728.

REFERENCES

Adler, J. N., & Colbert, J. A. (2013). Clinical decisions: medicinal use of marijuana—polling results. *New Engl J Med*, 368(22), e30. doi: 10.1056/NEJMclde1305159

Ahluwalia, J., Urban, L., Capogna, M., Bevan, S., & Nagy, I. (2000). Cannabinoid 1 receptors are expressed in nociceptive primary sensory neurons. *Neuroscience*, 100(4), 685–688. Retrieved from http://www.ncbi.nlm.nih.gov/pubmed/11036202

Altpeter, M., Schmall, V., Rakowski, W., Swift, R., & Campbell, J. (1994). *Alcohol and drug problems in the elderly: Instructor's guide [Project ADEPT curriculum for primary care physician training]*. Providence, RI.

Ashtari, M., Avants, B., Cyckowski, L., Cervellione, K. L., Roofeh, D., Cook, P., . . . Kumra, S. (2011). Medial temporal structures and memory functions in adolescents with heavy cannabis use. *J Psychiatr Res*, 45(8), 1055–1066. doi:10.1016/j.jpsychires.2011.01.004

Bailey, C. H., Giustetto, M., Huang, Y. Y., Hawkins, R. D., & Kandel, E. R. (2000). Is heterosynaptic modulation essential for stabilizing Hebbian plasticity and memory? *Nature Rev Neurosci*, 1(1), 11–20. doi:10.1038/35036191

Bhattacharyya, S., Crippa, J. A., Martin-Santos, R., Winton-Brown, T., & Fusar-Poli, P. (2009). Imaging the neural effects of cannabinoids: current status and future opportunities for psychopharmacology. *Curr Pharmaceut Design*, 15(22), 2603–2614. Retrieved from http://www.ncbi.nlm.nih.gov/pubmed/19689331

Bostwick, J. M., Reisfield, G. M., & DuPont, R. L. (2013). Clinical decisions: medicinal use of marijuana. *New Engl J Med*, 368(9), 866–868. doi: 10.1056/NEJMclde1300970

Braak, H., & Braak, E. (1991). Neuropathological stageing of Alzheimer-related changes. *Acta Neuropathol (Berl)*, 82(4), 239–259. Retrieved from http://www.ncbi.nlm.nih.gov/entrez/query.fcgi?cmd=Retrieve&db=PubMed&dopt=Citation&list_uids=1759558

Braak, H., & Braak, E. (1996). Evolution of the neuropathology of Alzheimer's disease. *Acta Neurol Scand Suppl*, 165, 3–12. Retrieved from http://www.ncbi.nlm.nih.gov/entrez/query.fcgi

?cmd=Retrieve&db=PubMed&dopt=Citation&l
ist_uids=8740983

Burns, H. D., Van Laere, K., Sanabria-Bohórquez, S.,
Hamill, T. G., Bormans, G., Eng, W., . . . Hargreaves,
R. J. (2007). [18F]MK-9470, a positron emission
tomography (PET) tracer for in vivo human PET
brain imaging of the cannabinoid-1 receptor.
Proc Natl Acad Sci USA, 104(23), 9800–9805.
doi: 10.1073/pnas.0703472104

Calignano, A., La Rana, G., Giuffrida, A., &
Piomelli, D. (1998). Control of pain initiation by
endogenous cannabinoids. Nature, 394(6690),
277–281. doi: 10.1038/28393

http://www.pubmedcentral.nih.gov/articlerender.
fcgi?artid=34324&tool=pmcentrez&rende
rtype=abstract" title="Are cannabinoids an
effective and safe treatment option in the
management of pain? A qualitative systematic
review" journalName="BMJ (Clin Res Ed)"
journalIssue="7303" vol="323">Campbell, F. A.,
Tramèr, M. R., Carroll, D., Reynolds, D. J., Moore,
R. A., & McQuay, H. J. (2001). Are cannabinoids
an effective and safe treatment option in the
management of pain? A qualitative systematic
review. BMJ (Clin Res Ed), 323(7303), 13–16.
Retrieved from http://www.pubmedcentral.nih.
gov/articlerender.fcgi?artid=34324&tool=pmcent
rez&rendertype=abstract

Carlson, G., Wang, Y., & Alger, B. E. (2002).
Endocannabinoids facilitate the induction of
LTP in the hippocampus. Nature Neurosci, 5(8),
723–724. doi: 10.1038/nn879

Chan, G. C., Hinds, T. R., Impey, S., & Storm,
D. R. (1998). Hippocampal neurotoxicity of
Delta9-tetrahydrocannabinol. J Neurosci, 18(14),
5322–5332. Retrieved from http://www.ncbi.nlm.
nih.gov/pubmed/9651215

Chevaleyre, V., & Castillo, P. E. (2003).
Heterosynaptic LTD of hippocampal GABAergic
synapses: a novel role of endocannabinoids in
regulating excitability. Neuron, 38(3), 461–472.
Retrieved from http://www.ncbi.nlm.nih.gov/
pubmed/12741992

Chevaleyre, V., & Castillo, P. E. (2004).
Endocannabinoid-mediated metaplasticity in
the hippocampus. Neuron, 43(6), 871–881.
doi: 10.1016/j.neuron.2004.08.036

Chevaleyre, V., Takahashi, K. A., & Castillo, P. E.
(2006). Endocannabinoid-mediated synaptic
plasticity in the CNS. Ann Rev Neurosci, 29, 37–76.
doi: 10.1146/annurev.neuro.29.051605.112834

Chiarlone, A., Bellocchio, L., Blázquez, C., Resel, E.,
Soria-Gómez, E., Cannich, A., . . . Guzmán, M.
(2014). A restricted population of CB1
cannabinoid receptors with neuroprotective

activity. Proc Natl Acad Sci USA, 111(22),
8257–8262. doi: 10.1073/pnas.1400988111

Collin, C., Davies, P., Mutiboko, I. K., & Ratcliffe, S.
(2007). Randomized controlled
trial of cannabis-based medicine in
spasticity caused by multiple sclerosis.
Eur J Neurology, 14(3), 290–296.
doi: 10.1111/j.1468-1331.2006.01639.x

Cousijn, J., Wiers, R. W., Ridderinkhof, K. R., van
den Brink, W., Veltman, D. J., & Goudriaan, A. E.
(2011). Grey matter alterations associated with
cannabis use: results of a VBM study in heavy
cannabis users and healthy controls. NeuroImage.
doi: 10.1016/j.neuroimage.2011.09.046

Crean, R. D., Crane, N. A., & Mason, B. J. (2011).
An evidence based review of acute and long-term
effects of cannabis use on executive cognitive
functions. J Addict Med, 5(1), 1–8. doi: 10.1097/
ADM.0b013e31820c23fa

DeCarlo, C. A., Tuokko, H. A., Williams, D.,
Dixon, R. A., & MacDonald, S. W. S. (2014).
BioAge: toward a multi-determined, mechanistic
account of cognitive aging. Ageing Res Rev, 18C,
95–105. doi: 10.1016/j.arr.2014.09.003

Devane, W. A., Dysarz, F. A., Johnson, M. R., Melvin,
L. S., & Howlett, A. C. (1988). Determination
and characterization of a cannabinoid receptor
in rat brain. Mol Pharmacol, 34(5), 605–613.
Retrieved from http://www.ncbi.nlm.nih.gov/
pubmed/2848184

Di Marzo, V., Bifulco, M., & De Petrocellis, L. (2004).
The endocannabinoid system and its therapeutic
exploitation. Nature Rev Drug Discov, 3(9),
771–784. doi: 10.1038/nrd1495

Donix, M., Burggren, A. C., Suthana, N. A., Siddarth,
P., Ekstrom, A. D., Krupa, A. K., . . . Bookheimer,
S. Y. (2010). Longitudinal changes in medial
temporal cortical thickness in normal subjects with
the APOE-4 polymorphism. NeuroImage, 53(1),
37–43. doi: 10.1016/j.neuroimage.2010.06.009

Dorard, G., Berthoz, S., Phan, O., Corcos, M., &
Bungener, C. (2008). Affect dysregulation
in cannabis abusers: a study in adolescents
and young adults. Eur Child Adolesc
Psychiatry, 17(5), 274–282. doi: 10.1007/
s00787-007-0663-7

[Editorial]. (1995). Deglamorising cannabis. Lancet,
346(8985), 1241. Retrieved from http://www.
ncbi.nlm.nih.gov/pubmed/7475708

Egertová, M., & Elphick, M. R. (2000). Localisation
of cannabinoid receptors in the rat brain using
antibodies to the intracellular C-terminal tail
of CB. J Compar Neurol, 422(2), 159–171.
Retrieved from http://www.ncbi.nlm.nih.gov/
pubmed/10842224

Eggan, S. M., & Lewis, D. A. (2007). Immunocytochemical distribution of the cannabinoid CB1 receptor in the primate neocortex: a regional and laminar analysis. *Cereb Cortex (New York: 1991)*, 17(1), 175–191. doi: 10.1093/cercor/bhj136

Ehrenreich, H., Rinn, T., Kunert, H. J., Moeller, M. R., Poser, W., Schilling, L., . . . Hoehe, M. R. (1999). Specific attentional dysfunction in adults following early start of cannabis use. *Psychopharmacology*, 142(3), 295–301. Retrieved from http://www.ncbi.nlm.nih.gov/pubmed/10208322

Elphick, M. R., & Egertová, M. (2001). The neurobiology and evolution of cannabinoid signalling. *Phil Trans R Soc London B*, 356(1407), 381–408. doi: 10.1098/rstb.2000.0787

Eubanks, L. M., Rogers, C. J., Beuscher, A. E., Koob, G. F., Olson, A. J., Dickerson, T. J., & Janda, K. D. (2006). A molecular link between the active component of marijuana and Alzheimer's disease pathology. *Mol Pharmaceutics*, 3(6), 773–777. doi: 10.1021/mp060066m

Freund, T. F., Katona, I., & Piomelli, D. (2003). Role of endogenous cannabinoids in synaptic signaling. *Physiological Rev*, 83(3), 1017–1066. doi: 10.1152/physrev.00004.2003

Fried, P., Watkinson, B., James, D., & Gray, R. (2002). Current and former marijuana use: preliminary findings of a longitudinal study of effects on IQ in young adults. *CMAJ*, 166(7), 887–891. Retrieved from http://www.pubmedcentral.nih.gov/articlerender.fcgi?artid=100921&tool=pmcentrez&rendertype=abstract

Gaoni, Y., & Mechoulam, R. (1964). Isolation, structure and partial synthesis of an active constituent of hashish. *J Am Chem Soc*, 86, 1646–1047.

Gély-Nargeot, M. C., Mure, C., Guérin-Langlois, C., Martin, K., & Descours, I. (1983). Effects of cognitive aging on memory performances. *Presse Médicale*, 29(15), 849–857. Retrieved from http://www.ncbi.nlm.nih.gov/pubmed/10827794

Gonzalez, R., Carey, C., & Grant, I. (2002). Nonacute (residual) neuropsychological effects of cannabis use: a qualitative analysis and systematic review. *J Clin Pharmacol*, 42(11 Suppl), 48S–57S. Retrieved from http://www.ncbi.nlm.nih.gov/pubmed/12412836

Grimby, A., & Berg, S. (1995). Stressful life events and cognitive functioning in late life. *Aging (Milan, Italy)*, 7(1), 35–39. Retrieved from http://www.ncbi.nlm.nih.gov/pubmed/7599246

Hampson, R. E., & Deadwyler, S. A. (1999). Cannabinoids, hippocampal function and memory. *Life Sciences*, 65(6–7), 715–723.

Retrieved from http://www.ncbi.nlm.nih.gov/pubmed/10462072

Hartung, B., Kauferstein, S., Ritz-Timme, S., & Daldrup, T. (2014). Sudden unexpected death under acute influence of cannabis. *Forensic Sci Int*, 237, e11–13. doi: 10.1016/j.forsciint.2014.02.001

Hohmann, A. G., Suplita, R. L., Bolton, N. M., Neely, M. H., Fegley, D., Mangieri, R., . . . Piomelli, D. (2005). An endocannabinoid mechanism for stress-induced analgesia. *Nature*, 435(7045), 1108–1112. doi: 10.1038/nature03658

Huestis, M. A., Gorelick, D. A., Heishman, S. J., Preston, K. L., Nelson, R. A., Moolchan, E. T., & Frank, R. A. (2001). Blockade of effects of smoked marijuana by the CB1-selective cannabinoid receptor antagonist SR141716. *Arch Gen Psychiatry*, 58(4), 322–328. Retrieved from http://www.ncbi.nlm.nih.gov/pubmed/11296091

Hultsch, D. F., Hertzog, C., Small, B. J., McDonald-Miszczak, L., & Dixon, R. A. (1992). Short-term longitudinal change in cognitive performance in later life. *Psychol Aging*, 7(4), 571–584. Retrieved from http://www.ncbi.nlm.nih.gov/pubmed/1466826

Iversen, L. (2003). Cannabis and the brain. *Brain*, 126(Pt 6), 1252–1270. Retrieved from http://www.ncbi.nlm.nih.gov/pubmed/12764049

Iversen, L. (2007). *The science of marijuana* (2nd ed.). Oxford: Oxford University Press.

Jager, G., & Ramsey, N. F. (2008). Long-term consequences of adolescent cannabis exposure on the development of cognition, brain structure and function: an overview of animal and human research. *Curr Drug Abuse Rev*, 1(2), 114–123. Retrieved from http://www.ncbi.nlm.nih.gov/pubmed/19630711

Johansson, B., Zarit, S. H., & Berg, S. (1992). Changes in cognitive functioning of the oldest old. *J Gerontology*, 47(2), P75–80. Retrieved from http://www.ncbi.nlm.nih.gov/pubmed/1538071

Kaufman, D. W., Kelly, J. P., Rosenberg, L., Anderson, T. E., & Mitchell, A. A. (2002). Recent patterns of medication use in the ambulatory adult population of the United States: the Slone survey. *JAMA*, 287(3), 337–344. Retrieved from http://www.ncbi.nlm.nih.gov/pubmed/11790213

Kishimoto, Y., & Kano, M. (2006). Endogenous cannabinoid signaling through the CB1 receptor is essential for cerebellum-dependent discrete motor learning. *J Neurosci*, 26(34), 8829–8837. doi: 10.1523/JNEUROSCI.1236-06.2006

Kreitzer, A. C. (2005). Neurotransmission: emerging roles of endocannabinoids. *Curr Biol*, 15(14), R549–551. doi: 10.1016/j.cub.2005.07.005

Lorenzetti, V., Solowij, N., Whittle, S., Fornito, A., Lubman, D. I., Pantelis, C., & Yücel, M. (2014). Gross morphological brain changes with chronic, heavy cannabis use. *Brit J Psychiatry, 206*(1), 77–78. doi: 10.1192/bjp.bp.114.151407

Lundqvist, T. (2010). Imaging cognitive deficits in drug abuse. *Curr Topics Behav Neurosci, 3*, 247–275. doi: 10.1007/7854_2009_26

Luszcz, M. A., & Bryan, J. (1999). Toward understanding age-related memory loss in late adulthood. *Gerontology, 45*(1), 2–9. Retrieved from http://www.ncbi.nlm.nih.gov/pubmed/9852374

Lyketsos, C. G., Garrett, E., Liang, K. Y., & Anthony, J. C. (1999). Cannabis use and cognitive decline in persons under 65 years of age. *Am J Epidemiol, 149*(9), 794–800. Retrieved from http://www.ncbi.nlm.nih.gov/pubmed/10221315

Lynch, M. E., & Campbell, F. (2011). Cannabinoids for treatment of chronic non-cancer pain; a systematic review of randomized trials. *Brit J Clin Pharmacol, 72*(5), 735–744. doi: 10.1111/j.1365-2125.2011.03970.x

Mackie, K. (2006). Cannabinoid receptors as therapeutic targets. *Ann Rev Pharmacol Toxicol, 46*, 101–122. doi: 10.1146/annurev.pharmtox.46.120604.141254

Marsicano, G., Wotjak, C. T., Azad, S. C., Bisogno, T., Rammes, G., Cascio, M. G., . . . Lutz, B. (2002). The endogenous cannabinoid system controls extinction of aversive memories. *Nature, 418*(6897), 530–534. doi: 10.1038/nature00839

Matsuda, L. A., Lolait, S. J., Brownstein, M. J., Young, A. C., & Bonner, T. I. (1990). Structure of a cannabinoid receptor and functional expression of the cloned cDNA. *Nature, 346*(6284), 561–564. doi: 10.1038/346561a0

Mechoulam, R., & Hanus, L. (2000). A historical overview of chemical research on cannabinoids. *Chem Physics Lipids, 108*(1–2), 1–13. Retrieved from http://www.ncbi.nlm.nih.gov/pubmed/11106779

Meier, M. H., Caspi, A., Ambler, A., Harrington, H., Houts, R., Keefe, R. S. E., . . . Moffitt, T. E. (2012). PNAS Plus: persistent cannabis users show neuropsychological decline from childhood to midlife. *Proc Natl Acad Sci, 109*(40), E2657–E2664. 1206820109–. Retrieved from http://www.pnas.org/cgi/content/abstract/1206820109v1

Miller, L. L., & Branconnier, R. J. (1983). Cannabis: effects on memory and the cholinergic limbic system. *Psychol Bull, 93*(3), 441–456. Retrieved from http://www.ncbi.nlm.nih.gov/pubmed/6306710

Moore, T. H. M., Zammit, S., Lingford-Hughes, A., Barnes, T. R. E., Jones, P. B., Burke, M., & Lewis, G. (2007). Cannabis use and risk of psychotic or affective mental health outcomes: a systematic review. *Lancet, 370*(9584), 319–328. doi: 10.1016/S0140-6736(07)61162-3

Murray, R. M., Morrison, P. D., Henquet, C., & Di Forti, M. (2007). Cannabis, the mind and society: the hash realities. *Nature Rev Neurosci, 8*(11), 885–895. doi: 10.1038/nrn2253

O'Leary, D. S., Block, R. I., Koeppel, J. A., Flaum, M., Schultz, S. K., Andreasen, N. C., . . . Hichwa, R. D. (2002). Effects of smoking marijuana on brain perfusion and cognition. *Neuropsychopharmacology, 26*(6), 802–816. doi: 10.1016/S0893-133X(01)00425-0

Pacher, P., Bátkai, S., & Kunos, G. (2006). The endocannabinoid system as an emerging target of pharmacotherapy. *Pharmacol Rev, 58*(3), 389–462. doi: 10.1124/pr.58.3.2

Pertwee, R. G. (2008). The diverse CB1 and CB2 receptor pharmacology of three plant cannabinoids: delta9-tetrahydrocannabinol, cannabidiol and delta9-tetrahydrocannabivarin. *Brit J Pharmacol, 153*(2), 199–215. doi: 10.1038/sj.bjp.0707442

Pillay, S. S., Rogowska, J., Kanayama, G., Gruber, S., Simpson, N., Pope, H. G., & Yurgelun-Todd, D. A. (2008). Cannabis and motor function: fMRI changes following 28 days of discontinuation. *Exper Clin Psychopharmacol, 16*(1), 22–32. doi: 10.1037/1064-1297.16.1.22

Pimplikar, S. W. (2009). Reassessing the amyloid cascade hypothesis of Alzheimer's disease. *Int J Biochem Cell Biol, 41*(6), 1261–1268. doi: 10.1016/j.biocel.2008.12.015

Pisanu, A., Acquas, E., Fenu, S., & Di Chiara, G. (2006). Modulation of Delta(9)-THC-induced increase of cortical and hippocampal acetylcholine release by micro opioid and D(1) dopamine receptors. *Neuropharmacology, 50*(6), 661–670. doi:10.1016/j.neuropharm.2005.11.023

Pope, H. G., Gruber, A. J., Hudson, J. I., Huestis, M. A., & Yurgelun-Todd, D. (2001). Neuropsychological performance in long-term cannabis users. *Arch Gen Psychiatry, 58*(10), 909–915. Retrieved from http://www.ncbi.nlm.nih.gov/pubmed/11576028

Pope, H. G., Gruber, A. J., & Yurgelun-Todd, D. (1995). The residual neuropsychological effects of cannabis: the current status of research. *Drug Alcohol Depend, 38*(1), 25–34. Retrieved from http://www.ncbi.nlm.nih.gov/pubmed/7648994

Pope, H. G., & Yurgelun-Todd, D. (1996). The residual cognitive effects of heavy marijuana use in college students. *JAMA, 275*(7), 521–527. Retrieved from http://www.ncbi.nlm.nih.gov/pubmed/8606472

Pruessner, J. C., Collins, D. L., Pruessner, M., & Evans, A. C. (2001). Age and gender predict volume decline in the anterior and posterior hippocampus in early adulthood. *J Neurosci, 21*(1), 194–200. Retrieved from http://www.ncbi.nlm.nih.gov/entrez/query.fcgi?cmd=Retrieve&db=PubMed&dopt=Citation&list_uids=11150336

Riedel, G., & Davies, S. N. (2005). Cannabinoid function in learning, memory and plasticity. *Handbook of Experimental Pharmacology*, (168), 445–477. Retrieved from http://www.ncbi.nlm.nih.gov/pubmed/16596784

Robinson, J. (2002). Decades of drug use: data from the '60s and '70s.

Rog, D. J., Nurmikko, T. J., Friede, T., & Young, C. A. (2005). Randomized, controlled trial of cannabis-based medicine in central pain in multiple sclerosis. *Neurology, 65*(6), 812–819. doi: 10.1212/01.wnl.0000176753.45410.8b

Rubino, T., Realini, N., Braida, D., Alberio, T., Capurro, V., Viganò, D., . . . Parolaro, D. (2009). The depressive phenotype induced in adult female rats by adolescent exposure to THC is associated with cognitive impairment and altered neuroplasticity in the prefrontal cortex. *Neurotoxicity Res, 15*(4), 291–302. doi:10.1007/s12640-009-9031-3

Substance Abuse and Mental Health Services Administration (SAMHSA) (2012). *Results from the 2012 National Survey on Drug Use and Health: summary of national findings.* Retrieved from http://www.samhsa.gov/data/NSDUH/2012SummNatFindDetTables/Index.aspx

Schaie, K. W. (1994). The course of adult intellectual development. *Am Psychol, 49*(4), 304–313. Retrieved from http://www.ncbi.nlm.nih.gov/pubmed/8203802

Schmetzer, A. D. (2000). Book review: Cannabis and cognitive functioning, by Nadia Solowij. *Ann Clin Psychiatry, 12,* 254–257.

Schwartz, R. H., Gruenewald, P. J., Klitzner, M., & Fedio, P. (1989). Short-term memory impairment in cannabis-dependent adolescents. *Am J Dis Child (1960), 143*(10), 1214–1219. Retrieved from http://www.ncbi.nlm.nih.gov/pubmed/2801665

Semple, D. M., McIntosh, A. M., & Lawrie, S. M. (2005). Cannabis as a risk factor for psychosis: systematic review. *J Psychopharmacol (Oxford, England), 19*(2), 187–194. Retrieved from http://www.ncbi.nlm.nih.gov/pubmed/15871146

Solowij, N., Michie, P. T., & Fox, A. M. (1995). Differential impairments of selective attention due to frequency and duration of cannabis use. *Biol Psychiatry, 37*(10), 731–739. doi: 10.1016/0006-3223(94)00178-6

Solowij, N., Stephens, R., Roffman, R. A., & Babor, T. (2002). Does marijuana use cause long-term cognitive deficits? *JAMA, 287*(20), 2653–2654; author reply 2654. Retrieved from http://www.ncbi.nlm.nih.gov/pubmed/12020296

Sullivan, J. M. (2000). Cellular and molecular mechanisms underlying learning and memory impairments produced by cannabinoids. *Learning Memory, 7*(3), 132–139. Retrieved from http://www.ncbi.nlm.nih.gov/pubmed/10837502

Troncoso, J. C., Sukhov, R. R., Kawas, C. H., & Koliatsos, V. E. (1996). In situ labeling of dying cortical neurons in normal aging and in Alzheimer's disease: correlations with senile plaques and disease progression. *J Neuropathol Exper Neurol, 55*(11), 1134–1142. Retrieved from http://www.ncbi.nlm.nih.gov/pubmed/8939196

Van Holst, R. J., & Schilt, T. (2011). Drug-related decrease in neuropsychological functions of abstinent drug users. *Curr Drug Abuse Rev, 4*(1), 42–56. Retrieved from http://www.ncbi.nlm.nih.gov/pubmed/21466500

Van Spall, H. G. C., Toren, A., Kiss, A., & Fowler, R. A. (2007). Eligibility criteria of randomized controlled trials published in high-impact general medical journals: a systematic sampling review. *JAMA, 297*(11), 1233–1240. doi: 10.1001/jama.297.11.1233

West, M. J. (1993). Regionally specific loss of neurons in the aging human hippocampus. *Neurobiol Aging, 14*(4), 287–293. Retrieved from http://www.ncbi.nlm.nih.gov/entrez/query.fcgi?cmd=Retrieve&db=PubMed&dopt=Citation&list_uids=8367010

Whitlow, C. T., Liguori, A., Livengood, L. B., Hart, S. L., Mussat-Whitlow, B. J., Lamborn, C. M., . . . Porrino, L. J. (2004). Long-term heavy marijuana users make costly decisions on a gambling task. *Drug Alcohol Depend, 76*(1), 107–111. doi: 10.1016/j.drugalcdep.2004.04.009

Wise, L. E., Thorpe, A. J., & Lichtman, A. H. (2009). Hippocampal CB(1) receptors mediate the memory impairing effects of Delta(9)-tetrahydrocannabinol. *Neuropsychopharmacology, 34*(9), 2072–2080. doi: 10.1038/npp.2009.31

Yoshida, T., Fukaya, M., Uchigashima, M., Miura, E., Kamiya, H., Kano, M., & Watanabe, M. (2006). Localization of diacylglycerol lipase-alpha around postsynaptic spine suggests close proximity between production site of an endocannabinoid, 2-arachidonoyl-glycerol, and presynaptic cannabinoid CB1 receptor. *J Neurosci, 26*(18), 4740–4751. doi: 10.1523/JNEUROSCI.0054-06.2006

Yücel, M., & Lubman, D. I. (2007). Neurocognitive and neuroimaging evidence of behavioural dysregulation in human drug addiction: implications for diagnosis, treatment and prevention. *Drug Alcohol Rev, 26*(1), 33–39. doi: 10.1080/09595230601036978

Yücel, M., Solowij, N., Respondek, C., Whittle, S., Fornito, A., Pantelis, C., & Lubman, D. I. (2008). Regional brain abnormalities associated with long-term heavy cannabis use. *Arch Gen Psychiatry, 65*(6), 694–701. doi: 10.1001/archpsyc.65.6.694

Yücel, M., Zalesky, A., Takagi, M. J., Bora, E., Fornito, A., Ditchfield, M., . . . Lubman, D. I. (2010). White-matter abnormalities in adolescents with long-term inhalant and cannabis use: a diffusion magnetic resonance imaging study. *J Psychiatry Neurosci, 35*(6), 409–412. doi: 10.1503/jpn.090177

Zajicek, J., Fox, P., Sanders, H., Wright, D., Vickery, J., Nunn, A., & Thompson, A. (2003). Cannabinoids for treatment of spasticity and other symptoms related to multiple sclerosis (CAMS study): multicentre randomised placebo-controlled trial. *Lancet, 362*(9395), 1517–1526. doi: 10.1016/S0140-6736(03)14738-1

Zhu, P. J., & Lovinger, D. M. (2007). Persistent synaptic activity produces long-lasting enhancement of endocannabinoid modulation and alters long-term synaptic plasticity. *J Neurophysiol, 97*(6), 4386–4389. doi: 10.1152/jn.01228.2006

SECTION B

MANIPULATIVE AND BODY-BASED PRACTICES

8

MASSAGE AND MOVEMENT THERAPIES

Claire D. Johnson and Bart N. Green

INTRODUCTION

Body-based practices are included as one of the five major categories of complementary and alternative medicine (CAM) in the classification system from National Center for Complementary and Alternative Medicine (NCCAM). The NCCAM definition states that "manipulative and body-based practices focus primarily on the structures and systems of the body, including the bones and joints, the soft tissues, and the circulatory and lymphatic systems" (Berman & Straus, 2004, 1; Leonard, 2008). One of the primary purposes of body-based therapies is to influence the structure of the body to improve function. Manual therapies have shown preliminary evidence to provide benefit for a wide variety of conditions, ranging from hip or knee osteoarthritis, back pain, neck pain, and headaches (Clar et al., 2014; French, Brennan, White, & Cusack, 2011). In addition to clinical effectiveness, some of the manual therapies may also show cost savings in managing musculoskeletal conditions when compared to other therapies (Tsertsvadze et al., 2014).

One of the most common body-based practices provided by a practitioner is massage. The Centers for Disease Control and Prevention's National Center for Health Statistics evaluated data from the National Health Interview Survey and found that massage was one of the most commonly used CAM therapies. Of the respondents in this survey, 5% reported using massage in 2002, which increased to 8.3% in 2007 (Barnes, Bloom, & Nahin, 2008). Other body-based therapies including movement-focused techniques, such as the Alexander technique and the Feldenkrais method, were not reportedly used as often as massage, reportedly by less than 1% of those surveyed (Barnes et al., 2008). Another study of the Medical Expenditure Panel Survey data analyzed trends in expenditures for ambulatory visits to CAM providers from 2002 to 2008. The study found that massage therapy accounted for 10%–14% of CAM services used by US adults (Davis, Martin, Coulter, & Weeks, 2013).

Some body-based practices are self-applied, but others, such as massage and movement-focused techniques, are delivered by trained and certified practitioners. These interactions between the practitioner and the patient are primarily physical through the power of touch, but may also include educational and psychosocial components. These methods may use touch to move or affect a body part or the whole body; the psychosocial components may include education, reassurance, and psychological support.

Human touch is considered by some to be a powerful component of the healing process (Edvardsson, Sandman, & Rasmussen, 2003; Elkiss & Jerome, 2012; Grzybowski, Stewart, & Weston, 1992; Veer, 1995). Touch can communicate a caring nature or impart healing properties. When a patient presents with a painful condition, the healthcare provider is often taught to touch the area of chief complaint. This helps to reassure the patient and increase satisfaction (Cocksedge, George, Renwick, & Chew-Graham, 2013; Khan, Hanif, Tabassum, Qidwai, & Nanji, 2014; Osmun, Brown, Stewart, & Graham, 2000) and it provides the practitioner with additional information about the patient's current condition. Touching the patient may not only improve the healer–patient relationship, it can give the provider essential information that may lead to more effective treatment. No matter what age a person is, touch is an important component of social interaction; it may be especially beneficial for the well-being of older adults (Bush, 2001).

This chapter describes the body-based therapies of massage and movement-focused therapies. This overview is not meant to be all inclusive or to represent all body-based therapies. For the purposes of this chapter, massage and movement-focused therapies are those delivered by a trained practitioner to a person for therapeutic purposes.

MASSAGE

Massage is the use of touch or force to areas and tissues of a patient for therapeutic purposes. Massage can be aimed at decreasing pain, increasing blood or lymph flow, increasing ranges of motion, or providing perceptive and sensory feedback. Massage is a broad category that includes many touch and body-based therapies. It is important to note that use of the term *massage* may be too general, as this term does not adequately describe the technique being used. One of the challenges of evaluating and reporting on massage therapies is that they are numerous and there is no centrally agreed-upon classification system. One classification system focuses on the phase of treatment (gentle, structural, movement) (Audette & Bailey, 2008), whereas another uses goals of treatment (relaxation, clinical, movement re-education, and energy work) (Sherman, Dixon, Thompson, & Cherkin, 2006). Various cultures and countries have developed their own styles, names, and targets for massage therapies; thus philosophical approaches may vary.

Although some health professions incorporate aspects of massage into their techniques (e.g., physical therapy, chiropractic, traditional Chinese medicine), massage is recognized as a separate practice in the United States and other countries through training, licensure, and credentials, depending upon the jurisdiction. Massage is a popular CAM therapy and is one of the most commonly used practitioner-based therapies (Barnes et al., 2008). According to a study of 2007 National Health Interview Survey data, 8.3% of US adults reported using massage, which was an increase in use compared to 2002 (Barnes et al., 2008). It is estimated that massage therapy contributes 10%–14% of CAM services used by adults (Davis et al., 2013). A systematic review of the literature showed that the range of older adults receiving massage over a 12-month period is between 1.5% and 16.2% (Harris, Cooper, Relton, & Thomas, 2014).

Education and Licensure

While it is estimated there are over 1300 massage therapy schools in the United States (Menard, 2014), the American Massage Therapy Association (AMTA) states that 350 of these are accredited massage therapy institutions, and that entering an accredited program generally requires a high school diploma. There are accrediting institutions that focus on massage, such as the Commission on Massage Therapy Accreditation (COMTA). COMTA is recognized by the US Department of Education as a specialized accrediting agency and maintains a list of accredited programs in massage therapy and bodywork (http://comta.org/). Other accrediting agencies that the AMTA lists include the National Accrediting Commission of Cosmetology Arts and Sciences (NACCAS), the Accrediting Commission of Career Schools and Colleges of Technology

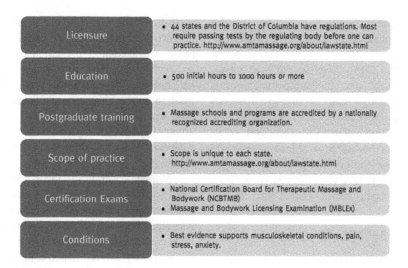

Licensure	• 44 states and the District of Columbia have regulations. Most require passing tests by the regulating body before one can practice. http://www.amtamassage.org/about/lawstate.html
Education	• 500 initial hours to 1000 hours or more
Postgraduate training	• Massage schools and programs are accredited by a nationally recognized accrediting organization.
Scope of practice	• Scope is unique to each state. http://www.amtamassage.org/about/lawstate.html
Certification Exams	• National Certification Board for Therapeutic Massage and Bodywork (NCBTMB) • Massage and Bodywork Licensing Examination (MBLEx)
Conditions	• Best evidence supports musculoskeletal conditions, pain, stress, anxiety.

FIGURE 8.1   Training and licensure for massage therapy.

(ACCSCT), and the Accrediting Bureau of Health Education Schools (ABHES) (Figure 8.1).

Some education programs are short (500 hours), while others may require more hours of training. However, the general trend is that massage therapy education programs continue to grow and improve. The preponderance of massage programs are considered vocational training and culminate in a certificate; however, others are more in depth and may lead to an associate degree (Menard, 2014). Most massage programs provide basic training in anatomy, physiology, kinesiology, safety, ethics, basic first responder emergency care, and classic, deep tissue, and sports massage.

Besides earning a certificate or degree, there may be other requirements to practice. This includes passing the Massage and Bodywork Licensing Exam (MBLEx) or the National Certification Board for Therapeutic Massage and Bodywork (NCBTMB) exam. Once the regional requirements are completed, certification by the National Certification Board for Therapeutic Massage and Bodywork may be required. After the massage therapist has earned the right to practice, many states require that the practitioner complete continuing education units (CEU) to stay informed of current practices.

Regulation for massage practice varies between states in the United States. While most states have a law that regulates massage therapy practice, there are still a few states where massage therapy is not regulated. There is a fair degree of inconsistency in the licensing laws and requirements. For example, Florida requires 500 hours from a board-approved massage therapy school and 24 hours of CEU biennially; Arizona requires 700 hours of schooling and 25 hours of CEU biennially; and New York requires 1000 hours of training and 36 hours of CEU triennially. (http://www.amtamassage.org/regulation/stateRegulations.html). A majority of states require one or more certification exams to practice in that state. The AMTA advocates for licensing massage therapy and has recommended elements for licensing laws (http://www.amtamassage.org/government/gr_overview.html).

Safety and Adverse Effects

Overall, massage is a relatively safe therapy (Grant et al., 2008). However there have been reports in the literature of a variety of unanticipated adverse events (K.E. Grant, 2003). The adverse effects associated with massage and body-based therapies often relate to the type of force used on the patient. Forceful treatments applied to a patient with bleeding tendencies or one who is susceptible to fracture or dislocation might cause injury. Reviews of the literature have suggested that adverse events directly resulting from massage are rare (Ernst, 2003).

A concern about safety is the ability of the practitioner to recognize concerning health signs and symptoms. With the duration and quality of massage education varying widely, there are therefore similar inconsistencies in the knowledge and skills of therapists (Menard, 2014). Also, massage clients may assume that the massage therapist has skills in diagnosis or may not mention areas of concern, or the therapist may miss red flags, resulting in delay of care for serious conditions. Since the risks associated with massage therapy are low (Yin, Gao, Wu, Litscher, & Xu, 2014), there has not been a great deal of study in this area, but one paper has reported that malpractice claims against massage therapists involve milder injury and occur less frequently than claims against medical doctors (Studdert et al., 1998). One method used to reduce unnecessary variation in care is to produce guidelines for practice; thus, the massage profession is working on such standards and guidelines (Grant et al., 2008).

Types of Massage

One of the most commonly known types of massage is classic massage. Classic massage, sometimes referred to as "Swedish" massage, applies firm but gentle force to tissues to increase circulation, decrease pain, and increase relaxation. Classic massage treats the whole body and is not necessarily aimed at targeted tissues like some of the other forms of massage. Terms associated with this type of massage include *effleurage* (stroking), *petrissage* (kneading), *tapotement* (percussion), and *friction* (rubbing) (Ernst, 2003; Sherman, et al., 2006).

There are many types of massage. Each massage therapist will have his or her own style and set of techniques that he or she was trained to use. Some massage therapists are trained in multiple techniques and may sometimes mix their therapies depending upon the needs of the client. While it is impossible to list them all, a brief overview of a range of popular massage techniques are listed here.

- *Acupressure* aims pressure at acupuncture points. This technique hypothetically stimulates the flow of energy through acupuncture meridians. A preliminary study suggests that ear acupressure may be helpful in reducing back pain (Yeh et al., 2014).
- *Craniosacral therapy* applies light touch to the head and sacrum. The hypothesis is that touch will help to restore optimal cerebrospinal fluid flow (Gehret, 2010).
- *Deep-tissue massage* aims to reduce pain and inflammation and rehabilitate injured tissue by focusing on the deep muscles and fascia. Studies have shown that deep-tissue massage may be effective for low back pain (Majchrzycki, Kocur, & Kotwicki, 2014) and improving blood pressure and heart rate (Kaye et al., 2008).

- *Myofascial release technique* directs force into dysfunctional muscle and fascial tissues to reduce restricted motion. Preliminary studies have shown that this type of massage may be helpful with fibromyalgia, chronic low back pain, tension headache, plantar heel pain, and lateral epicondylitis (Ajimsha, 2011; Ajimsha, Binsu, & Chithra, 2014; Ajimsha, Chithra, & Thulasyammal, 2012; Ajimsha, Daniel, & Chithra, 2014; Liptan, Mist, Wright, Arzt, & Jones, 2013).
- *Neuromuscular therapy* focuses pressure on soft tissue with the aim to balance the central nervous system and the musculoskeletal system. A preliminary study suggests that this type of treatment may assist motor symptoms in those with Parkinson's disease (Craig, Svircev, Haber, & Juncos, 2006).
- *Nimmo* technique is a myofascial technique focusing on trigger points and restoring motion and function (Cohen & Gibbons, 1998). Nimmo technique has been shown to improve muscle tone and to reduce pain and disability (Koo, Cohen, & Zheng, 2012).
- *Reflexology* targets pressure at areas of the feet that are hypothesized to correspond with health in other areas of the body (Gehret, 2010).
- Shiatsu applies pressure points along the energy meridians (Gehret, 2010). The goal of this Japanese style of massage is to balance *qi* (energy) and restore function.
- *Sports massage* is applied before athletic events to increase circulation and flexibility. Post-event, it is used to reduce inflammation and rehabilitate any injuries that may have occurred (Gehret, 2010).
- *Thai massage* involves deep, rhythmic pressure and stretching of the body into yoga-like poses. A preliminary study showed that Thai massage, in addition to other therapies, was helpful for people with knee osteoarthritis (Chiranthanut, Hanprasertpong, & Teekachunhatean, 2014).
- *Trigger point therapy* focuses on tender nodules and tight bands in muscles. These are focused areas of dysfunction to which pressure is applied. The aim is to reduce pain and restore function (Travell & Simons, 1983). Often, trigger point therapy is included in deep and sports massage therapy practices.
- *Tui na* is a type of Chinese massage therapy that uses various deep-tissue and focused techniques to promote blood circulation, relaxation, and *qi* (energy) movement (Yang, Zhao, & Wang, 2014).

Outcomes of Massage Therapy

There are many purported benefits of massage. Some people use massage to reduce stress and relieve muscle tension and there may also be benefits for people with anxiety, digestive problems, headaches, and other health concerns. While an exhaustive review of the medical literature pertaining to massage is beyond the scope of this chapter, we present a few summaries of studies that highlight some of the potential benefits of massage in this section.

Several studies have investigated the potential effects of massage on blood pressure. A clinical trial was performed on adults aged 52 to 66 years, with and without coronary artery disease. Blood pressure and heart rate variability were measured before, during, and after foot reflexology was applied. The study found beneficial effects for the patients with coronary artery disease (Lu, Chen, & Kuo, 2011). A randomized controlled trial evaluated the effects of massage on anxiety, blood pressure, and heart rate. Male patients in a coronary care unit were randomized to receive routine care, and the intervention group received a 60-minute massage. When both groups were compared, only the group that received massage showed reduced anxiety, improved blood pressure, and lower heart rate (Adib-Hajbaghery, Abasi, & Rajabi-Beheshtabad, 2014).

Massage has been used to alleviate pain and anxiety after cardiac surgery (Bauer et al., 2010). A randomized controlled trial of 113 patients who received coronary artery bypass graft surgery compared massage therapy to standard care with relaxation. Some patients were given massage therapy to areas that the patient designated as a concern, and another group of patients did not receive massage. By the fourth day, the patients who received massage showed significant improvement in rated pain, anxiety, tension, and relaxation compared to the control group.

Massage has been shown to have an effect on dementia. A preliminary study showed promising findings for a course of massage and ear acupuncture on sleep in elderly people with dementia (Rodriguez-Mansilla et al., 2013). Another study showed similar results for those with dementia in relation to pain, depression, and anxiety (Rodriguez-Mansilla et al., 2014). A study that evaluated hand massage in older adults with chronic pain showed a reduction in pain intensity compared to a regular care group (Cino, 2014).

Pain is often experienced by older adults and may interfere with function and quality of life. Chronic pain also is associated with depression (Turk, Okifuji, & Scharff, 1995) and neuropsychological performance (Weiner, Rudy, Morrow, Slaboda, & Lieber, 2006). Pain can create physical and psychological dependency on pharmaceutical medication; thus non-pharmaceutical options may be beneficial. Among older adults with pain, massage has been reported to be associated with fewer limitations due to physical or emotional problems, better emotional health, more energy, better social interactions, and better overall health (Munk, Kruger, & Zanjani, 2011; Munk & Zanjani, 2011).

Many people use massage for spinal pain. A preliminary study of 45 women with chronic neck pain receiving massage showed signs of improvement in pain after one treatment (Bakar et al., 2014). A larger study of 228 people with chronic neck pain showed clinically meaningful improvement with multiple 60-minutes massages per week for 4 weeks (Sherman et al., 2014). A systematic review described preliminary studies that support massage as an effective treatment when compared to other treatments or placebo. The study stated that the majority of current evidence addresses non-specific back pain and that benefits are mainly seen in the short term (Kumar, Beaton, & Hughes, 2013).

Balance and fall prevention is a priority as people age; therefore procedures that assist with mobility, balance, and proprioception are encouraged. An experimental study evaluated balance measures in 35 older adults. They found after a single 60-minute massage short-term positive effects on static and dynamic balance (Sefton, Yarar, & Berry, 2012a). A randomized trial evaluated balance and cardiovascular outcomes and found that six weekly 60-minute massages produced immediate and long-term benefits in posture and balance (Sefton, Yarar, & Berry, 2012b). Finally, a study of 28 subjects 65 to 95 years old showed improvement in functional tests (one leg balance, timed up and go, and lateral reach) after massage and mobilization (Vaillant et al., 2009).

The body of knowledge related to clinical research on the physiological and psychological effects of massage is ever developing. As with many of the provider-based CAM therapies, finding valid research studies is a challenge. Especially concerning body-based therapies, there are issues with study

Table 8.1. Examples of Research Studies Evaluating Massage for Common Problems

ARTICLE	CONDITION	PURPOSE	TYPE, STUDIES INCLUDED	OUTCOMES
Chaibi & Russell, 2014	Chronic headache	Evaluate manual therapy for frequency, duration, and intensity for patients with primary chronic headache.	SR, 6 randomized controlled trials (1 included massage)	The authors conclude that manual therapy (i.e., massage and physiotherapy) is effective in the management of patients with chronic headache.
Brosseau, Wells, Tugwell, et al., 2012	Neck pain	Update evidence-based clinical practice guideline on the use of massage for adults with neck pain.	Clinical practice guideline developed from 10 selected studies	Strength of evidence recommendations included that therapeutic massage, when compared to a control, will decrease pain and improve range of motion. The guideline recommends that massage is effective for short-term relief for subacute and chronic neck pain that is of mechanical origin.
Cheng & Huang, 2014	Neck pain	Evaluate massage therapy for neck pain.	SR and meta-analysis, 15 randomized controlled trials	Massage resulted in immediate effects on pain relief compared with inactive therapies. They found no evidence of massage improving function.
Ezzo et al., 2007	Neck pain	Evaluate massage for treatment of neck disorders	SR of trials of massage alone or in combination with other therapies, 19 trials	Twelve of 19 trials were rated low quality. Only six compared massage alone compared to other treatments. The authors were not able to make recommendations due to the study limitations.
Kong et al., 2013	Neck and shoulder pain	Evaluate the effectiveness of massage therapy for neck and/or shoulder pain and functional status	SR, 12 randomized trials	Massage for shoulder and neck pain showed significant immediate effects compared to inactive therapies. Massage did not show significant functional status improvement. Massage did not show superior effects compared to other active therapies.

Author	Condition	Purpose	Design	Findings
van den Dolder, Ferreira, & Refshauge, 2014	Shoulder pain	Evaluate effect of massage and/or exercise for shoulder conditions	SR, 23 papers (20 clinical trials)	Massage was effective for producing immediate moderate improvements for range of motion, pain, and functional scores. However, massage studies were rated as low-quality evidence.
Brosseau, Wells, Poitras, et al., 2012	Low back pain	Update evidence-based clinical practice guideline on the use of massage for adults with low back pain.	Clinical practice guideline was developed from 11 selected studies	Strength of evidence recommendations included that therapeutic massage, when compared to a control, will decrease pain and improve functional status. The guideline recommends that massage is effective for short-term relief for subacute and chronic low back pain and that effects are maintained if exercise and education are provided in combination.
Furlan, Imamura, Dryden, & Irvin, 2009	Low back pain	Evaluate effect of massage therapy on low back pain	SR, 13 randomized trials	Results showed massage was superior to sham for low back pain in two studies. Eight studies showed massage was similar to exercise therapy and superior to other therapies. One study of reflexology showed no effect on low back pain. Two studies compared massage techniques to each other for back pain. The authors conclude that there may be some benefit for massage for subacute and chronic nonspecific low back pain.
Li, Wang, Feng, Yang, & Sun, 2014	Fibromyalgia	Evaluate massage therapy for patients with fibromyalgia	SR, 9 randomized controlled trials	Massage improved pain, anxiety, and depression in patients with fibromyalgia. Massage therapy that was given 5 weeks or greater resulted in significant reduction in these three outcomes.
Yuan, Matsutani, & Marques, 2014	Fibromyalgia	Evaluate effects of different types of massage on patients with fibromyalgia	SR, 10 clinical randomized and non-randomized trials were selected	Myofascial release improved fibromyalgia symptoms (i.e., pain, anxiety and depression). Lymphatic drainage massage may be superior to connective tissue massage for stiffness and depression. Most massage types in the trials improved the quality of life.

(continued)

Table 8.1. Continued

ARTICLE	CONDITION	PURPOSE	TYPE, STUDIES INCLUDED	OUTCOMES
Liao, Chen, Wang, & Tsai, 2014	Hypertension	Evaluate effect of massage on patients with hypertension or prehypertension	Meta-analysis, 9 randomized controlled trials	Massage significantly reduced systolic and diastolic blood pressure compared with control treatments for patients with hypertension and prehypertension.
Yang, et al., 2014	Hypertension	Evaluate massage (*tui na*) for treatment of hypertension	SR, 7 randomized trials	*Tui na*, in addition to antihypertensive drugs, was superior to antihypertensive drugs alone. *Tui na* alone was not superior to antihypertensive drugs. The authors note heterogeneity and low methodological quality of the studies.
Bao et al., 2014	Cancer pain	Evaluate systematic reviews and meta-analyses on complementary and alternative medicine for cancer pain in adults.	SR, 27 systematic reviews, 5 of which were reviewed for massage effects on cancer pain	Of the studies that focused on massage therapy, three concluded that massage has a beneficial effect on cancer pain, one study showed no benefit for massage on pain for breast cancer. The authors conclude that the findings are conflicted.
Ernst, 2009	Cancer pain	Evaluate classic massage for cancer pain.	SR, 14 randomized controlled trials	Findings suggest that classic massage may reduce pain, nausea, anxiety, depression, anger, stress, fatigue, and improve quality of life. However, methodological quality of the studies was scored low.
Falkensteiner, Mantovan, Muller, & Them, 2011	Cancer pain	Review literature of massage therapy for pain, anxiety, and depression for palliative care for cancer patients	Narrative review of 6 clinical studies	Four of the five studies evaluating pain showed massage resulted in improved pain scores. Anxiety was measured in three of the studies with reduction in perceived anxiety.

Wilkinson, Barnes, & Storey, 2008	Cancer pain	Evaluate massage for symptom relief in patients with cancer	SR, 10 randomized controlled trials	Reduction in pain and nausea was found in some trials and most showed psychological symptom improvements (e.g., anxiety) and other psychological symptoms. Quality of life and depression were equivocal. The authors noted that the trials had methodological limitations.
Pan, Yang, Wang, Zhang, & Liang, 2014	Breast cancer side effects	Evaluate massage effects on breast cancer-related symptoms	SR, 18 randomized trials	Massage showed greater reduction in anger and fatigue for patients with breast cancer. There were no significant differences in depression, upper limb lymphedema, anxiety, pain, cortisol, or quality of life measures because of massage.
Lafferty, Downey, McCarty, Standish, & Patrick, 2006	End-of-life care	Evaluate massage and mind-body therapies for treatment at end of life	SR, 27 clinical trials, 8 included massage	Massage showed reduction in mental distress and reduced pain for end-of-life patients. The authors note study design issues in the studies.

SR = Systematic review.

designs and other factors, such as finding believable sham treatments that have no therapeutic effect, blinding participants, and recruitment (Berman & Straus, 2004; Mehling, DiBlasi, & Hecht, 2005). Massage is a practice that is individualized both with the practitioner and client; thus some factors are difficult to control in the research setting, such as force, stroke length and duration, patient expectation, and placebo effects (Mehling et al., 2005). As noted with many of the systematic reviews that evaluate clinical trials, quality of evidence is low or not meeting criteria to include in the review. However, in spite of these challenges, there is a growing interest in research of body-based therapies, especially massage. Included in Table 8.1 are examples of reviews of the literature that evaluate the effects of massage on various conditions experienced by older adults.

MOVEMENT-FOCUSED THERAPIES

Movement-focused therapies focus on movement, balance, and posture. With age, physical structure changes, and posture may become more stooped and less balanced, resulting in decreased function and increased risk of injury. Spinal kyphosis becomes more prominent as people age. A study comparing the posture of older to younger women found that spinal curvatures were more prominent in older subjects (Drzal-Grabiec, Snela, Rykala, Podgorska, & Banas, 2013). A study of men and women over 60 years old showed significant changes in body posture when compared to a control group (Drzal-Grabiec, Rykala, Podgorska, & Snela, 2012).

Some studies have suggested a link between posture and overall health. A study of older adults showed that one factor associated with greater risk of falling and osteoporotic fractures was hyperkyphosis (Kado, Huang, Nguyen, Barrett-Connor, & Greendale, 2007). A study of 596 women aged 47–92 years suggested that hyperkyphotic posture may be related to increased risks of future fractures (Huang, Barrett-Connor, Greendale, & Kado, 2006). A study of 1578 older (mean age 72.5 years) men and women evaluated functional activities and posture. Those who had hyperkyphotic posture were more likely to have functional limitations, such as difficulty bending, walking, climbing, and standing from sitting in a chair (Kado, Huang, Barrett-Connor, & Greendale, 2005). Thus, posture seems to have a relationship with function in aging. Others have summarized the relationship of posture in the elderly with

dysfunction including pulmonary function, physical function, fractures, falls, gastrointestinal problems, gynecologic problems, quality of life, and mortality (Kado, 2009).

There have been studies to determine if postural changes due to aging can be influenced with interventions. A study measured the posture of 250 women aged 50–59 over one year. Those who performed spinal extension exercises three times per week for one year had less kyphosis progress than those who did not perform the exercises (Ball, Cagle, Johnson, Lucasey, & Lukert, 2009). Another study measured the effects of exercise for older women on posture, strength, ranges of motion, and physical performance. Participants who engaged in group exercise two times a week over 12 weeks showed significant improvements in kyphosis and other outcomes (Katzman, Sellmeyer, Stewart, Wanek, & Hamel, 2007).

Some body-based therapies focus on posture and movement. Terms associated with these techniques include *somatic education, movement therapy,* or *posture-focused body-based therapies.* The integral relationship of structure and function are core components of these therapies. Each therapy has developed independently. Thus, there are differences in theories and protocols. However, each therapy focuses on the importance of sound posture and movement.

Some movement-focused therapies incorporate active patient engagement in the treatment and typically include touching by the therapist. Touch by the practitioner usually guides motion or gives postural cues; others use touch aimed for therapeutic purposes to modify tissue structure or function. Each technique requires training and certification in order to be recognized as a practitioner of the art. Although there are a myriad of movement-based therapies, the Alexander technique, Feldenkrais method, and Rolfing Structural Integration are perhaps the most well known.

Alexander Technique

Alexander technique is named after Fredrick Matthias Alexander. He experienced vocal problems during the early years of his acting career and because he was not able to find relief from medical treatments, he began developing procedures to address his problem (Jain, Janssen, & DeCelle, 2004). After he experienced an improvement, in the early 1900s he began teaching his techniques to others. Alexander technique instructors provide individualized lessons that focus on re-education of poor postural habits and motion. The lessons include education about posture, body awareness, movement, stretching muscles, reducing spasms, and visualization exercises (Little et al., 2008). The sessions include the practitioner touching the student and focus on retraining motion and proprioceptive training, and may include using objects (e.g., chairs or mirrors for visual feedback (Jain & Astin, 2001). To become a certified Alexander technique practitioner, approximately 1600 hours of training are required (www.amsatonline.org and www.stat.org.uk).

Although only a few high-quality studies exist (Ernst & Canter, 2003), there is some preliminary evidence for the effectiveness of Alexander technique (Woodman & Moore, 2012). A randomized controlled trial compared patients with chronic or recurrent low back pain that received Alexander technique to other groups receiving exercise and massage. This study showed that those who received Alexander technique and exercise showed retained improvement after one year (Little, et al., 2008). A randomized controlled trial compared Alexander technique to usual care for visually impaired older adults. The study did not find a significant effect of Alexander technique for falls, but found improvements in postural sway and improved mobility (Gleeson, Sherrington, Lo, & Keay, 2014). A randomized controlled trial compared Alexander technique to massage and a control group for patients with Parkinson's disease; those receiving the Alexander technique intervention improved for both depression and ratings on a self-assessment disability scale (Stallibrass, Sissons, & Chalmers, 2002).

Feldenkrais Method

Feldenkrais method originated from Moshé Feldenkrais. He had aggravated a knee injury and decided to rehabilitate himself (Jain & Astin, 2001). In the 1940s, he began writing books about his method, which focused on movement and posture. Feldenkrais method educates the patient to improve mobility and function (Lyttle, 1997). Feldenkrais sessions focus on the re-education of posture and movement, especially how the body interacts against the force of gravity. The one-on-one sessions for Feldenkrais technique use *functional integration*, which provides verbal instruction and touching by the practitioner to guide the student (Schlinger, 2006). Touch used by Feldenkrais is not forceful and is not aimed at specific tissues; instead, the practitioner's touch is meant to guide motion. Feldenkrais practitioners may be found in over 30 countries and require 800 to 1000 hours to be certified in the technique (www.feldenkrais.com) (Buchanan, Nelsen, & Geletta, 2014; Schlinger, 2006).

There are few studies that evaluate the clinical effects of the Feldenkrais method (Ernst, 2005). A randomized controlled trial evaluated patients with neck pain and visual impairment, comparing a control group to those who received Feldenkrais method. The results showed that those receiving the therapy had less pain than controls immediately after treatment and after one year (Lundqvist, Zetterlund, & Richter, 2014). A randomized study of adults 65 years and older compared those receiving Feldenkrais method to a wait-list control group. Those in the treatment group showed improved balance and mobility, and decreased fear of falling after the 5-week program (Ullmann, Williams, Hussey, Durstine, & McClenaghan, 2010). A randomized study compared a version of the Feldenkrais method to no intervention to measure balance and function in people 55 years and older (Vrantsidis et al., 2009). Significance was shown for two outcome measures (Modified Falls Efficacy Scale and gait speed) in favor of the intervention (Vrantsidis et al., 2009).

Rolfing Structural Integration

Rolfing was named after Ida Rolf, who developed the method she called *Structural Integration* (Jacobson 2011a, 2011b) during the 1920s. Her approach aimed to influence the structures of the body (e.g., head, torso, pelvis, extremities) so they would be aligned in relationship to gravity and the fascial planes of the body. It was thought that with alignment and balance, the body would function better (James, Castaneda, Miller, & Findley, 2009; Jones, 2004). One of the underlying assumptions for this technique is that fascia tightens, causing aberrant movement and imbalance, resulting in dysfunction and pain. Structural Integration focuses force on fascia, with the purpose of rebalancing and re-educating the body to improve natural motion and balance (Myers, 2004). Treatments include manipulation of fascia and retraining the body using active and passive movements. Treatments traditionally consist of 10 sessions, each focusing on a different region of the body. Sessions may include deep-tissue massage and manipulation, with a primary focus on rebalancing posture as it is affected by gravity, and re-education about body position, motion, and posture. For example, the first session focuses on breathing, myofascial therapy to the torso and neck, and mobilization of the pelvis and lower extremities (Adams et al., 2013). Although there is a protocol, each treatment focuses on the specific needs of the patient based upon his or her postural faults or previous fascial injuries. A Rolf practitioner must be trained and certified at the Rolf Institute of Structural Integration (Jones, 2004). The headquarters of the Rolf Institute is located in Colorado and has offices in Australia, Canada, Europe, Japan, and South America. Training is approximately 700 hours, and continuing education is required (www.rolf.org) to maintain certification.

Research studies on Structural Integration are sparse. Jacobson provides a brief summary of six clinical studies, none of which is a clinical controlled trial. The summary offers preliminary evidence that Structural Integration might be promising for neck pain, impaired balance, and chronic fatigue syndrome (Jacobson, 2011a).

SUMMARY

Massage and movement-focused therapies are provider-based CAM therapies. Although the NCCAM has classified manipulative and body-based therapies into one of the categories of CAM, there is no clear classification system of these practices. Massage and postural therapies typically use touch as a primary component of the therapy, but may incorporate other methods into treatment, including educational and psychological therapies. The primary focus of massage and movement-focused therapies is on structure and function; thus they are well-suited to physical conditions such as those that influence the circulatory, lymphatic, nervous, and musculoskeletal systems. There is a growing body of research and evidence, especially for massage. Current evidence shows that these therapies are safe and may be helpful for specific conditions in the aging population. Massage and movement therapies may relieve common conditions such as neck and back pain but may also help with prevention of injury (i.e., falls) and may improve mental health, such as through stress and anxiety reduction.

DISCLOSURE STATEMENTS

Claire Johnson is a professor at the National University of Health Sciences and is the Editor-in-Chief for the *Journal of Manipulative and Physiological Therapeutics*. She is a chiropractor and was previously a certified massage therapist. She is a member of the American Public Health Association and the American Chiropractic Association. She sits on the NCMIC Mutual Holding Company Board of Directors and the advisory committee for Medical Evidence Evaluation Advisory Committee (MEEAC), Division of Workers' Compensation, California. She is a contractor with the Association of Chiropractic Colleges and the World Federation of Chiropractic for peer review and scientific conference services. She has no other conflicts to disclose.

Bart Green is a chiropractor and serves as the Editor-in-Chief of the *Journal of Chiropractic Education* and is the Associate Editor in the publications department of the National University of Health Sciences. He provides continuing education lectures for chiropractors and receives compensation for these programs. He has no other conflicts to disclose.

REFERENCES

Adams, D., Dagenais, S., Clifford, T., Baydala, L., King, W. J., Hervas-Malo, M., . . . Vohra, S. (2013). Complementary and alternative medicine use by pediatric specialty outpatients. *Pediatrics, 131*(2), 225–232. doi: 10.1542/peds.2012-1220peds.2012-1220 [pii]

Adib-Hajbaghery, M., Abasi, A., & Rajabi-Beheshtabad, R. (2014). Whole body massage for reducing anxiety and stabilizing vital signs of patients in cardiac care unit. *Med J Islam Repub Iran, 28*, 47.

Ajimsha, M. S. (2011). Effectiveness of direct vs indirect technique myofascial release in the management of tension-type headache. *J Bodyw Mov Ther, 15*(4), 431–435. doi: 10.1016/j.jbmt.2011.01.021S1360-8592(11)00022-2 [pii]

Ajimsha, M. S., Binsu, D., & Chithra, S. (2014). Effectiveness of myofascial release in the management of plantar heel pain: a randomized controlled trial. *Foot (Edinb), 24*(2), 66–71. doi: 10.1016/j.foot.2014.03.005S0958-2592(14)00013-3 [pii]

Ajimsha, M. S., Chithra, S., & Thulasyammal, R. P. (2012). Effectiveness of myofascial release in the management of lateral epicondylitis in computer professionals. *Arch Phys Med Rehabil, 93*(4), 604–609. doi: 10.1016/j.apmr.2011.1 0.012S0003-9993(11)00914-2 [pii]

Ajimsha, M. S., Daniel, B., & Chithra, S. (2014). Effectiveness of myofascial release in the management of chronic low back pain in nursing professionals. *J Bodyw Mov Ther, 18*(2), 273–281. doi: 10.1016/j.jbmt.2013.0 5.007S1360-8592(13)00074-0 [pii]

Audette, J. F., & Bailey, A. (2008). *Integrative pain medicine: the science and practice of complementary and alternative medicine in pain management.* Totowa, NJ: Humana.

Bakar, Y., Sertel, M., Ozturk, A., Yumin, E. T., Tatarli, N., & Ankarali, H. (2014). Short term effects of classic massage compared to connective tissue massage on pressure pain threshold and muscle relaxation response in women with chronic neck pain: a preliminary study. *J Manipulative Physiol Ther, 37*(6), 415–421. doi: 10.1016/j.jmpt.2014.0 5.004S0161-4754(14)00110-9 [pii]

Ball, J. M., Cagle, P., Johnson, B. E., Lucasey, C., & Lukert, B. P. (2009). Spinal extension exercises prevent natural progression of kyphosis. *Osteoporos Int, 20*(3), 481–489. doi: 10.1007/s00198-008-0690-3

Bao, Y., Kong, X., Yang, L., Liu, R., Shi, Z., Li, W., . . . Hou, W. (2014). Complementary and alternative medicine for cancer pain: an overview of systematic reviews. *Evid Based Complement Alternat Med, 2014,* 170396. doi: 10.1155/2014/170396

Barnes, P. M., Bloom, B., & Nahin, R. L. (2008). Complementary and alternative medicine use among adults and children: United States, 2007. *Natl Health Stat Report*(12), 1–23.

Bauer, B. A., Cutshall, S. M., Wentworth, L. J., Engen, D., Messner, P. K., Wood, C. M., . . . Sundt, T. M., 3rd. (2010). Effect of massage therapy on pain, anxiety, and tension after cardiac surgery: a randomized study. *Complement Ther Clin Pract, 16*(2), 70–75. doi: 10.1016/j.ctcp.2009.0 6.012S1744-3881(09)00074-7 [pii]

Berman, J. D., & Straus, S. E. (2004). Implementing a research agenda for complementary and alternative medicine. *Annu Rev Med, 55,* 239–254. doi: 10.1146/annurev.med.55.091902.103657

Brosseau, L., Wells, G. A., Poitras, S., Tugwell, P., Casimiro, L., Novikov, M., . . . Cohoon, C. (2012). Ottawa Panel evidence-based clinical practice guidelines on therapeutic massage for low back pain. *J Bodyw Mov Ther, 16*(4), 424–455. doi: 10.1016/j.jbmt.2012.0 4.002S1360-8592(12)00116-7 [pii]

Brosseau, L., Wells, G. A., Tugwell, P., Casimiro, L., Novikov, M., Loew, L., . . . Cohoon, C. (2012).

Ottawa Panel evidence-based clinical practice guidelines on therapeutic massage for neck pain. *J Bodyw Mov Ther, 16*(3), 300–325. doi: 10.1016/j.jbmt.2012.04.001S1360-8592(12)00115-5 [pii]

Buchanan, P. A., Nelsen, N. L., & Geletta, S. (2014). United States Guild Certified Feldenkrais Teachers(R): a survey of characteristics and practice patterns. *BMC Complement Altern Med, 14,* 217. doi: 10.1186/1472-6882-14-2171472-6882-14-217 [pii]

Bush, E. (2001). The use of human touch to improve the well-being of older adults: a holistic nursing intervention. *J Holist Nurs, 19*(3), 256–270.

Chaibi, A., & Russell, M. B. (2014). Manual therapies for primary chronic headaches: a systematic review of randomized controlled trials. *J Headache Pain, 15,* 67. doi: 10.1186/1129-2377-15-671129-2377-15-67 [pii]

Cheng, Y. H., & Huang, G. C. (2014). Efficacy of massage therapy on pain and dysfunction in patients with neck pain: a systematic review and meta-analysis. *Evid Based Complement Alternat Med, 2014,* 1–13, 204360. doi: 10.1155/2014/204360

Chiranthanut, N., Hanprasertpong, N., & Teekachunhatean, S. (2014). Thai massage, and Thai herbal compress versus oral ibuprofen in symptomatic treatment of osteoarthritis of the knee: a randomized controlled trial. *Biomed Res Int, 2014,* 490512. doi: 10.1155/2014/490512

Cino, K. (2014). Aromatherapy hand massage for older adults with chronic pain living in long-term care. *J Holist Nurs, 32*(4), 304–313. doi: 10.1177/ 089801011452837 8089801011 4528378 [pii]

Clar, C., Tsertsvadze, A., Court, R., Hundt, G. L., Clarke, A., & Sutcliffe, P. (2014). Clinical effectiveness of manual therapy for the management of musculoskeletal and non-musculoskeletal conditions: systematic review and update of UK evidence report. *Chiropr Man Therap, 22*(1), 12. doi: 10.1186/2045-709X-22-122045-709X- 22-12 [pii]

Cocksedge, S., George, B., Renwick, S., & Chew-Graham, C. A. (2013). Touch in primary care consultations: qualitative investigation of doctors' and patients' perceptions. *Br J Gen Pract, 63*(609), e283–290. doi: 10.3399/ bjgp13X665251

Cohen, J. H., & Gibbons, R. W. (1998). Raymond L. Nimmo and the evolution of trigger point therapy, 1929–1986. *J Manipulative Physiol Ther, 21*(3), 167–172.

Craig, L. H., Svircev, A., Haber, M., & Juncos, J. L. (2006). Controlled pilot study of the effects of neuromuscular therapy in patients with Parkinson's disease. *Mov Disord, 21*(12), 2127–2133. doi: 10.1002/mds.21132

Davis, M. A., Martin, B. I., Coulter, I. D., & Weeks, W. B. (2013). US spending on complementary and alternative medicine during 2002–08 plateaued, suggesting role in reformed health system. *Health Aff (Millwood), 32*(1), 45–52. doi: 10.1377/hlthaff.2011.032132/1/45 [pii]

Drzal-Grabiec, J., Rykala, J., Podgorska, J., & Snela, S. (2012). Changes in body posture of women and men over 60 years of age. *Ortop Traumatol Rehabil, 14*(5), 467–475. doi: 10.5604/15093492.10125041012504 [pii]

Drzal-Grabiec, J., Snela, S., Rykala, J., Podgorska, J., & Banas, A. (2013). Changes in the body posture of women occurring with age. *BMC Geriatr, 13*, 108. doi: 10.1186/1471-2318-13-1081471-2318-13-108 [pii]

Edvardsson, J. D., Sandman, P. O., & Rasmussen, B. H. (2003). Meanings of giving touch in the care of older patients: becoming a valuable person and professional. *J Clin Nurs, 12*(4), 601–609. doi: 754 [pii]

Elkiss, M. L., & Jerome, J. A. (2012). Touch—more than a basic science. *J Am Osteopath Assoc, 112*(8), 514–517. doi: 112/8/514 [pii]

Ernst, E. (2003). The safety of massage therapy. *Rheumatology (Oxford), 42*(9), 1101–1106. doi: 10.1093/rheumatology/keg306keg306 [pii]

Ernst, E. (2009). Massage therapy for cancer palliation and supportive care: a systematic review of randomised clinical trials. *Support Care Cancer, 17*(4), 333–337. doi: 10.1007/s00520-008-0569-z

Ernst, E., & Canter, P. H. (2003). The Alexander technique: a systematic review of controlled clinical trials. *Forsch Komplementarmed Klass Naturheilkd, 10*(6), 325–329. doi: 7588675886 [pii]

Ernst, E., & Canter, P. H. (2005). The Feldenkrais method: a systematic review of randomised clinical trials. *Physikalische Medizin Rehabilitationsmedizin Kurortmedizin 15*(3), 151–156.

Ezzo, J., Haraldsson, B. G., Gross, A. R., Myers, C. D., Morien, A., Goldsmith, C. H., . . . Peloso, P. M. (2007). Massage for mechanical neck disorders: a systematic review. *Spine (Phila Pa 1976), 32*(3), 353–362. doi: 10.1097/01.brs. 0000254099. 07294.2100007632- 200702010-00012 [pii]

Falkensteiner, M., Mantovan, F., Muller, I., & Them, C. (2011). The use of massage therapy for reducing pain, anxiety, and depression in oncological palliative care patients: a narrative review of the literature. *ISRN Nurs, 2011*, 929868. doi: 10.5402/2011/929868

French, H. P., Brennan, A., White, B., & Cusack, T. (2011). Manual therapy for osteoarthritis of the hip or knee: a systematic review. *Man Ther, 16*(2), 109–117. doi: 10.1016/j.math.2010.10.011S1356-689X(10)00188-8 [pii]

Furlan, A. D., Imamura, M., Dryden, T., & Irvin, E. (2009). Massage for low back pain: an updated systematic review within the framework of the Cochrane Back Review Group. *Spine (Phila Pa 1976), 34*(16), 1669–1684. doi: 10.1097/BRS.0b013e3181ad7bd6

Gehret, K. (2010). *Body work: careers in massage therapy.* Sausalito, CA: Soulstice Media.

Gleeson, M., Sherrington, C., Lo, S., & Keay, L. (2014). Can the Alexander Technique improve balance and mobility in older adults with visual impairments? A randomized controlled trial. *Clin Rehabil, 29*(3), 244–260. doi: 0269215514542636 [pii]10.1177/0269215514542636

Grant, K. E. (2003). Massage safety: injuries reported in Medline relating to the practice of therapeutic massage—1965–2003. *J Bodyw Move Ther, 7*(4), 207–212. doi: 10.1016/S1360-8592(03)00043-3

Grant, K. E., Balletto, J., Gowan-Moody, D., Healey, D., Kincaid, D., Lowe, W., & Travillian, R. S. (2008). Steps toward massage therapy guidelines: a first report to the profession. *Int J Ther Massage Bodywork, 1*(1), 19–36.

Grzybowski, S. C., Stewart, M. A., & Weston, W. W. (1992). Nonverbal communication and the therapeutic relationship: leading to a better understanding of healing. *Can Fam Physician, 38*, 1994–1998.

Harris, P. E., Cooper, K. L., Relton, C., & Thomas, K. J. (2014). Prevalence of visits to massage therapists by the general population: a systematic review. *Complement Ther Clin Pract, 20*(1), 16–20. doi: 10.1016/j.ctcp.2013.11.001S1744-3881(13)00089-3 [pii]

Huang, M. H., Barrett-Connor, E., Greendale, G. A., & Kado, D. M. (2006). Hyperkyphotic posture and risk of future osteoporotic fractures: the Rancho Bernardo study. *J Bone Miner Res, 21*(3), 419–423. doi: 10.1359/JBMR.051201

Jacobson, E. (2011a). Structural integration, an alternative method of manual therapy and sensorimotor education. *J Altern Complement Med, 17*(10), 891–899. doi: 10.1089/acm.2010.0258

Jacobson, E. (2011b). Structural integration: origins and development. *J Altern Complement Med, 17*(9), 775–780. doi: 10.1089/acm.2011.0001

Jain, N., & Astin, J. A. (2001). Barriers to acceptance: an exploratory study of complementary/alternative medicine disuse.

J Altern Complement Med, 7(6), 689–696. doi: 10.1089/10755530152755243

Jain, S., Janssen, K., & DeCelle, S. (2004). Alexander technique and Feldenkrais method: a critical overview. *Phys Med Rehabil Clin N Am, 15*(4), 811–825, vi. doi: 10.1016/j.pmr.2004.04.0 05S1047965104000233 [pii]

James, H., Castaneda, L., Miller, M. E., & Findley, T. (2009). Rolfing structural integration treatment of cervical spine dysfunction. *J Bodyw Mov Ther, 13*(3), 229–238. doi: 10.1016/j.jbmt.2008.0 7.002S1360-8592(08)00139-3 [pii]

Jones, T. A. (2004). Rolfing. *Phys Med Rehabil Clin N Am, 15*(4), 799–809, vi. doi: 10.1016/j.pmr.2004. 03.008S1047965104000178 [pii]

Kado, D. M. (2009). The rehabilitation of hyperkyphotic posture in the elderly. *Eur J Phys Rehabil Med, 45*(4), 583–593. doi: R33092224 [pii]

Kado, D. M., Huang, M. H., Barrett-Connor, E., & Greendale, G. A. (2005). Hyperkyphotic posture and poor physical functional ability in older community-dwelling men and women: the Rancho Bernardo study. *J Gerontol A Biol Sci Med Sci, 60*(5), 633–637. doi: 60/5/633 [pii]

Kado, D. M., Huang, M. H., Nguyen, C. B., Barrett-Connor, E., & Greendale, G. A. (2007). Hyperkyphotic posture and risk of injurious falls in older persons: the Rancho Bernardo Study. *J Gerontol A Biol Sci Med Sci, 62*(6), 652–657. doi: 62/6/652 [pii]

Katzman, W. B., Sellmeyer, D. E., Stewart, A. L., Wanek, L., & Hamel, K. A. (2007). Changes in flexed posture, musculoskeletal impairments, and physical performance after group exercise in community-dwelling older women. *Arch Phys Med Rehabil, 88*(2), 192–199. doi: S0003-9993(06)01483-3 [pii]10.1016/j. apmr.2006.10.033

Kaye, A. D., Kaye, A. J., Swinford, J., Baluch, A., Bawcom, B. A., Lambert, T. J., & Hoover, J. M. (2008). The effect of deep-tissue massage therapy on blood pressure and heart rate. *J Altern Complement Med, 14*(2), 125–128. doi: 10.1089/ acm.2007.0665

Khan, F. H., Hanif, R., Tabassum, R., Qidwai, W., & Nanji, K. (2014). Patient attitudes towards physician nonverbal behaviors during consultancy: result from a developing country. *ISRN Family Med, 2014*, 1–6, 473654. doi: 10.1155/2014/473654

Kong, L. J., Zhan, H. S., Cheng, Y. W., Yuan, W. A., Chen, B., & Fang, M. (2013). Massage therapy for neck and shoulder pain: a systematic review and meta-analysis. *Evid Based Complement Alternat Med, 2013*, 1–10, 613279. doi: 10.1155/2013/613279

Koo, T. K., Cohen, J. H., & Zheng, Y. (2012). Immediate effect of nimmo receptor tonus technique on muscle elasticity, pain perception, and disability in subjects with chronic low back pain. *J Manipulative Physiol Ther, 35*(1), 45–53. doi: 10.1016/j.jmpt.2011.0 9.013S0161-4754(11)00231-4 [pii]

Kumar, S., Beaton, K., & Hughes, T. (2013). The effectiveness of massage therapy for the treatment of nonspecific low back pain: a systematic review of systematic reviews. *Int J Gen Med, 6*, 733–741. doi: 10.2147/IJGM.S50243ijgm-6-733 [pii]

Lafferty, W. E., Downey, L., McCarty, R. L., Standish, L. J., & Patrick, D. L. (2006). Evaluating CAM treatment at the end of life: a review of clinical trials for massage and meditation. *Complement Ther Med, 14*(2), 100–112. doi: S0965-2299(06)00028-8 [pii]10.1016/j. ctim.2006.01.009

http://books.google.com/books?id=gdur2zFd928 C&printsec=frontcover#v=onepage&q&f=false" title="Manipulative and body-based practices: an overview" journalName="Backgrounder">Leo nard, B. (2008). Manipulative and body-based practices: an overview. *Backgrounder.* Retrieved from http://books.google.com/books?id=gdur2 zFd928C&printsec=frontcover#v=onepage&q& f=false

Li, Y. H., Wang, F. Y., Feng, C. Q., Yang, X. F., & Sun, Y. H. (2014). Massage therapy for fibromyalgia: a systematic review and meta-analysis of randomized controlled trials. *PLoS One, 9*(2), e89304. doi: 10.1371/journal. pone.0089304PONE-D-13-45402 [pii]

Liao, I. C., Chen, S. L., Wang, M. Y., & Tsai, P. S. (2014). Effects of massage on blood pressure in patients with hypertension and prehypertension: a meta-analysis of randomized controlled trials. *J Cardiovasc Nurs.* doi: 10.1097/ JCN.0000000000000217.

Liptan, G., Mist, S., Wright, C., Arzt, A., & Jones, K. D. (2013). A pilot study of myofascial release therapy compared to Swedish massage in fibromyalgia. *J Bodyw Mov Ther, 17*(3), 365–370. doi: 10.1016/j. jbmt.2012.11.010S1360-8592(12)00240-9 [pii]

Little, P., Lewith, G., Webley, F., Evans, M., Beattie, A., Middleton, K., . . . Sharp, D. (2008). Randomised controlled trial of Alexander technique lessons, exercise, and massage (ATEAM) for chronic and recurrent back pain. *Br J Sports Med, 42*(12), 965–968. doi: 42/12/965 [pii]

Lu, W. A., Chen, G. Y., & Kuo, C. D. (2011). Foot reflexology can increase vagal modulation, decrease sympathetic modulation, and lower blood pressure in healthy subjects and patients with coronary artery disease. *Altern Ther Health Med, 17*(4), 8–14.

Lundqvist, L. O., Zetterlund, C., & Richter, H. O. (2014). Effects of Feldenkrais method on chronic neck/scapular pain in people with visual impairment: a randomized controlled trial with one-year follow-up. *Arch Phys Med Rehabil, 95*(9), 1656–1661. doi: 10.1016/j.apmr.2014.0 5.013S0003-9993(14)00408-0 [pii]

Lyttle, T. (1997). The Feldenkrais Method: application, practice and principles. *J Bodyw Move Ther, 1*(5), 262–269.

Majchrzycki, M., Kocur, P., & Kotwicki, T. (2014). Deep tissue massage and nonsteroidal anti-inflammatory drugs for low back pain: a prospective randomized trial. *Scientific World Journal, 2014*, 1–7, 287597. doi: 10.1155/2014/287597

Mehling, W. E., DiBlasi, Z., & Hecht, F. (2005). Bias control in trials of bodywork: a review of methodological issues. *J Altern Complement Med, 11*(2), 333–342. doi: 10.1089/acm.2005.11.333

Menard, M. B. (2014). Choose wisely: the quality of massage education in the United States. *Int J Ther Massage Bodywork, 7*(3), 7–24.

Munk, N., Kruger, T., & Zanjani, F. (2011). Massage therapy usage and reported health in older adults experiencing persistent pain. *J Altern Complement Med, 17*(7), 609–616. doi: 10.1089/ acm.2010.0151

Munk, N., & Zanjani, F. (2011). Relationship between massage therapy usage and health outcomes in older adults. *J Bodyw Mov Ther, 15*(2), 177–185. doi: 10.1016/j.jbmt.2010.0 1.007S1360-8592(10)00008-2 [pii]

Myers, T. W. (2004). Structural integration: developments in Ida Rolf's "recipe." *J Bodyw Move Ther, 8*(2), 131–142.

Osmun, W. E., Brown, J. B., Stewart, M., & Graham, S. (2000). Patients' attitudes to comforting touch in family practice. *Can Fam Physician, 46*, 2411–2416.

Pan, Y. Q., Yang, K. H., Wang, Y. L., Zhang, L. P., & Liang, H. Q. (2014). Massage interventions and treatment-related side effects of breast cancer: a systematic review and meta-analysis. *Int J Clin Oncol, 19*(5), 829–841. doi: 10.1007/s10147-013-0635-5

Rodriguez-Mansilla, J., Gonzalez Lopez-Arza, M. V., Varela-Donoso, E., Montanero-Fernandez, J., Gonzalez Sanchez, B., & Garrido-Ardila, E. M. (2014). The effects of ear acupressure, massage therapy and no therapy on symptoms of dementia: a randomized controlled trial.

Clin Rehabil. doi: 0269215514554240 [pii]10.1177/0269215514554240

Rodriguez-Mansilla, J., Gonzalez-Lopez-Arza, M. V., Varela-Donoso, E., Montanero-Fernandez, J., Jimenez-Palomares, M., & Garrido-Ardila, E. M. (2013). Ear therapy and massage therapy in the elderly with dementia: a pilot study. *J Tradit Chin Med, 33*(4), 461–467.

Schlinger, M. (2006). Feldenkrais Method, Alexander Technique, and yoga: body awareness therapy in the performing arts. *Phys Med Rehabil Clin N Am, 17*(4), 865–875. doi: S1047-9651(06)00047-7 [pii]10.1016/j.pmr.2006.07.002

Sefton, J. M., Yarar, C., & Berry, J. W. (2012a). Massage therapy produces short-term improvements in balance, neurological, and cardiovascular measures in older persons. *Int J Ther Massage Bodywork, 5*(3), 16–27.

Sefton, J. M., Yarar, C., & Berry, J. W. (2012b). Six weeks of massage therapy produces changes in balance, neurological and cardiovascular measures in older persons. *Int J Ther Massage Bodywork, 5*(3), 28–40.

Sherman, K. J., Cook, A. J., Wellman, R. D., Hawkes, R. J., Kahn, J. R., Deyo, R. A., & Cherkin, D. C. (2014). Five-week outcomes from a dosing trial of therapeutic massage for chronic neck pain. *Ann Fam Med, 12*(2), 112–120. doi: 10.1370/ afm.160212/2/112 [pii]

Sherman, K. J., Dixon, M. W., Thompson, D., & Cherkin, D. C. (2006). Development of a taxonomy to describe massage treatments for musculoskeletal pain. *BMC Complement Altern Med, 6*, 24. doi: 1472-6882-6-24 [pii]10.1186/1472-6882-6-24

Stallibrass, C., Sissons, P., & Chalmers, C. (2002). Randomized controlled trial of the Alexander technique for idiopathic Parkinson's disease. *Clin Rehabil, 16*(7), 695–708.

Studdert, D. M., Eisenberg, D. M., Miller, F. H., Curto, D. A., Kaptchuk, T. J., & Brennan, T. A. (1998). Medical malpractice implications of alternative medicine. *JAMA, 280*(18), 1610–1615. doi: jlm71042 [pii]

Travell, J. G., & Simons, D. G. (1983). *Myofascial pain and dysfunction: the trigger point manual.* Baltimore, MD: Williams & Wilkins.

Tsertsvadze, A., Clar, C., Court, R., Clarke, A., Mistry, H., & Sutcliffe, P. (2014). Cost-effectiveness of manual therapy for the management of musculoskeletal conditions: a systematic review and narrative synthesis of evidence from randomized controlled trials. *J Manipulative Physiol Ther, 37*(6), 343–362. doi: 10.1016/j.jmpt. 2014.05.001S0161-4754(14)00087-6 [pii]

Turk, D. C., Okifuji, A., & Scharff, L. (1995). Chronic pain and depression: role of perceived impact and perceived control in different age cohorts. *Pain, 61*(1), 93–101. doi: 0304-3959(94)00167-D [pii]

Ullmann, G., Williams, H. G., Hussey, J., Durstine, J. L., & McClenaghan, B. A. (2010). Effects of Feldenkrais exercises on balance, mobility, balance confidence, and gait performance in community-dwelling adults age 65 and older. *J Altern Complement Med, 16*(1), 97–105. doi: 10.1089/acm.2008.0612

Vaillant, J., Rouland, A., Martigne, P., Braujou, R., Nissen, M. J., Caillat-Miousse, J. L., . . . Juvin, R. (2009). Massage and mobilization of the feet and ankles in elderly adults: effect on clinical balance performance. *Man Ther, 14*(6), 661–664. doi: 10.1016/j.math.2009.03.004S1356-689X(09)00043-5 [pii]

van den Dolder, P. A., Ferreira, P. H., & Refshauge, K. M. (2014). Effectiveness of soft tissue massage and exercise for the treatment of non-specific shoulder pain: a systematic review with meta-analysis. *Br J Sports Med, 48*(16), 1216–1226. doi: 10.1136/bjsports-2011-090553bjsports-2011-090553 [pii]

Veer, J. V. (1995). The healing touch. *West J Med, 162*(4), 374.

Vrantsidis, F., Hill, K. D., Moore, K., Webb, R., Hunt, S., & Dowson, L. (2009). Getting grounded gracefully: effectiveness and acceptability of Feldenkrais in improving balance. *J Aging Phys Act, 17*(1), 57–76.

Weiner, D. K., Rudy, T. E., Morrow, L., Slaboda, J., & Lieber, S. (2006). The relationship between pain, neuropsychological performance, and physical function in community-dwelling older adults with chronic low back pain. *Pain Med, 7*(1), 60–70. doi: PME091 [pii]10.1111/j.1526-4637.2006.00091.x

Wilkinson, S., Barnes, K., & Storey, L. (2008). Massage for symptom relief in patients with cancer: systematic review. *J Adv Nurs, 63*(5), 430–439. doi: 10.1111/j.1365-2648.2008.04712.xJAN4712 [pii]

Woodman, J. P., & Moore, N. R. (2012). Evidence for the effectiveness of Alexander Technique lessons in medical and health-related conditions: a systematic review. *Int J Clin Pract, 66*(1), 98–112. doi: 10.1111/j.1742-1241.2011.02817.x

Yang, X., Zhao, H., & Wang, J. (2014). Chinese massage (Tuina) for the treatment of essential hypertension: a systematic review and meta-analysis. *Complement Ther Med, 22*(3), 541–548. doi: 10.1016/j.ctim.2014.03.008S0965-2299(14)00039-9 [pii]

Yeh, C. H., Morone, N. E., Chien, L. C., Cao, Y., Lu, H., Shen, J., . . . Suen, L. K. (2014). Auricular point acupressure to manage chronic low back pain in older adults: a randomized controlled pilot study. *Evid Based Complement Alternat Med, 2014*, 375173. doi: 10.1155/2014/375173

Yin, P., Gao, N., Wu, J., Litscher, G., & Xu, S. (2014). Adverse events of massage therapy in pain-related conditions: a systematic review. *Evid Based Complement Alternat Med, 2014*, 1–11, 480956. doi: 10.1155/2014/480956

Yuan, S. L., Matsutani, L. A., & Marques, A. P. (2014). Effectiveness of different styles of massage therapy in fibromyalgia: A systematic review and meta-analysis. *Man Ther*. doi: S1356-689X(14)00182-9 [pii]10.1016/j.math.2014.09.003

9

CHIROPRACTIC CARE

Claire D. Johnson and Bart N. Green

INTRODUCTION

The National Center for Health Statistics reports that the most common reasons US adults seek complementary and alternative medicine (CAM) treatment is for musculoskeletal problems, the most common among these being back (17.1%) and neck (5.9%) complaints (Barnes, Bloom, & Nahin, 2008). Chiropractic is recognized as one of the most commonly accessed CAM professions in the United States (Eisenberg et al., 1998; Kaptchuk & Eisenberg, 1998). Therefore, it is not surprising that of the body-based therapies, chiropractic is reported as the most commonly used practitioner-based therapy; 8.6% of adults 18 years and over used chiropractic in the past 12 months (Barnes et al., 2008). A recent analysis showed that in the United States, "[c]hiropractic care accounted for 77–82% of total ambulatory visits to complementary and alternative medicine providers from 2002 to 2008... " (Davis, Martin, Coulter, & Weeks, 2013, 49). In the United States, chiropractic is not only the largest

CAM profession, it is also the most regulated and most recognized, and it is the third largest healthcare profession (Christensen, Kollasch, & Hyland, 2010). There are approximately 70,000 chiropractic licenses in the United States alone (Christensen et al., 2010). Chiropractic is also an established health profession in many countries around the world (WFC, 2009).

The study by Eisenberg et al. (1998) showed that 11% of the US population had used chiropractic in the previous 12 months; more recent studies have suggested increasing trends in utilization. An analysis of 2006 Medical Expenditure Panel Survey data showed that 12.6 million US adults reported using chiropractic in the previous year (Davis, Sirovich, & Weeks, 2010). The estimate of how many older patients access chiropractic can be found in National Board of Chiropractic Examiners (NBCE) survey data in which chiropractors report the percentage of older patients in their practices (22.8% were aged 51–64, and 15.4% were 65 or older). Over one-third of chiropractic patients are older patients, as reported by practicing doctors of chiropractic (Christensen et al., 2010). A recent epidemiological study of US adults aged 65–99 receiving chiropractic spinal manipulation under Medicare showed that the number of chiropractic users were estimated to be between 1.6 and 1.8 million (6.2%–6.9% of Medicare Part B beneficiaries) (Whedon, Song, & Davis, 2013). Other studies have estimated chiropractic usage by older adults to be around 4.8% (Weigel et al., 2010).

Although chiropractic has evolved into a commonly used method when conservative approaches to musculoskeletal conditions, such as back and neck pain, are warranted, knowing the origins of chiropractic provides us with a better understanding of the theories behind this unique form of health care. Chiropractic began in the United States during the late 1890s. At that time, the concerns about medical "cures" (i.e., bleeding and purging) resulted in some irregular healers searching outside the traditional medical methods to re-establish health through methods that were more natural. Though his initial interest was in magnetic healing, Daniel David Palmer created chiropractic as an approach to healing that included manipulation, and offered this method as an alternative to medical cures available. One of the early underlying principles of chiropractic was that it was believed that the patient's body had an innate ability to heal itself, as long as interference was removed to allow the body to heal.

Conventional medicine was establishing its dominance and viewed other health professions as external or *irregular* practices. Therefore, chiropractic developed outside the conventional medical system and has often been associated as a CAM profession. At that time, any practitioner not trained in allopathic medicine was not recognized by medical associations; therefore, chiropractic evolved outside the institution of Western medicine. At the beginning of the twentieth century, legalization of the health professions was occurring in the United States. In the creation of a legal defense to clarify that chiropractors were not practicing medicine but instead their own form of health care, a unique lexicon was created from litigation (C. Johnson, 2010). Thus, to be recognized as a distinct profession with its own unique science, art, and philosophy, chiropractic schools and associations were adamant about using a distinct vocabulary to preserve professional identity. Terms in medicine such as *manipulation* would be *adjustment* in chiropractic; *joint dysfunction* would be *subluxation complex*. It is important

to note that a *chiropractic subluxation* does not mean the same in medical terminology; thus it is not a joint dislocation, but rather is a shorthand term for a more complex entity. The term *innate intelligence* was considered by some chiropractors to be the essential component of the body's ability to heal and regulate itself. The first chiropractic descriptions of innate intelligence were published years before similar terms, such as *homeostasis*, were coined and described in the medical literature (Cannon, 1932; Keating, 2002).

The early years of chiropractic emphasized the differences between the chiropractic approach and the biomedical approach. This distinction was primarily in the tools that medical doctors used most: drugs and surgery. Thus, the chiropractic profession has traditionally been a conservative profession and, for most of its existence, practitioners managed patient health through natural healing methods without the use of drugs or surgery. Theories for the basis of chiropractic care have advanced over the years. When it was establishing a foothold as a profession, the primary focus was to provide spinal manipulations (i.e., *adjustments*) to remove spinal dysfunction (i.e., *subluxations*). The thought was that if the nervous system was functioning properly, then the tissues of the body that were influenced by nerves would have a greater chance to heal or ward off disease. Since that time, the chiropractic profession's scope and practice have evolved to augment subluxation correction. Chiropractic care includes manipulation in addition to other therapies, such as exercise, physical modalities, and soft tissue mobilization, and methods, such as nutrition, education, and injury prevention. Thus, chiropractic care utilizes manipulation as part of a therapeutic regimen, but chiropractic care is not the equivalent of manipulation (Hawk, 1998). Doctors of chiropractic are trained to provide a variety of treatments, primarily aimed at musculoskeletal conditions, though some are trained more broadly to address other conditions.

The National Center for Complementary and Alternative Medicine (NCCAM) classification system that categorizes the CAM modalities places chiropractic under a body-based CAM approach (http://nccam.nih.gov/health/chiropractic/introduction.htm and http://nccam.nih.gov/health/whatiscam). However, there has been some confusion in the scientific literature regarding what the term *chiropractic* means. Sometimes, the term refers to spinal manipulation, even if the practitioner is not a chiropractor. In other cases, the term has been used to mean all of the broad approaches that a chiropractor might use in practice. Thus, it is important to distinguish how this term is being used when reviewing evidence in the literature and considering this profession.

The current state of the art of chiropractic shows that this profession has evidence for effectiveness for musculoskeletal conditions (Bronfort et al., 2011; Bronfort et al., 2012; Bronfort et al., 2014), can offer a focus on wellness and prevention (Dehen, Whalen, Farabaugh, & Hawk, 2010), has produced best practices recommendations for chiropractic care for older adults using a consensus process (Hawk, Schneider, Dougherty, Gleberzon, & Killinger, 2010), and has the ability to address the various components of the determinants of health (Johnson & Green, 2009). Chiropractic healing includes physical, psychosocial, emotional, and/or spiritual/metaphysical components and offers a holistic view of health (Johnson et al., 2008), which is strikingly similar to the World Health Organization's definition of health as "[a] state of complete physical, mental and social well-being, and not merely the absence of disease" (WHO, 2003)

EDUCATION AND PRACTICE

Chiropractic education is accredited on various levels. The Council on Chiropractic Education (CCE) is recognized by the US Department of Education. The CCE accredits 15 Doctor of Chiropractic (DC) degree programs at 18 locations within the United States. The CCE process helps to assure quality to various stakeholders, licensing and regulatory bodies, professional entities, and the public. Most chiropractic colleges are also accredited by regional accrediting bodies that confirm the integrity of the academic program. However, accreditation of the professional training processes by CCE and regional academic accreditation are separate processes (Coulter, Adams, Coggan, Wilkes, & Gonyea, 1998). Besides the CCE and regional vetting, the World Health Organization has published guidelines on chiropractic safety and training (http://apps.who.int/medicinedocs/en/d/Js14076e/).

Chiropractic training in the United States is standardized. According to the US Bureau of Labor Statistics, "Doctor of Chiropractic programs typically take 4 years to complete and require at least 3 years of undergraduate college education for admission" (http://www.bls.gov/ooh/healthcare/chiropractors.htm) (Figure 9.1). In many ways, chiropractic curricula are structured similarly to traditional medical school curricula (Coulter et al., 1998). Typically, the first years are didactic, followed by increasing clinical interaction, ending in clinical internships. As the student progresses toward graduation, he or she must pass various examinations within the institution as well as external exams. The National Board of Chiropractic Examiners (NBCE) (for the US) and the International Board of Chiropractic Examiners (outside the US) are the testing agencies for the chiropractic profession. The NBCE standardized examinations assess knowledge

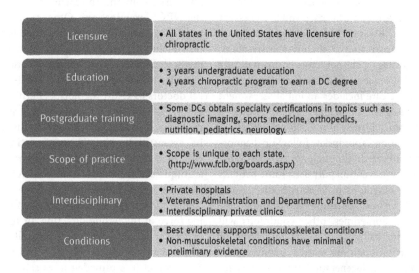

FIGURE 9.1   Characteristics of chiropractic licensure, education, and scope of practice.

and skills relevant to chiropractic in both basic and clinical science subjects. All of the US state licensing boards use the NBCE scores in their evaluation of a doctor to determine licensure. For those who graduate and wish to pursue a specialty, there are residency or postgraduate programs that allow DCs to focus clinical skills in areas of radiology, orthopedics, sports medicine, nutrition, and other topics.

Most relevant to the care of the aging patient is the extensive training that chiropractors receive on the common conditions of the neuromusculoskeletal system. Basic science courses include neurology, physiology, anatomy, and biomechanics. Clinical courses include history taking, physical examination, and the care of neuromusculoskeletal problems. Most chiropractic curricula have a designated course in geriatrics and include topics related to aging disorders throughout other courses. Clinical training is done under the supervision of a licensed practitioner. Typically, patients encountered are from the local community; however, many colleges have training opportunities with underserved or special needs clinics (Johnson, 2007). There are many opportunities during clinical training for the management of aging patients.

Doctors of chiropractic are licensed in each of the United States and in numerous other countries. Each jurisdiction's law delineates the scope of practice for its chiropractors (Chang, 2014). While there are many similarities in chiropractic practice across states, regions, and countries, it should be noted that variations in practice laws cause a range of practices. Regardless of the location of practice, each doctor of chiropractic is expected to practice within the scope of practice where they are licensed and to the extent to which he or she was trained, which includes diagnosis, referral, and management. How each state or province regulates its chiropractors is also typically written into the practice act or law for the region.

Chiropractic care includes an initial assessment of the presenting condition and typically includes a past health history, history of chief complaint, physical examination, and appropriate follow-up diagnostic studies if indicated. Although not typically done for screening or prevention purposes, some patients will require radiographs of various body regions. This may aid in clinical decision-making and to rule out pathology. Sometimes, other conditions will be found incidentally, which result in referral or co-management. Conditions such as abdominal aortic aneurysm, spinal degeneration, tumors, or osteoporosis are some of the potential findings (Taylor &

Bussieres, 2012). Because the most common complaints presenting to chiropractic offices are musculoskeletal, the examination tends to include vital signs, inspection, palpation, orthopedic tests, neurological exam, ranges of motion, and postural and gait analysis. Other examination procedures may also be included if indicated, such as eye/ear/mouth exam and heart/lung/abdomen exam.

Chiropractic care includes a variety of modalities, but the one most often associated with chiropractic is manipulation. Manipulation and mobilization of body parts are popular body-based practices used by adults (Barnes et al., 2008). Mobilization may include soft tissue work and passive movement of joint tissues, whereas manipulation is most commonly used to describe the skillful application of a rapid and controlled force to induce motion into joints. Manipulation is performed on areas of the body not functioning properly and is typically aimed at the spinal joints; however, other joints and areas may also be included, such as the temporomandibular joint and the upper and lower extremities. People commonly seek manipulation to treat back and neck pain, sciatica, pain in other joints, arthritis, some types of headaches, and a variety of other musculoskeletal problems (Green & Johnson, 2014; Morin & Aubin, 2014).

Doctors of chiropractic reportedly perform upwards of 90% of spinal manipulations in the United States (Shekelle, Adams, Chassin, Hurwitz, & Brook, 1992; Shekelle & Brook, 1991), which is congruent with the considerable amount of training in manipulation provided during the DC curriculum and the focus of manipulation in the NBCE examinations. Other types of licensed practitioners may be trained to provide manipulation, including osteopaths, physical therapists, and medical doctors; however, most authors do not consider osteopaths, physical therapists, or medical doctors as CAM therapists (Berman & Straus, 2004). The training for manipulation among these professions varies, but chiropractic is known for its extensive training in manipulation (Coulter et al., 1998). Each profession and jurisdiction has a unique scope for what type of practitioner may perform manipulation. Because force is applied to a joint, there is risk for over-applying force, providing force in the wrong direction, or in the wrong clinical situation. Therefore, only well-trained and licensed professionals should provide manipulation so that it is provided in as safe a manner as possible.

Chiropractic manipulation most often is performed by hand. Some believe that the doctor's direct contact of the patient is important, including patient response and the doctor's ability to feel and control the amount of force. Some chiropractic techniques include adjusting instruments or devices that help to aim the force to the specific body region. These may be handheld devices (e.g., the Activator instrument; Duarte et al., 2014) or mechanized tables that will allow an impulse to drop specific sections of the table thereby imparting force to the patient (Hessell, Herzog, Conway, & McEwen, 1990), or tables that focus specific distractive forces into the spine with the doctor's touch (Cox, Fromelt, & Shreiner, 1983; Kruse & Cambron, 2011). It is thought by some that these devices facilitate motion into the desired area but are perceived as gentler by the patient. Most chiropractors have been trained in a variety of manipulative techniques; thus if a patient requires less force, this can be controlled by hand or by using a device that will deliver a reduced amount of force.

In addition to manipulation, other common chiropractic treatment methods include mobilization, exercise therapy, adjunct therapies (ultrasound, heat/cold), muscle therapies (trigger point, massage, acupressure, vibration), nutritional counseling, bracing/supports/heel lifts/taping, traction, stress reduction/biofeedback, lifestyle modification/counseling (Brantingham et al., 2012; Brantingham et al., 2013; Bryans et al., 2011; Bryans et al., 2014; M. G. Christensen & National Board of Chiropractic Examiners, 2005; Lawrence et al., 2008).

While chiropractors are focused typically on decreasing pain and increasing function, they also include health and wellness methods in their practices. During the well-patient history and examination, patients are typically screened for basic functions. These include mobility, balance, posture, strength, reflexes, mental status, and other neurological functions. Prevention measures may include smoking cessation, improving diet, and increasing healthy exercise, as well as aiming to improve motion, function, and activities of daily living.

Most patients use chiropractic care as a complement to medicine, as opposed to using it as an alternative to medicine. Some healthcare teams have found that including a doctor of chiropractic is a good fit for the patients they serve. Therefore, many chiropractors can be found working in cooperative practices and interdisciplinary clinics (Meeker, 2000; Smith, Greene, & Meeker, 2002). Chiropractic services have also been incorporated for many years into various large healthcare settings such as private hospitals (Branson, 2009), the Veterans Administration (Dunn, Green, & Gilford, 2009; Green, Johnson, & Lisi, 2009), and the Department of Defense (Goldberg et al., 2009; Green, Johnson, Lisi, & Tucker, 2009). Most chiropractors enjoy working with other healthcare providers and value having others on the healthcare team for their patients. Since the scope of chiropractic is limited, they must rely on the rest of the healthcare network to take care of their patients' other needs. When caring for those with chronic pain, medication management—particularly the chronic use of opioids—is not the only option. Chiropractic care is a recommended non-pharmacological means to reduce pain and improve function for patients in chronic pain and can assist in better managing these patients (Dorflinger et al., 2014).

SAFETY AND SIDE EFFECTS

As with any treatment that is potentially helpful, providing the most effective and safest care should be a concern. While chiropractic care is generally regarded as effective and safe, there are known expected side effects, which include soreness or discomfort and sometimes a slight worsening of symptoms, but this typically is a short-term effect. Rarely, severe adverse or unexpected consequences of care may occur. Unanticipated adverse events associated with chiropractic care have been studied, and these events (e.g., injury, death) are considered quite rare (Biller et al., 2014; Boyle, Cote, Grier, & Cassidy, 2008; Cassidy et al., 2008; Choi, Boyle, Cote, & Cassidy, 2011; Rubinstein et al., 2007; Rubinstein et al., 2008). Nonetheless, measures should be taken by the doctor of chiropractic to reduce these occurrences. With a thorough history and physical examination, if any warning signs are present, the chiropractor should choose to refer or co-manage the case with another healthcare provider. There has been a movement to encourage patients and healthcare providers to communicate better about all the treatments that they are receiving in order to reduce adverse events and improve patient management. Patient safety is always the most important factor in health care, and improved patient–provider and provider–provider communication have been demonstrated to reduce misunderstandings, miscommunications, and error (Starmer et al., 2014; Stead et al., 2009).

Although chiropractic care does not include pharmaceutical medications, some practitioners will include nutritional counseling or supplements in their course of care. Also, if a patient is taking various types of over-the-counter or prescription medications, these may interact adversely with some aspects of chiropractic care. For example, patients taking nonsteroidal anti-inflammatory medications over an extended period are at a higher risk for gastric and arterial bleeding, and care should be delivered with this in mind (Bhala et al., 2013). As well, some medications cause musculoskeletal side effects. Some people who take statins to lower cholesterol may experience more muscle pain and present for chiropractic care (Ito, Maki, Brinton, Cohen, & Jacobson, 2014; Manocha, Bansal, Gumaste, & Brangman, 2013; Mansi, Frei, Pugh, Makris, & Mortensen, 2013). Thus chiropractors must be aware of side effects of other therapies that may be confounding the expected results from chiropractic care.

The safety of mobilization and manipulation is not free of risk; however, significant side effects from these treatments have low rates of occurrence, especially when compared to other treatment options, such as over-the-counter or pharmaceutical medications. A recent study showed that patients 66–99 years of age who had a musculoskeletal complaint and received chiropractic manipulation were less likely to have an injury as a side effect than patients who had a visit with their primary care provider (Whedon, Mackenzie, Phillips, & Lurie, 2014). Others have shown similar findings for chiropractic care in adult populations (Cassidy et al., 2009).

EVIDENCE
FOR CHIROPRACTIC CARE

Chiropractic has been studied in various ways, ranging from case studies to randomized trials. However, evaluating CAM therapies may be complicated, as the practice may not coincide with traditional biomedical research models (Berman & Straus, 2004). Nonetheless, there has been an increase in evaluation of the effectiveness of chiropractic in areas that benefit the aging population.

Back and Neck Pain

Approximately 43%–60% of the adult population report back or neck pain, and the prevalence of back pain continues to increase with age (Andersson & American Academy of Orthopaedic Surgeons., 2008). Direct medical costs associated with spine-related conditions are estimated at $193.9 billion for 2002–2004 and $14.0 billion for indirect costs (e.g., lost wages) per year (Andersson & American Academy of Orthopaedic Surgeons, 2008). People over 70 may have monthly back pain (25%) or neck pain (20%), with women reporting more pain than men (Hartvigsen, Frederiksen, & Christensen, 2006a). Back pain is associated with poor physical function and depression (Hartvigsen, Frederiksen, & Christensen, 2006b). A study by Weiner et al. (2003) of a large cohort of older adults found that low back pain was common (36%) and was associated with psychological barriers to performing functional tasks.

Chiropractic is well known for helping patients with back and neck pain (Bronfort, Haas, Evans, & Bouter, 2004; Bronfort, et al., 2011; Gross et al., 2010; Maiers et al., 2014). A recent study evaluated Medicare beneficiaries with back conditions and their use of chiropractic care (Weigel, Hockenberry, Bentler, & Wolinsky, 2013). The authors stated that "chiropractic treatment has comparable effects on functional outcomes when compared with medical treatment for all Medicare beneficiaries." When included with other therapies in systematic reviews, chiropractic care has shown clinical benefit and cost-effectiveness (Clar et al., 2014; Tsertsvadze et al., 2014). The authors of one large study concluded, "Chiropractic manipulation was found to be less costly and more effective than alternative treatment compared with either physiotherapy or GP care in improving neck pain" (Tsertsvadze et al., 2014, 343).

Evidence-based guidelines on the chiropractic treatment of neck pain in adults shows support for chiropractic care. Procedures that chiropractors use, including manipulation/mobilization, manual therapies, massage, and exercise, were found to show benefit for specific types of patients with neck pain (Bryans et al., 2014). An earlier study by the same group of researchers showed that "[e]vidence suggests that chiropractic care, including spinal manipulation, improves migraine and cervicogenic headaches" (Bryans et al., 2011).

Several guidelines include chiropractic or manipulation for patients presenting with back pain. Chou et al. (2007) published a guideline on therapies for acute and chronic low back pain and concluded, "good evidence of moderate efficacy for chronic or subacute low back pain are cognitive-behavioral therapy, exercise, spinal manipulation, and interdisciplinary rehabilitation" (Chou & Huffman, 2007). Examples of systematic reviews pertaining to the effectiveness of spinal manipulation and chiropractic care for back and neck pain are included in Table 9.1.

Bone Health

Doctors of chiropractic manage patients with coexisting conditions, such as osteoporosis. Various case reports have described the management of patients or conditions arising from osteoporosis. For example, a 74-year-old man presented with acute low back pain, generalized osteoporosis, and a compression fracture. The patient was managed under chiropractic care with activity modification, postural training, exercise, and soft tissue techniques. The patient's symptoms resolved and he returned to regular daily activities after 9 weeks, and no recurrence of symptoms were reported at 1 year follow-up. (Papa, 2012) Another case describes the chiropractic management of an 83-year-old man whose back pain was complicated by other conditions (i.e., leukemia, compression fractures, osteoporosis, and degenerative joint disease). The pain and functional rating scores were improved after 8 treatments and remained stable when measured at 4 months (Roberts & Wolfe, 2012).

Typically, red flags, including age and trauma, are indications for diagnostic imaging that will help to identify osteoporosis. Once diagnosed, the DC may manage the case if mild, or choose to co-manage or refer when there are complications or the osteoporosis is severe. The primary concern is that there may be a failure to diagnose and that fractures may not necessarily be caused by manipulation but rather are not diagnosed and are then aggravated by the manipulation (Haldeman & Rubinstein, 1992). Current diagnostic imaging guidelines clearly state the decision-making pathway for when to order imaging on patients that present with or without a complaint and are at risk for osteoporosis (Bussieres, Taylor, & Peterson, 2008; Taylor & Bussieres, 2012). Recommendations regarding bone health, such as monitoring diet and exercise and providing

screening for risk of osteoporosis, have been suggested as part of routine chiropractic care (Jamison, Geraghty, Keating, & Livingstone, 1988).

Function (Mobility, Balance, Proprioception)

Balance and mobility are important factors in healthy aging and injury prevention. A systematic review evaluated the current evidence for manual therapy to improve balance and prevent falls (Holt, Haavik, & Elley, 2012). They identified 11 trials that used manual therapy and found 9 trials showed statistical improvement in some of the outcomes. Holt et al. (Holt, Noone, Short, Elley, & Haavik, 2011) performed a study on chiropractic patients to discover the prevalence of fall risk factors. In their study of 12 chiropractic practices they measured 101 patients and found that falls and injuries followed existing data for this age group. The authors suggest that chiropractic clinics identify and implement interventions with fall risk factors for these patients. Several other studies have investigated the effect of chiropractic care on balance in aging adults (Hawk, Cambron, & Pfefer, 2009; Hawk, Hyland, Rupert, Colonvega, & Hall, 2006; Hawk, Pfefer, Strunk, Ramcharan, & Uhl, 2007; Palmgren, Sandstrom, Lundqvist, & Heikkila, 2006).

Because most patients will seek chiropractic care for aches and pains, chiropractors see the results of falls or other injuries. A report from an interdisciplinary team in Canada describes how doctors of chiropractic assist screening patients over 65 years of age for risk of falls through history taking, physical examination, and team efforts to prevent fall injuries. The multidisciplinary group (e.g., medicine, physical therapy, occupational therapy, and others, including chiropractic) focuses specifically on mobility and falls and provides screening, diagnosis, and management services to elderly and disabled patients (Bauman et al., 2014).

Neurological Disorders

Chiropractic care can be supportive, rehabilitative, and can be combined with conventional care for patients with neurological disorders. Various conditions may be identified in chiropractic practices. For example, patients with back pain may report to a chiropractic clinic and through clinical examination neurological diseases, such as Parkinson's disease, may be discovered (Burton, 2008). Chiropractic

Table 9.1. Systematic Reviews Pertaining to the Effectiveness of Spinal Manipulation and Chiropractic Care for Low Back and Neck Pain

AUTHOR	CONDITION	PURPOSE OF STUDY	TYPES OF STUDIES INCLUDED/ REVIEWED, INCLUSION CRITERIA	OUTCOMES
Hidalgo, Detrembleur, Hall, Mahaudens, & Nielens, 2014	LBP	To review the effectiveness of manipulation and soft tissue therapies for LBP	11 clinical trials including those for acute/subacute (<3 months) and chronic LBP	For acute/subacute LBP there was strong evidence favoring the use of SMT over sham for decreasing pain and increasing function. For chronic LBP there was moderate to strong evidence favoring SMT over sham for decreasing pain and improving function, moderate evidence favoring manipulation + mobilization/soft tissue therapies in combination with usual medical care over therapeutic exercise and back school for decreasing pain and improving function.
Walker, French, Grant, & Green, 2011	LBP	To determine the effects of combined chiropractic interventions on pain, disability, back-related function, overall improvement, and patient satisfaction in adults	12 RCTs comparing chiropractic care (SMT + other forms of therapy) to no care or other forms of care. Acute status, subacute status, and chronic status were included.	For acute and subacute LBP, chiropractic interventions improved short- and medium-term pain compared with other treatments; no significant difference in long-term pain. Short-term improvement in disability was greater in the chiropractic group compared to other therapies; no difference in medium- and long-term disability. For chronic LBP there was no difference for combined chiropractic interventions.
Rubinstein, van Middelkoop, Assendelft, de Boer, & van Tulder, 2011	LBP	To evaluate the effectiveness of SMT for treating chronic low back pain	26 RCTs	High-quality evidence for SMT having a significant, but not clinically relevant, short-term effect on pain relief and functional status in comparison with other interventions.

Author, Year	Condition	Purpose	Studies included	Findings
Lin, Haas, Maher, Machado, & van Tulder, 2011	LBP	To investigate the cost-effectiveness of guideline-endorsed treatments for LBP	26 economic studies done at the same time as RCTs investigating treatments endorsed by the guideline of the American College of Physicians and the American Pain Society	For subacute and chronic LBP, interdisciplinary rehabilitation, exercise, acupuncture, SMT or cognitive-behavioral therapy were cost-effective. For acute LBP there was insufficient evidence on the cost-effectiveness of SMT.
Lawrence et al., 2008	LBP and LBP-related leg pain	To review the literature pertaining to the use of SMT for LBP	12 guidelines, 64 RCTs, 13 systematic reviews/meta-analyses, and 11 cohort studies were included	For acute, subacute and chronic LBP there is evidence for the use of SMT to reduce symptoms and improve function. The addition of exercise to SMT is beneficial to outcomes. There is less evidence for the use of SMT for treating sciatica and/or radiculopathy.
Chou & Huffman, 2007	LBP with or without leg pain	To review the literature for benefits and harms associated with a variety of non-pharmacological therapies for treating LBP	40 SRs and 5 RCTs on acute (LBP < 4 weeks), subacute, and chronic LBP	For acute LBP, SMT and superficial heat demonstrated fair to good evidence for small to moderate. For subacute and chronic LBP there was good evidence that exercise, spinal manipulation, and interdisciplinary rehabilitation are moderately effective. Serious harms were rare. There is insufficient evidence on the efficacy of therapies for sciatica.
Bronfort et al., 2004	LBP and NP	To assess the efficacy of SMT and mobilization for LBP and NP	43 RCTs on acute and chronic LBP or NP	For acute LBP there is moderate evidence that SMT provides more short-term pain relief than mobilization and sham. For chronic LBP there is moderate evidence that SMT is similar to NSAIDs, and more effective than placebo in the short term and physical therapy in the long term. For acute NP the evidence was inconclusive, and for chronic NP there is moderate evidence that SMT and mobilization were superior to general practitioner management for short-term pain reduction and that SMT provided similar pain relief to high-technology rehabilitative exercise in the short and long terms.

(continued)

Table 9.1. Continued

AUTHOR	CONDITION	PURPOSE OF STUDY	TYPES OF STUDIES INCLUDED/REVIEWED, INCLUSION CRITERIA	OUTCOMES
Rubinstein, Terwee, Assendelft, de Boer, & van Tulder, 2013	LBP	To assess the effectiveness of SMT for acute LBP	20 RCTs for acute LBP	There is low- to very low–quality evidence suggesting no difference in effect for SMT when compared with inert interventions, sham SMT, or as adjunct therapy for the outcomes of pain and functional status. No serious complications were observed with SMT.
C. M. Goertz, Pohlman, Vining, Brantingham, & Long, 2012	LBP	To describe literature on patient-centered outcomes following a high-velocity low-amplitude SMT in patients with LBP	38 RCTs for nonspecific LBP	SMT imparted a small but consistent treatment effect at least as large as that seen in other conservative methods of care.
Michaleff, Lin, Maher, & van Tulder, 2012	LBP, NP	To investigate the cost-effectiveness of SMT compared to other treatment options for people with NP or back pain of any duration	6 cost effectiveness/cost utility analyses	SMT was a cost-effective treatment for NP and back pain if used alone or in combination with other therapies compared to general practitioner care, exercise, and physiotherapy.
Dagenais, Gay, Tricco, Freeman, & Mayer, 2010	LBP	To assess the scientific literature related to SMT for acute LBP	14 RCTs for acute LBP	Improvements in pain with SMT were superior to various controls in 3 studies and equivalent in 3 studies in the short term, equivalent in 4 studies in the intermediate term, and equivalent in 2 studies in the long term. Superior improvements in function with SMT were noted in 1 study and equivalent in 4 RCTs in the short term and equivalent in 1 study and inferior in 1 RCT in the long term.

(continued)

Study	Condition	Objective	Design	Findings
Schroeder, Kaplan, Fischer, & Skelly, 2013	NP	To compare SMT or mobilization of the cervical spine to physical therapy or exercise for reducing NP	6 RCTs for acute and chronic NP	For acute NP, reductions in pain severity were approximately the same for both the SMT/mobilization groups and the physical therapy groups; SMT patients were more satisfied with care in short- and long-term follow-ups. For chronic NP reductions in pain severity were approximately the same for both the SMT/mobilization groups and the physical therapy groups; there were no differences in patient satisfaction.
Huisman, Speksnijder, & de Wijer, 2013	NP	To determine the efficacy of thoracic SMT for reducing pain and disability in patients with NP	10 RCTs for mechanical NP	Thoracic SMT provided the same amount of pain reduction as control therapies and as cervical SMT. Thoracic SMT was more effective in treating NP when combined with therapeutic exercise and was more effective than traditional physiotherapeutic modalities such as heat and electrical stimulation.
Cross, Kuenze, Grindstaff, & Hertel, 2011	NP	To determine the effects of thoracic SMT on pain, range of motion, and self-reported function for NP	6 RCTs for acute or subacute mechanical NP	Short-term improvement in NP and range of motion were noted for thoracic SMT.
Walser, Meserve, & Boucher, 2009	NP and a variety of other musculoskeletal problems	To determine the effects of thoracic SMT on a variety of musculoskeletal problems, including NP	9 RCTs on mechanical NP	Significant pain reduction was associated with thoracic SMT in the high-quality studies reviewed. Improvements in cervical range of motion after thoracic SMT were also reported in studies of both high and fair quality.
Vernon & Humphreys, 2008	NP	To report on the change in NP noted after a single session of SMT, mobilization, and ischemic compression	9 clinical trials on NP	SMT studies yielded mean reductions in pain of 1.89 cm on a visual analog scale with effect sizes ranging from 0.33 to 2.3. Mobilization studies demonstrated effect sizes from 0.22 to 0.36.
Vernon, Humphreys, & Hagino, 2007	NP	To evaluate the magnitude of change in pain scores in studies evaluating SMT and mobilization for NP	16 RCTs investigating chronic NP not involving whiplash or arm/head pain	NP subjects showed clinical important improvements. SMT studies showed mean effect sizes of 1.63, 1.56, and 1.22 at 7, 12, and 55+ weeks, respectively.

Table 9.1. Continued

AUTHOR	CONDITION	PURPOSE OF STUDY	TYPES OF STUDIES INCLUDED/ REVIEWED, INCLUSION CRITERIA	OUTCOMES
Hurwitz et al., 2008	NP	To review the literature on the use, effectiveness, and safety of noninvasive interventions for NP associated with whiplash and also nonspecific NP	170 studies, including RCTs and SRs for effectiveness of interventions	4 RCTs showed active therapies involving mobilization were superior to other forms of care for whiplash. 6 RCTs on cervical SMT did not show a greater pain or disability reduction in the short or long term in subacute or chronic NP when compared to other treatments.
Gross et al., 2010	NP	To determine if SMT and mobilization relieve pain or improve function, and patient satisfaction in adults with mechanical NP	27 RCTs representing 32 studies, including acute, subacute, and chronic NP with or without headache or radiculopathy	There was moderate quality evidence for intermediate effects of SMT and mobilization for pain, function, and patient satisfaction. There was low-quality evidence for short-term effects of SMT improving pain.
Vincent, Maigne, Fischhoff, Lanlo, & Dagenais, 2013	NP	To determine the effectiveness of SMT/mobilization alone or in conjunction with exercise for nonspecific NP	18 RCTs of acute, subacute, and chronic NP	For acute neck pain, thoracic SMT and electrothermal therapy were beneficial in the short term and cervical SMT was beneficial in the long term. In acute and chronic NP, SMT combined with exercise was superior to SMT alone.

| Miller et al., 2010 | NP with or without cervicogenic headache or radiculopathy | To assess if SMT or mobilization combined with exercise improved pain, function, quality of life, global perceived effect, or patient satisfaction | 17 RCTs | Greater short-term pain relief was demonstrated in high-quality studies when SMT or mobilizations were combined with exercise over exercise alone. Moderate-quality studies support the combination of SMT or mobilization with exercise for pain reduction and improved quality of life over SMT/mobilization alone for chronic NP. Low-quality evidence shows clinically important long-term improvements in pain, function/disability, and global perceived effect when SMT and mobilization and exercise are compared to no treatment. |

LBP = low back pain; RCT = randomized controlled trial; SMT = spinal manipulative therapy; SR = systematic review; NP = neck pain.

care of patients with neurological disorders may be aimed at improving or maintaining function, for example through improving mobility, decreasing pain, improving posture, and increasing physical activity.

Mental Health

The factors that influence health behaviors of patients, including beliefs and attitudes and the encouragement of the chiropractor, may provide support to those who have movement or pain avoidance concerns. Chiropractors focus on restoring motion, reducing pain, and coaching the patient to return to daily activities quickly. It is recognized that pain behaviors may result in chronic pain and chronic pain behaviors. Thus, it is important to return people back to daily activity quickly. Mental health issues are not commonly treated by chiropractors; the NBCE reports a very small percentage of chiropractors stating that they treat psychological disorders (Christensen et al., 2010).

However, there is a proposed connection between the health of the body and the mind, and chiropractors often work with patients to become more aware of this relationship. Chiropractors provide education and care that helps patients reduce stressful aspects of their daily activities that may be negatively affecting their health. Managing stress, learning to use diaphragmatic breathing, meditation, mindfulness, and other forms of mind-body methods are often employed by chiropractors to assist patients with increase in function, pain management, and approach toward health. Chiropractic care also focuses on encouraging exercise, sleep hygiene, and helping patients perform activities they enjoy and increasing well-being.

Non-musculoskeletal Conditions

Although chiropractic is most known for helping musculoskeletal conditions, there have been claims that it can help with visceral conditions. For example, some have suggested that chiropractic may have a role in the assistance of urinary incontinence in the elderly (Keating, Jr., Schulte, & Miller, 1988). There have been no trials to demonstrate effectiveness; however, a case series of 21 patients ranging from 13 to 90 years of age describes chiropractic techniques to address stress urinary incontinence. The treatment consisted of manipulative therapy and myofascial trigger point therapy. They noted that for those who responded to treatment, their improvements were retained (Cuthbert & Rosner, 2012). Zhang et al. (2006) published a case series of chiropractic care for urinary incontinence in the elderly. Thirteen patients were monitored for incontinence over 8 weeks of care. The symptoms were self-reported and included decreased urinary frequency at night and improved bladder control (Zhang, Haselden, & Tepe, 2006). It is possible that the care influenced psychological or physiological mechanisms associated with urinary incontinence. However, without more controlled studies, it is not possible to know what mechanisms are involved.

Heart and Blood Pressure

A few studies have investigated the possible effects of chiropractic care and its influence on blood pressure. An early study evaluated the effects of chiropractic manipulation of the thoracic spine on blood pressure and anxiety (Yates, Lamping, Abram, & Wright, 1988). This exploratory study of 21 patients found significant short-term reduction in systolic and diastolic pressure and reduced anxiety. Another preliminary study evaluated the effect of chiropractic manipulation on blood pressure and found a statistical, although not clinical, significance in findings for young subjects (McKnight & DeBoer, 1988). Bakris et al. (2007) performed an 8-week pilot study to evaluate the effects of chiropractic manipulation of the upper cervical spine on heart rate and arterial blood pressure. They found that the experimental group had a significant drop in blood pressure compared to the control group. A matched-pair clinical trial by Dimmick et al. (Dimmick, Young, & Newell, 2006) evaluated the effects of chiropractic manipulation in normotensive subjects. They found there was a difference between groups in systolic blood pressure; however, this was a small non-randomized trial. A randomized trial by Goertz et al. (C. H. Goertz, Grimm, Svendsen, & Grandits, 2002) compared chiropractic manipulation with dietary changes to dietary changes alone and the effects on blood pressure for stage 1 hypertension. They found that there were no differences between groups at the end of this 4-week trial. It is not clear what the confounders might be in such studies. It is possible that chiropractic treatment reduces pain or has a calming effect, which may have an influence on blood pressure findings. However, larger experimental trials are needed before recommendations can be made.

Portal of Entry

Chiropractors may act as portal of entry or primary care practitioners, depending upon their location (Myburgh, Christensen, & Fogh-Schultz, 2014; Smith & Carber, 2009). Some have observed that chiropractors practicing in rural areas provide more care services than their urban counterparts (Lind, Diehr, Grembowski, & Lafferty, 2009). There have been reports of older adults presenting with serious conditions identified by their chiropractor and referred for medical management. For example, a 65-year-old patient who presented with back and abdominal pain was evaluated, but a suspicion of prostate cancer was raised. The patient was referred to a medical facility and studies confirmed prostate cancer. Thus, the chiropractor identified the condition and facilitated the patient's entry into the healthcare system (T. L. Johnson, Jr., 2010). For a case of a 69-year-old patient presenting with back pain, the chiropractor identified and referred the patient, who was confirmed to have renal cell carcinoma (Rectenwald, 2008). An 85-year-old woman with neck, back, and hip pain presented with musculoskeletal findings related to degenerative spinal disease and stenosis. During the chiropractic evaluation, additional neurological findings were noted, and the patient was immediately transported to the emergency department, where it was confirmed she was experiencing ischemic stroke (Liebich & Reinke, 2014). Thus, chiropractic care can be an important part of the healthcare network.

Overall Health and Patient Satisfaction

Chiropractic is known for consistently high patient satisfaction rates (Gaumer, 2006; Gemmell & Hayes, 2001; Verhoef, Page, & Waddell, 1997), and there is increased interest in the overall impact of chiropractic care on health and satisfaction. A study of Medicare beneficiaries looked at the effect of chiropractic care on functional measures, self-rated health measures, and satisfaction with care. The authors concluded there was a "protective effect of chiropractic care against 1-year declines in functional and self-rated health among Medicare beneficiaries with spine conditions, and indications that chiropractic users have higher satisfaction with follow-up care" (Weigel, Hockenberry, & Wolinsky, 2014, 542). Another study showed that chiropractic care for back complaints had a protective effect. This study of older Medicare beneficiaries showed protection against decline in activites of daily living (ADLs) and self-rated health (Weigel, Hockenberry, Bentler, & Wolinsky, 2014).

SUMMARY

Since its humble beginnings as an alternative to medical care in the late 1800s, the chiropractic profession has come a long way in developing its science and evidence base. With undergraduate and graduate training of approximately 7 or more years and licensure or recognition in many countries, chiropractors can provide a complementary approach to some of the many of the common presenting musculoskeletal conditions, such as back pain, neck pain, and headache. Overall, the procedures used in chiropractic care have been shown to be safe, and the strength of evidence for chiropractic effectiveness, predominantly in musculoskeletal conditions, continues to grow. Chiropractic approaches to the aging patient predominantly focus on structure and function (e.g., manipulation, education); however, chiropractic care can incorporate other aspects of prevention and wellness (e.g., exercise, rehabilitation, nutrition).

DISCLOSURE STATEMENTS

Claire Johnson is a professor at the National University of Health Sciences and is the Editor-in-Chief for the *Journal of Manipulative and Physiological Therapeutics*. She is a chiropractor and was previously a certified massage therapist. She is a member of the American Public Health Association and the American Chiropractic Association. She sits on the NCMIC Mutual Holding Company Board of Directors and the advisory committee for Medical Evidence Evaluation Advisory Committee (MEEAC), Division of Workers' Compensation, California. She is a contractor with the Association of Chiropractic Colleges and the World Federation of Chiropractic for peer review and scientific conference services. She has no other conflicts to disclose.

Bart Green is a chiropractor and serves as the Editor-in-Chief of the *Journal of Chiropractic Education* and is the Associate Editor in the publications department of the National University of Health Sciences. He provides continuing education lectures for chiropractors and receives compensation for these programs. He has no other conflicts to disclose.

REFERENCES

Andersson, G., & American Academy of Orthopaedic Surgeons. (2008). *The burden of musculoskeletal diseases in the United States: prevalence, societal, and economic cost.* Rosemont, IL: American Academy of Orthopaedic Surgeons.

Bakris, G., Dickholtz, M., Sr., Meyer, P. M., Kravitz, G., Avery, E., Miller, M., . . . Bell, B. (2007). Atlas vertebra realignment and achievement of arterial pressure goal in hypertensive patients: a pilot study. *J Hum Hypertens, 21*(5), 347–352. doi: 1002133 [pii]10.1038/sj.jhh.1002133

Barnes, P. M., Bloom, B., & Nahin, R. L. (2008). Complementary and alternative medicine use among adults and children: United States, 2007. *Natl Health Stat Report, 12,* 1–23.

Bauman, C. A., Milligan, J. D., Patel, T., Pritchard, S., Labreche, T., Dillon-Martin, S., . . . Riva, J. J. (2014). Community-based falls prevention: lessons from an Interprofessional Mobility Clinic. *J Can Chiropr Assoc, 58*(3), 300–311.

Berman, J. D., & Straus, S. E. (2004). Implementing a research agenda for complementary and alternative medicine. *Annu Rev Med, 55,* 239–254. doi: 10.1146/annurev.med.55.091902.103657

Bhala, N., Emberson, J., Merhi, A., Abramson, S., Arber, N., Baron, J. A., . . . Baigent, C. (2013). Vascular and upper gastrointestinal effects of non-steroidal anti-inflammatory drugs: meta-analyses of individual participant data from randomised trials. *Lancet, 382*(9894), 769–779. doi: 10.1016/S0140-6736(13)60 900-9S0140-6736(13)60900-9 [pii]

Biller, J., Sacco, R. L., Albuquerque, F. C., Demaerschalk, B. M., Fayad, P., Long, P. H., . . . Tirschwell, D. L. (2014). Cervical arterial dissections and association with cervical manipulative therapy: a statement for healthcare professionals from the american heart association/american stroke association. *Stroke, 45*(10), 3155–3174. doi: 10.1161/STR.00000000000000 16STR.0000000000000016 [pii]

Boyle, E., Cote, P., Grier, A. R., & Cassidy, J. D. (2008). Examining vertebrobasilar artery stroke in two Canadian provinces. *Spine (Phila Pa 1976), 33*(4 Suppl), S170–175. doi: 10.1097/ BRS.0b013e31816454e 000007632- 200802151-00018 [pii]

Branson, R. A. (2009). Hospital-based chiropractic integration within a large private hospital system in Minnesota: a 10-year example. *J Manipulative Physiol Ther, 32*(9), 740–748. doi: 10.1016/j.jmpt. 2009.10.014S0161-4754(09)00278-4 [pii]

Brantingham, J. W., Bonnefin, D., Perle, S. M., Cassa, T. K., Globe, G., Pribicevic, M., . . . Korporaal, C. (2012). Manipulative therapy for lower extremity conditions: update of a literature review. *J Manipulative Physiol Ther, 35*(2), 127–166. doi: 10.1016/j.jmpt.2012.0 1.001S0161-4754(12)00004-8 [pii]

Brantingham, J. W., Cassa, T. K., Bonnefin, D., Pribicevic, M., Robb, A., Pollard, H., . . . Korporaal, C. (2013). Manipulative and multimodal therapy for upper extremity and temporomandibular disorders: a systematic review. *J Manipulative Physiol Ther, 36*(3), 143–201. doi: 10.1016/j.jmpt. 2013.04.001S0161-4754(13)00053-5 [pii]

Bronfort, G., Evans, R., Anderson, A. V., Svendsen, K. H., Bracha, Y., & Grimm, R. H. (2012). Spinal manipulation, medication, or home exercise with advice for acute and subacute neck pain: a randomized trial. *Ann Intern Med, 156*(1 Pt 1), 1–10. doi: 10.7326/0003- 4819-156-1- 201201030- 00002156/1_Part_1/1 [pii]

Bronfort, G., Haas, M., Evans, R. L., & Bouter, L. M. (2004). Efficacy of spinal manipulation and mobilization for low back pain and neck pain: a systematic review and best evidence synthesis. *Spine J, 4*(3), 335–356. doi: 10.1016/j.spinee.2003 .06.002S1529943003001773 [pii]

Bronfort, G., Hondras, M. A., Schulz, C. A., Evans, R. L., Long, C. R., & Grimm, R. (2014). Spinal manipulation and home exercise with advice for subacute and chronic back-related leg pain: a trial with adaptive allocation. *Ann Intern Med, 161*(6), 381–391. doi: 10.7326/ M14-00061905126 [pii]

Bronfort, G., Maiers, M. J., Evans, R. L., Schulz, C. A., Bracha, Y., Svendsen, K. H., . . . Transfeldt, E. E. (2011). Supervised exercise, spinal manipulation, and home exercise for chronic low back pain: a randomized clinical trial. *Spine J, 11*(7), 585–598. doi: 10.1016/j.spinee.2011.0 1.036S1529-9430(11)00128-8 [pii]

Bryans, R., Decina, P., Descarreaux, M., Duranleau, M., Marcoux, H., Potter, B., . . . White, E. (2014). Evidence-based guidelines for the chiropractic treatment of adults with neck pain. *J Manipulative Physiol Ther, 37*(1), 42–63. doi: 10.1016/j.jmpt.20 13.08.010S0161-4754(13)00237-6 [pii]

Bryans, R., Descarreaux, M., Duranleau, M., Marcoux, H., Potter, B., Ruegg, R., . . . White, E. (2011). Evidence-based guidelines for the chiropractic treatment of adults with headache. *J Manipulative Physiol Ther, 34*(5), 274–289. doi: 10.1016/j.jmpt. 2011.04.008S0161-4754(11)00068-6 [pii]

Burton, R. R. (2008). Parkinson's disease without tremor masquerading as mechanical back pain; a case report. *J Can Chiropr Assoc, 52*(3), 185–192.

Bussieres, A. E., Taylor, J. A., & Peterson, C. (2008). Diagnostic imaging practice guidelines for musculoskeletal complaints in adults-an evidence-based approach-part 3: spinal disorders. *J Manipulative Physiol Ther, 31*(1), 33–88. doi: 10.1016/j.jmpt.2007.1 1.003S0161-4754(07)00314-4 [pii]

Cannon, W. B. (1932). *The wisdom of the body.* New York: W. W. Norton.

Cassidy, J. D., Boyle, E., Cote, P., He, Y., Hogg-Johnson, S., Silver, F. L., & Bondy, S. J. (2008). Risk of vertebrobasilar stroke and chiropractic care: results of a population-based case-control and case-crossover study. *Spine (Phila Pa 1976), 33*(4 Suppl), S176–183. doi: 10.1097/BRS. 0b013e318 164460000007632- 200802151- 00019 [pii]

Cassidy, J. D., Boyle, E., Cote, P., He, Y., Hogg-Johnson, S., Silver, F. L., & Bondy, S. J. (2009). Risk of vertebrobasilar stroke and chiropractic care: results of a population-based case-control and case-crossover study. *J Manipulative Physiol Ther, 32*(2 Suppl), S201–208. doi: 10.1016/j.jmpt.2008.1 1.020S0161-4754(08)00347-3 [pii]

Chang, M. (2014). The chiropractic scope of practice in the United States: a cross-sectional survey. *J Manipulative Physiol Ther, 37*(6), 363–376. doi: 10.1016/j.jmpt.2014.0 5.003S0161-4754(14)00091-8 [pii]

Choi, S., Boyle, E., Cote, P., & Cassidy, J. D. (2011). A population-based case-series of Ontario patients who develop a vertebrobasilar artery stroke after seeing a chiropractor. *J Manipulative Physiol Ther, 34*(1), 15–22. doi: 10.1016/j.jmpt.2010.1 1.001S0161-4754(10)00324-6 [pii]

Chou, R., & Huffman, L. H. (2007). Nonpharmacologic therapies for acute and chronic low back pain: a review of the evidence for an American Pain Society/American College of Physicians clinical practice guideline. *Ann Intern Med, 147*(7), 492–504. doi: 147/7/492 [pii]

Christensen, M.G., Kollasch, M.W., Hyland, J.K. (2010). *Practice analysis of chiropractic 2010.* Greeley: National Board of Chiropractic Examiners.

Christensen, M. G., & National Board of Chiropractic Examiners. (2005). *Job analysis of chiropractic 2005: a project report, survey analysis, and summary of the practice of chiropractic within the United States.* Greeley, CO: National Board of Chiropractic Examiners.

Clar, C., Tsertsvadze, A., Court, R., Hundt, G. L., Clarke, A., & Sutcliffe, P. (2014). Clinical effectiveness of manual therapy for the management of musculoskeletal and non-musculoskeletal conditions: systematic review and update of UK evidence report. *Chiropr Man Therap, 22*(1), 12. doi: 10.1186/2045-709X-22-122045- 709X-22-12 [pii]

Coulter, I., Adams, A., Coggan, P., Wilkes, M., & Gonyea, M. (1998). A comparative study of chiropractic and medical education. *Altern Ther Health Med, 4*(5), 64–75.

Cox, J. M., Fromelt, K. A., & Shreiner, S. (1983). Chiropractic statistical survey of 100 consecutive low back pain patients. *J Manipulative Physiol Ther, 6*(3), 117–128.

Cross, K. M., Kuenze, C., Grindstaff, T. L., & Hertel, J. (2011). Thoracic spine thrust manipulation improves pain, range of motion, and self-reported function in patients with mechanical neck pain: a systematic review. *J Orthop Sports Phys Ther, 41*(9), 633–642. doi: 10.2519/jospt.2011.36702620 [pii]

Cuthbert, S. C., & Rosner, A. L. (2012). Conservative chiropractic management of urinary incontinence using applied kinesiology: a retrospective case-series report. *J Chiropr Med, 11*(1), 49–57. doi: 10.1016/j.jcm.2011.1 0.002S1556-3707(12)00002-8 [pii]

Dagenais, S., Gay, R. E., Tricco, A. C., Freeman, M. D., & Mayer, J. M. (2010). NASS Contemporary concepts in spine care: spinal manipulation therapy for acute low back pain. *Spine J, 10*(10), 918–940. doi: 10.1016/j.spinee.2010.0 7.389S1529-9430(10)00942-3 [pii]

Davis, M. A., Martin, B. I., Coulter, I. D., & Weeks, W. B. (2013). US spending on complementary and alternative medicine during 2002–08 plateaued, suggesting role in reformed health system. *Health Aff (Millwood), 32*(1), 45–52. doi: 10.1377/hlthaff.2011.032132/1/45 [pii]

Davis, M. A., Sirovich, B. E., & Weeks, W. B. (2010). Utilization and expenditures on chiropractic care in the United States from 1997 to 2006. *Health Serv Res, 45*(3), 748–761. doi: 10.1111/j.1475-6773.2009.01067. xHESR1067 [pii]

Dehen, M. D., Whalen, W. M., Farabaugh, R. J., & Hawk, C. (2010). Consensus terminology for stages of care: acute, chronic, recurrent, and wellness. *J Manipulative Physiol Ther, 33*(6), 458–463. doi: 10.1016/j.jmpt.2010.0 6.007S0161-4754(10)00154-5 [pii]

Dimmick, K. R., Young, M. F., & Newell, D. (2006). Chiropractic manipulation affects the difference between arterial systolic blood pressures on the left and right in normotensive subjects. *J Manipulative Physiol Ther, 29*(1), 46–50. doi: S0161-4754(05)00348-9 [pii]10.1016/j.jmpt.2005.11.006

Dorflinger, L., Moore, B., Goulet, J., Becker, W., Heapy, A. A., Sellinger, J. J., & Kerns, R. D. (2014). A partnered approach to opioid management, guideline concordant care and the stepped care model of pain management. *J Gen Intern Med, 29*(Suppl 4), 870–876. doi: 10.1007/s11606-014-3019-2

Duarte, F. C., Kolberg, C., Barros, R. R., Silva, V. G., Gehlen, G., Vassoler, J. M., & Partata, W. A. (2014). Evaluation of peak force of a manually operated chiropractic adjusting instrument with an adapter for use in animals. *J Manipulative Physiol Ther, 37*(4), 236–241. doi: 10.1016/j.jmpt.2014.02.004S0161-4754(14)00058-X [pii]

Dunn, A. S., Green, B. N., & Gilford, S. (2009). An analysis of the integration of chiropractic services within the United States military and veterans' health care systems. *J Manipulative Physiol Ther, 32*(9), 749–757. doi: 10.1016/j.jmpt.2009.10.009S0161-4754(09)00273-5 [pii]

Eisenberg, D. M., Davis, R. B., Ettner, S. L., Appel, S., Wilkey, S., Van Rompay, M., & Kessler, R. C. (1998). Trends in alternative medicine use in the United States, 1990–1997: results of a follow-up national survey. *JAMA, 280*(18), 1569–1575. doi: joc80870 [pii]

Gaumer, G. (2006). Factors associated with patient satisfaction with chiropractic care: survey and review of the literature. *J Manipulative Physiol Ther, 29*(6), 455–462. doi: S0161-4754(06)00158-8 [pii]10.1016/j.jmpt.2006.06.013

Gemmell, H. A., & Hayes, B. M. (2001). Patient satisfaction with chiropractic physicians in an independent physicians' association. *J Manipulative Physiol Ther, 24*(9), 556–559. doi: S0161-4754(01)92370-X [pii]10.1067/mmt.2001.118980

Goertz, C. H., Grimm, R. H., Svendsen, K., & Grandits, G. (2002). Treatment of Hypertension with Alternative Therapies (THAT) Study: a randomized clinical trial. *J Hypertens, 20*(10), 2063–2068.

Goertz, C. M., Pohlman, K. A., Vining, R. D., Brantingham, J. W., & Long, C. R. (2012). Patient-centered outcomes of high-velocity, low-amplitude spinal manipulation for low back pain: a systematic review. *J Electromyogr Kinesiol, 22*(5), 670–691. doi: 10.1016/j.jelekin.2012.03.006S1050-6411(12)00056-9 [pii]

Goldberg, C. K., Green, B., Moore, J., Wyatt, M., Boulanger, L., Belnap, B., . . . Donaldson, D. S. (2009). Integrated musculoskeletal rehabilitation care at a comprehensive combat and complex casualty care program. *J Manipulative Physiol Ther, 32*(9), 781–791. doi: 10.1016/j.jmpt.2009.10.010S0161-4754(09)00274-7 [pii]

Green, B. N., & Johnson, C. D. (November 15–19, 2014). *Most common conditions presenting to the top provider-based complementary and alternative medicine therapies in the US adult population: 2012 National Health Interview Survey.* Paper presented at the 142nd Annual Meeting and Exposition of the American Public Health Association, New Orleans, LA. Retrieved November 21, 2014, from https://apha.confex.com/apha/142am/webprogram/Paper308630.html).

Green, B. N., Johnson, C. D., & Lisi, A. J. (2009). Chiropractic in U.S. military and veterans' health care. *Mil Med, 174*(6), vi–vii.

Green, B. N., Johnson, C. D., Lisi, A. J., & Tucker, J. (2009). Chiropractic practice in military and veterans health care: the state of the literature. *J Can Chiropr Assoc, 53*(3), 194–204.

Gross, A., Miller, J., D'Sylva, J., Burnie, S. J., Goldsmith, C. H., Graham, N., . . . Hoving, J. L. (2010). Manipulation or mobilisation for neck pain: a Cochrane Review. *Man Ther, 15*(4), 315–333. doi: 10.1016/j.math.2010.04.002S1356-689X(10)00073-1 [pii]

Haldeman, S., & Rubinstein, S. M. (1992). Compression fractures in patients undergoing spinal manipulative therapy. *J Manipulative Physiol Ther, 15*(7), 450–454.

Hartvigsen, J., Frederiksen, H., & Christensen, K. (2006a). Back and neck pain in seniors-prevalence and impact. *Eur Spine J, 15*(6), 802–806. doi: 10.1007/s00586-005-0983-6

Hartvigsen, J., Frederiksen, H., & Christensen, K. (2006b). Physical and mental function and incident low back pain in seniors: a population-based two-year prospective study of 1387 Danish Twins aged 70 to 100 years. *Spine (Phila Pa 1976), 31*(14), 1628–1632. doi: 0.1097/01.brs.0000222021.00531.ea00007632-200606150-00021 [pii]

Hawk, C. (1998). Chiropractic: more than spinal manipulation. *J Chiropr Humanit, 8,* 71–76.

Hawk, C., Cambron, J. A., & Pfefer, M. T. (2009). Pilot study of the effect of a limited and extended course of chiropractic care on balance, chronic pain, and dizziness in older adults. *J Manipulative Physiol Ther, 32*(6), 438–447. doi: 10.1016/j.jmpt.2009.06.008S0161-4754(09)00161-4 [pii]

Hawk, C., Hyland, J. K., Rupert, R., Colonvega, M., & Hall, S. (2006). Assessment of balance and risk for falls in a sample of community-dwelling adults aged 65 and older. *Chiropr Osteopat, 14,* 3. doi: 1746-1340-14-3 [pii]10.1186/1746-1340-14-3

Hawk, C., Pfefer, M. T., Strunk, R., Ramcharan, M., & Uhl, N. (2007). Feasibility study of short-term effects of chiropractic manipulation on older adults with impaired balance. *J Chiropr Med, 6*(4), 121–131. doi: 10.1016/j.jcme.2007.0 8.002S0899-3467(07)00102-4 [pii]

Hawk, C., Schneider, M., Dougherty, P., Gleberzon, B. J., & Killinger, L. Z. (2010). Best practices recommendations for chiropractic care for older adults: results of a consensus process. *J Manipulative Physiol Ther, 33*(6), 464–473. doi: 10.1016/j.jmpt.2010.0 6.010S0161-4754(10)00157-0 [pii]

Hessell, B. W., Herzog, W., Conway, P. J., & McEwen, M. C. (1990). Experimental measurement of the force exerted during spinal manipulation using the Thompson technique. *J Manipulative Physiol Ther, 13*(8), 448–453.

Hidalgo, B., Detrembleur, C., Hall, T., Mahaudens, P., & Nielens, H. (2014). The efficacy of manual therapy and exercise for different stages of non-specific low back pain: an update of systematic reviews. *J Man Manip Ther, 22*(2), 59–74. doi: 10.1179/2042618613Y.0000000041164 [pii]

Holt, K. R., Haavik, H., & Elley, C. R. (2012). The effects of manual therapy on balance and falls: a systematic review. *J Manipulative Physiol Ther, 35*(3), 227–234. doi: 10.1016/j.jmpt.2012.0 1.007S0161-4754(12)00028-0 [pii]

Holt, K. R., Noone, P. L., Short, K., Elley, C. R., & Haavik, H. (2011). Fall risk profile and quality-of-life status of older chiropractic patients. *J Manipulative Physiol Ther, 34*(2), 78–87. doi: 10.1016/j.jmpt.2010.1 2.010S0161-4754(10)00362-3 [pii]

Huisman, P. A., Speksnijder, C. M., & de Wijer, A. (2013). The effect of thoracic spine manipulation on pain and disability in patients with non-specific neck pain: a systematic review. *Disabil Rehabil, 35*(20), 1677–1685. doi: 10.3109/09638288.2012.750689

Hurwitz, E. L., Carragee, E. J., van der Velde, G., Carroll, L. J., Nordin, M., Guzman, J., . . . Haldeman, S. (2008). Treatment of neck pain: noninvasive interventions: results of the Bone and Joint Decade 2000–2010 Task Force on Neck Pain and Its Associated Disorders. *Spine (Phila Pa 1976), 33*(4 Suppl), S123–152. doi: 10.1097/BRS. 0b013e3181644 b1d00007632- 200802151- 00016 [pii]

Ito, M. K., Maki, K. C., Brinton, E. A., Cohen, J. D., & Jacobson, T. A. (2014). Muscle symptoms in statin users, associations with cytochrome P450, and membrane transporter inhibitor use: a subanalysis of the USAGE study. *J Clin Lipidol, 8*(1), 69–76. doi: 10.1016/j.jacl.2013.1 0.006S1933-2874(13)00306-1 [pii]

Jamison, J. R., Geraghty, B., Keating, G., & Livingstone, K. (1988). Osteoporosis screening and prevention in the chiropractic clinic. *J Manipulative Physiol Ther, 11*(5), 390–395.

Johnson, C. (2007). Poverty and human development: contributions from and callings to the chiropractic profession. *J Manipulative Physiol Ther, 30*(8), 551–556. doi: S0161-4754(07)00303-X [pii]10.1016/j. jmpt.2007.10.001

Johnson, C. (2010). Reflecting on 115 years: the chiropractic profession's philosophical path. *J Chiropr Humanit, 17*(1), 1–5. doi: 10.1016/j.echu. 2010.11.001S1556-3499(10)00034-3 [pii]

Johnson, C., Baird, R., Dougherty, P. E., Globe, G., Green, B. N., Haneline, M., . . . Smith, M. (2008). Chiropractic and public health: current state and future vision. *J Manipulative Physiol Ther, 31*(6), 397–410. doi: 10.1016/j.jmpt.2008.0 7.001S0161-4754(08)00178-4 [pii]

Johnson, C., & Green, B. N. (2009). Public health, wellness, prevention, and health promotion: considering the role of chiropractic and determinants of health. *J Manipulative Physiol Ther, 32*(6), 405–412. doi: 10.1016/j.jmpt.2009.0 7.001S0161-4754(09)00180-8 [pii]

Johnson, T. L., Jr. (2010). Abdominal and back pain in a 65-year-old patient with metastatic prostate cancer. *J Chiropr Med, 9*(1), 11–16. doi: 10.1016/j. jcm.2009.12.004S1556-3707(10)00005-2 [pii]

Kaptchuk, T. J., & Eisenberg, D. M. (1998). Chiropractic: origins, controversies, and contributions. *Arch Intern Med, 158*(20), 2215–2224.

Keating, J. C. (2002). The meanings of innate. *J Can Chiropr Assoc, 46*(1), 4–10.

Keating, J. C., Jr., Schulte, E. A., & Miller, E. (1988). Conservative care of urinary incontinence in the elderly. *J Manipulative Physiol Ther, 11*(4), 300–308.

Kruse, R. A., & Cambron, J. (2011). Chiropractic management of postsurgical lumbar spine pain: a retrospective study of 32 cases. *J Manipulative Physiol Ther, 34*(6), 408–412. doi: 10.1016/j.jmpt.2011.0 5.011S0161-4754(11)00119-9 [pii]

Lawrence, D. J., Meeker, W., Branson, R., Bronfort, G., Cates, J. R., Haas, M., . . . Hawk, C. (2008).

Chiropractic management of low back pain and low back-related leg complaints: a literature synthesis. *J Manipulative Physiol Ther,* *31*(9), 659–674. doi: 10.1016/j.jmpt.2008.1 0.007S0161-4754(08)00277-7 [pii]

Liebich, J. M., & Reinke, T. S. (2014). Presentation of an 85-year-old woman with musculoskeletal pain to a chiropractic clinic: a case of ischemic stroke. *J Chiropr Med,* *13*(1), 49–54. doi: 10.1016/j.jcm.20 14.01.005S1556-3707(14)00006-6 [pii]

Lin, C. W., Haas, M., Maher, C. G., Machado, L. A., & van Tulder, M. W. (2011). Cost-effectiveness of guideline-endorsed treatments for low back pain: a systematic review. *Eur Spine J,* *20*(7), 1024–1038. doi: 10.1007/s00586-010-1676-3

Lind, B. K., Diehr, P. K., Grembowski, D. E., & Lafferty, W. E. (2009). Chiropractic use by urban and rural residents with insurance coverage. *J Rural Health,* *25*(3), 253–258. doi: 10.1111/ j.1748-0361.2009.00227.xJRH227 [pii]

Maiers, M., Bronfort, G., Evans, R., Hartvigsen, J., Svendsen, K., Bracha, Y., . . . Grimm, R. (2014). Spinal manipulative therapy and exercise for seniors with chronic neck pain. *Spine J,* *14*(9), 1879–1889. doi: 10.1016/j.spinee.2013.1 0.035S1529-9430(13)01630-6 [pii]

Manocha, D., Bansal, N., Gumaste, P., & Brangman, S. (2013). Safety profile of high-dose statin therapy in geriatric patients with stroke. *South Med J,* *106*(12), 658–664. doi: 10.1097/ SMJ.00000000000 0002400007611- 201312000-00003 [pii]

Mansi, I., Frei, C. R., Pugh, M. J., Makris, U., & Mortensen, E. M. (2013). Statins and musculoskeletal conditions, arthropathies, and injuries. *JAMA Intern Med,* *173*(14), 1–10. doi: 10.1001/jamainternmed.2013.61841691918 [pii]

McKnight, M. E., & DeBoer, K. F. (1988). Preliminary study of blood pressure changes in normotensive subjects undergoing chiropractic care. *J Manipulative Physiol Ther,* *11*(4), 261–266.

Meeker, W. C. (2000). Public demand and the integration of complementary and alternative medicine in the US health care system. *J Manipulative Physiol Ther,* *23*(2), 123–126. doi: S0161-4754(00)90081-2 [pii]

Michaleff, Z. A., Lin, C. W., Maher, C. G., & van Tulder, M. W. (2012). Spinal manipulation epidemiology: systematic review of cost effectiveness studies. *J Electromyogr Kinesiol,* *22*(5), 655–662. doi: 10.1016/j.jelekin.2012.0 2.011S1050-6411(12)00042-9 [pii]

Miller, J., Gross, A., D'Sylva, J., Burnie, S. J., Goldsmith, C. H., Graham, N., . . . Hoving, J. L.

(2010). Manual therapy and exercise for neck pain: a systematic review. *Man Ther.,* *15*(4), 334–354. doi: S1356-689X(10)00034-2 [pii]10.1016/j.math.2010.02.007

Morin, C., & Aubin, A. (2014). Primary reasons for osteopathic consultation: a prospective survey in Quebec. *PLoS One,* *9*(9), e106259. doi: 10.1371/ journal.pone.0106259PONE-D-13-48201 [pii]

Myburgh, C., Christensen, H. W., & Fogh-Schultz, A. L. (2014). Chiropractor perceptions and practices regarding interprofessional service delivery in the Danish primary care context. *J Interprof Care,* *28*(2), 166–167. doi: 10.3109/13561820.2013.847408

Palmgren, P. J., Sandstrom, P. J., Lundqvist, F. J., & Heikkila, H. (2006). Improvement after chiropractic care in cervicocephalic kinesthetic sensibility and subjective pain intensity in patients with nontraumatic chronic neck pain. *J Manipulative Physiol Ther,* *29*(2), 100–106. doi: S0161-4754(05)00365-9 [pii]10.1016/j. jmpt.2005.12.002

Papa, J. A. (2012). Conservative management of a lumbar compression fracture in an osteoporotic patient: a case report. *J Can Chiropr Assoc,* *56*(1), 29–39.

Rectenwald, R. (2008). A case study of back pain and renal cell carcinoma. *J Chiropr Med,* *7*(1), 24–27. doi: 10.1016/j.jcme.2008.0 1.001S0899-3467(08)00005-0 [pii]

Roberts, J. A., & Wolfe, T. M. (2012). Chiropractic spinal manipulative therapy for a geriatric patient with low back pain and comorbidities of cancer, compression fractures, and osteoporosis. *J Chiropr Med,* *11*(1), 16–23. doi: 10.1016/j.jcm.2011.0 5.001S1556-3707(11)00167-2 [pii]

Rubinstein, S. M., Leboeuf-Yde, C., Knol, D. L., de Koekkoek, T. E., Pfeifle, C. E., & van Tulder, M. W. (2007). The benefits outweigh the risks for patients undergoing chiropractic care for neck pain: a prospective, multicenter, cohort study. *J Manipulative Physiol Ther,* *30*(6), 408–418. doi: S0161-4754(07)00178-9 [pii]10.1016/j. jmpt.2007.04.013

Rubinstein, S. M., Leboeuf-Yde, C., Knol, D. L., de Koekkoek, T. E., Pfeifle, C. E., & van Tulder, M. W. (2008). Predictors of adverse events following chiropractic care for patients with neck pain. *J Manipulative Physiol Ther,* *31*(2), 94–103. doi: 10.1016/j.jmpt.2007.1 2.006S0161-4754(07)00339-9 [pii]

Rubinstein, S. M., Terwee, C. B., Assendelft, W. J., de Boer, M. R., & van Tulder, M. W. (2013). Spinal manipulative therapy for acute low back pain: an update of the cochrane review. *Spine*

(Phila Pa 1976), 38(3), E158–177. doi: 10.1097/
BRS.0b013e31827dd89d

Rubinstein, S. M., van Middelkoop, M., Assendelft, W. J., de Boer, M. R., & van Tulder, M. W. (2011). Spinal manipulative therapy for chronic low-back pain: an update of a Cochrane review. Spine (Phila Pa 1976), 36(13), E825–846. doi: 10.1097/BRS. 0b013e3182197 fe100007632- 201106010- 00016 [pii]

Schroeder, J., Kaplan, L., Fischer, D. J., & Skelly, A. C. (2013). The outcomes of manipulation or mobilization therapy compared with physical therapy or exercise for neck pain: a systematic review. Evid Based Spine Care J, 4(1), 30–41. doi: 10.1055/s-0033-134160504030 [pii]

Shekelle, P. G., Adams, A. H., Chassin, M. R., Hurwitz, E. L., & Brook, R. H. (1992). Spinal manipulation for low-back pain. Ann Intern Med, 117(7), 590–598.

Shekelle, P. G., & Brook, R. H. (1991). A community-based study of the use of chiropractic services. Am J Public Health, 81(4), 439–442.

Smith, M., & Carber, L. A. (2009). Survey of US chiropractors' perceptions about their clinical role as specialist or generalist. J Chiropr Humanit, 16(1), 21–25. doi: 10.1016/j.echu.2010.0 2.009S1556-3499(10)00010-0 [pii]

Smith, M., Greene, B. R., & Meeker, W. (2002). The CAM movement and the integration of quality health care: the case of chiropractic. J Ambul Care Manage, 25(2), 1–16.

Starmer, A. J., Spector, N. D., Srivastava, R., West, D. C., Rosenbluth, G., Allen, A. D., . . . Landrigan, C. P. (2014). Changes in medical errors after implementation of a handoff program. N Engl J Med, 371(19), 1803–1812. doi: 10.1056/ NEJMsa1405556

Stead, K., Kumar, S., Schultz, T. J., Tiver, S., Pirone, C. J., Adams, R. J., & Wareham, C. A. (2009). Teams communicating through STEPPS. Med J Aust, 190(11 Suppl), S128–132. doi: ste11186_fm [pii]

Taylor, J. A., & Bussieres, A. (2012). Diagnostic imaging for spinal disorders in the elderly: a narrative review. Chiropr Man Therap, 20(1), 16. doi: 10.1186/ 2045-709X-20- 162045-709X- 20-16 [pii]

Tsertsvadze, A., Clar, C., Court, R., Clarke, A., Mistry, H., & Sutcliffe, P. (2014). Cost-effectiveness of manual therapy for the management of musculoskeletal conditions: a systematic review and narrative synthesis of evidence from randomized controlled trials. J Manipulative Physiol Ther, 37(6), 343–362. doi: 10.1016/j.jmpt. 2014.05.001S0161-4754(14)00087-6 [pii]

Verhoef, M. J., Page, S. A., & Waddell, S. C. (1997). The Chiropractic Outcome Study: pain, functional ability and satisfaction with care. J Manipulative Physiol Ther, 20(4), 235–240.

Vernon, H., & Humphreys, B. K. (2008). Chronic mechanical neck pain in adults treated by manual therapy: a systematic review of change scores in randomized controlled trials of a single session. J Man Manip Ther, 16(2), E42–52.

Vernon, H., Humphreys, K., & Hagino, C. (2007). Chronic mechanical neck pain in adults treated by manual therapy: a systematic review of change scores in randomized clinical trials. J Manipulative Physiol Ther, 30(3), 215–227. doi: S0161-4754(07)00059-0 [pii]10.1016/j. jmpt.2007.01.014

Vincent, K., Maigne, J. Y., Fischhoff, C., Lanlo, O., & Dagenais, S. (2013). Systematic review of manual therapies for nonspecific neck pain. Joint Bone Spine, 80(5), 508–515. doi: 10.1016/j.jbspin.2012 .10.006S1297-319X(12)00257-6 [pii]

Walker, B. F., French, S. D., Grant, W., & Green, S. (2011). A Cochrane review of combined chiropractic interventions for low-back pain. Spine (Phila Pa 1976), 36(3), 230–242. doi: 10.1097/ BRS. 0b013e318202ac7300007632- 201102010- 00008 [pii]

Walser, R. F., Meserve, B. B., & Boucher, T. R. (2009). The effectiveness of thoracic spine manipulation for the management of musculoskeletal conditions: a systematic review and meta-analysis of randomized clinical trials. J Man Manip Ther, 17(4), 237–246.

Weigel, P., Hockenberry, J. M., Bentler, S. E., Obrizan, M., Kaskie, B., Jones, M. P., . . . Wolinsky, F. D. (2010). A longitudinal study of chiropractic use among older adults in the United States. Chiropr Osteopat, 18, 34. doi: 10.1186/1746-1340-18-341746-1340-18- 34 [pii]

Weigel, P. A., Hockenberry, J., Bentler, S., & Wolinsky, F. D. (2013). Chiropractic use and changes in health among older medicare beneficiaries: a comparative effectiveness observational study. J Manipulative Physiol Ther, 36(9), 572–584. doi: 10.1016/j.jmpt.2013.0 8.008S0161-4754(13)00233-9 [pii]

Weigel, P. A., Hockenberry, J., Bentler, S. E., & Wolinsky, F. D. (2014). The comparative effect of episodes of chiropractic and medical treatment on the health of older adults. J Manipulative Physiol Ther, 37(3), 143–154. doi: 10.1016/j.jmpt.2013.1 2.009S0161-4754(14)00032-3 [pii]

Weigel, P. A., Hockenberry, J. M., & Wolinsky, F. D. (2014). Chiropractic use in the medicare population: prevalence, patterns, and associations with 1-year changes in health and satisfaction with care. *J Manipulative Physiol Ther*, 37(8), 542–551. doi: 10.1016/j.jmpt.2014.0 8.003S0161-4754(14)00144-4 [pii]

Weiner, D. K., Haggerty, C. L., Kritchevsky, S. B., Harris, T., Simonsick, E. M., Nevitt, M., & Newman, A. (2003). How does low back pain impact physical function in independent, well-functioning older adults? Evidence from the Health ABC Cohort and implications for the future. *Pain Med*, 4(4), 311–320. doi: 3042 [pii]

WFC. (2009). List of Chiropractic Colleges. Retrieved from http://www.wfc.org/website/ index.php?option=com_content&view=article&i d=141&Itemid=140&lang=en

Whedon, J. M., Mackenzie, T. A., Phillips, R. B., & Lurie, J. D. (2014). Risk of traumatic injury associated with chiropractic spinal manipulation in Medicare Part B beneficiaries aged 66–99. *Spine (Phila Pa 1976)*, 40(4), 264–270. doi: 10.1097/ BRS.0000000000000725

Whedon, J. M., Song, Y., & Davis, M. A. (2013). Trends in the use and cost of chiropractic spinal manipulation under Medicare Part B. *Spine J*, 13(11), 1449–1454. doi: 10.1016/j.spinee.2013.0 5.012S1529-9430(13)00521-4 [pii]

WHO. (2003). WHO definition of health. Retrieved December 15, 2014, from http://www.who.int/ about/definition/en/print.html

Yates, R. G., Lamping, D. L., Abram, N. L., & Wright, C. (1988). Effects of chiropractic treatment on blood pressure and anxiety: a randomized, controlled trial. *J Manipulative Physiol Ther*, 11(6), 484–488.

Zhang, J., Haselden, P., & Tepe, R. (2006). A case series of reduced urinary incontinence in elderly patients following chiropractic manipulation. *J Chiropr Med*, 5(3), 88–91. doi: 10.1016/S0899-3467(07)60139- 6S0899-3467 (07)60139-6 [pii]

SECTION C

WHOLE MEDICAL SYSTEMS

10

HOMEOPATHIC TREATMENT OF OLDER ADULTS

Michael Teut

INTRODUCTION

Homeopathy is one of the most frequently used yet also controversial forms of complementary and alternative medicine (CAM). It was founded more than 200 years ago by the German physician Samuel Hahnemann, who aimed to develop an effective, safe, and reliable drug therapy. At his time, Hahnemann was a strong opponent of many usual care treatments, which he considered harmful, such as blood letting and enemas (Teut et al., 2008). The therapeutic system of homeopathy is based on the ancient "principle of similars": homeopathic preparations of substances that cause symptoms in healthy individuals are used to stimulate healing responses in patients who display similar symptoms when ill. A single homeopathic remedy is then selected, based on a patient's total spectrum of symptoms. Classical homeopathy can be understood as a complex therapeutic system, consisting of homeopathic drugs and therapeutic communication, as well as lifestyle advice. Over the last 200 years, the practice

of homeopathy has spread all over the world and is highly prevalent today, especially in India (13.4% of all physicians), Brazil (4%), Germany (1.5%), and France (0.8%) (Dinges, 2012). Today homeopathy is often used in the treatment of chronic diseases to complement conventional treatments, aiming to reduce potentially harmful drugs and side effects (Teut et al., 2008).

The efficacy of homeopathic drugs, compared to placebo controls, is an ongoing focus of debate; meta-analyses of studies with higher quality have shown controversial results (for discussion, see Lüdtke and Ruetten 2008). On the other hand, pragmatic outcome research derived from clinical homeopathic practice has shown relevant results and reductions of disease severity in patients with mostly chronic disease conditions (Witt et al., 2005; Witt et al., 2008).

The discussion of the potential of homeopathic treatment, especially in geriatric patients in the United States, can be traced back to the 1940s. In the *Journal of the American Institute of Homeopathy,* several articles highlighted the use and the practical application of homeopathy in older patients (e.g., Shettel, 1946; Eisfelder, 1951; Lutz, 1963). Most of the homeopaths provided practical advice about homeopathic drug treatment, along with critical reflections on the use and dangers of usual care treatments. Most of those contemporary homeopaths believed that their treatment might help older adults to maintain a better state of health and live longer compared to conventional medical care. As early as the nineteenth century, homeopathic literature includes interesting information about the treatment of geriatric disease conditions. A good example is a therapeutic manual about the treatment of psychiatric diseases and conditions from the German homeopathic physician G. H. G. Jahr (1866) that contains a very detailed guideline for the treatment of cognitive impairments and dementia.

Only recently were the first clinical trials and systematic evaluations of homeopathy in older adults carried out.

PREVALENCE

The prevalence of visiting a homeopath in general populations was reviewed by Cooper et al. (2013), who summarized the findings of a total of 20 surveys and reported a prevalence of 1.5% (range 0.2–2.9). To date, only a few surveys have evaluated the prevalence of homeopathic use in older adults. Büssing et al. (2011) reported that 21% of older German adults reported having used homeopathy in the past 5 years. In a recent German study, 8% reported having made use of homeopathic medicines (Schnabel et al., 2014). For the United States, Cheung et al. (2007) reported a prevalence of 2.5% in community-dwelling older adults. An Australian survey of older patients at a rural health-screening clinic showed a 1-year prevalence of 3% in males and 15% in females (Wilkinson & Jelinek, 2009).

What are the reasons that older adults use homeopathy? Little is known about this, so far. A qualitative study in Germany showed that older adults often rely on complementary and alternative therapies that they learned to use in their childhood from their parents. They had knowledge and experiences about self-medications dating back to the days of their childhood, which were available during World War II and in the postwar period, in contrast to conventional medicine, which was less available and less well developed. For example, most participants remembered the time before the regular use of antibiotics (Stöckigt et al. 2013).

COMPARISONS OF HOMEOPATHY WITH PLACEBO INTERVENTIONS

The Core-Hom database (2014), which is the most complete database of clinical studies in homeopathy to date, does not contain clinical studies comparing the effects of homeopathic drugs versus placebos in geriatric conditions or older adults specifically.

COMPARISONS OF HOMEOPATHY WITH ACTIVE INTERVENTIONS

The Core-Hom database in 2014 only contained two clinical studies comparing homeopathy with active control therapies in geriatric conditions or older adults:

1. Issing et al. (2005) investigated the effect of Vertigoheel, a homeopathic complex remedy containing Cocculus indicus D4, Conium maculatum D3, Ambra grisea D6, and Petroleum D8, in a randomized double-blind controlled non-inferiority trial in older German adults between 60 and 80 years of age with artherosclerosis-related vertigo against a standardized Ginkgo biloba extract. A total of 170 patients participated in this trial. The primary outcome was measured after 6 weeks with a dizziness score. Compared to baseline, both interventions improved the vertigo status, and the group comparison showed that Vertigoheel was not inferior to ginkgo biloba, and that treatments were well tolerated in both groups.

2. In a clustered randomized pilot study, our research team in Berlin investigated the outcome of a 12-month integrative medicine intervention compared to usual care in older adults living in shared apartment communities, including the assistance of professional nurses and caregivers (Teut et al., 2013). The intervention took place over 12 months and consisted of individualized homeopathic treatment, modification of conventional medication if needed, weekly 60-minute exercise group (walking, ergometer training, muscular strength, motor skills, balance and coordination training, as well as group communication), naturopathic care (training of nurses about the use of herbal teas, naturopathic wraps and compresses, and the application of massage oils), and freshly prepared fruit or vegetable

juices. The usual care group (UC) received conventional care by family physicians, specialists, nurses, physiotherapists, and occupational therapists. A total of eight shared apartment communities were included; four were allocated to integrative medicine (29 patients) and four to UC (29 patients). After 12 months, improvements with medium effect sizes (≥ 0.3) were noted in activities of daily living, quality of life, well-being, and specific affective and social functioning outcomes. Smaller or no effects were observed for cognitive impairments, risk of falls, and motor and process skills. In the integrative medicine group the mean number of conventional drugs per patient was reduced from 6.8 ± 3.3 at baseline to 4.8 ± 1.5 after 12 months, whereas it remained stable in the UC group (baseline: 8.3 ± 5.0; 12 months: 8.5 ± 5.7). The intervention itself was found to be feasible but elaborate and time-consuming. This exploratory pilot study showed that for a full-scale trial the outcomes of activities of daily living and quality of life seem to be the most promising for future research. As always in small exploratory trials, the results must be interpreted with care; larger confirmatory trials are necessary to validate the effects.

PROSPECTIVE OBSERVATIONAL STUDIES

In a subgroup analysis of a prospective, multicenter cohort study of our research team, including a total of 3981 patients treated by homeopathic physicians in primary care practices in Germany and Switzerland (Witt et al., 2005; Witt et al., 2008), data were analyzed from all patients above 70 years of age who were consulting the physician for the first time (Teut et al., 2010). The main outcome measures were assessment by patient of the severity of complaints (numeric rating scales) and quality of life (SF-36) and by the physician of the severity of diagnoses (numeric rating scales) at baseline, and after 3, 12, and 24 months. A total of 83 patients were included in the subgroup analysis (41% men, mean age 73.2 ± [SD] 3.1 years; 59% women, 74.3 ± 3.8 years); 98.6% of all diagnoses were chronic with an average duration of 11.5 ± 11.5 years; 82% of the patients were taking medication at baseline. The most frequent diagnoses were hypertension (20.5%, disease duration 11.1 ± 7.5 years) and sleep disturbances (15.7%, 22.1 ± 25.8 years). The severity of complaints decreased significantly between baseline and 24 months in both patients' (from 6.3

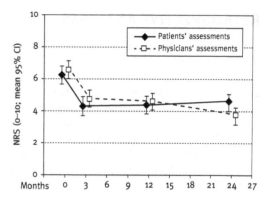

FIGURE 10.1   Disease severity in study population of older adults (> 70 years) under homeopathic treatment over 24 months on a numeric rating scale (NRS).

(Teut et al. 2010).

[95% CI: 5.7–6.8] to 4.6 [4.0–5.1]) and physicians' assessments (from 6.6 [6.0–7.1] to 3.7 [3.2–4.3]; Figure 10.1); quality of life (SF 36) and the number of medicines taken did not change significantly. The most frequently prescribed homeopathic drugs were Causticum, Phosphorus, and Lycopodium (Figure 10.2).

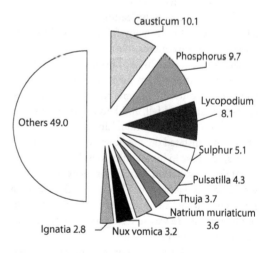

FIGURE   10.2   Most   frequently   prescribed homeopathic drugs in the study sample of older adults (> 70 years; in %).

(Teut et al. 2010).

RETROSPECTIVE ANALYSES

Teut (2006) reported a retrospective data analysis of 120 older adults treated with homeopathic drugs in a German geriatric hospital department over a period of 2 years. One-third of all treated patients had neurological disorders (mostly dementia and apoplectic insults). Seventy-two percent of all pre- scribed homeopathic drugs were of low potency. The most often prescribed homeopathic remedies were Nicotiana tabacum (6.3% of all prescriptions) and Acidum phosphoricum (5.3%).

A CASE STUDY

Mr. B., 79 years old, has been suffering for 7 years from memory loss as a result of mixed type demen- tia. Two years ago his wife was no longer able to care for him at home, as he had become increasingly restless and disoriented. He was then submitted to a geronto-psychiatry ward, where he completely lost his orientation, became aggressive, and beat up a nurse at the facility. After this episode, Mr. B. received neuroleptic treatment with risperidone and dipiperon and was moved to a senior living community where he finally settled down after some initial difficulties.

At the time of the homeopathic consultation he suffered from side effects of the neuroleptic medica- tion: he was no longer able to walk, was rigid and akinetic, and suffered from a constant tremor in his hands. In the months leading up to the consul- tation there had been many falls, which ultimately restricted his movements so much that he was bed- ridden. A recent reduction of his neuroleptic medi- cation (risperidone from 2 mg/day to 1 mg/day) had failed because he became increasingly restless, started walking and fell, and had to get stitches for a wound on his face. To calm him down, his family physician reinstated the previous dose of the neuro- leptics, resulting in his inability to walk.

At the consultation, he was not aware of who and where he was. He said that "none would really help him here." At night he slept very deeply and could not be roused. He was suffering from complete uri- nary and fecal incontinence.

In his past he was a worker who transported heavy sacks of coals to households for heating. He used to be a very strong man physically. Mr. B was also very social; he loved to drink beer with friends and sit in the pub. His wife has been visiting him several times a week, meetings that he enjoyed.

Medication per day was allopurinol 300 mg, torase- mide 5 mg, ferrous glycin sulfate 100 mg, risperi- done 2 mg, and dipiperone 5 ml.

Based on his individual symptoms, the patient received additionally the homeopathic medicine Lycopodium LM6, five drops daily. But his state of health worsened in the following 4 weeks and he had to be admitted to the hospital after he tried to get out of his bed and fell. Due to aggressive behavior, the hospital increased his neuroleptic medication again, and he was sent back completely bedridden and totally apathetic and unresponsive.

In the following homeopathic consultation he received the homeopathic drug Opium LM6, 5 drops daily. Dipiperone, ferrous glycin sulfate, and allopurinol were stopped and risperidone was reduced to 1 mg/day. In addition, he received physical therapy with walking exercise and daily short training intervals on an ergometer device (Motomed®).

Over the following 6 months, he learned to walk again, to eat his meals without help, was capable of carrying on a simple conversation, and his aggres- sive behavior was greatly reduced. After another 6 months, he surprised everybody when he dis- cussed a soccer game he watched on TV. These results remained stable for the 12 months he was under homeopathic treatment.

This case study shows that in many complex geri- atric problems only complex interventions make sense: the homeopathic medication Opium LM6 may have helped to improve his health, but only together with dose reductions of the neuroleptic medication and exercise training was the health sta- tus of this patient improved.

DISCUSSION

Only very few clinical trials have previously investi- gated the clinical use of homeopathic interventions in older adults. The data do not yet allow us to draw any definite conclusions. However, based on the data, the following hypotheses would be helpful for planning further trials:

1. Additional homeopathic treatment may help to reduce disease severity (Teut, 2010) and increase quality of life, activities of daily living, and general well-being in older adults (Teut, 2013).

2. Including homeopathic treatment in geriat- ric medical care may help to reduce polymedica- tion (compare Teut, 2013) and to find solutions for

difficult disease conditions and symptoms (Issing, 2005; Teut, 2011).

3. The spectrum of treated medical conditions and the medications used may differ significantly between settings (e.g., self-reliant older adults living at home, home care service user, or patients living in a nursing home).

SUMMARY

Homeopathic medical therapy may play a beneficial role in the long-term care of older adults with chronic diseases. Further studies on comparative effectiveness are needed to evaluate this hypothesis.

DISCLOSURE STATEMENT

Michael Teut received grant supports from Homöopathie-Stiftung des Deutschen Zentravereins homöopathischer Ärzte, omoeon e.V. and the Karl und Veronica Carstens-Stiftung.

REFERENCES

Büssing, A., Ostermann, T., Heusser, P., & Matthiessen, P. F. (2011). Usage of alternative medical systems, acupuncture, homeopathy and anthroposophic medicine, by older German adults. *Zhong Xi Yi Jie He Xue Bao*, 9(8), 847–856.

Cheung, C. K., Wyman, J. F., & Halcon, L. L. (2007). Use of complementary and alternative therapies in community-dwelling older adults. *J Altern Complement Med*, 13(9), 997–1006.

Cooper, K. L., Harris, P. E., Relton, C., Thomas, K. J. (2013). Prevalence of visits to five types of complementary and alternative medicine practitioners by the general population: a systematic review. *Complement Ther Clin Pract*, 19(4), 214–220.

CORE-Hom database. (2014). A database on clinical outcome research in homeopathy. Karl und Veronica Carstens Foundation. Retrieved November 18, 2014, from http://www.carstens-stiftung.de/core-hom/login.php

Dinges, M. (2012). Entwicklung der Homöopathie seit 30 Jahren. *Zeitschrift für Klassische Homöopathie*, 56(3), 137–148

Eisfelder, H. W. (1951). Homeopathy in geriatric practice. J Am Inst Homeopathy, 44(7), 145–146.

Issing W, Klein P, Weiser M. The homeopathic preparation Vertigoheel versus Ginkgo biloba in the treatment of vertigo in an elderly population: a double-blinded, randomized, controlled clinical trial. *J Altern Complement Med*. 2005 Feb;11(1), 155–160.

Jahr, G. H. G. (1866). Die Geisteskrankheiten. Dritter Band. In *Die Therapie nach den Grundsätzen der Homöopathie*. Leipzig: T. O. Weigel.427–453.

Lüdtke, R., & Rutten, A. L. (2008). The conclusions on the effectiveness of homeopathy highly depend on the set of analyzed trials. *J Clin Epidemiol*, 61(12), 1197–1204.

Lutz, G. A. (1963). Homeopathic remedies for geriatric patients. *J Am Inst Homeopathy*, 56, 402–403.

Schnabel, K., Binting, S., Witt, C. M., & Teut, M. (2014). Use of complementary and alternative medicine by older adults: a cross-sectional survey. *BMC Geriatr*, 26, 14:38.

Shettel, R. (1946). The relationship of geriatrics, pre-clinical medicine and homeopathy. *J Am Inst Homeopathy*, 39, 333–335

Stöckigt, B., Teut, M., & Witt, C. M. (2013). CAM use and suggestions for medical care of senior citizens: a qualitative study using the World Café Method. *Evid Based Complement Alternat Med*, 2013;2013:951245.

Teut, M. (2006). Integration der Homöopathie in die geriatrische Akut-Klinik. *Allgemeine Homöopathische Zeitung*, 251, 5–10.

Teut, M., Dahler, J., Lucae, C., Koch, U. (2008). *Kursbuch Homöopathie*. München: Elsevier.

Teut, M., Lüdtke, R., Schnabel, K., Willich, S. N., & Witt, C. M. (2010). Homeopathic treatment of elderly patients: a prospective observational study with follow-up over a two year period. *BMC Geriatr*, 22(10), 10.

Teut, M., Schnabel, K., Baur, R., Kerckhoff, A., Reese, F., Pilgram, N., Berger, F., Lucdtke, R., & Witt, C. M. (2013). Effects and feasibility of an Integrative Medicine program for geriatric patients-a cluster-randomized pilot study. *Clin Interv Aging*, 8, 953–961.

Wilkinson, J. M., & Jelinek, H. (2009). Complementary medicine use among attendees at a rural health screening clinic. *Complement Ther Clin Pract*, 15(2), 80–84.

Witt, C. M., Lüdtke, R., Baur, R., & Willich, S. N. (2005). Homeopathic medical practice: long-term results of a cohort study with 3981 patients. *BMC Public Health*, 5, 115.

Witt, C. M., Lüdtke, R., Mengler, N., & Willich, S. N. (2008). How healthy are chronically ill patients after eight years of homeopathic treatment? Results from a long term observational study. *BMC Public Health*, 17(8), 413.

11

AYURVEDA FOR HEALTHY AGING AND HEALTH-RELATED CONDITIONS

Shirley Telles, Sachin Kumar Sharma, Arti Yadav, and Acharya Balkrishna

PREVALENCE AND HEALTH ISSUES RELATED TO AGING

The worldwide population of elderly persons is increasing at present and is expected to reach up to 13.3% (1.2 billion) in 2025 (Sewaraj, 2006). At present, India stands second to China in its elderly population; 7% of the Indian population is aged 65 years and older, and this proportion is expected to rise to 10% by 2030. The National Sample Survey Organisation data underline that at any time almost 50% of the elderly may be ill, and 75% of them may have multiple diseases (Swanholm & Scheurer, 1955). The geriatric age group is more likely to have health problems, such as osteoporosis, cardiovascular disease, cancer, diabetes, and neurodegenerative disorders such as Alzheimer's disease (Pradeep, Indoriya, Chakrapany, & Rahul, 2014).

GENERAL CONCEPTS OF AYURVEDA RELATED TO HEALTH AND AGING

Basic Concepts in Ayurveda

Ayurveda defines three dynamic pathophysiological entities (*doshas*) as the basis for all body functions. The three *doshas* are called (in Sanskrit) *vata, pitta,* and *kapha. Kapha dosha* governs the nervous and musculoskeletal systems (Charaka Samhita, 2000; Sushruta Samhita, 2000; Valiathan, 2003). At the cellular level, *vata dosha* is associated with mechanisms regulating cell growth, differentiation, and cell death. The *vata dosha* also controls the movements of cells, molecules, nutrients, and wastes (Prasher et al., 2008; Sharma, 2011). The *pitta dosha* is responsible for processes involving change, such as digestion, metabolism, energy production, and

• 171

the maintenance of immunity (Charaka Samhita, 2000; Sushruta Samhita, 2000; Valiathan, 2003). At the cellular level, the *pitta dosha* is associated with the actions of enzymes, growth factors, hormones, and the reactions required for energy homeostasis and the maintenance of basal metabolism (Prasher et al., 2008; Sharma, 2011). The *kapha dosha* acts to form and maintain the mass, shape, and flexibility of the body (Charaka Samhita, 2000; Sushruta Samhita, 2000; Valiathan, 2003). At the cellular level, anabolic processes such as the biosynthesis of macromolecules and the coordination of gene and protein function may be associated with the *kapha dosha* (Prasher et al., 2008; Sharma, 2011; Sharma & Chandola, 2011).

Ayurveda states that diseases result from systemic imbalances and malfunctions of the three *doshas*. As mentioned earlier, specific diseases originate from interactions between abnormal *doshas* and weakened *dhatus* (life-sustaining tissues) (Svoboda, 1992; Balachandran & Govindarajan, 2005). For example, vitiation of *kapha dosha* is a common cause of cancer and diabetes; however, the *dhatus* that are affected differ (Sahu & Mishra, 2004; Acharya, 1992).

In Ayurveda, one's basic "body constitution" is termed *prakriti*. *Prakriti* arises due to a unique combination of fixed amounts of the three *doshas* (Sumantran & Tillu, 2012). Hence, *prakriti* determines individuality. Ayurveda recognizes seven types of *prakritis*, based on different combinations of the three *doshas*. Experimental analysis of the *prakriti* concept has revealed statistically significant correlations between an individual's *prakriti* and the expression of specific genes and biochemical parameters (Prasher et al., 2008). Another study found correlations between *prakriti* and HLA gene polymorphisms (Patwardhan, Joshi, & Chopra, 2005). Although one's *prakriti* is fixed, one's *doshas* are in dynamic equilibrium, and the optimal function of each *dosha* and normal interactions between *doshas* are essential for good health. Accordingly, individuals with "balanced" *doshas* (*sama prakriti*) are less susceptible to disease than individuals with abnormal *doshas*.

Ayurveda and Rejuvenation

In Ayurveda, *rasayana* drugs are described for their anti-aging effects. *Charaka Samhita* (*Chikitsa sthana* i/i/8) describes the anti-aging properties of *rasayanas* by stating, "Labhopayo hi shastanam rasadinam

rasayanam Rasayana." by courtesy of this, *rasayanas* are agents that are supportive to the qualitative (functional and constitutional) improvements of tissues that alter with aging. Such a qualitatively improved tissue would have optimal functions and therefore withstand premature aging consequent to its impaired quality. Hence qualitative up-gradation and stabilization of cells is a primary function of *rasayanas*, which leads to their anti-aging effects. Another Ayurveda text, *Sharangdhara Samhita*, suggests the use of *rasayana* in early aging (*jaravyadhi*), aging (*jara*), and disease (*vyadhi*) by stating, "rasayanam cha tajghyeyam yajjaravyadhi vinashanam." Hence *rasayana* preparations have beneficial effects in conditions in which a suboptimal quality of health could lead to premature aging and suboptimal functioning. Therefore *rasayana* preparations are proposed to promote tissue longevity through novel mechanisms, such as the reduction of the toxin/metabolic waste load within the cell through reduced production or increased scavenging, thus ensuring efficient use of energy within the cell and requiring less substrate consumption, leading to a reduced energy requirement and less waste production (Singh, Narsimhamurthy, & Singh, 2008).

The Concept of Disease in Ayurveda

Imbalances or disturbed interactions between *doshas* are considered a major cause of disease. An abnormal *dosha* can be inhibited, excessive, or disturbed (Svoboda, 1992). Indeed, the type and nature of disease is primarily determined by the *dosha* that is affected. For example, inflammatory diseases are associated with vitiation of the *pitta dosha* (Svoboda, 1992), whereas obesity and metabolic syndrome are associated with vitiation of the *kapha dosha* (Sharma, 2011; Sharma & Chandola, 2011). A specific illness manifests when the vitiated *dosha(s)* interact with weaknesses in specific organs. Conversely, pathogenic factors can also trigger abnormality of the *doshas* and can weaken the *dhatus* (the tissues that sustain life) (Svoboda, 1992). Diseases, such as cancer, affect the entire body and usually involve vitiation of all three *doshas* (Svoboda, 1992; Balachandran & Govindarajan, 2005).

Other Factors Contributing to Disease According to Ayurveda

In addition to the concepts of *doshas* and *prakriti*, the Ayurvedic concept of *agni* is important. *Agni* (digestive power) is the main entity responsible for metabolic and change-related processes at physiological and cellular levels. When *agni* is strong, the digestion of food is normal, and even vitiated *doshas* can be converted into nontoxic components (Trivedi, 1986). "Incompatible foods" (called *Viruddha Ahara*) can disturb *agni* and lead to the vitiation of *doshas*. It is believed that certain beneficial foods can be harmful if ingested in certain combinations or in specific situations. For example, fruits and milk are individually beneficial but in combination are difficult to digest and can vitiate the *kapha dosha* and lead to *agnimandya* (i.e., weak *agni*) (Acharya, 1992). A complex interplay between the diet and host factors regulates *agni* and is in turn influenced by *agni*. Hence, the nature and composition of the diet, quantity of food, timing of food intake, and the intrinsic properties of food are important. In addition, an individual's ability to digest and process food depends on host factors such as the *prakriti*, status of *doshas*, *agni*, tolerance, and digestion (Svoboda, 1992; Trivedi, 1986; Acharya, 1992). Hence, a feedback loop mechanism links diet and host factors with the strength and activity of *agni*. Long-term consumption of incompatible foods can impair this feedback mechanism and increase the susceptibility for various diseases (Svoboda, 1992; Trivedi, 1986; Acharya, 1992). A weakened *agni* can also result in decreased immune surveillance. Therefore, the maintenance of *agni* at optimum levels is important for avoiding disease (Trivedi, 1986; Acharya, 1992).

Ayurveda gives considerable importance to the collection of "toxic matter believed to be due to poor digestion" called *ama*, in the onset of disease (Svoboda, 1992, pp 160–161). Typically, *ama* manifests as a sticky, white coating of the tongue, which is believed to obstruct various internal microchannels and is associated with characteristic symptoms such as the loss of taste sensation, local or general inflammation, fatigue, heaviness, pain, abdominal discomfort, lethargy, indigestion, and constipation (Acharya, 1992; Svoboda, 1992). Since *ama* is considered to be the basis of disease, it must be fully removed before one can rectify vitiated *dosha(s)* (Acharya, 1992). Accordingly, the strengthening of *agni* and complete digestion of *ama* are the principal goals of Ayurvedic treatment. Hence, therapies such as purgation, enema, or therapeutic emesis lead to the complete removal of *ama* and the correction of imbalances in the *doshas* (Mitra, 2006). Improved *agni* results in complete digestion of *ama*, and causes

the condition known as *nirama* (free from *ama*). The *nirama* stage is favorable for additional treatments, which aim at resolving vitiated or depleted *doshas* and *dhatus* and reversing the disease pathology if possible (Mitra, 2006). Notably, the *panchakarma* (cleansing of the body) procedures for eliminating vitiated *doshas* are only effective if preexisting *ama* is completely removed (Mitra, 2006). The obstruction of micro-channels by *ama* is responsible for loss of homeostasis, inflammation, and tissue damage (Srinivasulu, 2010). Accordingly, Ayurveda believes that *ama* is the root cause of several diseases since it blocks important micro-channels (*srotas*) that nourish the tissues (*dhatus*).

AYURVEDA AND AGE-RELATED HEALTH CONDITIONS

Ayurveda, Obesity, and Associated Premorbid Conditions

Prameha is a syndrome described in ancient Ayurvedic texts that includes conditions such as obesity, prediabetes, diabetes mellitus, and metabolic syndrome (Sharma & Chandola, 2011). There are 20 subtypes of *prameha* due to the interaction of the three *doshas* and 10 *dushyas* (disturbed functioning of the principles that support the various bodily tissues); several of these subtypes have sweet urine, whereas some of them have different colored urine, highlighting the inflammatory conditions involved in metabolic syndrome. This disease has close ties to *sthaulya* (i.e., obesity).

Ayurveda and Diabetes

With regard to diabetes mellitus, *sahaja prameha* and *jatah pramehi* are comparable to type 1 diabetes, while *apathyanimittaja prameha* is comparable to type 2 diabetes. Various dietary, lifestyle, and psychological factors are involved in the etiology of *prameha*. There are several approaches to the management of diabetes in Ayurveda, including poly-herbal and single herb preparations. One such example is fenugreek (*Trigonella foenum-graecum; methika* in Sanskrit), which is one of the oldest medicinal plants, originating in India and Northern Africa. The possible hypoglycemic and antihyperlipidemic properties of oral fenugreek seed powder have been suggested by the results of preliminary animal and human trials (Sauvaire et al., 1998).

The hypoglycemic effects of fenugreek have been attributed to several mechanisms demonstrated in vitro (Sauvaire et al., 1998). The amino acid 4-hydroxyisoleucine in fenugreek seeds increased glucose-induced insulin release in human and rat pancreatic islet cells (Sauvaire et al., 1998). This amino acid appeared to act only on pancreatic beta cells, since the levels of somatostatin and glucagon were not altered. In studies on human participants, fenugreek reduced the area under the plasma glucose curve and increased the number of insulin receptors, although the mechanism for this effect is unclear (Raghuram, Sharma, Sivakumar, & Sahay, 1994). In humans, fenugreek seeds exert hypoglycemic effects by stimulating glucose-dependent insulin secretion from pancreatic beta cells (Ajabnoor & Tilmisany, 1988), as well as by inhibiting the activities of alpha-amylase and sucrose (Amin, Abdul-Ghani, & Suleiman, 1987).

Another example is *Syzygium jambolanum* (called *jambu* in Sanskrit), commonly known as black plum and originally indigenous to India. It has been used in various complementary and alternative systems of medicine and, before the discovery of insulin, as an anti-diabetic medication in Europe. The brew, prepared by boiling the seeds of *Syzygium jambolanum* in water, has been used in various traditional systems of medicine to manage hyperglycemia (Baliga, Fernandes, Thilakchand, D'Souza, & Rao, 2013).

In summary, there are herbs with proven benefits in diabetes mellitus, though their mechanism of action remains to be understood. Also, in Ayurveda a whole-system approach (involving the diet and routine) is emphasized.

Ayurveda and Cardiac Health

Raised cholesterol is estimated to be responsible for 18% of cerebrovascular disease and 56% of ischemic heart disease (WHO, 2002). Overall, these diseases account for about 4.4 million deaths (7.9% of the total deaths reported). *Lekhana basti* (a therapeutic enema) is aimed at creating a state in which nourishment is not desired (*apatarpana*). *Basti* is the fastest way to reach *apatarpana*. In a randomized controlled trial (Auti, Thakar, Shukla, & Ravishankar, 2013), patients were divided into two groups, of which group A was treated with *Lekhana basti* and group B was administered a polyherbal preperation, that

is, *Triphala Guggulu*,[1] for 21 days. Patients treated with *Lekhana basti* showed a decrease of about 5% in serum cholesterol, 9.1% in serum low density lipoprotein (LDL), and 0.4% in serum apolipoprotein B. *Lekhana basti* was found to have a significant effect in reducing the symptoms of accumulation of fats, called *medodushti*, and in the reduction of weight, body mass index (BMI), body fat percentage, body circumferences such as chest, abdomen, hip, pelvis, mid-thigh circumference, and skin-fold thickness (e.g., biceps, triceps, mid-arm, and abdominal skinfold thickness). *Medohara* and *Lekhaniya* (anti-obesity and hypolipidemic preparations) can increase the understanding about the prevention and management of conditions like dyslipidemia and its complications (Kumari, Pushpan, & Nishteswar, 2013). Drugs possessing *tikta rasa* (bitter taste), and those which are *ushna veerya* (exothermic), or have *laghu* and *ruksha guna* (light and dry qualities), were noted to be useful (Kumari, Pushpan, & Nishteswar, 2013). *Terminalia arjuna* (*arjuna* in Sanskrit) is widely used in Ayurveda for various cardiovascular ailments. The bark has been reported to contain several bioactive compounds (Maulik & Talwar, 2012). Several studies have reported its antioxidant, anti-ischemic, antihypertensive, and antihypertrophic effects, which have relevance to its therapeutic potential in cardiovascular diseases. Several clinical studies have reported its efficacy in patients with ischemic heart disease, hypertension, and heart failure (Maulik & Talwar, 2012). *Withania somnifera* (*Ashwagandha* in Sanskrit) is categorized as a *rasayana*, and is described to promote health and longevity, while *Terminalia arjuna* is primarily for the treatment of cardiac disorders (Sandhu, Shah, Shenoy, Chauhan, Lavekar, & Padhi, 2010).

Withania somnifera (*ashwagandha*) may therefore be useful for generalized weakness and to improve speed and lower limb muscular strength and neuromuscular coordination. *Terminalia arjuna* (*arjuna*) may prove useful to improve cardiovascular endurance and lower systolic blood pressure. *Terminalia arjuna* (*arjuna*) also has strong hypolipidemic and antioxidant properties. The bark extracts of *Terminalia arjuna* decrease platelet activation and may possess antithrombotic properties.

In summary, specific therapeutic procedures and herbal preparations can promote cardiac health and manage age-related cardiac disorders.

---

1. Emblica officinalis (Amalaki in Sanskrit), Terminalia chebula (Haritaki), Terminalia bellerica (Bibhitaki), Piper longum (Pippali), Commiphora mukul (Guggulu).

Ayurveda and Cancer

Present knowledge states that abnormalities involving epigenetic regulation, diet, environmental factors, and changes in immune functions can influence the outcome in cancer. Ayurveda also considers diet and environmental factors as important regulators of the digestive power and immunity, which in turn can influence the risk of cancer. The concept of a positive correlation between cancer and metabolic syndrome (Hanahan & Weinberg, 2011; Hirsch et al., 2010; Mantovani, Allavena, Sica, & Balkwill, 2008) has some similarities to the Ayurvedic view that interactions between vitiated *doshas* and weak tissues (*dhatus*) lead to systemic malfunctions that can manifest as cancer, involving specific organs. Certain anti-inflammatory drugs (Shacter, & Weitzman, 2002; Shishodia, Harikumar, Dass, Ramawat, & Aggarwal, 2008; Surh, Chun, Cha, Han, Keum, Park, Lee, 2001) and anti-diabetic drugs (Bundscherer, Reichle, Hafner, Meyer, & Vogt, 2009; Cabarcas, Hurt, & Farrar, 2010; Varga, Czimmerer, & Nagy, 2011) are effective against cancer because of the "indirect" involvement of inflammation and dyslipidemia in carcinogenesis. Ayurveda also uses "indirect" approaches to treat cancer because therapies aim to eliminate vitiated *doshas*, rejuvenate body functions, and restore immunity, through rejuvenating treatments (*rasayanaprayoga*).

The severity and clinical presentation of cancer vary, as each person has different patterns of dynamic changes in the functioning of the *dhatus* (life-sustaining tissues) (Sahu, & Mishra, 2004).

As mentioned earlier, abnormal *doshas*, weakened *dhatus*, and weakened *agni* are major risk factors that weaken the immune system and predispose an individual to cancer. Cancer is associated with poor diet (Galland, 2010; Kalogeropoulos, Panagiotakos, Pitsavos, Chrysohoou, Rousinou, Toutouza, & Stefanadis, 2010; Mencarelli et al., 2011), abnormal lipid metabolism (Bierhaus et al., 2001; Braun, Bitton-Worms, & Leroith, 2011; Bundscherer, Reichle, Hafner, Meyer, & Vogt, 2009; Cabarcas, Hurt, & Farrar, 2010; Chuu 2011; Harvey, Lashinger, & Hursting, 2011; Havel, 2002; Im & Osborne, 2011; Khaidakov et al., 2011; Modica, Murzilli, Salvatore, Schmidt, & Moschetta, 2008; Puglisi & Fernandez, 2008; Stryjecki & Mutch, 2011; Sun & Kashyap, 2011; Tsimikas & Miller, 2011; Vacca, Degirolamo, Mariani-Costantini, Palasciano, &

Moschetta, 2011; and Varga, Czimmerer, & Nagy, 2011;and Wang, Chen, Wang, Yu, Forman, & Huang, 2008), *kapha dosha* imbalance (Sharma, 2011; Sharma & Chandola, 2011), and metabolic syndrome (Braun, Bitton-Worms, & Leroith, 2011; Harvey, Lashinger, & Hursting, 2011; Havel 2002; Stryjecki & Mutch, 2011; Sun, & Kashyap, 2011). Instead of using targeted therapies for destruction of the tumors, Ayurvedic drugs or modes of treatment attempt to correct metabolic defects and restore normal tissue functions (this is called *sama dhatu parampara*). Like most forms of traditional medicine, Ayurvedic medicine is holistic; thus it rejuvenates the body's support systems (*rasayanaprayoga*) and forms a significant component of cancer therapy (Balachandran & Govindarajan, 2005; Charaka Samhita, 2000; Svoboda, 1992; Valiathan, 2003).

Ayurveda and Osteoporosis

Osteoporosis affects the entire skeleton. It is a metabolic disease of the bones, characterized by low bone mass and microarchitectural deterioration of the skeleton, leading to increased bone fragility with a consequent increase in the risk of fractures. In Ayurveda, it can be correlated with *asthi-majjakshaya* (a decrease in bone and bone-marrow). The treatment includes *basti* (a therapeutic enema), which is the main therapy for *asthi-* (bone) related diseases (Gupta, Shah, & Thakar, 2012). Also, the herb *Cissus quadrangularis* (*granthiman* in Sanskrit) is used to strengthen the bone by traditional practitioners of Ayurveda. It is administered orally. In a clinical trial, 12 patients with osteoarthritis treated with the therapeutic enema (*majjia-basti*) along with capsules of *Cissus quadrangularis* (*granthiman*) pulp showed definite benefits in pain, tenderness, general debility, and bone mineral density (Gupta, Shah, & Thakar, 2012).

Withania somnifera (*ashwagandha*) contains withanolides such as withaferin A (WFA), which acts as a proteasomal inhibitor (PI) and binds to the specific catalytic β subunit of the 20S proteasome (Khedgikar et al., 2013). It exerts a positive effect on osteoblasts by increasing osteoblast proliferation and differentiation. WFA was shown to increase expression of the osteoblast-specific transcription factor and mineralizing genes, promote osteoblast survival, and suppress inflammatory cytokines (Khedgikar et al., 2013). WFA treatment reduces the number of osteoclasts by decreasing the expression

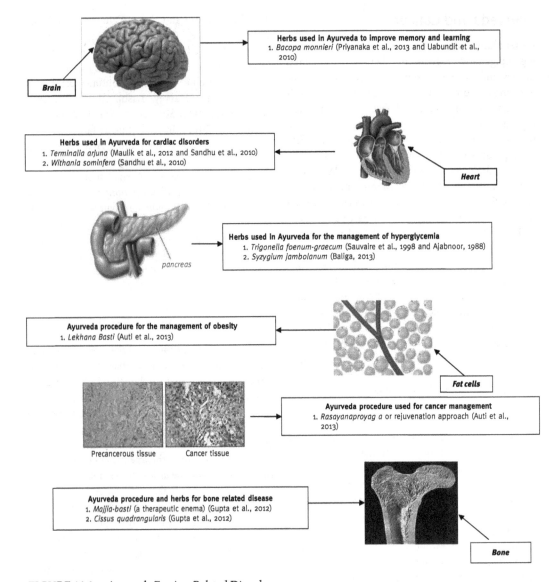

FIGURE 11.1   Ayurveda For Age-Related Disorders

of tartarate-resistant acid phosphatase and the receptor activator of nuclear factor kappa-B (RANK), and also indirectly by decreasing osteoprotegrin/RANK ligand ratio (Khedgikar et al., 2013). Oral administration of WFA to osteopenic ovariectomized mice increased osteoprogenitor cells in the bone marrow and increased expression of osteogenic genes (Khedgikar et al., 2013). WFA supplementation improves trabecular micro-architecture of the long bones, increases biomechanical strength parameters of the vertebrae and femur, and decreases bone turnover markers (osteocalcin and TNFα) and expression of skeletal osteoclastogenic genes. It also increases new bone formation and the expression of osteogenic genes in the femur as compared with placebo groups. These data suggest that WFA stimulates bone formation by facilitating proteasomal machinery and acts as a bone anabolic agent.

In summary, there are specific treatments (a therapeutic enema) and herbs that can help to prevent and manage osteoporosis in the aged.

Ayurveda and Alzheimer's Dementia

Aged people are more prone to developing neurodegenerative diseases. Neuronal degeneration due to increased formation of reactive oxygen species, combined with loss of antioxidant enzyme activities, is increased by the aging process. In Ayurveda the approach is multiple treatments as well as specific herbs. An example of the latter is *Bacopa monnieri* (*brahmi* in Sanskrit), a plant belonging to the family *Scrophulariaceae*, which has been used in Ayurveda to improve intelligence and memory (Priyanka, Singh, Mishra, & ThyagaRajan, 2013).

The results of a study comparing *Bacopa monnieri* (*brahmi*) with a known pharmacological agent used for dementia (i.e., donepezil) suggests that both *Bacopa monnieri* and donepezil exert distinct age-related effects on cell-mediated immune responses through selective modulation of antioxidant enzyme activities and intracellular targets that may influence the therapeutic efficacy of these drugs in neurodegenerative diseases (Priyanka, Singh, Mishra, & ThyagaRajan, 2013).

Another study determined the effect of an alcoholic extract of *Bacopa monnieri* on cognitive functions and neurodegeneration in an animal model of Alzheimer's disease (Uabundit, Wattanathorn, Mucimapura, & Ingkaninan, 2010). *Bacopa monnieri* extract improved the performance in a maze task. The reduction of neurons and cholinergic neuron densities was also mitigated. *Bacopa monnieri* is a potential cognitive enhancer and neuroprotectant against Alzheimer's disease. There are other treatment approaches, but since *Bacopa monnieri* is possibly the best known, it is mentioned here.

SUMMARY

In summary, Ayurveda has a whole-system approach to promote positive health throughout life and hence to promote healthy aging. While the concepts in Ayurveda involve terms not used in conventional medicine (e.g., *tridoshas, prakriti*), the basic principles are in line with recent approaches to lifestyle modification to promote healthy aging and to manage disorders associated with aging if they occur. The benefits have been summarized in the Figure 11.1.

DISCLOSURE STATEMENT

The authors state that there are no conflicts of interest.

REFERENCES

Acharya, Y. T. (1992). *Caraka samhita* (Chi 15/3–5, pp. 150; 212; 512; 518; 525). Varanasi, India: Chaukhamba Surbharati.

Ajabnoor, M. A., & Tilmisany, A. K. (1988). Effect of Trigonella foenum graceum on blood glucose levels in normal and alloxan-diabetic mice. *J Ethnopharmacol, 22*(1), 45–49.

Amin, R., Abdul-Ghani, A. S., & Suleiman, M. S. (1987). Effect of Trigonella feonum graecum on intestinal absorption. Proceedings of the 47th Annual Meeting of the American Diabetes Association (Indianapolis USA). *Diabetes, 36,* 211a.

Auti, S. S., Thakar, A. B., Shukla, V. J., & Ravishankar, B. (2013). Assessment of Lekhana Basti in the management of hyperlipidemia. *Ayu, 34*(4), 339–345. doi: 10.4103/0974-8520.127683

Balachandran, P., & Govindarajan, R. (2005). Cancer: an ayurvedic perspective. *Pharmacol Res, 51*(1), 19–30.

Baliga, M. S., Fernandes, S., Thilakchand, K. R., D'souza, P., & Rao, S. (2013). Scientific validation of the antidiabetic effects of Syzygium jambolanum DC (black plum), a traditional medicinal plant of India. *J Altern Complem Med, 19*(3), 191–197. doi: 10.1089/acm.2011.0752

Bierhaus, A. 1., Schiekofer, S., Schwaninger, M., Andrassy, M., Humpert, P. M., Chen, J., . . . Nawroth, P. P. (2001). Diabetesassociated sustained activation of the transcription factor nuclear factor-κB, *Diabetes, 50*(12), 2792–2808.

Braun, S., Bitton-Worms, K., & Leroith, D. (2011). The link between the metabolic syndrome and cancer. *Int J Biol Sci, 7*(7), 1003–1015.

Bundscherer, A., Reichle, A., Hafner, C., Meyer, S., & Vogt, T. (2009). Targeting the tumor stroma with peroxisome proliferator activated receptor (PPAR) agonists. *Anti-Cancer Agents Med Chem, 9*(7), 816–821.

Cabarcas, S. M., Hurt, E. M., & Farrar, W. L. (2010). Defining the molecular nexus of cancer, type 2 diabetes and cardiovascular disease. *Curr Mol Med, 10*(8), 741–755.

Charaka samhita (text with English translation). (2000). Varanasi, India: Chaukhamba Orientalia.

Chuu, C. P. (2011). Modulation of liver X receptor signaling as a prevention and therapy for colon cancer. *Med Hypoths, 76*(5), 697–699. doi: 10.1016/j.mehy.2011.01.037

Galland, L. (2010). Diet and inflammation. *Nutr Clin Practice, 25*(6), 634–640. doi: 10.1177/0884533610385703

Gupta, A. K., Shah, N., & Thakar, A. B. (2012). Effect of majja basti (therapeutic enema) and asthi shrinkhala (Cissus quadrangularis) in the management of osteoporosis (asthi-majjakshaya). *Ayu, 33*(1), 110–113. doi: 10.4103/0974-8520.100326

Hanahan, D., & Weinberg, R. A. (2011). Hallmarks of cancer: the next generation. *Cell, 144*(5), 646–674.

Harvey, A. E. Lashinger, L. M. & Hursting, S. D. (2011). The growing challenge of obesity and cancer: an inflammatory issue. *Ann NY Acad Sci, 1229*(1), 45–52.

Havel, P. J. (2002). Control of energy homeostasis and insulin action by adipocyte hormones: leptin, acylation stimulating protein, and adiponectin. *Curr Opin Lipidol, 13*(1), 51–59.

Hirsch, H. A., Iliopoulos, D., Joshi, A., Zhang, Y., Jaeger, S. A., Bulyk, . . . Struhl, K. (2010). A transcriptional signature and common gene networks link cancer with lipid metabolism and diverse human diseases. *Cancer Cell, 17*(4), 348–361.

Im, S. S. & Osborne, T. F. (2011). Liver X receptors in atherosclerosis and inflammation. *Circ Res, 108*(8), 996–1001. doi: 10.1161/CIRCRESAHA.110.226878.

Kalogeropoulos, N., Panagiotakos, D. B., Pitsavos, C., Chrysohoou, C., Rousinou, G., Toutouza, M., & Stefanadis, C. (2010). Unsaturated fatty acids are inversely associated and n-6/n-3 ratios are positively related to inflammation and coagulation markers in plasma of apparently healthy adults. *Clin Chim Acta, 411*(7–8), 584–591. doi: 10.1016/j.cca.2010.01.023

Khaidakov, M., Mitra, S., Kang, B. Y., Wang, X., Kadlubar, S., Novelli, G., . . . Mehta, J. L. (2011). Oxidized LDL receptor 1 (OLR1) as a possible link between obesity, dyslipidemia and cancer. *PLoS One, 6*(5):e20277. doi: 10.1371/journal.pone.0020277

Khedgikar, V., Kushwaha, P., Gautam, J., Verma, A., Changkija, B., Kumar, A., . . . Trivedi, R. (2013). Withaferin A: a proteasomal inhibitor promotes healing after injury and exerts anabolic effect on osteoporotic bone. *Cell Death Disease, 4,* e778. doi: 10.1038/cddis.2013.294.

Kumari, H., Pushpan, R., & Nishteswar, K. (2013). Medohara and Lekhaniya dravyas (anti-obesity and hypolipidemic drugs) in Ayurvedic classics: a critical review. *Ayu, 34*(1), 11–16. doi: 10.4103/0974-8520.115437.

Mantovani, A., Allavena, P., Sica, A., & Balkwill, F. (2008). Cancerrelated inflammation. *Nature, 454*(7203), 436–444.

Maulik, S. K., & Talwar, K. K. (2012). Therapeutic potential of Terminalia arjuna in cardiovascular disorders. *Am J Cardiovasc Drugs, 12*(3), 157–163. doi: 10.2165/11598990

Mencarelli, A., Distrutti, E., Renga, B., D'Amore, C., Cipriani, S., Palladino, G., . . . Fiorucci, S. (2011). Probiotics modulate intestinal expression of nuclear receptor and provide counter-regulatory signals to inflammation-driven adipose tissue activation. *PLoS ONE, 6*(7), e22978. doi: 10.1371/journal.pone.0022978

Mitra, J. (2006). *Ashtanga samgraha.* Varanasi, India: Chowkhambha Sanskrit Series Office.

Modica, S., Murzilli, S., Salvatore, L., Schmidt, D. R., & Moschetta, A. (2008). Nuclear bile acid receptor FXR protects against intestinal tumorigenesis. *Cancer Res, 68*(23), 9589–9594. doi: 10.1158/0008-5472.CAN-08-1791

Patwardhan, B., Joshi, K., & Chopra, A. (2005). Classification of human population based on HLA gene polymorphism and the concept of Prakriti in Ayurveda. *J Altern Complem Med, 11*(2), 349–353.

Pradeep, S., Indoriya, G. S., Chakrapany, S., & Rahul, P. (2014). Geriatric health care through nutraceuticals of morinda citrifolia l.: a review. *Ayushdhara, 1*(2), 33–39.

Prasher, B., Negi, S., Aggarwal, S., Mandal, A. K., Sethi, T. P., Deshmukh, S. R., . . . Mukerji, M. (2008). Whole genome expression and biochemical correlates of extreme constitutional types defined in Ayurveda. *J Transl Med, 6,* 48. doi: 10.1186/1479-5876-6-48

Priyanka, H. P., Singh, R. V., Mishra, M., & ThyagaRajan, S. (2013). Diverse age-related effects of Bacopa monnieri and donepezil in vitro on cytokine production, antioxidant enzyme activities, and intracellular targets in splenocytes of F344 male rats. *Int Immunopharmacol, 15*(2), 260–274. doi: 10.1016/j.intimp.2012.11.018

Puglisi, M. J., & Fernandez, M. L. (2008). Modulation of C-reactive protein, tumor necrosis factor-α, and adiponectin by diet, exercise, and weight loss. *J Nutrition, 138*(12), 2293–2296. doi: 10.3945/jn.108.097188

Raghuram, T. C., Sharma, R. D., Sivakumar, B., & Sahay, B. K. (1994). Effect of fenugreek seeds on intravenous glucose disposition in non-insulin dependent diabetic patients. *Phytother Res, 8*(2), 83–86.

Sahu, M., & Mishra, L. C. (2004). Benign growths, cysts, and malignant tumors. In *Scientific Basis of Ayurvedic Therapies* (pp. 273–305). Washington DC: CRC Press.

Sandhu, J. S., Shah, B., Shenoy, S., Chauhan, S., Lavekar, G. S., & Padhi, M. M. (2010). Effects of Withania somnifera (Ashwagandha) and Terminalia arjuna (Arjuna) on physical performance and cardiorespiratory endurance in healthy young adults. *Int J Ayurveda Res, 1*(3), 144–149. doi: 10.4103/0974-7788.72485

Sauvaire, Y., Petit, P., Broca, C., Manteghetti, M., Baissac, Y., Fernandez-Alvarez, J., . . . Ribes G. (1998). 4- Hydroxyisoleucine: a novel amino acid potentiator of insulin secretion. *Diabetes, 47*(2), 206–210.

Sewaraj, I. (2006). *Preventive geriatric, I.R.M.S.* New Delhi: NIHFW.

Shacter, E., & Weitzman, S. A. (2002). Chronic inflammation and cancer. *Oncology, 16*(2), 217–226.

Sharma, H., & Chandola, H. M. (2011). Ayurvedic concept of obesity, metabolic syndrome, and diabetes mellitus. *J Altern Complem Med, 17*(6), 549–552.

Sharma, M. H. (2011). Contemporary Ayurveda. In M. S. Micozzi, (Ed.), *Fundamentals of Complementary and Alternative Medicine* (4th ed., pp. 495–508). St. Louis: Saunders Elsevier.

Shishodia, S., Harikumar, K. B., Dass, S., Ramawat, K. G., & Aggarwal, B. B. (2008). The guggul for chronic diseases: ancient medicine, modern targets. *Anticancer Res, 28*(6), 3647–3664.

Singh, R. H., Narsimhamurthy, K., & Singh, G. (2008). Neuronutrient impact of Ayurvedic Rasayana therapy in brain aging. *Biogerontology, 9*(6), 369–374. doi: 10.1007/s10522-008-9185-z

Srinivasulu, M. (2010). *Concept of ama in Ayurveda.* Varanasi, India: Choukhambha Sanskrit Series Office.

Stryjecki, C., & Mutch, D. M. (2011). Fatty acid-gene interactions, adipokines and obesity. *Eur J Clin Nutr, 65*(3), 285–297.

Sumantran, V. N, & Tillu, G. (2012). Cancer, inflammation, and insights from Ayurveda. *Evid Based Compl Altern Med, 2012,* 1–11. doi: 10.1155/2012/306346

Sun, G., & Kashyap, S. R. (2011). Cancer risk in type 2 diabetes mellitus: metabolic links and therapeutic considerations. *J Nutr Metab, 2011,* 708183. doi: 10.1155/2011/708183

Surh, Y. J., Chun, K. S., Cha, H. H., Han, S. S., Keum, Y. S., Park, K. K., & Lee, S. S. (2001). Molecular mechanisms underlying chemopreventive activities of anti-inflammatory phytochemicals: down-regulation of COX-2 and iNOS through suppression of NF-κB activation. *Mutation Res, 480*(481), 243–268.

Sushruta samhita (text with English translation). (2000). Varanasi, India: Chaukhamba Visvabharati.

Svoboda, R. E. (1992). *Ayurveda life health and longevity.* New Delhi: Penguin Books India.

Swanholm, C. E., John, H. S., & Scheurer, P. J. (1955). A survey of alkaloid in Hawaiian plants pacific region, *Pacific Sci, 13,* 295–305.

Trivedi, R. P. (1986). *Agni atisara grahani koshtha vata prakaranani.* Varanasi, India: Baidyanath.

Tsimikas, S., & Miller, Y. I. (2011). Oxidative modification of lipoproteins: mechanisms, role in inflammation and potential clinical applications in cardiovascular disease. *Curr Pharmaceut Design, 17*(1), 27–37.

Uabundit, N., Wattanathorn, J., Mucimapura, S., & Ingkaninan, K. (2010). Cognitive enhancement and neuroprotective effects of Bacopa monnieri in Alzheimer's disease model. *J Ethnopharmacol, 127*(1), 26–31. doi: 10.1016/j.jep.2009.09.056

Vacca, M., Degirolamo, C., Mariani-Costantini, R., Palasciano, G., & Moschetta, A. (2011). Lipid-sensing nuclear receptors in the pathophysiology and treatment of the metabolic syndrome. *Wiley Interdisc Rev, 3*(5), 562–587. doi: 10.1002/wsbm.137

Valiathan, M. S. (2003). *The legacy of Charaka.* Chennai, India: Orient Longman.

Varga, T., Czimmerer, Z., & Nagy, L. (2011). PPARs are a unique set of fatty acid regulated transcription factors controlling both lipid metabolism and inflammation. *Biochimica Biophysica Acta, 1812*(8), 1007–1022. doi: 10.1016/j.bbadis.2011.02.014

Wang, Y. D., Chen, W. D., Wang, M., Yu, D., Forman, B. M. & Huang, W. (2008). Farnesoid X receptor antagonizes nuclear factor κB in hepatic inflammatory response. *Hepatology, 48*(5), 1632–1643. doi: 10.1002/hep.22519

WHO. (2002). WHO global infobase online. Retrieved from http://www.who.int/infobase/report.aspx?rid=112 and ind=CHO.

GLOSSARY OF THE SANSKRIT TERMS USED IN THE TEXT

Agni: Fire; the force residing within the body that creates digestion; responsible for the transformation of one substance into another; metabolism. *Agni* is contained within *pitta*.

Agnimandya: Slow or weak digestive power or digestion capacity.

Ama: Toxic residue that is left behind as a byproduct of poor digestion.

Arjuna: *Terminalia arjuna*; an herb used in Ayurveda for cardiovascular problems.

Ashwagandha: *Withania somnifera*; an herb used in Ayurveda for rejuvenation.

Asthi: Bone

Brahmi: *Bacopa monnieri*; an herb described in Ayurveda for neurodegenerative disorders.

Charaka Samhita: Considered the greatest of all the classical texts on Ayurveda; written by Charaka, it contains the teachings of the sage Agnivesa, one of the six students of the great sage Atreya. Charaka was himself a great physician.

Dhatus: Seven fundamental elements that support the basic structure and functioning of the body. The seven *dhatus* described in Ayurveda are *rasa* (lymph), *rakta* (blood), *mamsa* (muscles), *medha* (fat), *asthi* (bone), *majja* (marrow of bone and spinal) and *shukra* (semen).

Doshas: Three main forces that govern the body (*väta, pitta,* and *kapha*).

Granthiman: *Cissus quadrangularis*, an herb described in Ayurveda for bone-related disease.

Gunas: Three basic qualities of nature: *sattva, rajas,* and *tamas*.

Jambu: Black plum, which is useful for diabetes.

Kapha: The force behind the structure and stability of the body. Its elements are water and earth; qualities are heavy, cold, moist, static, smooth, and soft. Also a term for mucus.

Kshaya: Decrease

Laghu: Light

Lekhana: Herbs that reduce fatty tissue and support weight loss.

Majja: One of the seven *dhatus,* or tissues; consists of the nervous system and anything that fills an empty space within the body, such as the brain, spinal cord, bone marrow.

Medodushti: Symptoms of accumulation of fats.

Medohara: Reduces blood lipids.

Methika: Fenugreek, useful for diabetes.

Nirama: Without *ama,* or free from toxic matter.

Ojas: The subtle immune system; the essence that gives strength and endurance to tissues and mind; the force that keeps the tissues healthy. Primarily composed of earth and water (qualities similar to *kapha*), produced from the essence of *shukra*. When strong, no disease can affect the body. The energetic template of *kapha*.

Panchakarma: Panchkarma is Ayurveda's primary purification and detoxification treatment, which includes five procedures.

Pitta: The force in the body that is responsible for digestion and metabolism; its elements are fire along with a small amount of water; its principal quality is heat, although it is also light, slightly oily, unstable, and sharp.

Prakriti: Pure potential for matter (unmanifested potential); the soul's *guna* (*sattva, rajas,* or *tamas*) in its seed form.

Prameha: Polyuria (excessive urinary volume) and diabetes. There are 20 types of *prameha*. Not all types of *prameha* are diabetes, but diabetes is a type of *prameha*.

Rasa: Taste

Rasayanaprayoga: An Ayurveda therapy prescribed for the elimination of vitiated doshas, rejuvenation of body functions, and restoration of immunity.

Rasayanas: Rejuvenative tonic; nourishes all *dhatus* and builds *ojas*. A specialized form of tonification that follows purification such as *panchakarma*; a special term meaning "that which promotes longevity by preventing aging and by making the body young." Also called *pashatkarma*.

Ruksha: Rough or dry quality.

Sama: Balanced or a state of equilibrium.

Sharangdhara Samhita: One of the three supplemental (or "lesser") classical books on Ayurveda (the other two are the *Ashtanga Samgraha* and the *Madhava Nidanam*). Written by Sarangadhara (1200–1500 C.E.), it is famous for its reference to pulse diagnosis and is the first to mention this art.

Srota: Channels in the body; some are gross and some are subtle. In some texts, *srota* is used synonymously with *nadi*. The ears are also called *srota*.

Sthaulya: Obesity

Tikta: Bitter

Tri: The number three (3).

Ushna Veerya: Exothermic

Vata: The force within the body responsible for motion; its elements are air and ether; its qualities are light, cold, dry, mobile, subtle, and rough.

Vyadhi: Disease

REFERENCE

Laursen, M., & Talbert, R. (2004). *Glossary of sanskrit terms for the Ayurvedic practitioner*. Retrieved from https://www.google.co.in/? gws_rd=ssl#q=Glossary+of+ Sanskrit+Terms+for+the+ Ayurvedic+Practitioner.

12

AGING AND MENTAL HEALTH FROM AN INTEGRATIVE EAST–WEST PERSPECTIVE

Sonya E. Pritzker, Shelley Ochs, Edward Kwok-ho Hui, and Ka-Kit Hui

INTRODUCTION

Integrative East–West medicine is a patient-centered and evidence-based approach that judiciously incorporates principles and therapeutic modalities from traditional Chinese medicine with a biopsychosocial perspective and a sharp focus on disease prevention and health promotion. In addition to drawing upon evidence in nutritional science as well as biomedical research, integrative East–West medicine relies heavily on Chinese medicine in both theory and practice. In approaching mental health in aging patients, integrative East–West medicine incorporates Chinese medicine's emphasis on balance, trust in the body's ability to heal itself, and the connectedness of mind, body, and spirit (Hui, Hui, & Johnston, 2006). In practical terms, this means that integrative East–West medicine, like Chinese medicine, treats individual patients holistically, taking into account mental, physical, and spiritual experience in the diagnosis and treatment of "imbalances," as opposed to specific illnesses and diseases.

Integrative East–West medicine thus draws upon the diagnostic toolkit of Chinese medicine, wherein patients are assessed individually in terms of the full scope of their life circumstances, physical symptoms, and clinical presentation. This is especially relevant in the aging patient, as older persons often have an increased disease burden, take more medications with increased risk of adverse response, and typically face more social, cultural, and economic challenges. The US healthcare system, moreover, remains based on an acute care model that is ill equipped to deal with the chronic, overlapping conditions that the aging patient often confronts. Both prevention and treatment in integrative East–West medicine start from the premise that healing is possible at any age.

The role of age in integrative East–West clinical assessment is important, as in Chinese medicine, a person's age is understood to correlate directly to his or her "essence," or homeostatic reserve. Such reserve can be built up or broken down by eating habits, self-care or self-destructive behaviors, and other lifestyle choices. A person's ability to regenerate body tissue, to cope with uncertainty and stress, or to think through complex problems is therefore intimately intertwined with both the amount and the quality of his or her essence. The key to note here is that in Chinese medicine, although essence naturally declines as we age, we can replenish or deplete it through our life choices. Attentive care toward a physical imbalance, for example, can help bolster the manner in which we cope with emotional stress. Likewise, a physical stressor can quite quickly overcome our emotional reserves, causing emotional volatility and/or declining ability to think clearly in other areas of our lives. In Chinese medicine, stress can thus be understood as anything—either positive or negative—that is more than what the body can handle at a given time. In this sense, any event can be emotionally stressful, whether it is a walk to the corner, a drive in rush-hour traffic, the death of a spouse, or the high-pitched ring of a new cell phone.

From this description, it is clear that in Chinese medicine, mental health is inherently linked to physical health, as both emerge from the same core essence or reserve. The "mind" in Chinese medicine is thus deeply interwoven with physical, social, and spiritual experience. That said, mental health, both emotional and cognitive, has long been considered in Chinese medicine. For example, Chinese medicine's notion of "depression" (*yuzheng*) points to an overall state of depressed energy and flow, which can be experienced as pain or fatigue, rather than anything emotional. It also sometimes refers to the condition of "emotional stagnation," wherein sadness, irritability, and lassitude prevail. It does not always completely overlap, however, with "depression" as it is understood in contemporary biomedical psychiatry. Though some similar symptoms are present, Chinese medicine's emphasis on the individual experiencing the symptoms—in terms of his or her physical, emotional, and spiritual experience as well as lifestyle and habits—dictates that the same overarching syndrome in different patients can indicate different underlying patterns.

Integrative East–West medicine incorporates, above all, the Chinese medical perspective on the importance of understanding the whole individual in the support of mental health at any age. There is considerable overlap here with the biopsychosocial perspective in psychiatry, as well as with the patient-centered movement toward personalized care (Pritzker, Katz, & Hui, 2013). In this chapter, we provide a brief overview of prevention, diagnosis, and treatment of mental health in aging patients from the integrative East–West perspective. Throughout the chapter, we incorporate relevant research. A short case study demonstrating the integrative East–West approach to the care of an aging patient with a complex set of complaints, including fatigue, memory difficulties, and depressed mood is also included.

PREVENTION

Overview

Preventing disease and maintaining optimal wellness are important goals in both the traditional medicine of China and integrative East–West medicine. In premodern Chinese medical texts, this was often expressed though the metaphor of the "superior physician" who is able to recognize and treat minor signs or symptoms of discomfort or suboptimal functioning before progression to full-blown pathological disorders. Chinese medical advice regarding mental health overlaps in significant ways with modern research on the relationship between social support, healthy intimate relationships, positive personal belief systems, and health outcomes (Lavretsky, 2010; Uchino, 2006). Ge Hong (284–364 C.E.), a pivotal figure in the early history of Chinese medicine, asserted that the key to health and longevity lies in moderating human desires for the following: fame and reputation, sensory stimulation and sexual activity, wealth, rich foods, and emotional stimulation. Ge Hong is considered to have exemplified these ideals in his own life, as he refused high government office, choosing instead to pursue a quiet life of contemplation and medical practice. Sun Simiao (581–682 C.E.), also known as "the sage of medicine," was renowned as both a physician and master of inner cultivation techniques such as meditation and visualization. He emphasized the deleterious effects of troubling emotions and negative moods on the mind–body complex, with statements such as "excessive thinking harms the heart" and "excessive rumination about the past harms the will and drive." Sun Simiao's reference to "the heart" here, it is important to note, points to one of the most fundamental principles of Chinese medicine: that the organs or "organ-networks," including the heart, spleen, lungs, kidney, and liver, each incorporate both mental and physical phenomena in human experience. The heart is thus understood both as the organ in the chest responsible for the circulation of blood, as well as the hub of consciousness, "mental vitality," memory, and spirit (Wiseman & Feng, 1998). Although space does not allow a detailed explanation of each organ-network, it is important to keep in mind that the organ-networks comprise a complex nexus of structures and functions that often overlaps with biomedical understandings of the same-name organ but also includes mental and emotional aspects that are distinctly Chinese. Therefore, in the prevention, diagnosis, and treatment of mental health disorders at any age, Chinese medicine always maintains a dual focus on both body and mind.

This holistic view of the person finds continuity in the forms of integrative medicine practiced in China today, including "traditional Chinese medical geriatrics." Within this subdiscipline of Chinese medicine, there is a proactive orientation toward encouraging older persons to maintain social relationships and cultivate positive mental attitudes. The emphasis on behavior and mental habits extends to the prevention and treatment of mental health concerns or mild disorders. Chinese medicine practitioners are in a unique position to prevent mental health disorders because the standard intake, part of the "four examinations" in Chinese medicine, will always include detailed questions about the individual's prevailing moods and feelings. These mental–emotional aspects of the person are evaluated within the holistic rubric of mind–body patterns or imbalances described in Chinese medicine. Prevention is then tailored to the particular pattern of imbalance that could, if left untreated, progress into a diagnosable mental disorder. For practitioners and advocates of Chinese medicine, this exemplifies its advantages: subclinical symptoms can be addressed in order to prevent diseases and disorders. In addition to treating subclinical symptoms with acupuncture and herbal medicine, however, one of the common ways in which practitioners of Chinese medicine address prevention is by recommending certain lifestyle modifications or self-help practices, some of which are described in the following sections.

Exercise and Social Activity

In Chinese culture, *yang-sheng*, or cultivating life, refers to a wide variety of practices that are utilized for maintaining and increasing wellness (Farquhar & Zhang, 2012). These practices are considered essential for healthy aging. In contemporary China, as well as many parts of the United States

with a concentrated population of older persons of Chinese descent, a visit to a public park early in the morning provides an ample sampling of these practices. Groups of men and women ranging from age 40 to age 80 and even beyond can be seen engaged in ballroom dancing, tai chi, various forms of qi gong that may include tapping or massaging the acupuncture channels, walking backward, writing poems on the pavement with a large brush and water, or dancing with red flags and drums. The social environment of the park provides both encouragement for physical exercise and emotional enjoyment for those who attend. In the United States, senior centers and other neighborhood gathering spots may also serve this function for clients. Mild exercise in a socially supportive environment is considered to be the most essential form of disease prevention for seniors in Chinese medicine. Several research studies have specifically examined tai chi practice in older adults, and have found that tai chi is associated with improvements in sleep quality, fatigue, and depressive symptoms (Irwin et al., 2014), improved depressed mood over time (Li et al., 2014), and enhanced cognitive function in older adults (Wayne et al., 2014). Research has also shown that tai chi is useful in the treatment of geriatric depression (Lavretsky et al., 2011).

Nutrition

In contrast to Western nutrition, which makes generalized food recommendations based on the examination of the components of specific foods, Chinese medicine takes a holistic perspective on each individual patient. Dietary recommendations in Chinese medicine are thus tailored to the patient based on constitution, lifestyle, environment, climate, and season in order to cultivate balance (Wongvibulsin, Lee, & Hui, 2012). Warming foods are often prescribed for patients with cold imbalances such as loose stool and fatigue, for example, while cooling foods are given to people suffering from heat conditions such as night sweats and fever. While the physical temperature of the food is taken into account, the temperature of certain foods according to Chinese medicine often has more to do with the environment in which the food was grown and the season during which it generally thrives. Furthermore, it is not the type of food alone that is relevant; the entire process, from food production to digestion, is essential. How, where, and when the food is grown or raised, how it is prepared, how and when it is consumed, and the body's response to the food are all important factors. Chinese medicine likewise stresses the importance of the appropriate timing of meals, taking the time to enjoy food, and not multitasking while eating (Wongvibulsin et al., 2012).

Sleep

In Chinese medical theory, sleep is essential for rejuvenating all of the organ-networks, particularly the liver, heart, and kidneys. Good sleeping habits are emphasized in order to ensure the optimal functioning of the entire organism. The quality of sleep is just as significant as the quantity of sleep; therefore any sleep pattern that does not leave one feeling refreshed in the morning would be addressed as a clinical problem.

According to the circadian rhythm theory derived from the traditional Chinese medicine "clock," each organ-network is most active during a set 2-hour time period each day. This is the most important time for both biological and psychological functions pertaining to each particular network. Because the "wood/gall bladder" time of 11 p.m. to 1 a.m. is considered to be essential for replenishing the blood—understood as the source of nourishment for other organ functions—in the body, wellness advice emphasizes getting to sleep before 11 p.m. This is particularly true for elderly patients, who tend to become "blood deficient" due to the normal aging process. Signs of blood deficiency, which may be improved by an earlier bedtime, include poor concentration, irritability, dry skin, poor circulation, and muscle tightness.

Other recommendations for improving sleep include not eating or watching TV 2 hours before bed, taking a walk after dinner, and soaking the feet and lower legs in hot water for 20 minutes before bed. Sleeping on the right side of the body is also advised, so that the "blood returns to the liver," allowing it to be properly nourished. Liver functions include vision, mood regulation, suppleness of the muscles and tendons, and overall stamina.

Massage

One of the common effects of daily stress from a Chinese medical perspective is physical tension at various sites of the body, especially the neck and back. Mental and emotional experiences thus leave traces on the body, which can result in physical pain and other illnesses. Regular massage at specific points on the neck, arms, legs, and feet can help to relieve these traces, or "knots," encouraging the free circulation of *qi*—the vital and active substance responsible for maintaining all physiologic activity in the body (Wiseman & Feng, 1998). In addition to administering light massage, integrative East–West practitioners often give patients specific prescriptions for self-massage that can easily be done on a daily basis. It is important to note here that massage in Chinese medicine, in addition to being a chief treatment modality, can and should be done as a preventive measure. There are particular acupuncture points or "acupoints" that are useful for preventive mental health in aging patients. These include Large Intestine 4, Liver 3, Stomach 36, Pericardium 6, Spleen 6, and Conception Vessel 17 (see Figure 12.1).

DIAGNOSIS

Overview

In integrative East–West medicine, physicians always examine multiple psychological, social, and biological dimensions in the diagnosis of individual patients at particular moments in time. Both diagnosis and treatment are accordingly individualized and constantly modified. Integrative East–West medicine further draws heavily upon the fact that the Chinese medicine practitioner identifies "energetic blockages, discerns functional dysregulation, and gauges homeostatic reserve to arrive at a pathophysiological pattern unique to the patient and at that particular point in time" (Hui et al., 2006). This is accomplished through a detailed intake as well as an extensive qualitative examination of the pulse, including both rate and overall "shape," and the tongue, including tongue shape, coating texture, and color. The "pattern" (*zheng*) diagnosis that results from this process is achieved through a balanced assessment of the patient's symptoms and tongue and pulse readings, as well as consideration of the patient's psychosocial circumstances, everyday environment, preferences, and emotions.

What this means is that any illness is understood as a constellation of patterns and presentations that together reflect the unique interaction of constitutional, environmental, lifestyle, and psychosocial processes in each individual. In Chinese medicine, diagnosis is thus made as an assessment of the particular "set" of disharmonies affecting a given individual at that particular point in time. These disharmonies are ascertained through a combination

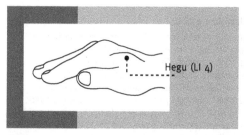

Large Intestine 4 (LI 4)

This point is located at the highest spot of the muscle when the thumb and the index fingers are brought close together. *This point is good for stress, headaches, toothaches, facial pain and neck pain. However, as a word of precaution, it can induce labor and must never be used during pregnancy*

Hegu (LI 4)

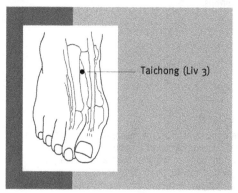

Liver (LI 3)

You need to take off your shoe to find this point. It is located about two finger widths above the place where the skin of your big toe and next toe joins. *This is an excellent area to stimulate for stress, low back pain, high blood pressure, limb pain, insomnia, and emotional upset.*

Taichong (Liv 3)

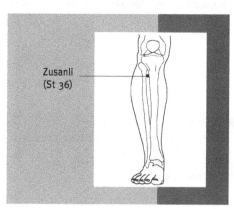

Stomach 36 (St 36)

Find the point by measuring four finger widths down from the bottom of your knee cap. Then, cut across toward the outside of your leg. You'll find it about one finger breadth from the outer boundary of your shin bone. If you are in the right place, a muscle should pop out as you move your foot up and down. *You can find this point useful for fatigue and depression as well as knee pain and gastrointestinal discomfort.* This point is frequently stimulated for health promotion and longevity.

Zusanli (St 36)

FIGURE 12.1   Useful acupoints for older patients and mental health.

of diagnostic techniques, including detailed history taking, close observation, tongue and pulse diagnosis, and palpation. Diagnosis is continually being refined, moreover, because a patient is ideally reassessed using the same four examinations during each visit. In Chinese medicine, pattern diagnosis therefore emerges out of an interaction between doctor and patient and, while it may incorporate biological tests, never depends on such results alone. The physician him or herself thus becomes the most important diagnostic tool in Chinese medicine, relying upon his or her senses of sight, smell, and touch, as well as his or her skills as a listener,

to make an assessment of the patient. In this scenario, every aspect of the doctor–patient encounter becomes clinically relevant.

In diagnosing mental health disturbances in the aging patient, each individual can be diagnosed with one or several pattern diagnoses that form an individual pattern. There are general guidelines, however, for relating Chinese medical patterns to any diagnoses that the patient has received from psychologists or psychiatrists. Next, we briefly describe how several common biomedical categories of mental imbalance relevant to aging patients might be approached from a Chinese medical perspective.

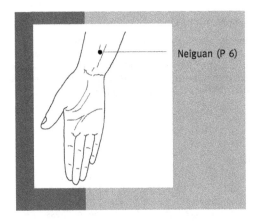

Pericardium 6 (P 6)

Turn your hand over so that your palm is facing up to the ceiling. Locate the crease where your wrist and hand connect. This is the point located about three fingers breadth above that crease, and is midway between the two large bones in your arm. *This point can help provide relief or nausea, anxiety, carpal tunnel syndrome, upset stomach, motion sickness, and headaches and is even used for regulation of heart palpitations.*

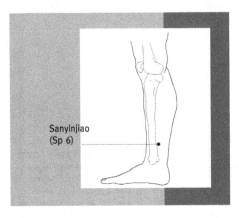

Spleen (6 Sp 6)

Find the bony mound on the inside of your leg close to your ankle. From the top of this bump measure four finger widths up your leg, and push at the area just slightly behind the leg bone. *This point is for menstrual cramping, fatigue, insomnia and menopause symptoms (i.e., night sweats and hot flashes). Avoid during pregnancy.*

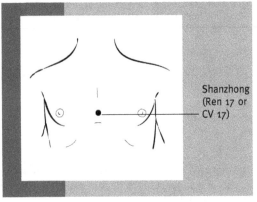

Conception Vessel 17 (CV 17 or Ren 17)

This point is located midway between the nipples. *This point is useful for asthma, bronchitis, chest pain, breast pain, palpitation, acid reflux, indigestion, insufficient and anxiety.*

FIGURE 12.1   Continued

Depression

"Depression," as defined by the *Diagnostic and Statistical Manual of Mental Disorders* (5th edition; *DSM-5*), is a very particular constellation of symptoms, including depressed mood, diminished interest or pleasure, significant weight loss or gain, feelings of worthlessness and guilt, and inability to think or concentrate, among others (American Psychiatric Association & DSM-5 Task Force, 2013). In Chinese medicine, these symptoms are all recognized as pathological, but instead of grouping them together as "depression," they all are understood as indexes of deeper underlying patterns related to the flow of *qi* throughout the body. These patterns, moreover, are tied to long-term constitutional factors, as well as other physical symptoms. They are often grouped together in different "syndromes" or "patterns," each of which resembles depression in some ways, but each syndrome is approached differently in terms of treatment. One of the major underlying causes of all depression-like syndromes in Chinese medicine is an interruption in the smooth flow of emotions throughout the body, a function related to the liver organ-network in Chinese medicine. This flow can be disrupted in many different ways over time, including unfulfilled desires, blood loss, faulty diet, insufficient exercise, anger, and, relevant to the current chapter, aging (Flaws & Lake, 2001). In approaching a patient who is exhibiting signs of depression, it is therefore critical to understand the specific symptoms in great detail, including their history and relation to major life events such as physical trauma or emotional disappointment. Some depressed patients will have considerably more irritability than others, who may complain of more sadness and apathy or overall weakness and fatigue. Some patients will have dry skin, while others will present with chronic excess phlegm in the nose and throat. Understanding the particular constellation of symptoms—both emotional and physical—in an individual will lead to vastly different, personally tailored diagnoses.

Anxiety

Generalized anxiety disorder is defined by the *DSM-5* as excessive anxiety and worry about a wide range of items that are difficult to control (American Psychiatric Association & DSM-5 Task Force, 2013). Symptoms of restlessness, easy fatigue, difficulty concentrating, irritability, muscle tension, or sleep disturbance may present in different patients. Again, though all of these symptoms are considered pathological in Chinese medicine, each patient may be diagnosed with a different pattern, depending on their particular history and presentation. Chinese medicine pays particularly close attention to whether the symptoms of anxiety manifest more as fear and fright or general worry. In general, however, anxiety syndromes or patterns are related to overall weakness and overstimulation of the emotions (Flaws & Lake, 2001). When the emotions are chronically overstimulated, the heart, liver, and spleen organ-networks are all affected, leading to a "disturbance in the flow of *qi* and blood" in the

body as well as an overall "depletion and detriment" (Flaws & Lake, 2001, p. 369). If the patient is experiencing sudden episodes of fear, for example, a deficiency of heart *qi* is often implicated (Flaws & Lake, 2001). If there is concurrent depression and irritability, the liver is included in the diagnosis. Chronic dizziness, insomnia, ringing in the ears, and long-term fright may indicate an overall deficiency of fluids. For confirming any of these diagnoses, however, as in any condition, the patient suffering from anxiety must be evaluated in terms of both physical and emotional or mental symptoms. The presence of concurrent low back or knee soreness is relevant, for example, as is the consistency and timing of urination.

Dementia

Aging patients suffering from dementia often present with impaired memory, significant trouble with decision-making and other executive functions, and limited social functioning. Chinese medicine approaches the underlying causes of what are often understood to be patterns of "feeblemindedness," "impaired memory," "deranged speech," and/or "withdrawal and mania" (Flaws & Lake, 2001, p. 292). All of these patterns can be closely tied to the natural decline in essence as well as organ function in older aged individuals. Again, the other physical and mental symptoms, as well as the patient's history, matter greatly in diagnosis. One common diagnosis for patents reporting challenges in thinking clearly, confusion, and easy fright is "kidney essence insufficiency," which also commonly occurs with physical symptoms such as knee and back soreness, overall lack of strength, and a deep, weak pulse (Flaws & Lake, 2001, p. 292). If there is also vertigo and severe insomnia, as well as emaciation and night sweats, an overall insufficiency of *yin*—the cooling, receptive complement to the more active *yang*—is further implicated. There are several other possible diagnoses here, but the key to remember, as with depression or anxiety, is that dementia in each patient is different from an integrative East–West perspective.

TREATMENT

Generally speaking, therapies in integrative East–West medicine aim to restore a patient's homeostatic reserve and achieve the dynamic balance that is central to a healthy state. The treatment plan, in addition to self-care recommendations such as lifestyle and nutritional modification, might include acupuncture, bodywork/acupressure, and body–mind exercises such as tai chi. Acupuncture is utilized in part due to the fact that a growing body of research is emerging that provides support for this modality through biomolecular mechanisms involving multiple neurotransmitters and neural pathways (Hui, Marina, Liu, Rosen, & Kwong, 2010). Furthermore, there is accumulating evidence that suggests the clinical efficacy of acupuncture and integrative care for a wide variety of mental health conditions, in both aging patients as well as in primary care. Despite controversy over research methodology, acupuncture has consistently been shown to be as effective or more effective than conventional antidepressants or therapy in treating depression (Arvidsdotter, Marklund, & Taft, 2014; Mukaino, Park, White, & Ernst, 2005; Schnyer, 2011), especially in combination with conventional care (Chen et al., 2014). Acupuncture likewise has been shown to have a positive effect in the treatment of dementia and cognitive impairment (Chou, Chu, & Lin, 2009; Wang et al., 2012; Zhang et al., 2013).

Acupuncture points can also be stimulated through means other than acupuncture needles, for example trigger point injections, transcutaneous electrical nerve stimulation, and bodywork/acupressure recommendations that can be reviewed with patients and/or caregivers. Therefore, acupuncture in East–West medicine is used not so much as a therapeutic technique but rather as a conceptual framework that guides treatment choices with the goal of stimulating the body's own endogenous healing and regulatory mechanisms. This can be especially important in older persons, who might already have infrastructure decline and decreased homeostatic reserve that will preclude the use of more invasive treatment modalities like pharmacotherapy and surgical procedures. Acupoints particularly useful in the older patient and in mental health are the same as those recommended earlier for preventive massage (see Figure 12.1).

Therapy in East–West medicine also focuses on the deactivation of myofascial trigger and tender points, which sometimes overlap with acupuncture points and are useful in the treatment of both pain and non-pain symptoms and conditions. Myofascial pain syndromes and fibromyalgia, which occupy opposite ends of the spectrum as localized and generalized forms of soft tissue dysfunction, are exceedingly common but are not widely recognized by many clinicians (Ge, Wang, Danneskiold-Samsoe, Graven-Nielsen, & Arendt-Nielsen, 2010; Giamberardino, Affaitati, Fabrizio, & Costantini, 2011). Both dry and wet needling, for example which is trigger point injection with various substances (most commonly local anesthetics), can be used. The research database is growing, with some well-designed studies demonstrating efficacy with respect to the control of symptoms and quality-of-life measures with massage and bodywork (Cherkin et al., 2011; Kutner et al., 2008; Mehling et al., 2007). Integrative East–West medicine also utilizes bodywork techniques, in particular stretching and massage, delivered either by trained clinicians, or by family/caregivers or by the patients themselves.

In treating mental health issues in patients at any age, particular habits and pursuits, whether occupational or recreational, may need to be curtailed or discontinued. Physical activity and exercise, so often generically prescribed, should be tailored appropriately to the individual to optimize the body's response and to avoid injury. Likewise, nutritional recommendations based on the principles of Chinese medicine, wherein recommended foods and eating regimens for each patient might vary according to the nature of his or her condition and constitution, should also be provided (Wongvibulsin et al., 2012).

CASE STUDY

An 85-year-old woman presents with long-standing fatigue. She cannot date its onset but reports that it has been problematic for several years. Her appetite is preserved and her weight is stable. She doesn't feel terribly refreshed when she wakes up in the morning and feels exhausted most of the time. However, she is able to perform most activities of daily living. She reports some increasing short-term memory difficulties and endorses occasional depressed mood attributed to loneliness. Aside from intermittent achiness in the lumbar region and chronic low-level discomfort in her replaced left knee, she is free of pain.

Her medical history is notable for hypertension, generalized osteoarthritis, osteoporosis with history of vertebral compression fracture, hearing impairment, hypothyroidism, and history of major depression requiring hospitalization around the time of her husband's death six years previously. She is status post total abdominal hysterectomy, left knee replacement, and appendectomy. Her medications include alendronate, levothyroxine, calcium and vitamin D supplements, glucosamine/chondroitin sulfate, and, as needed, psyllium. She does not smoke, and drinks a glass and a half of wine with dinner. Two sisters had dementia of Alzheimer's type. There is hearing impairment, mild ankle swelling, soreness in the lumbar region, gait impairment without history of falls but some degree of fear of falling, constipation improved with psyllium, and urge urinary incontinence.

Physical examination is notable for oropharynx with moist mucosa and well-fitting dentures, no thyromegaly, chest and abdomen within normal limits, moderate kyphosis with tenderness to palpation of soft tissues in the lumbosacral and bilateral hip and gluteal regions, inability to arise from seated position without use of arms, and slow casual gait with use of single point cane. She scores 26 of 30 on the Folstein Mini-Mental State Examination, losing 3 points for recall and 1 point for attention/calculation. Clock drawing is normal. With respect to Chinese medical physical examination, the pulse is floating-empty and slightly rapid, which may indicate insufficiency of *qi* and/or blood, and the tongue is slightly pale with minimal coating, which indicates minor blood deficiency and possibly spleen *qi* deficiency. Complete blood count, comprehensive metabolic panel, vitamin B_{12}, and thyroid function are all within normal limits, and lumbar spine plain films reveal degenerative changes.

From a conventional medical perspective, this patient's fatigue is without organic etiology, and reassurance with recommendation for increased socialization and physical activity will be important. There is likely a mild dysthymia for which antidepressant pharmacotherapy or referral for psychotherapy potentially could be considered. Her hearing impairment should be optimized with hearing aids, and her venous insufficiency can be managed with recommendation for leg elevation and compression stockings. Aggressive efforts to prevent further cognitive decline, especially with her strong family history, and injurious falls, for which her frailty and osteoporosis place her at high risk, will also be paramount. From a Chinese medical perspective, her presentation with its constellation of symptoms and physical examination support diagnoses of kidney and spleen deficiency as well as liver *qi* stagnation. Stimulation of specific acupuncture points, herbal formulas, and dietary recommendations to support the kidney and spleen organ systems and soothe or regulate the liver *qi* can be prescribed.

Aspects of this individual's past medical history and current presentation demonstrate age-related infrastructure decline. Osteoporosis is often a disease of the aged in the absence of secondary factors, and osteoarthritis has affected one of her knees as well as the spine. The significant family history of dementia is notable given this patient's deficits in memory on simple office testing and speaks to prenatal and genetic influences on this individual's constitution. Further inquiry might reveal other "insults," aside from the mentioned passing of her husband and subsequent depressive episode, sustained by the patient over the years. Definitions of frailty continue to evolve, but most would agree that it is characterized by " . . . excess vulnerability to stressors, with reduced ability to maintain or regain homeostasis after a destabilizing event" and common phenotypic manifestations include bone fragility, muscle weakness, vulnerability to infection, high risk of delirium, and severely diminished physical capabilities without regard to individual disease or disease states (Walston et al., 2006). The inadequacy of the disease-based approach in the individual with multimorbidity and/or several geriatric syndromes is highlighted by these new insights into the nature of health and disease. Although researchers continue in their efforts to define and characterize frailty and allostatic load, specific interventions beyond physical activity, appropriate dietary intake, and stress management are still lacking. Chinese medicine, with its diagnostic elucidation of a pathophysiological pattern that is a dynamic and global snapshot of the sick individual, offers the framework with which to approach such individuals. The emphasis on the preservation and strengthening of endogenous resistance in the prevention of chronicity of ill health is paramount.

For this patient, reassurance is probably not enough from the patient's perspective with respect to her primary concern of fatigue, so recommendations to increase physical activity and engage in activities to take her mind off this concern will hopefully be of help. Her risk of progression from amnestic mild cognitive impairment to dementia is increased, and this will need to be followed closely. While preventive pharmacotherapy has not proven successful, it will be reasonable to recommend exercise of mind and increased socialization. Adaptation of self and environment to her gait disturbance might be enhanced by regular practice of tai chi, which has been effective in decreasing fear of falling and falling itself in such individuals.

The focus of treatment from the Chinese medical perspective would be to strengthen the weakened kidney system, accomplished through administration of specific acupuncture point prescriptions, as well as recommendation for appropriate lifestyle and dietary changes, including regular gentle exercise, self-massage at points such as those included in Figure 12.1, eating of warm foods at regular times, and sleep before 11 p.m.

SUMMARY

In conclusion, we hope to have demonstrated the ways in which the integrative East–West approach to aging and mental health can help better address symptoms at an earlier stage in disease progression, when they may be barely discernible from a conventional perspective. The goal is to address *most* problems in the primary care setting and to avoid the development of serious illness. When it comes to treating mental health issues in aging patients, a focus on identifying lifestyle and dietary factors and harnessing the patient's own ability to get well can potentially limit the likelihood of fragmented implementation of diagnostic evaluation and pharmacologic treatments that may lead to therapeutic failure and potential iatrogenic harm (Tu, Johnston, & Hui, 2009). This approach can be then supplemented with therapeutic modalities such as acupuncture, acupuncture-like stimulation, bodywork, and trigger point management. Extensive study of Chinese medicine, while encouraged, is not required. A great deal of the approach described here can be effectively delivered in the context of a typical primary care office visit, including recommended self-massage at the acupoints depicted in Figure 12.1, and referral to tai chi and other light exercise programs. For more complex cases, referral to a licensed integrative physician is recommended. Patients often welcome an integrative approach, moreover, leading to greater adherence and a greater likelihood of therapeutic success (Jong, van de Vijver, Busch, Fritsma, & Seldenrijk, 2012; Wolever et al., 2011).

DISCLOSURE STATEMENTS

The authors of this paper, Drs. Pritzker, Hui, Ochs, and Hui, have no conflicts to disclose. Dr. K. Hui is the Founder and Director of the UCLA Center for East-West Medicine (CEWM), and Drs. Pritzker and Hui are employed by CEWM.

REFERENCES

American Psychiatric Association & DSM-5 Task Force. (2013). *Diagnostic and statistical manual of mental disorders* (5th ed.; *DSM-5*). Washington, DC: American Psychiatric Association.

Arvidsdotter, T., Marklund, B., & Taft, C. (2014). Six-month effects of integrative treatment, therapeutic acupuncture and conventional treatment in alleviating psychological distress in primary care patients: follow up from an open, pragmatic randomized controlled trial. *BMC Complement Altern Med, 14*, 210. doi: 10.1186/1472-6882-14-210

Chen, J., Lin, W., Wang, S., Wang, C., Li, G., Qu, S., . . . Xiao, W. (2014). Acupuncture/electroacupuncture enhances anti-depressant effect of Seroxat: the Symptom Checklist-90 scores. *Neural Regen Res, 9*(2), 213–222. doi: 10.4103/1673-5374.125353

Cherkin, D. C., Sherman, K. J., Kahn, J., Wellman, R., Cook, A. J., Johnson, E., . . . Deyo, R. A. (2011). A comparison of the effects of 2 types of massage and usual care on chronic low back pain: a randomized, controlled trial. *Ann Intern Med, 155*(1), 1–9. doi: 10.7326/ 0003-4819-155-1- 201107050-00002

Chou, P., Chu, H., & Lin, J. G. (2009). Effects of electroacupuncture treatment on impaired cognition and quality of life in Taiwanese stroke patients. *J Altern Complement Med, 15*(10), 1067–1073.

Farquhar, J., & Zhang, Q. (2012). *Ten thousand things: nurturing life in contemporary Beijing.* New York: Zone Books.

Flaws, B., & Lake, J. (2001). *Chinese medical psychiatry: a textbook and clinical manual* (1st ed.). Boulder, CO: Blue Poppy Press.

Ge, H. Y., Wang, Y., Danneskiold-Samsoe, B., Graven-Nielsen, T., & Arendt-Nielsen, L. (2010). The predetermined sites of examination for tender points in fibromyalgia syndrome are frequently associated with myofascial trigger points. *J Pain, 11*(7), 644–651. doi: 10.1016/j.jpain.2009.10.006

Giamberardino, M. A., Affaitati, G., Fabrizio, A., & Costantini, R. (2011). Effects of treatment of myofascial trigger points on the pain of fibromyalgia. *Curr Pain Headache Rep, 15*(5), 393–399. doi: 10.1007/s11916-011-0205-3

Hui, K. K., Hui, E. K., & Johnston, M. F. (2006). The potential of a person-centered approach in caring for patients with cancer: a perspective from the UCLA center for East-West medicine. *Integr Cancer Ther, 5*(1), 56–62. doi: 10.1177/1534735405286109

Hui, K. K., Marina, O., Liu, J., Rosen, B. R., & Kwong, K. K. (2010). Acupuncture, the limbic system, and the anticorrelated networks of the brain. *Auton Neurosci, 157*(1–2), 81–90. doi: 10.1016/j.autneu.2010.03.022

Irwin, M. R., Olmstead, R., Carrillo, C., Sadeghi, N., Breen, E. C., Witarama, T., . . . Nicassio, P. (2014). Cognitive behavioral therapy vs. tai chi for late life insomnia and inflammatory risk: a randomized controlled comparative efficacy trial. *Sleep, 37*(9), 1543–1552. doi: 10.5665/sleep.4008

Jong, M. C., van de Vijver, L., Busch, M., Fritsma, J., & Seldenrijk, R. (2012). Integration of complementary and alternative medicine in primary care: what do patients want? *Patient Educ Couns, 89*(3), 417–422. doi: 10.1016/j.pec.2012.08.013

Kutner, J. S., Smith, M. C., Corbin, L., Hemphill, L., Benton, K., Mellis, B. K., . . . Fairclough, D. L. (2008). Massage therapy versus simple touch to improve pain and mood in patients with advanced cancer: a randomized trial. *Ann Intern Med, 149*(6), 369–379.

Lavretsky, H. (2010). Spirituality and aging. *Aging Health, 6*(6), 749–769. doi: 10.2217/ahe.10.70

Lavretsky, H., Altstein, L., Olmstead, R., Ercoli, L., Riparetti-Brown, M., St. Cyr, N., & Irwin, M. R. (2011). Complementary use of tai chi chih augments escitalopram treatment of geriatric depression: a randomized controlled trial. *Am J Geriatr Psychiatry, 19*(10), 839–850. doi: 10.1097/JGP.0b013e31820ee9ef

Li, Y., Su, Q., Guo, H., Wu, H., Du, H., Yang, G., . . . Niu, K. (2014). Long-term tai chi training is related to depressive symptoms among Tai Chi practitioners. *J Affect Disord, 169*, 36–39. doi: 10.1016/j.jad.2014.07.029

Mehling, W. E., Jacobs, B., Acree, M., Wilson, L., Bostrom, A., West, J., . . . Hecht, F. M. (2007). Symptom management with massage and acupuncture in postoperative cancer patients: a randomized controlled trial. *J Pain Symptom Manage, 33*(3), 258–266. doi: 10.1016/j.jpainsymman.2006.09.016

Mukaino, Y., Park, J., White, A., & Ernst, E. (2005). The effectiveness of acupuncture for depression: a systematic review of randomised controlled trials. *Acupunct Med, 23*(2), 70–76.

Pritzker, S. E., Katz, M., & Hui, K. K. (2013). Person-centered medicine at the intersection of East and West. *Eur J Person-Centered Med, 1*(1), 209–215. doi: 10.5750/ejpch.v1i1.653

Schnyer, R. N. (2011). Commentary on the Cochrane Review of acupuncture for depression. *Explore (NY), 7*(3), 193–197. doi: 10.1016/j.explore.2011.02.013

Tu, B., Johnston, M., & Hui, K. K. (2009). Elderly patient refractory to multiple pain medications successfully treated with integrative East-West medicine. *Int J Gen Med, 1*, 3–6.

Uchino, B. N. (2006). Social support and health: a review of physiological processes potentially underlying links to disease outcomes. *J Behav Med, 29*(4), 377–387. doi: 10.1007/s10865-006-9056-5

Walston, J., Hadley, E. C., Ferrucci, L., Guralnik, J. M., Newman, A. B., Studenski, S. A., . . . Fried, L. P. (2006). Research agenda for frailty in older adults: toward a better understanding of physiology and etiology: summary from the American Geriatrics Society/National Institute on Aging Research Conference on Frailty in Older Adults. *J Am Geriatr Soc, 54*(6), 991–1001. doi: 10.1111/j.1532-5415.2006.00745.x

Wang, Z., Nie, B., Li, D., Zhao, Z., Han, Y., Song, H., . . . Li, K. (2012). Effect of acupuncture in mild cognitive impairment and Alzheimer disease: a functional MRI study. *PLoS One, 7*(8), e42730. doi: 10.1371/journal.pone.0042730

Wayne, P. M., Walsh, J. N., Taylor-Piliae, R. E., Wells, R. E., Papp, K. V., Donovan, N. J., & Yeh, G. Y. (2014). Effect of tai chi on cognitive performance in older adults: systematic review and meta-analysis. *J Am Geriatr Soc.* doi: 10.1111/jgs.12611

Wiseman, N., & Feng, Y. (1998). *A practical dictionary of Chinese medicine* (1st ed.). Brookline, MA: Paradigm Publications.

Wolever, R. Q., Webber, D. M., Meunier, J. P., Greeson, J. M., Lausier, E. R., & Gaudet, T. W. (2011). Modifiable disease risk, readiness to change, and psychosocial functioning improve with integrative medicine immersion model. *Altern Ther Health Med, 17*(4), 38–47.

Wongvibulsin, S., Lee, S. S., & Hui, K. K. (2012). Achieving balance through the art of eating: demystifying Eastern nutrition and blending it with Western nutrition. *J Tradit Complement Med, 2*(1), 1–5.

Zhang, H., Zhao, L., Yang, S., Chen, Z., Li, Y., Peng, X., . . . Zhu, M. (2013). Clinical observation on effect of scalp electroacupuncture for mild cognitive impairment. *J Tradit Chin Med, 33*(1), 46–50.

PART III

STRESS-REDUCING INTERVENTIONS

SECTION A

BIOLOGICALLY BASED PRACTICES

13

POTENTIAL USE OF PLANT ADAPTOGENS IN AGE-RELATED DISORDERS

Alexander Panossian and Patricia L. Gerbarg

Health is the ability to adapt to one's environment.

George Canguilhem (1943)

INTRODUCTION

Adaptogens derived from plants are extracts containing metabolic regulators that enable cells and living organisms to adapt to a multitude of stressors, including heat, cold, hypoxia, chemical toxins, heavy metals, radiation, physical load, and emotional stress. Commonly recognized adaptogenic plants are *Rhodiola rosea* (Arctic root), *Schizandra chinensis, Eleutherococcus senticosus* (acanthopanax or Siberian ginseng), *Panax ginseng,* and *Withania somnifera* (ashwaganda). This chapter focuses on the first three—*R. rosea, S. chinensis,* and *E. senticosus*—which have been used for thousands of years in Europe and Asia to increase energy, endurance, sexual performance, and fertility, as well as to treat inflammation, injuries, and infections. Animal and human studies confirm that individually and in combination, these phytomedicinals improve physical and mental performance and endurance under stress. They show promising benefits in age-related disorders, including age-associated cognitive decline, memory decline, neurodegenerative disorders, hypoxia/ischemia, fatigue, cardiovascular disease, and cancer (see reviews by Gerbarg & Brown, 2013; Panossian, 2013; Panossian et al., 1999; Panossian & Wagner, 2011; Panossian & Wikman, 2009, 2010, 2014).

This chapter begins with an overview of aging and regulatory pathways as targets for anti-aging treatments. Potential benefits of adaptogens and their mechanism of action associated with key mediators of stress response and adaptation to stress will be reviewed, including the following:

- Up-regulation of transcription factor, heat shock factor HSF1, which initiates production of a molecular chaperon, heat shock protein Hsp70 (Panossian et al., 2009; Panossian et al., 2012);
- Modulation of membrane receptors, such as glycoprotein protein coupled receptors (GPCR) and their signaling pathways (Panossian et al., 2013; Panossian et al., 2014);
- Forkhead box O (FOXO) family transcription factors, which play critical roles in the cell cycle,

cell death, metabolism, and oxidative stress resistance (Wiegant et al., 2009);

- Down-regulation of apoptotic signaling protein—stress-activated protein kinase p-JNK and stress-activated increase of cortisol (Panossian et al., 2007);
- Protection against free radical reactive oxygen species (ROS) damage to cell membranes, proteins, and DNA (Boon-Niermeijer et al., 2000; Boon-Niermeijer et al., 2012; Schriner et al. 2009; Wiegant et al., 2008).

The overview of molecular mechanisms is followed by a review of clinical studies in elderly populations and studies in younger adults with findings relevant to mental health and diseases of aging. Case vignettes and future directions will be discussed. Clinical guidelines, and the risks and benefits of adaptogen preparations have been presented in other publications by Brown, Gerbarg and Graham (2004), Brown, Gerbarg and Muskin (2008, 2009) Gerbarg and Brown (2013, 2015).

MOLECULAR MECHANISMS AS TARGETS FOR ANTI-AGING INTERVENTIONS

Age-associated disorders derive from decreasing abilities to cope with stress, to maintain cellular and system homeostasis (dynamic equilibrium/balance), and to sustain physiological functions. Common diseases of aging are associated with neurodegeneration (age-associated cognitive decline, Alzheimer's disease, Parkinson's disease, and senile dementia), atherosclerosis (cardiovascular and cerebrovascular diseases), immune regulation (cancer, autoimmune, and chronic inflammatory diseases) and endocrine/metabolic dysfunction (diabetes and obesity). The mean life span of all living organisms is genetically determined. During senescence, disease development involves the interactions of numerous cell types, proteins, and molecules on various levels of regulation of defense response and homeostasis maintenance. Therefore, there are many potential molecular targets for interventions that could prevent, delay, or slow the progression of age-related diseases.

Four key regulatory levels are the metabolomic, proteomic, transcriptomic, and genomic. The proteomic level includes the regulation of the number and activity of receptor proteins and the biosynthesis and activity of enzymes, chaperones, and transcription factors. Upstream levels of regulation are the transcriptional and gene-expression levels associated with the activation (up-regulation) and inhibition (down-regulation) of DNA array cascades. When a cell is deficient, for example, in a receptor protein, up-regulation increases the synthesis and transport of that protein into the cell membrane and, thus, the responsivity of the cell is restored, re-establishing homeostasis. Down-regulation decreases the expression of genes and the synthesis of corresponding proteins, for example, when a cell is overstimulated by a neurotransmitter, hormone, or drug for a prolonged period of time, and expression of the receptor protein is reduced in order to decrease sensitivity to stress and to protect the cell.

One current therapeutic strategy is directed toward correcting failures in specific signaling pathways that are known to ameliorate and postpone aging by multiple gene activation. At the transcriptional level of regulation there are two molecular targets related to complimentary longevity pathways: the HSF1/Hsp70 and the FOXO pathways. Modulating these two pathways may delay the onset of neurodegenerative diseases, cognitive decline, cardiovascular disease, cancer, and diabetes via multi-gene effects.

AGING AND LONGEVITY REGULATORY PATHWAYS: HSF1, HSP70, JNK, AND FOXO

Senescence is associated with the gradual loss of cell functions degrading the ability of innate defense systems to adapt to environmental stressors and maintain homeostasis. The free radical or oxidative stress theory of aging (Bondy & Maiese, 2010) postulates that organisms are continuously exposed to reactive oxygen species, which are generated as byproducts of normal cellular metabolism. When innate antioxidant systems (glutathione peroxidase, superoxide dismutase, and catalase) incompletely neutralize ROS, cumulative cellular oxidative damage to macromolecules, including lipid peroxidation and oxidation of DNA and proteins, induces irreversible functional changes and age-associated diseases. However, antioxidant therapies alone have not proven to increase life span. Inconclusive results from antioxidant trials suggest that reducing ROS damage alone is insufficient

(Steinberg & Witztum, 2002). It may be necessary to specifically target defective cellular defense and repair mechanisms.

Stress-induced generation of ROS results in destructive interactions with many proteins, including those that trigger genetic programs of cellular senescence and cell death (apoptosis). Loss of function, cumulative damage to proteins, and toxic protein aggregates initiate age-related changes leading to illness, senescence, and decreased life span. In aging cells, significantly reduced expression of heat shock protein Hsp70 and its precursor, heat shock transcription factor HSF1, correlates with a decreased ability to cope with stress (Heidari et al., 1994; Heydari et al., 2000). When cells are exposed to protein damage, HSF1 initiates the production of molecular chaperone Hsp70 (Heiadri et al., 2000), which repairs proteins by folding denatured polypeptides and supports the degradation of irreversibly damaged proteins and their aggregates. In addition, Hsp70 directly protects cells against entry into apoptic pathways. In brain cells, the inhibition of HSF1 and Hsp70 expression occurs in Alzheimer's disease (Bhat et al., 2004) and is associated with the accumulation of protein aggregates of β-amyloid peptide and cytoskeletal protein (Winklhofer et al., 2008). Age-related decline of hepatic Hsp70 expression contributes to reduced liver detoxification (Gagliano et al., 2007) and protection from toxic substances (Lindquist & Craig, 1988). Attenuation of Hsp70 is associated with up-regulation of stress-activated protein kinase (JNK) dependent apoptosis and progression of cancer. In most humans, decline in induction of Hsp70 by stress is associated with aging and age-related disease (Singh et al., 2007). Remarkably, Hsp70 does not decrease with age in some individuals who live more than 100 years (Ambra et al., 2004)

In young organisms, the balance between pro- and anti-aging JNK-mediated programs is shifted in favor of Hsp70 (see Figure 13.1). Despite strong oxidative stresses, a young cell can survive and divide because stress-activated Hsp70 blocks JNK-stimulated apoptosis. Increased levels of Hsp70 correlate with increased life span. In contrast, with aging, when induction of Hsp70 is depressed, the balance shifts in favor of the aging and apoptosis programs. Consequently, even weak oxidative stress can induce the degeneration of neuronal cells and the progression of aging-related diseases. The ability to respond rapidly to stress by generating increased Hsp70 correlates with high adaptability and increased life span (Minois et al., 2001).

Oxidative stress can trigger two signaling pathways through the activation of JNK kinase: the aging program by up-regulation of p-53 transcription factor and the anti-aging program, which is Hsp70-dependent. At young ages, activation of HSF1-Hsp70 inhibits JNK-mediated aging, senescence, and apoptosis pathway. At older ages down-regulation of HSF1-Hsp70 response attenuates inhibition of JNK-induced aging, senescence and apoptosis. ADAPT-232 upregulates HSF1-Hsp70 In vitro and in vivo; down-regulates JNK in vivo; and inhibits aging, senescence, and apoptosis in vivo. Exercise can up-regulate Hsp70

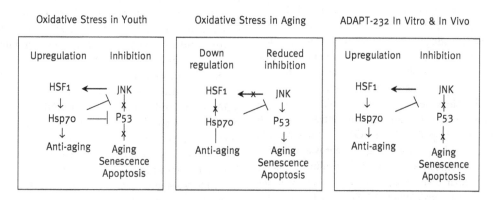

FIGURE 13.1   Oxidative stress: Effects of age and ADAPT-232 on longevity regulatory pathways.

HSF1 = Heat shock factor 1; Hsp70 = Heat shock protein 70; JNK = JN kinase; p-53 transcription factor = P-53; ↓ or ← for activation; x for blocking; | for inhibition; bold text for the prevailing process.

contributing to maintenance of muscle fiber integrity, regeneration and recovery. Conversely, Hsp70 expression is reduced during muscle inactivity and aging. Malfunction of HSP70 generation may drive muscle atrophy, contractile dysfunction, and reduced regeneration. Beneficial effects of the activation of Hsp70 biosynthesis in skeletal muscle have been established in animal studies, suggesting Hsp70 as a key therapeutic target for conditions that negatively affect skeletal muscle mass and function (Morton et al., 2014; Senf, 2013).

A forkhead family transcription factor FOXO3 suppresses tumors (down-regulation of FOXO3A activity is often seen in cancer). Genotype FOXO3A is strongly associated with human longevity (Flachsbart et al., 2009; Willcox et al., 2008). FOXO is activated by oxidative stress, DNA damage, nutrient deprivation, cytokines, and hypoxia; it is inhibited by insulin, growth factors, and stress-activated Jun-N-terminal kinase (INK). FOXO3 can be inhibited and translocated out of the nucleus into the cytoplasm by proteins (e.g., protein kinase B [Akt/PKB]) in the phosphatidylinositol 3-kinase (PI3K) signaling pathway. During stress, FOXO transcription factors translocate to the nucleus, where they transactivate genes involved in resistance to oxidative stress and energy metabolism in worms, as well as genes implicated in the repair of damaged DNA, glucose metabolism, autophagy, cell cycle arrest, and apoptosis in mammals. Hsp70 controls FOXO/DAF-16 activity by promoting FOXO export out of the nucleus. DAF-16 is a key FOXO transcription factor that controls innate immunity in *Caenorhabditis elegans*.

Age-related attenuation of the HSF1/Hsp70 pathway enables the deposition of toxic beta-amyloid fibrils, activating the FOXO pathway. Up-regulation of HSF1 pathways may reduce protein aggregate deposition, possibly preventing or delaying the onset of neurodegenerative diseases, and may be beneficial in ischemia, reperfusion injury, inflammation, and sepsis. The concomitant activation of both the HSF1/Hsp70 and the FOXO pathways could reduce oxidative stress (e.g., cerebrovascular disease, cancer, osteoarthritis, etc.), insulin resistance, and cellular division dysfunction (in cancer). *The simultaneous modulation of HSF1 and FOXO pathways by adaptogens is a unique opportunity to synergistically balance and preserve cellular repair and defense systems.*

EFFECT OF ADAPTOGENS ON LIFE SPAN, HSP70, HSF1, JNK, NEUROPEPTIDE Y AND FOXO SIGNALING PATHWAYS

The adaptogens *R. rosea*, *S. chinensis*, and *E. senticossus*, alone and in combination (ADAPT-232), up-regulate transcription factor HSF1, and initiate increased production of molecular chaperon Hsp70 in vitro and in vivo (Asea et al., 2013; Chiu & Ko, 2004; Hernández-Santana et al., 2014; Lee et al., 2009; Li et al., 2014; Panossian et al., 2009; Panossian et al., 2010; Prodius et al. 1997) (see Figure 13.1). Adaptogens also inhibit stress activated protein kinase JNK (Panossian et al., 2007), a key mediator of apoptosis and aging (Figure 13.1). In addition, adaptogens cause the activation of FOXO by the translocation of transcription factor DAF-16 from the cytoplasm into the nucleus (Wiegant et al., 2009). Pre-treatment Schizandrin B, an active constituent of *S. chinensis*, induces increases in Hsp25 and Hsp70 expression in rat hearts and protects against myocardial ischemia-reperfusion injury (Chiu & Ko, 2004). The hepatic cytoprotective action of Schisandrin B against acetaminophen-induced liver injury is mediated, at least in part, by the induction ·of HspP27 and Hsp70 in mice. Oral administration of Schisandrin B increased Hsp27 and Hsp70 gene and protein expression in a dose-dependent manner (Li et al., 2014).

ADAPT-232 and its active constituent, salidroside, stimulated the expression and release of HSF1 and downstream release of Hsp70 in isolated neurolgia cells (Panossian et al., 2009; Panossian et al., 2010). Furthermore, ADAPT-232-induced expression and release of Hsp70 from glioma cells was dependent on HSF1 and a stress hormone, neuropeptide Y (NPY). Based on these findings, it was hypothesized that HSF1 and NPY could be primary upstream molecular targets for adaptogens in neuroglia cells [Panossian et al., 2012]. ADAPT-232 and salidroside act on NPY expression via a mechanism dependent on up-regulation of HSF1. The concomitant activation of both NPY and Hsp70 is specific to adaptogens (Asea et al., 2013). The activation of NPY by ADAPT-232 initiates Hsp70 expression in neuroglia cells, which support the homeostasis of neuronal cells. The stimulation and release of NPY and Hsp70 into systemic circulation gives rise to adaptive and stress-protective effects via the central nervous, autonomic, endocrine, immune, cardiovascular, and gastrointestinal systems. Both NPY and Hsp70 play important roles in the regulation of aging and pathogenesis of age-related diseases (Calderwood et al., 2009; Kuo & Zukowska, 2007). These studies suggest that the stimulation and release of NPY and Hsp70 into systemic circulation is a defense response triggered by ADAPT-232, which increases adaptation to stress and longevity in animal models. NPY is also involved in the regulation of the hypothalamic-pituitary-adrenal (HPA) axis, energy homeostasis, secretion of Hsp70, cytoprotection, and immunity.

R. rosea, S. chinensis, E. senticossus, W. somnifera, and *P. ginseng* have been shown to extend life span and survival under stress in the nematode *Caenorhabditis elegans* (Kumar et al., 2013; Lee et al., 2007; Wiegant et al., 2009), fruit fly *Drosophila melanogaster* (Gospodaryov et al., 2013; Jafari et al., 2007; Schriner et al., 2009; Schriner et al., 2013), and yeast *Saccharomyces cerevisiae* (Bayliak & Lushchak, 2011). Salidrosides (rhodioloside) and other extracts of *R. rosea* and *S. chinensis* were found to be the most active inhibitors of stress-induced phosphorylated kinase (p-SAPK/p-JNK) (Figure 13.1). Oral supplementation with salidroside or extracts of *E. senticosus, S. chinensis,* and *R. rosea* over a 7-day period in rabbits subjected to restraint stress significantly decreased immobilization stress-induced elevation of p-SAPK/p-JNK. In the nematode *C. elegans,* adaptogens induced the translocation of the DAF-16 transcription factor from the cytoplasm into the nucleus, suggesting a reprogramming of transcriptional activities favoring synthesis of proteins involved in stress resistance and longevity (Wiegant et al., 2009). Based on these observations, it was suggested that adaptogens are experienced as mild to moderate stressors and thereby induce increased stress resistance and a longer life span.

Thus, the proposed strategy of therapeutic intervention in age-associated diseases is directed toward correcting failures in specific signaling pathways that are known to ameliorate and postpone aging by the activation of multiple genes. At the transcriptional level, two anti-aging molecular targets are the HSF1 and FOXO pathways (Perez et al., 2012). Modulating these two pathways may delay the onset of neurodegenerative diseases and other age-related illnesses.

DNA MICROARRAY ANALYSIS PREDICTS THE POTENTIAL INDICATION OF ADAPTOGENS IN AGING-ASSOCIATED DISORDERS

Natural aging and adaptation to environmental challenges are multistep processes involving interactions of many molecular networks through intracellular and extracellular communications (signaling pathways). At the transcriptional level, two complimentary longevity pathways, HSF1 and FOXO, have been described. Additional pathways are presumably involved in the development of age-related disorders. DNA microarray analysis of mechanisms of action found that *R. rosea* up- or down-regulated 1063 genes, *S. chinensis* 1091 genes, and *E. senticossus* 1075 genes. Overlaps within the analysis identified 261 genes that are up- or down-regulated by all three adaptogens (Panossian et al., 2013). Analysis of downstream actions of these 261 genes provides information on the possible influence of adaptogens on cellular and physiological functions, predicting possible effects on disease pathogenesis, including age-associated disorders (see Box 13.1 and Table 13.1). Data were analyzed using QIAGEN's Ingenuity® Pathway Analysis (IPA®, QIAGEN Redwood City, www.qiagen.com/ingenuity).

Adaptogens down-regulate the expression of genes encoding adenylate cyclase and up-regulate gene expression for phosphodiestherase. Therefore, it was hypothesized that adaptogens reduce the cyclic adenosine monophosphate (cAMP) level in brain cells. Low levels of c-AMP down-regulate protein kinase A (PKA) activity. PKA functions include the regulation of glycogen, sugar, and lipid metabolism. The effects of PKA activation vary with the cell type; for example, in adipocytes PKA stimulates lipases, while in myocytes (skeletal muscle) and hepatocytes PKA increases glucose formation (by stimulating glycogenolysis and inhibiting glycogenesis) and its catabolic transformation to pyruvate (glycolysis). This provides free energy in the form of adenosyl triphosphate (ATP) and nicotine adenine dinucleotide, reduced (NADH), which are important in stress response. The regulation of cAMP levels and PKA activity is a key mechanism of energy homeostasis and represents a metabolic switch between catabolism and anabolism. Down-regulation of cAMP and

PKA by adaptogens decreases stress-induced catabolic transformations. PKA is presumably responsible for the stress-induced protective energy-saving effects of adaptogens. This energy-saving effect favors ATP-consuming anabolic transformations. The inhibition of adenylate cyclase by adaptogens can increase intracellular ATP levels and prevent ATP from being converted to cAMP. This increased store of ATP might represent an energy source for other ATP-dependent enzymatic reactions required for metabolism (Panossian et al., 2013). *These findings are consistent with the plausible mechanism of ATP generation by adaptogens and their potential benefits in fatigue and age-related diseases.*

Prefrontal cortex neurons contain hyperpolarization-activated channels that can open when exposed to cAMP during stress. Excessive opening of these channels impairs cognitive function. It has been hypothesized that cAMP inhibitors can inactivate these channels, enabling more normal neuronal function, reconnecting hyperpolarized cells to the neural network, and thus improving working memory, which is essential for abstract thinking, planning, and executive functions (Wang et al., 2011). This hypothesis is consistent with studies in which adaptogens improved cognitive function in humans (see Table 13.2) (Panossian & Wikman, 2010).

Adaptogens affect G-protein signaling phosphatidylinositol and phospholipase C pathways. All tested adaptogens up-regulate the *PLCB1* gene, which encodes phosphoinositide-specific phospholipase C (PLC), and the *PI3KC2G* gene, which encodes (PI3Ks) (Panossian et al., 2013). When activated by a G-protein, phospholipase C (PLC) catalyzes the hydrolysis of phosphatidylinositol 4,5-bisphosphate (PIP2) into diacylglycerol (DAG) and inositol-1,4,5-triphosphate (IP_3). IP_3 is involved in a variety of cellular signaling pathways associated

Table 13.1. Clinical Trials of Adaptogens Relevant to Age-Related Conditions: Cognitive Function, Memory, Fatigue, Stress, Depression

ADAPTOGEN DOSE/ DAY DURATION	DESIGN/ TOTAL SUBJECTS	PRIMARY OUTCOMES	JADAD SCORE*	REFERENCE	COMMENTS
R. rosea SHR-5 170 mg/d 2 weeks	DBRPC, CO 56 healthy MDs night duty stress [24–35 y]	↓Mental fatigue; ↑perceptive and cognitive functions, concentration, speed of audiovisual perception	4	Darbinyan, et al. (2000)	Benefits did not persist at 6 weeks, possibly due to cumulative fatigue
R. rosea SHR-5 50 mg b.i.d. 20 days	DBRPC 40 students exam stress [17–19y]	↓Mental fatigue; ↑perception, ↑well-being, ↑physical fitness ($p < 0.01$)	3	Spasov, et al. (2000)	
Rhodiola rosea SHR-5 370 mg or 555 mg single dose	DBRPC 3 groups 161 healthy military cadets [19–21 y]	↑Capacity for mental work, ↑anti-fatigue vs control ($p < 0.001$); no significant difference between two dosage groups	3	Shevtsov, et al. (2003)	
ADAPT-232 Single dose 3 caps	DBPC, CO 60 healthy adults	↑ Short-term memory, speed, accuracy in computerbased and psychometric tests	1	Bogatova et al. (1994)	
ADAPT-232 Single dose	DBPC, CO, 5 Russian cosmonauts	↑ Working capacity during training 90-day isolation	1	Bogatova et al. (1997)	
R. rosea (Rodaxon)	DPRPC 60 foreign high school students	↑Physical fitness, ↓mental fatigue, ↓anxiety	1	Spasov et al. (2000)	
Rhodosin R. rosea 100 mg 20 days	DBRPC 60 adult students adaptation to academic load	↑physical fitness, ↓mental fatigue ($p < 0.01$) and ↑well-being ($p < 0.05$)	1	Spasov et al. (2000)	
Rodelim (R. rosea, E. senticosus, S. chinensis) 100 mg single dose	DBRPC 60 adults	Improved mental working capacity in computer and correction tests against a background of fatigue	1	Rooslyakova et al. (2000)	

(continued)

Table 13.1. Continued

ADAPTOGEN DOSE/ DAY DURATION	DESIGN/ TOTAL SUBJECTS	PRIMARY OUTCOMES	JADAD SCORE*	REFERENCE	COMMENTS
ADAPT-232 single dose 270 mg vs. placebo	DBRPC 40 women chronic psychology-cal stress [20–68 y]	Stressful test of attention pre- and 2 hours post-ADAPT 270 mg: ↑ Mental speed and accuracy during mental fatigue	5	Aslanyan et al. (2010)	
E. senticosus 2 mg eleutherosides (B and E) 2 months	RDBPC 96 adults Chronic fatigue syndrome [21–65 y]	↓Fatigue in both groups. E. senticosus better effects than placebo in subjects with less severe fatigue & fatigue ≥ 5 y	5	Hartz et al. (2004)	
R. rosea SHR-5 228 mg twice daily 4 wks	RDBPC 60 adults Stress-induced fatigue/ burnout [20–55 y]	R. rosea significant improvements in fatigue, burnout, cognitive function, attention, accuracy, cortisol response to awakening stress	5	Olsson et al. (2009)	
R.rosea WS*1375 200 mg twice/d 4 wks	OL 101 adults Life stress sympotoms	↓Stress symptoms, perceived stress, fatigue, Numbers Connecting Test, disability, Clinical Global Impression	1	Edwards, et al. (2012)	
R.rosea, vitamins, minerals Vigodana®12 wks	OL 120 adults Physical and cognitive deficiencies [50–89 y]	Improvements in physical and cognitive deficiencies ($p < 0.001$) and speed digital connection test ($p < 0.001$)	0	Fintelman & Gruenwald (2007)	
R. rosea Rhodax® 340 mg/d 10 wks	OL 10 adults generalized anxiety disorder [34–55 y]	Significant ↓anxiety and depression ratings	0	Bystritsky et al. (2008)	
R. rosea extract New cultivation in Canada. 42 days	DBRPC 48 Nursing students (18–55 y)	Fatigue worsened with R. rosea compared to placebo. No data on amount of rest between work shifts.	0	Punja et al. (2014)	Poor quality. Lacks quality control extraction and standardization
R. rosea SHR-5 170 or 340 mg twice/d 6 weeks	DBRPC 91 patients mild to moderate depression [18–70 y]	SHR-5 significant ↓depression, insomnia, emotional instability, somatization; ↑self-esteem ($p < 0.001$)	5	Darbinyan et al. (2007)	

with phenomena as diverse as depression and tumor growth. DAG activates protein kinase C (PKC), which phosphorylates numerous other proteins and plays an important role in tumor growth. PI3K is a key upstream mediator of signal transduction, regulation of NF-kB-mediated defense responses, and apoptosis. PI3K is required for long-term enhancement of neurotransmission, which potentiates memory and learning (Karpova et al., 2006; Yang et al., 2008).

Adaptogens up-regulate *SERPINI1* gene (serpin peptidase inhibitor, neuroserpin), which is involved in the development and function of the nervous system. Neuroserpin controls axon growth and thereby supports neurotransmission. It plays an important role in synapse development and regulates synaptic plasticity, suggesting involvement in learning and memory (Kinghorn et al., 2006). Moreover, neuroserpin inhibits the activity of tissue plasminogen activator (tPA), which influences cell migration, blood clotting, and inflammation (Yepes & Lawrence, 2004).

All tested adaptogens down-regulated the *CETP* gene (Panossian et al., 2013), which encodes cholesteryl ester transfer protein, a lipid plasma protein that facilitates the transport of cholesterol esters and triglycerides between low-density lipoproteins (LDL) and high-density lipoproteins (HDL). Pharmacological inhibition of *CETP* alleviates atherosclerosis and other cardiovascular diseases, as well as metabolic syndrome (Barter et al., 2003).

Adaptogens down-regulate the *ESR1* gene (Panossian et al., 2013). *ESR1* encodes estrogen receptor alpha (ERα), a nuclear receptor belonging to a large family of transcription factors, transducing hormonal signals and regulating expression of target genes. ERs are over-expressed in approximately 70% of breast cancers (Deroo & Korach, 2006). Pharmacological down-regulation of *ESR1* may be beneficial in the treatment and prevention of cancers of the breast, ovaries, colon, prostate, and endometrium (Ascenzi et al., 2006).

CLINICAL EVIDENCE OF ADAPTOGEN EFFECTS IN AGE-ASSOCIATED DISORDERS

Adaptogens have been used to prevent or delay adverse effects of aging on energy, cognitive function, memory, physical endurance, sexual function, cancer, and infections. Documented benefits include enhanced energy, mental and physical performance under stress in healthy adults; reduced

damage from cardiac and cerebrovascular ischemia, hypoxia, and trauma in animal models; and anticarcinogenic effects and protection of hepatocytes and bone marrow from chemotherapy toxicities in animals with human cancer cell transplants (Brown & Gerbarg, 2004, 2009, 2011). Support for the use of adaptogens in age-related diseases derives from traditional medicines, clinical experience, in vitro and animal studies, extrapolation from studies in younger adults, and a limited number of studies in elderly subjects.

Adaptogen Studies and Case Illustrations in Elderly Adults

In a 12-week open efficacy and safety study, *R. rosea* extract in combination with vitamins and minerals (Vigocana®) was given to 120 adults, including 38 women and 37 men between the ages of 50 and 89 years, who had physical and cognitive deficiencies in concentration, memory, and stress tolerance (Fintelmann & Gruenwald, 2007). Statistically significant improvements occurred in physical and cognitive deficiencies ($p < 0.001$) and speed of digital connection test completion ($p < 0.001$). No adverse events occurred, and 99% of patients and physicians rated safety as "good" or "very good." These findings warrant replication in a randomized, controlled trial (RCT). The results are consistent with clinical observations by the author (PG), who found consistent improvements in alertness, concentration, mental clarity, memory, mood, and energy in elderly patients as the following cases illustrate. No adverse effects occurred in these cases.

Case #1: Professor Z.

An eminent 70-year-old physicist, Professor Z., was experiencing increasing difficulties remembering the details of scientific papers he had read over the years. After contacting Dr. Gerbarg, he began taking *R. rosea* 20 minutes before meals: 300 mg every morning plus 150 mg at noon. After 6 weeks he reported substantial improvements in his ability to rapidly recall the authors, dates, and titles of the many publications he enjoyed citing during his lectures and in response to students' questions.

Case #2: Mrs. V.

Mrs. V., a 95-year-old, was an avid reader, musician, and conversationalist. She became annoyed when her increasing mental and physical fatigue forced her to take afternoon naps. To her, a 3-hour nap was a waste of precious time. Taking *R. rosea* 100 mg in the morning and at noon enabled her to stay mentally alert throughout the day and to keep up with her reading schedule so that she could discuss the latest historical or biographical tome she had assigned her friends and relatives to read.

Parkinson's Disease

Parkinson's disease (PD), the second most common neurodegenerative disorder, results from loss of dopaminergic (DA) neurons in substantia nigra pars compacta. Current medical treatments have limited effects on the underlying degenerative cascade of events. In a mouse model of PD, salidroside protected dopaminergic neurons, in a dose-dependent manner, against MPTP/MPP$^+$-induced toxicity by reducing the production of ROS-NO, decreasing cytochrome-c, inhibiting capsase-3, -6, and -9, reducing alpha-synuclein aggregation, and other mechanisms (Wang, Hong, Chen, et al., 2014). Salidroside increases the expression and release of Hsp70 and neuropeptide Y from neuroglia cells (Panossian et al., 2012). Human studies of adaptogen combinations are needed to verify clinical observations that they can be safe and beneficial in the treatment of PD, as in the following case.

Case #3: Mrs. R.

A retired, 75-year-old schoolteacher, Mrs. R. enjoyed an active lifestyle that included golf, bridge, socializing, and playing with her grandchildren until she developed Parkinson's disease. After 5 years, despite treatment with Levodopa, her symptoms progressed to the point where she rarely spoke or rose from sitting in a chair. She developed cognitive decline and secondary depression. She responded to *R. rosea* 540 mg every morning (no change in Levodopa doses). Mrs. R. began talking spontaneously, recovered her energy and drive to about 80% of her premorbid level, and resumed most of her former activities.

Adaptogens in Cardiovascular Disease

Adaptogens are widely used in traditional Chinese medicine (TCM), including *P. ginseng, E. senticosus, S. chinensis,* and *R. rosea* and related subspecies, such as *Rhodiola sacra* and *Rhodiola kirilowii,* for treatment of ischemic heart disease (IHD) and angina pectoris. The heterogeneity of TMC formulas and wide variations in the quality of studies make comparisons difficult. Nevertheless, a systematic review of 13 randomized controlled trials of formulations containing *R. sacra* and *R. kirilowii* found that the overall effectiveness of *Rhodiola* formulations was higher than control groups with significant differences in symptomatic and ECG improvements (Yu, Qin, Wang, et al., 2014). Studies included *Rhodiola* versus other TCMs, *Rhodiola* versus routine Western medicines (RWM), and *Rhodiola* plus RWM. The authors concluded that *Rhodiola* formulas may have positive benefits as solo treatments or in combination with RWM for IHD, but better quality studies are needed.

Chronic stress contributes to the development of cardiovascular disease over time. An RCT of 40 military personnel (aged 25–50 years) experiencing chronic work stress with stress reactive type-cardiostressor-arterial blood pressure ≥ 140/80 and resting heart rate ≥ 80 beats/minute, but with no cardiovascular disease, provided twice daily lifestyle counselling for 30 days to all subjects (Ciumaşu-Rîmbu, Popa, & Vulpoi, 2012). In addition, the active treatment group received ADAPT, a fixed combination of *E. senticosus, S. chinensis,* and *R. rosea* extracts twice daily. After 30 days, the group that had been given adaptogens showed improved tolerance to a novel stressor with significantly lower systolic blood pressure, diastolic blood pressure, and resting heart rate compared to controls. In a double-blind RCT of 20 hypertensive digitalized subjects aged 65 and older, those who were given *E. senticosus* 300 mg/day showed greater improvements in social functioning ($p = 0.02$) on the Health Related Quality of Life measure compared with those given placebo at 4-week testing (Cicero, Derosa, Briolante, et al., 2004). However, the differences between groups attenuated at 8-week testing. There were no adverse events, changes in blood pressure, or changes in serum digitalis levels.

Adaptogen Effects on Stress Tolerance, Fatigue, Cognitive Function, Memory, Depression

In studies of students, adult workers, physicians, military cadets, and cosmonauts under stress, high-quality adaptogen preparations showed benefits for fatigue, cognitive functions, memory, accuracy, speed, work capacity, anxiety, mood, and well-being (Gerberg & Brown 2013; Brown, Gerbarg, & Muskin 2009; Panossian 2013; Panossian & Wikman, 2009, 2010). Table 13.2 summarizes studies published after 1990. The large body of adaptogen studies, including those with less rigorous methodologies published between 1945 and 1990, has been reviewed (Brown, Gerbarg, & Ramazanov 2002; Brown et al., 2004; Panossian & Wagner, 2011). Although adaptogens have not been studied for post-traumatic stress disorder (PTSD), they have shown benefits in studies of stress tolerance, anxiety, and depression. Their capacity to help balance stress response systems suggests a potential role in the prevention and treatment of PTSD. Anecdotally, one author (PG) has found that some patients with long-standing PTSD report that *R. rosea* reduces over-reactivity, anxiety, depression, and sleep problems.

CURRENT LIMITATIONS AND FUTURE DIRECTIONS

An important limitation in the assessment of studies of herbal preparations in general is the variability of composition and activity of bioactive constituents due to genetic and environmental (climate, soil characteristics, plant infections, fertilization) factors. Differences in processing raw materials, extraction, distillation, purification, and storage also affect the final composition and activity. Batch-to-batch reproducibility is not usually evaluated. Discrepancies among studies are attributable to variations in herbal extracts, study populations, and methodologies. In order to improve reproducibility and efficacy of herbal preparations, further progress is needed in the accurate identification of rootstocks, good manufacturing and good agricultural practice (GMP-GAP)–based production, and sufficiently characterized and properly specified products.

Perhaps the most promising areas for adaptogen studies are diseases associated with aging and stress-induced disorders including fatigue (from all causes), depression (monotherapy or antidepressant augmentation), PTSD, neuroprotection (brain aging, cognitive decline, Parkinson's disease, cerebrovascular insufficiency, and dementia), attention, cancer (to augment chemotherapy and protect liver and bone marrow from chemotherapy toxicity), menopause, physical and mental performance enhancement, high altitude tolerance, and space flight (Brown et al., 2004; Brown et al., 2009; Gerbarg, Illig, & Brown 2015). The identification of new targets for the prevention and treatment of age-related diseases, through omics and systems biology studies, will contribute to longevity and quality of life.

DISCLOSURE STATEMENTS

Author P. Gerbarg reports no conflicts of interest in relation to this article. A. Panossian is an employee but not a shareholder of Swedish Herbal Institute, a research and development–based company producing herbal preparations.

ACKNOWLEDGMENTS

The authors wish to thank Richard P. Brown, MD, for reviewing this manuscript and providing case material.

REFERENCES

Ambra, R., Mocchegiani, E., Giacconi, R., et al. (2004). Characterization of the HSP70 response in lymphoblasts from aged and centenarian subjects and differential effects of in vitro zinc supplementation. *Exp Gerontol, 39*(10), 1475–1484.

Ascenzi, P., Bocedi, A., & Marino, M. (2006). Structure-function relationship of estrogen receptor alpha and beta: impact on human health. *Mol Aspects Med, 27,* 299–402.

Asea, A., Kaur, P., Panossian, A., & Wikman, K. G. (2013). Evaluation of molecular chaperons Hsp72 and neuropeptide Y as characteristic markers of adaptogenic activity of plant extracts. *Phytomedicine, 20,* 1323–1329.

Aslanyan, G., Amroyan, E., Gabrielyan, E., Panossian, A., &Wikman, G. (2010). Double-blind, placebo-controlled, randomised study of the single dose effects of ADAPT-232 on cognitive functions. *Phytomedicine, 17,* 494–499.

Barter, P. J., Brewer, H. B., Jr., Chapman, M. J., Hennekens, C. H., Rader, D. J., & Tall, A. R. (2003). Cholesteryl ester transfer protein: a novel target for raising HDL and inhibiting atherosclerosis. *Arterioscler Thromb Vasc Biol, 23,* 160–167.

Bayliak, M. M, & Lushchak, V. I. (2011). The golden root, Rhodiola rosea, prolongs lifespan but decreases oxidative stress resistance in yeast Saccharomyces cerevisiae. *Phytomedicine, 18*(14), 1262–1268. doi: 10.1016/j.phymed.2011.06.010.

Bhat, R. V., Budd Haeberlein, S. L., & Avila, J. (2004). Glycogen synthase kinase 3: a drug target for CNS therapies. *J Neurochem, 89*(6), 1313–1317.

Bogatova, R. I., & Malozemov, V. V. (1994). *Experimental research on the estimation of influence of single dose of phytoadaptogens on short-term memory: report on ADAPT 232.* Moscow: Institute of Medical and Biological Problems (IMBP), pp. 1–151.

Bogatova, R. I., Shlyakova, L. V., Salnitsky, V. P., Wikman, G. (1997). Evaluation of the effect of a single dose of a phytoadaptogen on human subjects' work ability during long isolation. *Aerospace Environ Med, 31,* 51–54.

Bondy, S., & Maiese, K. (Eds.) (2010). *Aging and age-related disorders.* New York: Humana Press.

Boon-Niermeijer, E. K., van den Berg, A., Vorontsova, O. N., Bayda, L. A., Malyshev, I. Y., & Wiegant, F. A. C. (2012). Enhancement of adaptive resistance against a variety of chronic stress conditions by plant adaptogens: protective effects on survival and embryonic development of Lymnaea stagnalis. *Adaptive Med,* 4(4): 233–244.

Boon-Niermeijer, E. K., van den Berg, A., Wikman, G., Wiegant, F. A. (2000). Phyto-adaptogens protect against environmental stress-induced death of embryos from the freshwater snail Lymnaea stagnalis. *Phytomedicine, 7,* 389–399.

Brown, R. P., & Gerbarg, P. L. (2011). Integrative treatments in brain Injury. In J. M. Silver, S. C. Yudofsky, & T. W. McAllister (Eds.), *Neuropsychiatry of traumatic brain injury* (3rd ed., pp. 599–622). Washington, DC: American Psychiatric Press.

Brown, R. P., Gerbarg, P. L., & Graham, B. (2004). *The Rhodiola revolution.* New York: Rodale Press.

Brown, R. P., Gerbarg, P. G., & Muskin, P. R. (2008). In A. Tasman, J. Kay, & J. Lieberman (Eds.), *Alternative treatments in psychiatry* (3rd ed., pp. 2318–2353). London: John Wiley & Sons.

Brown, R. P., Gerbarg, P. L., & Muskin, P. R. (2009). *How to use herbs, nutrients, and yoga in mental health care.* New York: W. W. Norton.

Brown, R. P., Gerbarg, P. L., & Ramazanov, Z. (2002). A phytomedical review of Rhodiola rosea. *Herbalgram, 56,* 40–62.

Bystritsky, A., Kerwin, L., & Feusner, J. D. (2008). A pilot study of Rhodiola rosea (Rhodax) for generalized anxiety disorder (GAD). *J Altern Complement Med, 14*(2), 175–180. doi: 10.1089/ acm.2007.7117.

Calderwood, S. K., Murshid, A., & Prince, T. (2009). The shock of aging: molecular chaperones and the heat shock response in longevity and aging: a mini-review. *Gerontology, 55*(5), 550–558.

Chiu, P. Y., & Ko, K. M. (2004). Schisandrin B protects myocardial ischemia-reperfusion injury partly by inducing Hsp25 and Hsp70 expression in rats. *Mol Cell Biochem, 266*(1–2), 139–144. PubMed PMID: 15646035.

Cicero, A. F., Derosa, G., Brillante, R., Bernardi, R., Nascetti, S., & Gaddi, A. (2004). Effects of Siberian ginseng (Eleutherococcus senticosus maxim.) on elderly quality of life: a randomized clinical trial. *Arch Gerontol Geriatr Suppl, 9,* 69–73.

Ciumaşu-Rîmbu, M., Popa, L., & Vulpoi, C. (2012). Neuropeptide Y stimulation as primary target for preventive measures of maladaptative cardiovascular reactions in occupational chronic stress exposure. *Rev Med Chir Soc Med Nat Iasi, 116*(3), 790–793.

Darbinyan, V., Aslanyan, G., Amroyan, E., Gabrielyan, E., Malmstrom, C., & Panossian, A. (2007). Clinical trial of Rhodiola rosea L. extract SHR-5 in the treatment of mild to moderate depression. *Nord J Psychiatr, 61,* 343–348.

Deroo, B. J., & Korach, K. S. (2006). Estrogen receptors and human disease. *J Clin Invest, 116,* 561–567.

Droge, W. (2002). Free radicals in the physiological control of cell function. *Physiol Rev, 82,* 47–95.

Edwards, D., Heufelder, A., & Zimmermann, A. (2012). Therapeutic effects and safety of Rhodiola rosea extract WS® 1375 in subjects with life-stress symptoms—results of an open-label study. *Phytother Res, 6,* 1220–1225.

Fintelmann, V., & Gruenwald, J. (2007). Efficacy and tolerability of a Rhodiola rosea extract in adults with physical and cognitive deficiencies. *Adv Ther 24,* 929–939.

Flachsbart, F., Caliebe, A., Kleindorp, R., Blanché, H., von Eller-Eberstein, H., Nikolaus, S., Schreiber, S., & Nebel, A. (2009). Association of FOXO3A variation with human longevity confirmed in

German centenarians. *Proc Natl Acad Sci USA* *106*(8), 2700–2705.

Gagliano, N., Grizzi, F., & Annoni, G. (2007). Mechanisms of aging and liver functions. *Dig Dis*, *25*(2),118–123.

Gerbarg, P. L., & Brown, R. P. (2013). Phytomedicines for prevention and treatment of mental health disorders. In Phillip R. Muskin, Patricia L. Gerbarg, and Richard P. Brown (Eds.), *Complementary and integrative therapies for psychiatric disorders. Psychiatric Clinics of North America, 36*(1), 37–47. doi: 10.1016/j. psc.2012.12.004.

Gerbarg, P. L., & Brown, R. P. (2015) Therapeutic nutrients, herbs, and hormones. In David D'Addona, Barry Fogel, and Donna Greenberg (Eds.) *Psychiatric care of the medical patient* (4th ed.). New York: Oxford University Press.

Gerbarg, P., Illeg, P., & Brown, R. P. (2015). Rhodiola rosea. In Alain Cuerrier & Kwesi Ampong-Nyarko (Eds.), Traditional herbal medicines for modern times (vol. 14, pp. 225-252). New York: Taylor & Francis

Gospodaryov, D. V., Yurkevych, I. S., Jafari, M., Lushchak, V. I., Lushchak, O. V. (2013). Lifespan extension and delay of age-related functional decline caused by Rhodiola rosea depends on dietary macronutrient balance. *Longev Healthspan*, *2*(1), 5.

Hartz, A. J., Bentler, S., Noyes, R., Hoehns, J., Logemann, C., Sinift, S., Butani, Y., Wang, W., Brake, K., Ernst, M., and Kautzman, H. (2004). Randomized controlled trial of Siberian ginseng for chronic fatigue. *Psychol. Med, 34*, 51–56.

Hernández-Santana, A., Pérez-López, V., Zubeldia, J. M., Jiménez-del-Rio, M. (2014). A Rhodiola rosea root extract protects skeletal muscle cells against chemically induced oxidative stress by modulating heat shock protein 70 (HSP70) expression. *Phytother Res, 28*(4), 623–628.

Heydari, A. R., Takahashi, R., Gutsmann, A., You, S., Richardson, A. (1994). Hsp70 and aging. *Experientia, 50*(11–12), 1092–1098. Review. PubMed PMID: 7988669.

Heydari, A. R., You, S., Takahashi, R., Gutsmann-Conrad, A., Sarge, K. D., Richardson, A. (2000). Age-related alterations in the activation of heat shock transcription factor 1 in rat hepatocytes. *Exp Cell Res, 256*(1), 83–93. PubMed PMID: 10739655.

Jafari, M., Felgner, J. S., Bussel, I. I., Hutchili, T., Khodayari, B., Rose, M. R., Vince-Cruz, C., Mueller L. D. (2007). Rhodiola: a promising anti-aging Chinese herb. *Rejuvenation Res, 10*(4), 587–602.

Karpova, A., Sanna, P. P., and Behnisch, T. (2006). Involvement of multiple phosphatidylinositol 3-kinase-dependent pathways in the persistence of late-phase long term potentiation expression. *Neuroscience, 137,* 833–841.

Kayani, A. C., Morton, J. P., McArdle, A. (2008). The exercise-induced stress response in skeletal muscle: failure during aging. *Appl Physiol Nutr Metab, 33*(5), 1033–1041.

Kinghorn, K. J., Crowther, D. C., Sharp, L. K., Nerelius, C., Davis, R. L., Chang, H. T., Green, C., Gubb, D. C., Johansson, J., & Lomas, D. A. (2006). Neuroserpin binds Abeta and is a neuroprotective component of amyloid plaques in Alzheimer disease. *J Biol Chem, 281,* 29268–29277.

Kregel, K. C., & Zhang, H. J. (2007). An integrated view of oxidative stress in aging: basic mechanisms, functional effects, and pathological considerations. *Am J Physiol Regul Integr Comp Physiol, 292,* R18–R36.

Kumar, R., Gupta, K., Saharia, K., Pradhan, D., & Subramaniam, J. R. (2013). Withania somnifera root extract extends lifespan of Caenorhabditis elegans. *Ann Neurosci, 20*(1), 13–16.

Kuo, L. E., Abe, K., & Zukowska, Z. (2007). Stress, NPY and vascular remodeling: implications for stress-related diseases. *Peptides, 28*(2), 435–440.

Lee, F. T., Kuo, T. Y., Liou, S. Y., & Chien, C. T. (2009). Chronic Rhodiola rosea extract supplementation enforces exhaustive swimming tolerance. *Am J Chin Med, 37*(3), 557–572.

Lee, J. H., Choi, S. H., Kwon, O. S., Shin, T. J., Lee, J. H., Lee, B. H., Yoon, I. S., Pyo, M. K., Rhim, H., Lim, Y. H., Shim, Y. H., Ahn, J. Y., Kim, H. C., Chitwood, D. J., Lee, S. M., & Nah, S. Y. (2007). Effects of ginsenosides, active ingredients of Panax ginseng, on development, growth, and life span of Caenorhabditis elegans. *Biol Pharm Bull, 30*(11), 2126–2134.

Li, L., Zhang, T., Zhou, L., Zhou, L., Xing, G., Chen, Y., & Xin, Y. (2014). Schisandrin B attenuates acetaminophen-induced hepatic injury through heat-shock protein 27 and 70 in mice. *J Gastroenterol Hepatol, 29*(3), 640–647.

Lindquist, S., & Craig, E. A. (1988). The heat-shock proteins. *Annu Rev Genet, 22,* 631–677.

Minois, N., Khazaeli, A. A., & Curtsinger, J. W. (2001). Locomotor activity as a function of age and life span in Drosophila melanogaster overexpressing HSP70. *Exp Gerontol, 36*(7), 1137–1153.

Morton, J. P., Kayani, A. C., McArdle, A., & Drust, B. (2009). The exercise-induced stress response of skeletal muscle, with specific emphasis on humans. *Sports Med, 39*(8), 643–662.

Narimanian, M., Badalyan, M., Panosyan, V., Gabrielyan, E., Panossian, A., Wikman, G., & Wagner, H. (2005). Impact of Chisan® (ADAPT-232) on the quality-of-life and its efficacy as an adjuvant in the treatment of acute non-specific pneumonia. *Phytomedicine, 12*(10), 723–729.

Olsson, E. M., von Scheele, B., & Panossian, A. G. (2009). A randomised, double-blind, placebo-controlled, parallel-group study of the standardised extract shr-5 of the roots of Rhodiola rosea in the treatment of subjects with stress-related fatigue. *Planta Med, 75,* 105–112.

Panossian, A., Hambartsumyan, M., Hovanissian, A., Gabrielyan, E., & Wikman, G. (2007). The adaptogens Rhodiola and Schizandra modify the response to immobilization stress in rabbits by suppressing the increase of phosphorylated stress-activated protein kinase, nitric oxide and cortisol. *Drug Targets Insights, 1,* 39–54. http://www.la-press.com/ the-adaptogens-rhodiola-and-schizandra-modify-the-response-to-immobili-a260.

Panossian, A., Hamm, R., Kadioglu, O., Wikman, G., & Efferth, T. (2013). Synergy and antagonism of active constituents of ADAPT-232 on transcriptional level of metabolic regulation of isolated neuroglia cells. *Front Neurosci, 7,* 16. doi: 10.3389/fnins.2013.00016. http://www.frontiersin.org/Journal/Abstract.aspx?s=744&name=neuroendocrine_science&ART_DOI=10.3389/fnins.2013.00016.

Panossian, A., Hamm, R., Kadioglu, O., Wikman, G., & Efferth, T. (2014). Mechanism of action of Rhodiola, salidroside, tyrosol and triandrin in isolated neuroglial cells: an interactive pathway analysis of the downstream effects using RNA microarray data. *Phytomedicine, 21,* 1325–1348.

Panossian, A., & Wagner, H. (2011). Adaptogens: a review of their history, biological activity, and clinical benefits. *HerbalGram, 90,* 52–63.

Panossian, A., & Wikman, G. (2009). Evidence-based efficacy of adaptogens in fatigue, and molecular mechanisms related to their stress-protective activity. *Curr Clin Pharmacol, 4*(3), 198–219.

Panossian, A., & Wikman, G. (2010). Effects of adaptogens on the central nervous system and the molecular mechanisms associated with their stress-protective activity. *Pharmaceuticals, 3*(1), 188–224. doi: 10.3390/ph3010188; http://www.mdpi.com/1424-8247/3/1/188/pdf.

Panossian, A., Wikman, G., Kaur, P., & Asea, A. (2009). Adaptogens exert a stress protective effect by modulation of expression of molecular chaperons. *Phytomedicine, 16*(6–7), 617–622.

Panossian, A., Wikman, G., Kaur, P., & Asea A. (2010). Molecular chaperones as mediators of stress protective effect of plant adaptogens. In A. Asea & B. K. Pedersen (Eds.), *Heat shock proteins and whole body physiology 5,* 351–364.

Panossian, A., Wikman, G., Kaur, P., & Asea, A. (2012) Adaptogens stimulate neuropeptide Y and Hsp72 expression and release in neuroglia cells. *Front Neurosci, 6,* 6. doi: 10.3389/fnins.2012.00006. http://www.frontiersin.org/neuroendocrine_science/10.3389/fnins.2012.00006/full

Panossian, A., Wikman, G., & Wagner, H. (1999). Plant adaptogens. III. Earlier and more recent aspects and concepts on their mode of action. *Phytomedicine 6,* 287–300.

Perez, F. P., Moinuddin, S. S., Ulain Shamim, Q., Joseph, D. J., Morisaki, J., & Zhou, X. (2012). Longevity pathways: HSF1 and FoxO pathways, a new therapeutic target to prevent age-related diseases. *Curr Aging Sci, 5*(2), 87–95.

Prodius, P. A., Manukhina, E. B., Bulanov, A. E., Vikman, G., & Malyshev, I. I. (1997). [Adaptogen ADAPT modulates synthesis of inducible stress protective protein HSP 70 and increases organism resistance to heat shock]. *Biull Eksp Biol Med, 123*(6), 629–631 (Russ.).

Rooslyakova, N. A., Bogatova, R. I., Verishvili, M. O., & Wikman, G. (2000). The effect of single dose of Rodelim pystoadaptogen on the performance of operators under intense activity. In *Abstract book of scientific conference biologically active food supplements and natural medicines in prophylaxis, treatment and rehabilitation* (pp. 157–160). Moscow: .

Schaffler, K., Wolf, O. T., & Burkart, M. (2013). No benefit adding eleutherococcus senticosus to stress management training in stress-related fatigue/weakness, impaired work or concentration, a randomized controlled study. *Pharmacopsychiatry, 46*(5), 181–190. doi: 10.1055/s-0033-1347178.

Schriner, S. E., Abrahamyan, A., Avanessian, A., Bussel, I., Maler, S., Gazarian, M., Holmbeck, M. A., & Jafari, M. (2009). Decreased mitochondrial superoxide levels and enhanced protection against paraquat in Drosophila melanogaster supplemented with Rhodiola rosea. *Free Radic Res, 43*(9), 836–843.

Schriner, S. E., Lee, K., Truong, S., Salvadora, K. T., Maler, S., Nam, A., Lee, T., & Jafari, M. (2013). Extension of Drosophila lifespan by Rhodiola rosea through a mechanism independent from dietary restriction. *PLoS One, 8*(5), e63886.

Sen, S. M., Dodd, S. L., McClung, J. M., & Judge, A. R. (2008). Hsp70 overexpression inhibits NF-kappa B and Foxo3a transcriptional activities and prevents skeletal muscle atrophy. *FASEB J*, 22, 3836–3845.

Senf, S. M. (2013). Skeletal muscle heat shock protein 70: diverse functions and therapeutic potential for wasting disorders. *Front Physiol*, 4, 330.

Senf, S. M., Dodd, S. L., & Judge, A. R. (2010). FOXO signaling is required for disuse muscle atrophy and is directly regulated by Hsp70. *Am J Physiol Cell Physiol*, 298(1), C38–45.

Senf, S. M., Dodd, S. L., McClung, J. M., & Judge, A. R. (2008). Hsp70 overexpression inhibits NF-kappaB and Foxo3a transcriptional activities and prevents skeletal muscle atrophy. *FASEB J*, 22(11), 3836–3845.

Shevtsov, V. A., Zholus, I., Shervarly, V. I., et al. (2003). A randomized trial of two different doses of a SHR-5 Rhodiola rosea extract versus placebo and control of capacity for mental work. *Phytomedicine*, 10(2–3), 95–105.

Singh, R., Kolvraa, S., & Rattan, S. I. (2007). Genetics of human longevity with emphasis on the relevance of HSP70 as candidate genes. *Front Biosci*, 12, 4504–4513.

Singh, V., & Aballay, A. (2009). Regulation of DAF-16-mediated Innate Immunity in Caenorhabditis elegans. *J Biol Chem*, 284(51), 35580–35587.

Spasov, A. A., Mandrikov, V. B., Miranova, I. A, et al. (2000). The effect of the preparation rodakson on the psychophysiological and physical adaptation of students to an academic load. *Eksp Klin Farmakol*, 63(1), 76–78.

Spasov, A. A., Wikman, G. K., Mandrikov, V. B., et al. (2000). A double-blind placebo-controlled pilot study of the stimulating and adaptogenic effect of Rhodiola rosea SHR-5 extract on the fatigue of students caused by stress during an examination period with a repeated low-dose regimen. *Phytomedicine*, 7(2), 85–89.

Steinberg, D., & Witztum, J. L. (2002). Is the oxidative modification hypothesis relevant to human atherosclerosis? Do the antioxidant trials conducted to date refute the hypothesis? *Circulation*, 105, 2107–2111.

Tardif, J. C., Gregoire, J., L'Allier, P. L., et al. (2008). Effects of the antioxidant succinobucol (AGI-1067) on human atherosclerosis in a randomized clinical trial. *Atherosclerosis*, 197(1), 480–486.

Wang, S., He, H., Chen, L., Zhang, W., Zhang, X., & Chen, J. (2014). Protective effects of salidroside in the MPTP/MPP+-induced model of Parkinson's disease through ROS-NO-related mitochondrion pathway. *Mol Neurobiol*, .

Wang M[1], Gamo NJ, Yang Y, Jin LE, Wang XJ, Laubach M, Mazer JA, Lee D, Arnsten AF. Neuronal basis of age-related working memory decline. Nature. 2011 Jul 27;476(7359):210-3. doi: 10.1038/nature10243.

Wiegant, F. A. C., Limandjaja, G., de Poot, S. A. H., Bayda, L. A., Vorontsova, O. N., Zenina, T. A., Langelaar Makkinje, M., Post, J. A., & Wikman, G. (2008). Plant adaptogens activate cellular adaptive mechanisms by causing mild damage. In L. Lukyanova, N. Takeda, & P. K. Singal (Eds.), *Adaptation biology and medicine: health potentials* (vol. 5, pp. 319–332). New Delhi: Narosa.

Wiegant, F. A. C., Surinova, S., Ytsma, E., et al. (2009). Plant adaptogens increase lifespan and stress resistance in C. elegans. *Biogerontology*, 10(1), 27–42.

Willcox, B. J., Donlon, T. A., He, Q., Chen, R., Grove, J. S., Yano, K., Masaki, K. H., Willcox, D. C., Rodriguez, B., & Curb, J. D. (2008). FOXO3A genotype is strongly associated with human longevity. *Proc Natl Acad Sci USA*, 105(37), 13987–13992.

Winklhofer, K. F., Tatzelt, J., Haass. (2008). The two faces of protein misfolding: gain- and loss-of function in neurodegenerative diseases. *EMBO J*, 27(2), 336–349.

Yang, P. C., Yang, C. H., Huang, C. C., & Hsu, K. S. (2008). Phosphatidylinositol 3-kinase activation is required for stress protocol-induced modification of hippocampal synaptic plasticity. *J Biol Chem*, 283, 2631–2643.

Yepes, M., & Lawrence, D. A. (2004). Neuroserpin: a selective inhibitor of tissue-type plasminogen activator in the central nervous system. *Thromb Haemost*, 91, 457–464.

Yu, L., Qin, Y., Wang, Q., Zhang, L., Liu, Y., Wang, T., Huang, L., Wu, L., & Xiong, H. (2014). The efficacy and safety of Chinese herbal medicine, Rhodiola formulation in treating ischemic heart disease: a systematic review and meta-analysis of randomized controlled trials. *Complement Ther Med*, 22(4), 814–825. doi: 10.1016/j.ctim.2014.05.001.

SECTION B

MIND–BODY MEDICINE

14

MIND–BODY TECHNIQUES TO IMPROVE COPING AND STRESS RESPONSE

Ronald M. Glick and Esther G. Teverovsky

BACKGROUND

For the holistic practitioner, there are basic topics that are discussed with patients, independent of the reason bringing them in for care. High on the list are diet, exercise, and stress management. The premise is that the health conditions that one experiences with age and as part of the Western lifestyle are not necessarily inevitable. No one is surprised to learn that chronic stress contributes to the risk of developing heart disease, cancer, and other health conditions. The mechanisms conferring these risks are often quite similar to those seen over time in normal aging and include systemic inflammation, telomere shortening, and a shift from parasympathetic to sympathetic predominance, among others. Chapter 1 of this volume reviews these pathways in more detail. There are medications that block inflammation, but unfortunately, adverse effects often outweigh the benefits. We have yet to discover a telomere-lengthening pill.

Lazarus defines stress as "a condition or feeling experienced when a person perceives that demands exceed the personal and social resources the individual is able to mobilize" (1966). Eliminating stress for anyone, particularly older adults, is not realistic, given health issues, family stressors, and financial concerns, among many others. Our goal, in this regard, is to help improve a person's coping abilities. Before turning to specific approaches, it is helpful to consider what questions we would like to answer.

How do individuals manage stress? As a part of the care of older adults, it is reasonable to ask how they manage stress. In the hierarchy of responses, on the low end are things like, "I'm so wiped out, I just veg out in front of the TV," or "a stiff drink." When patients give us a blank stare, we need to take a step back and inquire more about the stressors in their lives. Commonly, individuals can easily provide a list of their concerns and problems, but they may not be able to identify their resources in managing stress. While this discussion is focused on "mind–body techniques," there are many positive and adaptive responses that relate to Lazarus's definition of stress, referring to the perception of demands outweighing resources. As such, many activities, such as golf with friends, gardening, church activity groups, and bridge club, can enhance an individual's resources and ability to cope. Regular religious practice, such as communal worship and spiritual meditation, may energize and provide support for many individuals. Physical exercise can be an excellent stress reliever, but may be less available to those with pain or significant health problems. When patients are unsure as to what may be the most helpful for them, we have the opportunity to direct them to programs in their communities.

Do we explore stress management by itself or as part of wider lifestyle changes? As people age, they have diminished ability to maintain homeostasis and decreased functional reserve. It makes intuitive sense that the greatest benefit will come from an interaction of lifestyle changes. The Dean Ornish Programs have looked at the combined effects of these interventions. Similarly, in the complementary, alternative, and integrative medicine world, we are familiar with whole-systems approaches, such as Ayurveda and traditional Chinese medicine, which may combine dietary, mind–body, exercise, energetic, and spiritual approaches. With regard to the mind–body aspect, typically, interventions have been studied in isolation, rather than as part of an integrative program. Enticingly, a small open trial showed a reversal of memory impairments among individuals with Alzheimer's disease who participated in comprehensive lifestyle changes that included changes to diet, yoga, and meditation (Bredesen, 2014). Lifestyle interventions are discussed further in Chapter 2 of this volume.

Are there comorbid or concurrent conditions, which travel with stress, and for which mind–body approaches may provide some benefit? Certainly, insomnia, anxiety, and depression come to mind as conditions associated with high levels of chronic stress. From the standpoint of disabling conditions, pain is certainly worth exploring, given the prevalence of osteoarthritis and other chronic pain conditions among older adults. Also, it will be important to note whether mind–body practice can impact on chronic health conditions such as hypertension, metabolic syndrome, or diabetes.

How are mind–body approaches best studied? For Western medical treatments, the gold standard of research is the randomized controlled double blind trial. While one tries to follow this design for complementary approaches, as complex interventions, there are many challenges in design. The methodological flaws and marked variability noted in systematic reviews and meta-analyses point to these complexities. Considerations, important both for designing studies as well as for understanding the information include the following:

- For yoga, tai chi, and meditation, there are many forms of each. Although the similarities are often greater than the differences, this disparity adds complexity both to design as well as the ability to generalize from one approach to another.
- As with any interpersonally oriented program, the skill and other qualities of the instructor can make a large difference on outcomes.
- What is an appropriate "dose" of treatment (i.e., how many sessions, how long does each session last, how many times per week, for how many weeks)?
- Does the program encourage practice between sessions, and if so, how is compliance measured and related to treatment outcomes?
- Does one study a specific disease-based population or healthy individuals? Similarly, does one study community-dwelling older adults or those in group settings? To what extent can one generalize results from one population to another?
- What is an appropriate control or comparison group?
- Depending on the research question, is it better to present the intervention practice to novices, or to experienced or master-level practitioners?

These last two issues merit further discussion. Within the RCT design, optimally, one would control for the "active" or therapeutic component of the treatment maintaining the other non-salient aspects. This becomes a challenge for complex interventions such as yoga or TC in which it would be fruitless to try to parse out what is "therapeutic." Yeh and colleagues address this hypothetical challenge to find a control lacking the active ingredient for a TC study (Yeh, Kaptchuk, & Shmerling, 2010): "Is it rhythmic exercise, deliberate and deep breathing, contemplative concentration, group relaxing imagery, a charismatic teacher, or some synergistic combination of these elements? If so, would the matched control include awkward movements, halted breathing, participant isolation, unpleasant imagery, or a tepid teacher? Would the resulting intervention be credible, valid, or even genuinely inactive?"

The advantages of working with individuals without prior experience with a modality include greater generalizability to the population at large and the ability to study the intervention with randomization to an appropriate control. In particular, for identifying physiological mechanisms, one may see more dramatic changes with master-level practitioners, such as yogis and Buddhist monks, as compared with novices to the modality. Indeed, across measures of cardiac functionality and functional neuroimaging, adept practitioners have enhanced changes compared with novices (Lutz, Greischar, Perlman, & Davidson, 2009).

One final issue pertains to how we, as the consumers, best interpret scientific research. Investigators may be less likely to submit the results of a negative trial for publication, and journals may be less inclined to publish an inconclusive or negative study. Additionally, as studies of mind–body practices or other complementary therapies may have limited funding support, the sample size in these trials may be low. This combination of bias in submission and publication and small numbers of participants may lead to positive findings that would not hold up under more rigorous study. Consequently, caution is recommended in drawing more general conclusions.

What is a mind–body practice, and which practices do we include in this discussion? Primarily, we are focusing on personal or group activities that enhance resilience and coping, primarily through their impact on stress-management abilities. The decision as to which practices to include and exclude can be somewhat circular and confusing. Is jogging a mind–body practice? Certainly, many individuals describe a "zen-like" or mindful state that occurs with long-distance running, but the primary effect is seen to be physiologically related to the aerobic activity. Conversely, many of the benefits from yoga and TC relate to the physical exercise component, but we are in agreement with the National Center for Complementary and Integrative Health (NCCIH) that these are best considered as mind–body practices. Hypnosis and prayer are discussed elsewhere in this text. Yoga and paced breathing also have dedicated chapters, but we include yoga in this discussion, given its central role in mind–body practice. While other activities may have a mind–body effect, we are focusing on three Eastern-derived practices: yoga, meditation, and tai chi.

YOGA

Yoga refers to a family of practices that developed as a part of India's culture and philosophy. Literally, the term means "joining" or "yoking together," referring to mind, body, and spirit. Historically, its popularity in the West has been focused on the *asanas*, or poses. *Pranayama*, or yogic breathing, is typically taught along with the physical exercise. Other aspects include meditation, which is discussed later in this chapter, and a more spiritual aspect. Yoga falls within the wider Ayurvedic system of healing, in the same way that tai chi and qi gong are a part of traditional Chinese medicine (TCM). There are a number of forms of yoga, with the most common being Hatha. As with Yang style tai chi, given its wide exposure, many individuals start out with Hatha yoga and then explore other forms of practice. Particularly for older adults, who may be sedentary, may have lost mobility, and may have concurrent arthritic conditions, it is important to start slowly and work closely with the instructor, in order to avoid injury.

Yoga has been shown to have a direct impact on psychological stress. In a sample of university employees, yoga led to greater feelings of self-confidence during stressful situations as compared with wait-list controls (Hartfiel, Havenhand, Khalsa, Clarke, & Krayer, 2011). Even a single yoga class was able to decrease scores on the perceived stress scale, and this effect was more pronounced after 8 weeks of instruction (Huang, Chien, & Chung, 2013). In a sample of individuals older than age 60, twice-weekly yoga practice led to a variety of improved health-related outcomes, including decreased stress (Halpern, Cohen, Kennedy, Reece, Cahan, & Baharav, 2014).

In addition, yoga has a direct impact on the immune and stress response systems. In a sample of individuals with chronic illnesses, yoga decreased glucocorticoids, increased beta-endorphins, and decreased IL-6 and TNF-alpha. In a study by Eda et al., salivary beta-defensin 2 was increased in older adults after the completion of a 90-minute yoga practice (Eda, Shimizu, Suzuki, Tanabe, Lee, & Akama, 2013). This is relevant because beta-defensin 2 is an important part of the body's defense against respiratory illnesses and because its levels have been tied with stress and immune function (Usui, Yoshikawa, Orita, Ueda, Katsura, Fujimoto et al., 2011). Yoga has also been shown to increase heart rate variability and to decrease blood pressure (Huang, Chien, &

Chung, 2013; Papp, Lindfors, Storck, & Wandell, 2013; Tyagi & Cohen, 2014).

Yoga has shown a positive impact on sleep, a clinically relevant outcome that is closely associated with stress (Hall, Matthews, Kravitz, Gold, Buysse, Bromberger, et al., 2009; Ohayon, 2005). This is particularly important among older adults because sleep quality decreases greatly with age. Some populations have rates of insomnia approaching 50%, and insomnia is presumed to be one pathway through which stress adversely impacts health (Foley, Monjan, Brown, Simonsick, Wallace, & Blazer, 1995; Maggi, Langlois, Minicuci, Grigoletto, Pavan, Foley, et al., 1998). Among a geriatric sample, those practicing yoga for 6 months showed decreased self-reported sleep latency, increased total time spent asleep, and improved feelings of being rested in the morning (Manjunath & Telles, 2005). Improved sleep among those practicing yoga has been found both in community-dwelling elders and in those in assisted-living facilities (Chen, Chen, Chao, Hung, Lin, & Li, 2009; Chen, Chen, Lin, Fan, Lin, & Li, 2010). Among a sample of older adults with insomnia, yoga improved sleep quality, sleep latency, sleep efficiency, and sleep duration (Halpern, Cohen, Kennedy, Reece, Cahan, & Baharav, 2014).

When stress is at high levels, it increases risk for and severity of psychiatric illnesses. The impact of yoga on stress may account for the efficacy of yoga in ameliorating certain psychiatric illnesses. In a systematic review, Cramer et al. note that current evidence supports the use of yoga as an ancillary treatment for depression (Cramer, Lauche, Langhorst, & Dobos, 2013). They suggest that more and better-designed studies examining the influence of yoga on those with identified depressive disorders are needed in order to strengthen the evidence basis for yoga as a treatment for depression. Among a general group of older people, several studies show lower ratings on depression and anxiety inventories after a yoga intervention (Chen, Chen, Chao, Hung, Lin, & Li, 2009; Chen, Chen, Lin, Fan, Lin, & Li, 2010; Halpern, Cohen, Kennedy, Reece, Cahan, & Baharav, 2014). Among individuals with dementia, both depressed mood and problem behaviors were shown to decrease among those participating in yoga (Chen, Wang, Li, & Chen, 2011).

Yoga has been found to be useful in people with a variety of aging-related diseases. Among people with chronic pain conditions, including lower back pain, osteoarthritis, rheumatoid arthritis, and headache, yoga resulted in decreased pain and improved functioning (Field, 2011). To date, relatively little attention has been directed at yoga as an intervention for chronic pain in older populations. In a small sample ($n = 21$) of individuals with osteoarthritis and a mean age of 80, chair yoga improved physical functioning but did not directly impact pain or mood (Park, McCaffrey, Dunn, & Goodman, 2011).

A recent systematic review examining yoga use by cancer survivors found that 11 of the 13 articles demonstrated improvement in physical or psychological functioning (Sharma, Haider, & Knowlden, 2013). Yoga appears beneficial in blood-pressure control in hypertension (Tyagi & Cohen, 2014). Similarly, it can enhance glycemic control among diabetic patients, in addition to resulting in decreased BMI, improved lipid profiles, and decreased markers of oxidative stress (Hegde, Adhikari, Kotian, Pinto, D'Souza, & D'Souza, 2011; Shantakumari, Sequeira, & El deeb, 2013). Yoga improves balance, which may decrease the risk of falls (Schmid, Van Puymbroeck, & Koceja, 2010; Tiedemann, O'Rourke, Sesto, & Sherrington, 2013).

TAI CHI AND QI GONG

There are many parallels between tai chi (TC) and yoga, and in fact there was likely cross-talk between Chinese and Indian cultures, leading to shared concepts. As an example, in TCM, the Upper Dan Tien is the center of *shen*, or spirit, located identically with the third-eye *chakra*, which is connected to intuition and perception. The similarities extend to mindful awareness of the body, a focus on breathing practice, connection with the earth, and employing movement as a meditative practice. Another commonality is the range of practice, from more vigorous, to greater slowness and stillness. Many cultures have a word for vital force or energy, including *qi* in TCM thinking, *prana* in Indian philosophy, and *ruach* in Hebrew.

Is TC an exercise, a form of martial arts, or a mind–body practice? The short answer is yes. There are five main schools or family styles of TC. Yang style, particularly Yang 24 short form, is the most widely practiced in the West. The full name, *tai chi chuan*, is loosely translated as "supreme ultimate fist." It has been a part of health practice and Chinese martial arts for close to a millennium. A 2007 National Health Interview Survey (NHIS) estimated that 2.3 million individuals in the United States participated in TC practice over the prior year (Barnes, Bloom, & Nahin, 2008). Qi gong is a parallel practice, which overlaps significantly with TC. One difference is intention. TC was developed as a martial arts form, and some styles are true to this origin, with ballistic movements and weapons forms, using items such as swords in the practice. Qi gong is considered more a means to balance the energetic aspects of the body's organs. In practice, particularly as taught in senior settings, the similarities are greater than the differences. They share slow rhythmic movements, focus on breathing, and mindful awareness. In many studies, the activity described incorporates components of both, and for the purpose of this discussion, qi gong is subsumed under the heading of TC.

Aerobic exercise is known to have beneficial effects on mental and physical health, as well as slowing the physiologic aspects of aging. It follows that a person who wants to remain healthy will maintain regular physical exercise. According to the 2012 NHIS, approximately 45% of adults in the United States aged 65–74 are "sufficiently active" (CDC, 2013). This refers to participating in 150–300 minutes per week of moderate-intensity physical activity. Anyone who has made a New Year's resolution or has started on an exercise regimen can vouch for the difficulties in maintaining a program over time.

TC offers several features that may be helpful in engaging older adults and encouraging them to maintain regular practice. Classes are widely available in community centers and senior programs and generally are inexpensive. Once participants get past the initial period, they seem to "get it" and find the practice enjoyable, in contrast to the boredom or repetitiveness one may experience with other forms of exercise. The presence of senior-oriented programs circumvents the concern seen with other recreational activities, such as a spa aerobics class, of needing to keep up with younger, more agile participants. Many individuals are reluctant to consider more contemplative forms of mind–body practice. For them, the physical activity is engaging. Finally, given the isolation that many older adults experience, the group setting may provide collegial support.

TC enhances immunity, as measured by response to influenza or varicella vaccination, as well as impact on inflammatory cytokines (Ho, Wang, Ng, Ho, Ziea, Wong et al., 2013; Morgan, Irwin, Chung, & Wang, 2014). In experienced TC practitioners, decreased signs of oxidative damage were noted, along with a greater percentage of normal rather than damaged DNA, as compared with a matched

group from the community (Goon, Noor Aini, Musalmah, Yasmin Anum, & Wan Ngah, 2008). Taken together, these health benefits can keep a person physiologically younger and can help maintain physical activity.

TC appears to have health-promoting effects on cardiorespiratory function, as well as providing symptomatic improvement in a number of disease states. A meta-analysis by Taylor-Piliae found significant benefit of TC on aerobic capacity, often preventing the decline seen with age (Taylor-Piliae, 2008). Blood pressure reduction is seen in hypertensive patients with TC (Wang, Feng, Yang, Liu, Teng, Li, et al., 2013). While studies of diabetic patients did not show improvement in the primary outcome of glycemic control, they did indicate enhanced lipid profile (Yan, Gu, & Pan, 2013).

Studies have also shown benefit for osteoarthritis with improvement in pain and physical activity (Ye, Cai, Zhong, Cai, & Zheng, 2014). A moderate body of research has shown benefit for lower extremity strength, stability of gait, and risk for falls (Hackney & Wolf, 2014).

Like other mind–body practices, TC appears to exert a prominent effect on autonomic and hormonal pathways. This includes a decrease in sympathetic activity and increased parasympathetic predominance in heart rate variability monitoring in both cardiac patients and healthy practitioners (Lu & Kuo, 2003; Sato, Makita, Uchida, Ishihara, & Masuda, 2010). TC also decreases cortisol (Campo, Light, O'Connor, Nakamura, Lipschitz, LaStayo et al., 2014; Nedeljkovic, Ausfeld-Hafter, Streitberger, Seiler, & Wirtz, 2012). In two studies, one of which was conducted with older adults, TC decreased several biomarkers of oxidative stress (Rosado-Perez, Ortiz, Santiago-Osorio, & Mendoza-Nunez, 2013; Rosado-Perez, Santiago-Osorio, Ortiz, & Mendoza-Nunez, 2012).

What are the psychological effects or benefits of TC, particularly for older adults? Several systematic reviews have explored this question (Abbott & Lavretsky, 2013; Blake & Hawley, 2012; Jimenez, Melendez, & Albers, 2012; Lee & Ernst, 2012). Consistent improvement has been seen across studies in general measures of quality of life, self-efficacy, and mood. For specific trials treating depression as well as other study populations, TC elicits significant improvement in mood. Similarly, consistent reduction in perceived stress and anxiety ratings has been seen across studies. TC also has a strong benefit on sleep quality. Given these findings, it would be of particular importance in gerontology to know if TC can enhance cognitive function. Studies have been mixed, with some showing improvement in cognitive and memory tasks as compared to exercise or attention-control groups, and further research in this area is needed. A meta-analysis found a large effect size of TC on cognitive function as compared to a non-intervention control and a moderate effect size as compared with an exercise comparator (Wayne, Walsh, Taylor-Piliae, Wells, Papp, Donovan, et al., 2014).

While studies of TC on propensity for falls and osteoarthritis have been conducted on older adults, other research typically involves mixed-age groups. Irwin and colleagues at UCLA have performed a series of trials on older adults. They use a specific form called tai chi chih (TCC), and they have demonstrated that this can be readily learned and practiced by seniors and has a significant mind–body effect. Consistent with the findings noted earlier, gleaned from more diverse age groups, they have found wide benefits from their program. On the mechanistic end, TCC enhances cellular immunity in response to the varicella vaccine, decreases cortisol release, decreases the inflammatory markers IL-6 and NF-κB, and decreases sympathetic activity, including pre-ejection period and systolic BP (Black, Irwin, Olmstead, Ji, Crabb Breen, & Motivala, 2014; Campo, Light, O'Connor, Nakamura, Lipschitz, LaStayo et al., 2014; M. Irwin, Pike, & Oxman, 2004; M. R. Irwin & Olmstead, 2012; M. R. Irwin, Olmstead, & Oxman, 2007; M. R. Irwin, Pike, Cole, & Oxman, 2003; Motivala, Sollers, Thayer, & Irwin, 2006). Clinically, individuals with insomnia showed significant improvement in sleep quality and older adults with depression who were not responsive to an antidepressant, and who showed a significant response to TCC, not seen in the control group (M. R. Irwin, Olmstead, Carrillo, Sadeghi, Breen, Witarama et al., 2014; M. R. Irwin, Olmstead, & Motivala, 2008; Lavretsky, Alstein, Olmstead, Ercoli, Riparetti-Brown, Cyr, et al., 2011).

MEDITATION

The word *meditation* refers to a variety of contemplative practices that have arisen out of many world cultures. Various meditation techniques have the goals of promoting relaxation; developing loving-kindness; increasing a sense of connectedness with nature, other people, or the divine; or increasing life energy. In order to do this, individuals shift their focus in order to self-regulate their minds. Common forms of meditation vary in the nature of that focus. Attention may be directed to breathing, mantras, and/or non-judgmentally monitoring sensations and perceptions as they appear and recede.

The practice of meditation has been helpful for individuals in managing psychological stress. A meta-analysis showed that there is a low level of evidence that mindfulness-based stress reduction (MBSR) decreased psychological stress. The same study did not show evidence for mantra-based meditation (Goyal, Singh, Sibinga, Gould, Rowland-Seymour, Sharma, et al., 2014). In a study that is relevant to geriatric populations in particular, the authors found that MBSR decreased stress among dementia caregivers when compared with caregiver education and support (Whitebird, Kreitzer, Crain, Lewis, Hanson, & Enstad, 2013).

There are multiple studies that show a direct effect of meditation on physiological markers of stress and aging. Studies have shown improved heart rate variability among practitioners of meditation and those being trained in it (Bantornwan, Watanapa, Hussarin, Chatsiricharoenkul, Larpparisuth, Teerapornlertratt, et al., 2014; Krygier, Heathers, Shahrestani, Abbott, Gross, & Kemp, 2013; Peressutti, Martin-Gonzalez, & Mesa, 2010). Meditation has also been shown to decrease blood pressure and attenuate the blood pressure response to stress (Nyklicek, Mommersteeg, Van Beugen, Ramakers, & Van Boxtel, 2013). Studies are mixed on the impact of meditation on changes in salivary cortisol levels (Malarkey, Jarjoura, & Klatt, 2013; Nyklicek, Mommersteeg, Van Beugen, Ramakers, & Van Boxtel, 2013). Among dementia caregivers, those trained in Kirtan Kriya meditation (KKM) had decreased levels of certain pro-inflammatory cytokines (NF-κB) and increased activity of interferon response factors (Black, Cole, Irwin, Breen, St Cyr, Nazarian, et al., 2013).

Telomeres are a particularly important physiological marker because of their relationship with both stress and aging. When compared with non-meditating controls, female long-term practitioners of loving-kindness meditation showed longer telomeres (Hoge, Chen, Orr, Metcalf, Fischer, Pollack, et al., 2013). Individuals participating in a 3-month, intensive meditation retreat had higher levels of telomerase compared with matched, wait-list controls (Jacobs, Epel, Lin, Blackburn, Wolkowitz, Bridwell, et al., 2011). Lavretsky and colleagues found that dementia caregivers who did Kirtan Kriya meditation had increased immune cell telomerase activity, compared with a group that listened to relaxing music. This study is particularly relevant because the participants were practicing meditation for 12 minutes/day (as opposed to 6 hours in the Jacobs study) and because the participants were generally older (mean age 61).

There is preliminary evidence that meditation improves sleep. In the meta-analysis mentioned earlier, the confidence interval to suggest that mindfulness meditation can improve sleep was −3% to 24% (Goyal, Singh, Sibinga, Gould, Rowland-Seymour, Sharma, et al., 2014). Several different subpopulations have shown improved sleep with meditation, including organ transplant patients (Gross, Kreitzer, Thomas, Reilly-Spong, Cramer-Bornemann, Nyman, et al., 2010), those with anxiety disorders (Hoge, Bui, Marques, Metcalf, Morris, Robinaugh, et al., 2013), and those taking antidepressants (Britton, Haynes, Fridel, & Bootzin, 2012). In a study looking specifically at those with insomnia, MBSR outperformed eszopiclone, a benzodiazepine receptor agonist, in improving sleep latency, as measured by wrist actigraphy and scores on the Pittsburgh Sleep Quality Index (Gross, Kreitzer, Reilly-Spong, Wall, Winbush, Patterson, et al., 2011). Because insomnia is prevalent among older adults, and because treatment with sedative/hypnotics has risks of side effects among this population, it would be useful to see future work address the effectiveness of meditation to treat insomnia in older adults. This point is brought home by a study that found a correlation between cumulative benzodiazepine exposure and the development of Alzheimer's disease (Billioti de Gage, Moride, Ducruet, Kurth, Verdoux, Tournier, et al., 2014).

Meditation is shown to have a meaningful impact on a number of measures of psychiatric well-being. In two studies, depressive symptoms decreased among dementia caregivers who are taught to meditate (Lavretsky, Epel, Siddarth, Nazarian, Cyr, Khalsa, et al., 2013; Whitebird, Kreitzer, Crain, Lewis, Hanson, & Enstad, 2013). Meditation may also decrease anxiety symptoms, although to our knowledge this has not been shown specifically in geriatric populations. A meta-analysis showed reduction of depressive and anxiety symptoms among individuals with anxiety and mood disorders who engaged in mindfulness-based therapy (Hofmann, Sawyer, Witt, & Oh, 2010).

Mindfulness meditation has become a core component of several psychotherapeutic modalities and has shown effectiveness in treating psychiatric illnesses. Dialectical behavioral therapy is one of the only evidence-based treatments for borderline personality disorder, and mindfulness practice is one of the four skill modules central to this approach. Mindfulness-based cognitive therapy (MBCT) is a psychotherapeutic modality designed to integrate ideas from cognitive behavioral therapy and mindfulness meditation. Among individuals with the diagnosis of depression who do not respond fully to first-line depression treatments, it has been shown to decrease symptoms (Britton, Haynes, Fridel, & Bootzin, 2012; Chiesa, Mandelli, & Serretti, 2012; Geschwind, Peeters, Huibers, van Os, & Wichers, 2012). Among individuals with anxiety disorders, studies have shown that MBCT improves symptoms of post-traumatic stress disorder, panic disorder, and generalized anxiety disorder (Kim, Lee, Choi, Suh, Kim, Kim, et al., 2009; King, Erickson, Giardino, Favorite, Rauch, Robinson, et al., 2013). A meta-analysis found that mindfulness-based therapies were associated with decreased pain, depression, anxiety, and symptom severity among individuals with somatization disorders (Lakhan & Schofield, 2013).

There are some exciting findings relating to meditation and late-life cognitive changes. Compared with controls, people who engage in regular meditation have increased hippocampal volume and gray matter concentration (Holzel, Ott, Gard, Hempel, Weygandt, Morgen, et al., 2008; Luders, Phillips, Clark, Kurth, Toga, & Narr, 2012). When individuals are taught meditation, they show increased left hippocampal volume compared with wait-list controls (Holzel, Carmody, Vangel, Congleton, Yerramsetti, Gard, et al., 2011). One pilot study of individuals with mild cognitive impairment found that MBSR increased functional connectivity between the posterior cingulate and the bilateral medial prefrontal cortex and left hippocampus. It also found a trend toward less bilateral hippocampal volume atrophy (Wells, Yeh, Kerr, Wolkin, Davis, Tan, et al., 2013). A recent systematic review examining the impact of meditation on cognition found preliminary evidence that meditation can have a positive impact on attention, memory, executive function, processing speed, and general cognition. However, methodological issues in a large number of these studies make interpretation somewhat difficult, and future work is needed (Gard, Holzel, & Lazar, 2014).

SUMMARY

There is growing evidence that a variety of mind–body interventions have positive impacts on the individuals who practice them. Certainly, more research in the area will help us to identify which interventions, practiced with which duration and frequency, can be most helpful for which group of individuals.

By definition, mind–body approaches impact favorably on stress measures and coping. The interventions discussed also impact on health in a number of other ways. If medicine had a "pill" that did all of these things, it might be considered malpractice not to prescribe it. Beneficial effects of mind–body practice include the following:

- Reducing manifestations of health problems common among older adults, such as diabetes and hypertension;
- Improving sleep, which is often disrupted in older adults, with potential impact on physical and mental health;
- Improving coping and function and decreasing stress associated with chronic pain;
- Reducing symptoms of anxiety and depression;
- Reducing stress response, as measured by heart rate variability or cortisol secretion;
- Reducing the release of inflammatory cytokines and enhancing immune functioning;
- Increasing telomerase activity;
- Enhancing function and at times structure in brain centers associated with decreased stress response.

It is clear that these interventions already are being used widely. Although national data are limited, an informal survey of senior centers within our own community (Pittsburgh, PA) revealed that yoga and TC classes are fairly ubiquitous. Pittsburgh is probably in the middle of the road, with some communities embracing such programming to a greater degree. As research and consumer interest increase, we anticipate that mind–body programs with seniors in mind will become more readily available in smaller communities. Our patients describe interest in participating in such programs, although they also experience several barriers. Among these limitations are issues with transportation, their own caregiving responsibilities, finances, and reticence to trying something new. With regard to formal meditation instruction, we found fewer resources in our own community, and these programs were not specific to an older adult population.

Patients born after World War II are more likely to have some experience with mind–body practice. For them, rather than the uncertainty of a new practice, they may be open to re-engaging in something they found helpful or enjoyable in the past. Many have had experience with yoga or meditation, given their popularity over the last several decades. TC may resonate for those with experience with martial arts or those who describe themselves as "too hyper for meditation."

Given the changes in health care, there are increasing opportunities to include mind–body programming within the clinic setting. As the geriatric clinic in our university-based healthcare system develops as a medical home, we are in the early stages of creating a mindfulness meditation program. Our hope is to do so in a sustainable way and to help our patients maintain high levels of functioning. It will be important to track quality assurance outcomes for such model programs, including quality of life, physical symptoms, and psychological symptoms.

As with other areas of medicine, the challenge is translating from our knowledge of what can be helpful to what our patients actually can carry out. Can we lead the horse to water? Surprisingly, in our experience, older adults are commonly open and willing to participate in programming that sounds interesting to them, and mind–body practice appears to have a draw. As with the horse, the challenge is to get them to drink, or to participate and continue their participation. Obviously, any benefit is contingent on continued involvement. If compliance with antihypertensive medication is any indication, we shouldn't expect that patients will continue for the health benefit alone. In a study of MBSR for older adults with chronic low back pain, not only did they find benefit during the acute phase of the study, but patients continued the practice, noting ongoing benefits with pain, stress levels, and overall well-being (Morone, Lynch, Greco, Tindle, & Weiner, 2008). Hopefully, this more direct benefit will keep people motivated.

The greatest promise with mind–body practice relates to studies assessing the effects on cognitive functioning and risk for dementia. As the population ages, perhaps greater than our fear of decline in physical health is the concern of dementia. If further studies confirm that mind–body practices can improve cognition or prevent dementia, it will be compelling to both providers and patients. Additionally, given the anticipated personal and societal costs of dementia care, this could take on public health significance.

DISCLOSURE STATEMENT

Dr. Glick and Dr. Teverovsky have no conflicts to disclose.

REFERENCES

Abbott, R., & Lavretsky, H. (2013). Tai Chi and Qigong for the treatment and prevention of mental disorders. *Psychiatr Clin North Am*, 36(1), 109–119. doi: 10.1016/j.psc.2013.01.011

Bantornwan, S., Watanapa, W. B., Hussarin, P., Chatsiricharoenkul, S., Larpparisuth, N., Teerapornlertratt, T., et al. (2014). Role of meditation in reducing sympathetic hyperactivity and improving quality of life in lupus nephritis patients with chronic kidney disease. *J Med Assoc Thailand*, 97(Suppl 3), S101–107.

Barnes, P. M., Bloom, B., & Nahin, R. (2008). *CDC National Health Statistics Report #12. Complementary and alternative medicine use among adults and children: United States, 2007.* http://www.cdc.gov/nchs/data/nhsr/nhsr012.pdf

Billioti de Ga ge, S., Moride, Y., Ducruet, T., Kurth, T., Verdoux, H., Tournier, M., et al. (2014). Benzodiazepine use and risk of Alzheimer's disease: case-control study. *BMJ*, 349, g5205. doi: 10.1136/bmj.g5205

Black, D. S., Cole, S. W., Irwin, M. R., Breen, E., St Cyr, N. M., Nazarian, N., et al. (2013). Yogic meditation reverses NF-B and IRF-related transcriptome dynamics in leukocytes of family dementia caregivers in a randomized controlled trial. *Psychoneuroendocrinology*, 38(3), 348–355.

Black, D. S., Irwin, M. R., Olmstead, R., Ji, E., Crabb Breen, E., & Motivala, S. J. (2014). Tai chi meditation effects on nuclear factor-kappaB signaling in lonely older adults: a randomized controlled trial. *Psychother Psychosom*, 83(5), 315–317. doi: 10.1159/000359956

Blake, H., & Hawley, H. (2012). Effects of Tai Chi exercise on physical and psychological health of older people. *Curr Aging Sci*, 5(1), 19–27.

Bredesen, D. E. (2014). Reversal of cognitive decline: a novel therapeutic program. *Aging (Albany NY)*, 6(9), 707–717.

Britton, W. B., Haynes, P. L., Fridel, K. W., & Bootzin, R. R. (2012). Mindfulness-based cognitive therapy improves polysomnographic and subjective sleep profiles in antidepressant users with sleep complaints. *Psychother Psychosom*, 81(5), 296–304.

Campo, R. A., Light, K. C., O'Connor, K., Nakamura, Y., Lipschitz, D., LaStayo, P. C., et al. (2014). Blood pressure, salivary cortisol, and inflammatory cytokine outcomes in senior female cancer survivors enrolled in a tai chi chih randomized controlled trial. *J Cancer Surviv*. doi: 10.1007/s11764-014-0395-x

CDC. (2013). Early release of selected estimates based on data from the January–September 2012 National Health Interview Survey. http://www.cdc.gov/nchs/data/nhis/earlyrelease/earlyrelease201303.pdf

Chen, K. M., Chen, M. H., Chao, H. C., Hung, H. M., Lin, H. S., & Li, C. H. (2009). Sleep quality, depression state, and health status of older adults after silver yoga exercises: cluster randomized trial. *Int J Nurs Studies*, 46(2), 154–163.

Chen, K. M., Chen, M. H., Lin, M. H., Fan, J. T., Lin, H. S., & Li, C. H. (2010). Effects of yoga on sleep quality and depression in elders in assisted living facilities. *J Nurs Res*, 18(1), 53–61.

Chen, K. M., Wang, H. H., Li, C. H., & Chen, M. H. (2011). Community vs. institutional elders' evaluations of and preferences for yoga exercises. *J Clin Nurs*, 20(7–8), 1000–1007.

Chiesa, A., Mandelli, L., & Serretti, A. (2012). Mindfulness-based cognitive therapy versus psycho-education for patients with major depression who did not achieve remission following antidepressant treatment: a preliminary analysis. *J Alt Compl Med*, 18(8), 756–760.

Cramer, H., Lauche, R., Langhorst, J., & Dobos, G. (2013). Yoga for depression: a systematic review and meta-analysis. *Depression Anxiety*, 30(11), 1068–1083.

Eda, N., Shimizu, K., Suzuki, S., Tanabe, Y., Lee, E., & Akama, T. (2013). Effects of yoga exercise on salivary beta-defensin 2. *Eur J Applied Physiol*, 113(10), 2621–2627.

Field, T. (2011). Yoga clinical research review. *Complement Ther Clin Pract*, 17(1), 1–8. doi: 10.1016/j.ctcp.2010.09.007

Foley, D. J., Monjan, A. A., Brown, S. L., Simonsick, E. M., Wallace, R. B., & Blazer, D. G. (1995). Sleep complaints among elderly persons: an epidemiologic study of three communities. *Sleep*, 18(6), 425–432.

Gard, T., Holzel, B. K., & Lazar, S. W. (2014). The potential effects of meditation on age-related cognitive decline: a systematic review. *Ann NY Acad Sci*, 1307, 89–103.

Geschwind, N., Peeters, F., Huibers, M., van Os, J., & Wichers, M. (2012). Efficacy of mindfulness-based cognitive therapy in relation to prior history of depression: randomised controlled trial. *Br J Psychiatry, 201*(4), 320–325.

Goon, J. A., Noor Aini, A. H., Musalmah, M., Yasmin Anum, M. Y., & Wan Ngah, W. Z. (2008). Long term Tai Chi exercise reduced DNA damage and increased lymphocyte apoptosis and proliferation in older adults. *Med J Malaysia, 63*(4), 319–324.

Goyal, M., Singh, S., Sibinga, E. M., Gould, N. F., Rowland-Seymour, A., Sharma, R., et al. (2014). Meditation programs for psychological stress and well-being: a systematic review and meta-analysis. *JAMA Intern Med, 174*(3), 357–368.

Gross, C. R., Kreitzer, M. J., Reilly-Spong, M., Wall, M., Winbush, N. Y., Patterson, R., et al. (2011). Mindfulness-based stress reduction versus pharmacotherapy for chronic primary insomnia: a randomized controlled clinical trial. *Explore, 7*(2), 76–87.

Gross, C. R., Kreitzer, M. J., Thomas, W., Reilly-Spong, M., Cramer-Bornemann, M., Nyman, J. A., et al. (2010). Mindfulness-based stress reduction for solid organ transplant recipients: a randomized controlled trial. *Alt Ther Health Med, 16*(5), 30–38.

Hackney, M. E., & Wolf, S. L. (2014). Impact of Tai Chi Chu'an practice on balance and mobility in older adults: an integrative review of 20 years of research. *J Geriatr Phys Ther, 37*(3), 127–135. doi: 10.1519/JPT.0b013e3182abe784

Hall, M. H., Matthews, K. A., Kravitz, H. M., Gold, E. B., Buysse, D. J., Bromberger, J. T., et al. (2009). Race and financial strain are independent correlates of sleep in midlife women: the SWAN sleep study. *Sleep, 32*(1), 73–82.

Halpern, J., Cohen, M., Kennedy, G., Reece, J., Cahan, C., & Baharav, A. (2014). Yoga for improving sleep quality and quality of life for older adults. *Alt Ther Health Med, 20*(3), 37–46.

Hartfiel, N., Havenhand, J., Khalsa, S. B., Clarke, G., & Krayer, A. (2011). The effectiveness of yoga for the improvement of well-being and resilience to stress in the workplace. *Scand J Work Env Hea, 37*(1), 70–76.

Hegde, S. V., Adhikari, P., Kotian, S., Pinto, V. J., D'Souza, S., & D'Souza, V. (2011). Effect of 3-month yoga on oxidative stress in type 2 diabetes with or without complications: a controlled clinical trial. [Erratum appears in Diabetes Care. 2012 Apr;35(4):939]. *Diabetes Care, 34*(10), 2208–2210.

Ho, R. T., Wang, C. W., Ng, S. M., Ho, A. H., Ziea, E. T., Wong, V. T., et al. (2013). The effect of t'ai chi exercise on immunity and infections: a systematic review of controlled trials. *J Alt Compl Med, 19*(5), 389–396. doi: 10.1089/acm.2011.0593

Hofmann, S. G., Sawyer, A. T., Witt, A. A., & Oh, D. (2010). The effect of mindfulness-based therapy on anxiety and depression: a meta-analytic review. *J Consult Clin Psychol, 78*(2), 169–183. doi: 10.1037/a0018555

Hoge, E. A., Bui, E., Marques, L., Metcalf, C. A., Morris, L. K., Robinaugh, D. J., et al. (2013). Randomized controlled trial of mindfulness meditation for generalized anxiety disorder: effects on anxiety and stress reactivity. *J Clin Psychiatry, 74*(8), 786–792.

Hoge, E. A., Chen, M. M., Orr, E., Metcalf, C. A., Fischer, L. E., Pollack, M. H., et al. (2013). Loving-Kindness Meditation practice associated with longer telomeres in women. *Brain Behav Immun, 32*, 159–163.

Holzel, B. K., Carmody, J., Vangel, M., Congleton, C., Yerramsetti, S. M., Gard, T., et al. (2011). Mindfulness practice leads to increases in regional brain gray matter density. *Psychiatry Res, 191*(1), 36–43.

Holzel, B. K., Ott, U., Gard, T., Hempel, H., Weygandt, M., Morgen, K., et al. (2008). Investigation of mindfulness meditation practitioners with voxel-based morphometry. *Social Cogn Affect Neurosci, 3*(1), 55–61.

Huang, F. J., Chien, D. K., & Chung, U. L. (2013). Effects of Hatha yoga on stress in middle-aged women. *J Nurs Res, 21*(1), 59–66.

Irwin, M., Pike, J., & Oxman, M. (2004). Shingles immunity and health functioning in the elderly: tai chi chih as a behavioral treatment. *Evid-Based Compl Alt Med, 1*(3), 223–232. doi: 10.1093/ecam/neh048

Irwin, M. R., & Olmstead, R. (2012). Mitigating cellular inflammation in older adults: a randomized controlled trial of Tai Chi Chih. *Am J Geriatr Psychiatry, 20*(9), 764–772. doi: 10.1097/JGP.0b013e3182330fd3

Irwin, M. R., Olmstead, R., Carrillo, C., Sadeghi, N., Breen, E. C., Witarama, T., et al. (2014). Cognitive behavioral therapy vs. tai chi for late life insomnia and inflammatory risk: a randomized controlled comparative efficacy trial. *Sleep, 37*(9), 1543–1552. doi: 10.5665/sleep.4008

Irwin, M. R., Olmstead, R., & Motivala, S. J. (2008). Improving sleep quality in older adults with moderate sleep complaints: a randomized controlled trial of Tai Chi Chih. *Sleep, 31*(7), 1001–1008.

Irwin, M. R., Olmstead, R., & Oxman, M. N. (2007). Augmenting immune responses to varicella zoster virus in older adults: a randomized, controlled trial of Tai Chi. *J Am Geriatr Soc, 55*(4), 511–517. doi: 10.1111/j.1532-5415.2007.01109.x

Irwin, M. R., Pike, J. L., Cole, J. C., & Oxman, M. N. (2003). Effects of a behavioral intervention, Tai Chi Chih, on varicella-zoster virus specific immunity and health functioning in older adults. *Psychosom Med, 65*(5), 824–830.

Jacobs, T. L., Epel, E. S., Lin, J., Blackburn, E. H., Wolkowitz, O. M., Bridwell, D. A., et al. (2011). Intensive meditation training, immune cell telomerase activity, and psychological mediators. *Psychoneuroendocrinology, 36*(5), 664–681.

Jimenez, P. J., Melendez, A., & Albers, U. (2012). Psychological effects of Tai Chi Chuan. *Arch Gerontol Geriatr, 55*(2), 460–467. doi: 10.1016/j.archger.2012.02.003

Kim, Y. W., Lee, S. H., Choi, T. K., Suh, S. Y., Kim, B., Kim, C. M., et al. (2009). Effectiveness of mindfulness-based cognitive therapy as an adjuvant to pharmacotherapy in patients with panic disorder or generalized anxiety disorder. *Depression Anxiety, 26*(7), 601–606.

King, A. P., Erickson, T. M., Giardino, N. D., Favorite, T., Rauch, S. A., Robinson, E., et al. (2013). A pilot study of group mindfulness-based cognitive therapy (MBCT) for combat veterans with posttraumatic stress disorder (PTSD). *Depress Anxiety, 30*(7), 638–645. doi: 10.1002/da.22104

Krygier, J. R., Heathers, J. A., Shahrestani, S., Abbott, M., Gross, J. J., & Kemp, A. H. (2013). Mindfulness meditation, well-being, and heart rate variability: a preliminary investigation into the impact of intensive Vipassana meditation. *Int J Psychophysiol, 89*(3), 305–313.

Lakhan, S. E., & Schofield, K. L. (2013). Mindfulness-based therapies in the treatment of somatization disorders: a systematic review and meta-analysis. *PLoS One, 8*(8), e71834. doi: 10.1371/journal.pone.0071834

Lavretsky, H., Alstein, L. L., Olmstead, R. E., Ercoli, L. M., Riparetti-Brown, M., Cyr, N. S., et al. (2011). Complementary use of tai chi chih augments escitalopram treatment of geriatric depression: a randomized controlled trial. *Am J Geriatr Psychiatry, 19*(10), 839–850. doi: 10.1097/JGP.0b013e31820ee9ef

Lavretsky, H., Epel, E. S., Siddarth, P., Nazarian, N., Cyr, N. S., Khalsa, D. S., et al. (2013). A pilot study of yogic meditation for family dementia caregivers with depressive symptoms: effects on mental health, cognition, and telomerase activity. *Int J Geriatr Psychiatry, 28*(1), 57–65.

Lazarus, R. S. (1966). *Psychological stress and the coping process.* New York: McGraw Hill.

Lee, M. S., & Ernst, E. (2012). Systematic reviews of t'ai chi: an overview. *Br J Sports Med, 46*(10), 713–718. doi: 10.1136/bjsm.2010.080622

Lu, W. A., & Kuo, C. D. (2003). The effect of Tai Chi Chuan on the autonomic nervous modulation in older persons. *Med Sci Sports Exerc, 35*(12), 1972–1976. doi: 10.1249/01.mss.0000099242.10669.f7

Luders, E., Phillips, O. R., Clark, K., Kurth, F., Toga, A. W., & Narr, K. L. (2012). Bridging the hemispheres in meditation: thicker callosal regions and enhanced fractional anisotropy (FA) in long-term practitioners. *Neuroimage, 61*(1), 181–187.

Lutz, A., Greischar, L. L., Perlman, D. M., & Davidson, R. J. (2009). BOLD signal in insula is differentially related to cardiac function during compassion meditation in experts vs. novices. *Neuroimage, 47*(3), 1038–1046. doi: 10.1016/j.neuroimage.2009.04.081

Maggi, S., Langlois, J. A., Minicuci, N., Grigoletto, F., Pavan, M., Foley, D. J., et al. (1998). Sleep complaints in community-dwelling older persons: prevalence, associated factors, and reported causes. *J Am Geriatr Society, 46*(2), 161–168.

Malarkey, W. B., Jarjoura, D., & Klatt, M. (2013). Workplace based mindfulness practice and inflammation: a randomized trial. *Brain Behav Immun, 27*(1), 145–154. doi: 10.1016/j.bbi.2012.10.009

Manjunath, N. K., & Telles, S. (2005). Influence of Yoga and Ayurveda on self-rated sleep in a geriatric population. *Indian J Med Res, 121*(5), 683–690.

Morgan, N., Irwin, M. R., Chung, M., & Wang, C. (2014). The effects of mind-body therapies on the immune system: meta-analysis. *PLoS One, 9*(7), e100903. doi: 10.1371/journal.pone.0100903

Morone, N. E., Lynch, C. S., Greco, C. M., Tindle, H. A., & Weiner, D. K. (2008). "I felt like a new person": the effects of mindfulness meditation on older adults with chronic pain: qualitative narrative analysis of diary entries. *J Pain, 9*(9), 841–848. doi: 10.1016/j.jpain.2008.04.003

Motivala, S. J., Sollers, J., Thayer, J., & Irwin, M. R. (2006). Tai Chi Chih acutely decreases sympathetic nervous system activity in older adults. *J Gerontol A Biol Sci Med Sci, 61*(11), 1177–1180.

Nedeljkovic, M., Ausfeld-Hafter, B., Streitberger, K., Seiler, R., & Wirtz, P. H. (2012). Taiji practice attenuates psychobiological stress reactivity: a randomized controlled trial in healthy subjects. *Psychoneuroendocrinology, 37*(8), 1171–1180. doi: 10.1016/j.psyneuen.2011.12.007

Nyklicek, I., Mommersteeg, P. M., Van Beugen, S., Ramakers, C., & Van Boxtel, G. J. (2013). Mindfulness-based stress reduction and physiological activity during acute stress: a randomized controlled trial. *Health Psychol, 32*(10), 1110–1113.

Ohayon, M. M. (2005). Prevalence and correlates of nonrestorative sleep complaints. *Arch Intern Med, 165*(1), 35–41.

Papp, M. E., Lindfors, P., Storck, N., & Wandell, P. E. (2013). Increased heart rate variability but no effect on blood pressure from 8 weeks of hatha yoga: a pilot study. *BMC Research Notes, 6*, 59.

Park, J., McCaffrey, R., Dunn, D., & Goodman, R. (2011). Managing osteoarthritis: comparisons of chair yoga, Reiki, and education (pilot study). *Holistic Nurs Pract, 25*(6), 316–326.

Peressutti, C., Martin-Gonzalez, J. M., J, M. G.-M., & Mesa, D. (2010). Heart rate dynamics in different levels of Zen meditation. *Int J Cardiol, 145*(1), 142–146.

Rosado-Perez, J., Ortiz, R., Santiago-Osorio, E., & Mendoza-Nunez, V. M. (2013). Effect of Tai Chi versus walking on oxidative stress in Mexican older adults. *Oxid Med Cell Longev, 2013*, 298590. doi: 10.1155/2013/298590

Rosado-Perez, J., Santiago-Osorio, E., Ortiz, R., & Mendoza-Nunez, V. M. (2012). Tai chi diminishes oxidative stress in Mexican older adults. *J Nutr Health Aging, 16*(7), 642–646.

Sato, S., Makita, S., Uchida, R., Ishihara, S., & Masuda, M. (2010). Effect of Tai Chi training on baroreflex sensitivity and heart rate variability in patients with coronary heart disease. *Int Heart J, 51*(4), 238–241.

Schmid, A. A., Van Puymbroeck, M., & Koceja, D. M. (2010). Effect of a 12-week yoga intervention on fear of falling and balance in older adults: a pilot study. *Arch Phys Med Rehabil, 91*(4), 576–583.

Shantakumari, N., Sequeira, S., & El deeb, R. (2013). Effects of a yoga intervention on lipid profiles of diabetes patients with dyslipidemia. *Indian Heart J, 65*(2), 127–131.

Sharma, M., Haider, T., & Knowlden, A. P. (2013). Yoga as an alternative and complementary treatment for cancer: a systematic review. *J Alt Compl Med, 19*(11), 870–875.

Taylor-Piliae, R. E. (2008). The effectiveness of Tai Chi exercise in improving aerobic capacity: an updated meta-analysis. *Med Sport Sci, 52*, 40–53. doi: 10.1159/000134283

Tiedemann, A., O'Rourke, S., Sesto, R., & Sherrington, C. (2013). A 12-week Iyengar yoga program improved balance and mobility in older community-dwelling people: a pilot randomized controlled trial. *J Gerontol A, 68*(9), 1068–1075.

Tyagi, A., & Cohen, M. (2014). Yoga and hypertension: a systematic review. *Alt Ther Health Med, 20*(2), 32–59.

Usui, T., Yoshikawa, T., Orita, K., Ueda, S. Y., Katsura, Y., Fujimoto, S., et al. (2011). Changes in salivary antimicrobial peptides, immunoglobulin A and cortisol after prolonged strenuous exercise. *Eur J Appl Physiol, 111*(9), 2005–2014. doi: 10.1007/s00421-011-1830-6

Wang, J., Feng, B., Yang, X., Liu, W., Teng, F., Li, S., et al. (2013). Tai chi for essential hypertension. *Evid Based Compl Alt Med, 2013*, 215254. doi: 10.1155/2013/215254

Wayne, P. M., Walsh, J. N., Taylor-Piliae, R. E., Wells, R. E., Papp, K. V., Donovan, N. J., et al. (2014). Effect of tai chi on cognitive performance in older adults: systematic review and meta-analysis. *J Am Geriatr Soc, 62*(1), 25–39. doi: 10.1111/jgs.12611

Wells, R. E., Yeh, G. Y., Kerr, C. E., Wolkin, J., Davis, R. B., Tan, Y., et al. (2013). Meditation's impact on default mode network and hippocampus in mild cognitive impairment: a pilot study. *Neurosci Lett, 556*, 15–19.

Whitebird, R. R., Kreitzer, M., Crain, A. L., Lewis, B. A., Hanson, L. R., & Enstad, C. J. (2013). Mindfulness-based stress reduction for family caregivers: a randomized controlled trial. *Gerontologist, 53*(4), 676–686.

Yan, J. H., Gu, W. J., & Pan, L. (2013). Lack of evidence on Tai Chi-related effects in patients with type 2 diabetes mellitus: a meta-analysis. *Exp Clin Endocrinol Diabetes, 121*(5), 266–271. doi: 10.1055/s-0033-1334932

Ye, J., Cai, S., Zhong, W., Cai, S., & Zheng, Q. (2014). Effects of tai chi for patients with knee osteoarthritis: a systematic review. *J Phys Ther Sci, 26*(7), 1133–1137. doi: 10.1589/jpts.26.1133

Yeh, G. Y., Kaptchuk, T. J., & Shmerling, R. H. (2010). Prescribing tai chi for fibromyalgia—are we there yet? *N Engl J Med, 363*(8), 783–784. doi: 10.1056/NEJMe1006315

15

YOGA AS AN INTEGRATIVE INTERVENTION IN HEALTHY AGING AND AGE-RELATED DISORDERS

Shirley Telles, Nilkamal Singh, Arti Yadav, and Acharya Balkrishna

HEALTHY AGING AND A POSSIBLE ROLE FOR YOGA

Introduction

By 2042 in India, the proportion of people aged 60 and older will exceed that of people aged 0–14 (United Nations Population Division, 2008). The aging of the population in India will bring with it an increase in the burden of chronic disease. In addition, the rapid economic growth in these countries, accompanied by rapid urbanization, may also contribute to the increase in non-communicable diseases. Urbanization is associated with unhealthy nutrition and physical inactivity, leading to obesity and increases in the prevalence of chronic diseases such as diabetes (Wang, Du, Zhai, & Popkin, 2007; Wang, Kong, Wu, Bai, & Burton, 2005). The rate of diabetes in India is expected to increase 150.5%, from 31.7 million to 79.4 million, over the same period between 2000 and 2030 (International Diabetes Federation, 2008). Ischemic heart disease

and stroke are two other leading causes of mortality and disease burden in people aged 60 and older (Mathers, Lopez, & Murray, 2006).

Regression results reveal that the health status of the older adult population was significantly worse in India. The presence of chronic disease significantly worsened health, and even more so if people had more than one chronic disease. Although smoking, heavy drinking, and inadequate physical activity all had negative effects on health, only inadequate physical activity was significant when other covariates were controlled for (WHO, 2002–2003).

More than half of the burden of non-communicable disease occurs in the 45-plus age group in China and India. One of the major determinants of the change in disease burden over the next two decades in India is the rapidly aging population. For most Group I causes (communicable, maternal, perinatal, and nutritional conditions), demographic and epidemiological changes are acting in the same direction to reduce total DALYs (DALY = disability adjusted life year). For Group

II (non-communicable diseases), demographic changes tend to greatly increase DALYs. DALYs per thousand people aged 45 and older will decline. This suggests that although the size of the older population will be larger, the older population will be healthier.

In summary, by 2030, older adults will bear two-thirds of the total disease burden worldwide, and nearly half of them will be in India.

An Overview of Healthy Aging

The concept of aging suggests decline, both physical and mental. Yet in recent years the phrases "healthy aging" and "successful aging" have found their way into the media as well as into research protocols.

Successful aging has a low risk of disease and disease-related disability, high mental and physical function, and active engagement with life. Similarly, in his definition of healthy aging, Vaillant (2002) describes the importance of physical, social, and emotional health, suggesting that aging well also involves the ability to forgive, to feel grateful, and to experience joy.

Research in the area of aging has been successful in providing evidence of the physiological changes that occur with increasing chronological age. These physiological changes include, among others, changes in cardiovascular structure (DiBello et al., 1993), a slow progressive decline in body mass (Bray, 1979), and a decrease in the strength per unit of muscle mass (Frontera, Hughes, Lutz, & Evans, 1991; Reed, Pearlmutter, Yochum, Meredith, & Mooradian, 1991). The research data suggest that these physiological decrements may contribute to a reduction in the overall quality of life of the older adult population (Buchner, Larson, Wagner, Koepsell, & DeLateur, 1996). For both the older adult and an adult of middle age, the answer is that many of the age-related physiological changes respond quite well to an intervention that involves a whole-systems approach, modifying the physical (e.g., diet, level of activity), mental, and emotional patterns and even possibly influencing the spiritual dimension of life.

The focus of prevention research has been primarily on methods of developing and maintaining good health, preserving the quality of life of the older adult population, and improving those systems that contribute to the successful completion of the activities of daily living (ADLs). The musculoskeletal and cardiorespiratory systems respond favorably to a variety of interventions. Similarly, Saltin (1986) and Spina et al. (1993) found that relative to a sedentary person, the older adult who has maintained an active lifestyle, while presenting with a lower maximal heart rate, has a significantly larger stroke volume. As such, the active older adult has the advantage of a larger maximal cardiac output, which serves in part to compensate for the age-related decrease in maximal heart rate.

Also, consider the role of the physical activity component in the prevention of osteoporosis. The skeletal system gives a framework for muscles and tendons to have origins and insertions, without which movement would not be able to be generated. This relationship between degradation and deposition shifts from one that favors deposition to one that is more degradative, with women losing bone mineral more rapidly than men (36 grams/decade vs. 30 grams/decade, respectively; as reported by Riggs & Melton, 1992). The older adult is at greater risk for a variety of fractures. Though this age-related change in bone health seems like a dire forecast for the aging adult's later years, it need not be the case: much like the muscular system, the skeletal systems responds quite well to regular physical activity.

Cognitive decline, particularly loss of memory associated with aging, is a concern. The scientific consensus is that many older adults experience decline in their cognitive abilities, and Alzheimer's disease accounts for some portion of this decline (Nolan & Blass, 1992; Wilson, Bennett, & Swartzendruber, 1997). The areas of cognition most likely to show age-related decrements are declarative or episodic memory (i.e., the ability to learn and retain new information) and mental-processing skills such as perceptual speed. This refers to the speed with which simple perceptual comparisons can be completed, usually measured with timed tasks that require substituting symbols or making same/different judgments about pairs of visual stimuli (Wilson, Bennett, & Swartzendruber, 1997).

There is growing evidence to support the idea that neural plasticity continues across the life span, suggesting that cognitive and physical stimulation help to maintain perceptual and memory skills. The activities involved information processing as a central feature, not merely engaging in physical exercise. Activities included reading newspapers, magazines, and books; and playing games such as cards, checkers, crosswords, or other puzzles. On an average, a person who was at the 90th percentile for frequent cognitive activity at baseline was 47% less likely to develop Alzheimer's disease compared to a person who engaged in infrequent activity (10th percentile) (Friedland et al., 2001). It was concluded that the diversity as well as the intensity of the intellectual activities carried out in young to middle adulthood was reduced in the patients who later developed dementia (Friedland et al., 2001). The mental component of yoga, which involves understanding and incorporating universally applicable principles, encourages thought and debate and keeps the practitioner cognitively engaged.

Depressive illness, recognizable in older adults by symptoms that include sad, downcast moods, tearfulness, recurrent thoughts of death or suicide, diminished pleasure, feelings of hopelessness or worthlessness, restlessness, indecisiveness, and lack of initiative, is one example of a common spectrum of psychiatric symptoms in late life that are often under-diagnosed (Reynolds, Alexopoulos, & Katz, 2002). Depression can be triggered from environmental circumstances such as loneliness, bereavement, retirement, disability of a spouse, and feeling unwanted or no longer useful (Cummings, 1998). Depression in older adults can also be caused by medical conditions or can be a response to physical illness (Frazer, Leicht, & Baker, 1996; Weintraub, Furlan, & Katz, 2002).

Increasing evidence demonstrates that a variety of forms of psychotherapy and psychological interventions are as effective in older adults compared to the response of younger adults (Pinquart & Soerensen, 2001; Zarit & Knight, 1996).

While maintaining emotional stability, having an adaptive coping style, and being actively engaged with life are intrinsic factors of successful aging (Perls, Silver, & Lauerman, 1999; Rowe & Kahn, 1998 and Vaillant, 2002), it is interesting to note that diverse studies have shown that yoga practice increases the ability to cope with circumstances that cannot be altered. Yoga philosophy is especially important in this. Another important factor is social support.

The relation between social support and health has been of interest for many years. Data from a sample of 2829 noninstitutionalized people aged 55 to 85 years showed that having fewer feelings of loneliness and greater feelings of mastery are directly associated with a reduced mortality risk, when other possible factors are controlled for (Penninx, van Tilburg, Kriegsman, Deeg, Boeke, & van Eijk, 1997). Also, people who received a moderate level of emotional support and those with high levels of emotional support had reduced mortality risks compared to those with low levels of emotional support. Receiving a high level of instrumental support was related to a higher risk of death. The interaction between disease status and social support or personal coping resources on mortality could not be shown.

There is an important connection between spirituality and late life health. On the positive side, spiritual activities predict longevity. For example, in a meta-analytic study analyzing 29 articles, researchers concluded that individuals who scored higher on measure of religious involvement were almost 30% less likely to have died during the period represented by the study than those scoring lower on religious involvement measures, even after accounting for health, gender, race, health behavior, and social support (McCullough, Hoyt, Larson, Koenig, & Thoresen, 2000).

Managing Specific Conditions Associated with Aging Through Yoga: A Review of the Literature

This article will review the existing literature related to the use of yoga for health issues most commonly encountered in older people. Two early studies described the effect of transcendental meditation (TM) on the aging process. The first study (Alexander, Langer, Newman, Chandler, Davies, 1989) assessed 73 residents of homes for the elderly (mean age = 81 years). Participants were randomly assigned to TM, mindfulness training, or relaxation; the TM group improved the most in terms of paired associate learning, cognitive flexibility, mental health, systolic blood pressure, and ratings of behavioral flexibility, aging, and treatment efficacy. After 3 years the TM group showed a 100% survival rate.

In another study (n = 84, mean age = 53 years) there was a significant correlation between length of time practicing TM and the biological age, with short-term practitioners having a biological age that was 5.0 years younger (than the chronological age) while long-term TM practitioners' biological age was 12.0 years younger (Wallace, Dillbeck, Jacobe, & Harrington, 1982).

More recently the effect of mindfulness on cellular aging and telomerase length in particular has been studied (Epel, Daubenmier, Moskowitz, Folkman, & Blackburn, 2009). Mindfulness is believed to directly increase positive arousal states and to reduce stress arousal associated changes in telomere length and cellular aging.

HYPERTENSION

Uncontrolled hypertension is believed to be responsible for 62% of cerebrovascular disease and 49% of ischemic heart disease in older persons (Chobanian et al., 2003).

Yoga as an Intervention A systematic search of the literature was carried out based on a search of multiple databases, including Academic Search Premier, AltHealthWatch, Biosis/Biological Abstracts, CINAHL Plus with Full Text, Cochrane Library, Embase, MEDLINE, PsycINFO, PsycARTICLES, Natural Standard, and Web of Science (Hagins, States, Selfe & Innes, 2013). Additional studies were identified by searching bibliographies of reviews, and selected uncontrolled studies of yoga and blood pressure.

When the results of all 17 studies which had 22 comparisons, were examined and pooled, yoga was associated with a small but significant decline in both systolic and diastolic blood pressure (−4.17 and −3.26 mmHg, respectively). Further, the effects of yoga on blood pressure varied according to the type of yoga intervention and with the comparison group, but not by duration of yoga practice.

When the analysis was restricted to studies using interventions incorporating three elements of yoga practice (postures, meditation, and breathing), larger reductions of −8.17 (systolic) and −6.14 (diastolic) mmHg were observed. Declines of this magnitude are of clear clinical and prognostic significance (Chobanian et al., 2003).

Yoga was also associated with a significant decline in systolic (−7.96 mmHg) and diastolic blood pressure (−5.52 mmHg) relative to no treatment, but not when compared to exercise or other types of interventions. The overall quality of studies included in this meta-analysis was poor.

OSTEOPOROSIS

Osteoporosis is one of the most common skeletal disorders. Fracture of the hip specifically has been shown to be a major problem, leading to increased morbidity and mortality in older persons (Wolinsky, Fitzgeral, & Stump, 1997). The development of osteopenia and osteoporosis is strongly related to the changes in bone turnover that occur with aging. One study showed that rates of bone formation (BAP) and resorption are high in elderly women, with bone resorption increasing more than bone formation, and acting as the major determinant of bone mass (Garnero, Sornay-Rendu, Chapuy, & Delmas, 1996).

Yoga as an Intervention Considering that yoga practice increases muscular strength of specific groups (Dash, & Telles, 2001) and muscle endurance for repetitive tasks (Telles, Sharma, Yadav, Singh, & Balkrishna, 2014), it has been suggested that yoga may, like other forms of exercise, lead to beneficial effects in managing osteoporosis and osteopenia, such as the ability to retard bone loss and prevent fractures. Biochemical markers of bone formation and resorption may play an important role in monitoring therapy.

On an average, participants in a 12-week yoga program showed improvement in bone turnover (Judith Balk, Gluck, Bernardo, & Catov, 2009). In addition, minutes spent practicing yoga positively correlated with increase in bone formation and negatively correlated with increase in bone resorption. These markers trended in the hypothesized directions, toward improvement and reduced risk for osteoporosis. Interestingly, other weight-bearing exercise (e.g., walking) did not show this correlation as strongly.

There are also anecdotal and clinical reports of the benefits of yoga practice in reducing osteopenia (Balkrishna, 2007).

SLEEP AND SLEEP DISORDERS

Epidemiologic studies indicate that about 60% of older adults have sleep complaints most of the time (Foley et al., 1995). The three most commonly reported sleep disturbance symptoms are difficulty initiating sleep, difficulty maintaining sleep, and early morning awakening (Ohayon, 2002). That could result in tiredness, fatigue, depression, greater anxiety, irritability, pain sensitivity, muscle tremors, immunosuppression, and lack of daytime alertness (Pandi-Perumal et al., 2002).

Yoga as an Intervention Eight senior activity centers were randomly assigned to either the Silver yoga experimental group or a wait-list control group (Chen et al., 2009). A cluster randomized trial was used. A total of 139 participants were recruited from eight senior activity centers and were randomly assigned to either the experimental ($n = 62$) or the control ($n = 66$) group. One hundred and thirty participants completed the 6-month study (attrition rate: 6.47%). The 70-minute Silver yoga program, which included warm-up techniques, hatha yoga gentle stretching, relaxation, and guided-imagery meditation, was implemented in four randomly selected senior activity centers as the experimental intervention. The participants in the wait-list control group participated in the regular activity programs in the senior centers (such as singing, arts and crafts)

The level of state depression of the participants was measured by the Taiwanese Depression Questionnaire (TDQ) (Lee, Yang, Lai, Chiu, & Chau, 2000); the SF-12 Healthy Survey, Chinese version (Ware, Snow, Kosinski, & Gandek, 1993), was used to assess somatic symptoms.

After Silver yoga, participants' daytime dysfunction and depression state decreased and subjective sleep quality, PSQI total score, physical health perception, and mental health perception improved. Similar positive changes did not occur in the control group. These results are in agreement with a three-armed (yoga, Ayurveda, control) trial conducted on community home–dwelling seniors (Manjunath, & Telles, 2005). At 6 months the subjective sleep quality, PSQI total score, physical health perception, and mental health perception of the participants in the experimental group were significantly better than those participants in the control group, and the sleep latency, daytime dysfunction, and depression state of the participants in the experimental group were significantly less than those participants in the control group.

An overall enhancement of self-perception in both the physical and mental health status of the participants in the experimental group was supported by Wood (1993) in that the yogic stretching and breathing program had a markedly invigorating effect on perceptions of both mental and physical energy in a group of 71 adults with ages ranging from 21 to 76 years. Finally, a decrease in depression found in this group of older adults was consistent with various previous studies (Manjunath & Telles, 2004; Pilkington, Kirkwood, Rampes, & Richardson, 2005; Waelde

& Thompson, 2004; Woolery, Myers, Sternlieb, & Zeltzer, 2004).

Through the progression of a sequence of static physical postures, yoga uses stretching to improve joint flexibility and muscular strength, massage blood vessels, and improve blood circulation (Luskin et al., 2000). A 15-minute guided-imagery meditation was incorporated at the end of the Silver yoga program to facilitate a state of relaxation (Chen, Tseng, Ting, & Huang, 2007). The senior participants experienced stretching and relaxing in the program, and their bodies and minds were challenged and relaxed at the same time, which might be the possible reason for the enhanced sleep quality and self-perception of health status, and the decreased depression of the participants.

STROKE

Stroke is one of the most prevalent conditions worldwide, causing devastating impairments and negative consequences for survivors (Saposnik & Estol, 2011).

Yoga as an Intervention

The process used for this literature review was highly structured and involved systematic searching of relevant databases included major biomedical, nursing, and specialist complementary therapy databases including MEDLINE, EMBASE, AMED, CISCOM, CINAHL, PsycINFO, PubMed, Web of Science, Science Direct, EBSCO, Scopus British Nursing Index, and the Cochrane Library (Lazaridou, Philbrook, & Tzika, 2013). Yoga is a useful tool for the rehabilitation process after stroke. All studies in the systematic review focused on mood, fatigue, stress, cognitive ability, and quality of life after stroke. This review shows that yoga in the context of stroke rehabilitation has seldom been addressed. Therefore, this systematic review highlights the lack of definitive evidence of yoga's efficacy in stroke rehabilitation and suggests that this topic warrants future investigation. Methodological limitations of the studies included in this review were small sample sizes, limited descriptions of the randomized process when applicable, lack of reporting sampling methods, reasons for dropouts, and insufficient description of specific yoga or meditative practices.

Physical changes in the form of improved mobility, motor coordination, and cognitive changes in the form of improvement of speech impairments seem to be the main components that stroke survivors could benefit from (Lynton, Kligler, & Shiflett, 2007).

Through the methods of body posture, breath training, and consciousness meditation, overall well-being could be improved, with positive benefits to the nervous system (Streeter, Gerbarg, Saper, Ciraulo, & Brown, 2012), endocrine system (Nidhi, Padmalatha, Nagarathna, & Amritanshu, 2013), cardiovascular system (Papp, Lindfors, Storck, & Wandell, 2013), respiratory system (Santaella et al., 2011), and immunity (Arora & Bhattacharjee, 2008).

After meditation practice, results showed that the density of gray matter increased in regions governing distinctly different activities, such as memory, self-awareness, and compassion. Additionally, gray matter decreased in the amygdala, the part of the brain associated with fear and stress (Lazar et al., 2005). In a more recent study, relaxation techniques seem to affect the genes involved in controlling how the body handles free radicals, inflammation processes, and cell death (Bhasin et al., 2013).

Interestingly, there was no identified study exploring the neurobiology and plasticity of stroke patients after yoga or a mindfulness-based intervention.

Emotional liability is another component following stroke where mindfulness could have beneficial effects.

Additionally, hatha yoga practices could help in limb rehabilitation in stroke survivors. Mindfulness and yoga practices might improve post-stroke hemiparesis, (Bastille & Gill-Body, 2004), although more focused research is needed to determine their effectiveness.

DEMENTIA

Preventing Loss of Independence through Exercise (PLIÉ) is a novel, integrative exercise program for individuals with dementia that combines elements of different conventional and complementary exercise modalities (e.g., tai chi, yoga, Feldenkrais, and dance movement therapy) and focuses on training procedural memory for basic functional movements (e.g., changing from sitting to standing) while increasing mindful body awareness and facilitating social connection. This study presents analyses of qualitative data collected during a 36-week cross-over pilot clinical trial in 11 individuals. Qualitative data included exercise instructors' written notes, which were prepared after each class and also following biweekly telephone calls with caregivers and monthly home visits; three video-recorded classes; and written summaries prepared by research assistants following pre- and post-intervention quantitative assessments. Data were extracted for each study participant and placed on a timeline for a month of observation. Data were coded and analyzed to identify themes that were confirmed and refined through an iterative, collaborative process by the entire team, including a qualitative researcher and the exercise instructors. Three overall themes emerged: (1) functional changes included increasing body awareness, movement memory, and functional skills; (2) emotional changes included greater acceptance of resting, sharing of personal stories and feelings, and a positive attitude toward exercise; (3) social changes included more coherent social interactions and making friends. These qualitative results suggest that the PLIÉ program may be associated with beneficial functional, emotional, and social changes for individuals with mild to moderate dementia. Further study of the PLIÉ program in individuals with dementia is warranted (Wu et al., 2015).

Another study examined the effects of brief daily yogic meditation on mental health, cognitive functioning, and immune cell telomerase activity in family dementia caregivers with mild depressive symptoms (Lavretsky et al., 2013). Thirty-nine family dementia caregivers [mean age 60.3 years old (SD = 10.2)] were randomized to practicing Kirtan Kriya or listening to relaxation music for 12 minutes per day for 8 weeks. The severity of depressive symptoms and mental and cognitive functioning were assessed at baseline and follow-up. Telomerase activity in peripheral blood mononuclear cells (PMBC) was examined in peripheral PBMC pre-intervention and post-intervention.

The meditation group showed significantly lower levels of symptoms of depression and greater improvement in mental health and cognitive functioning compared with the relaxation group. In the meditation group, 65.2% showed 50% improvement on the Hamilton Depression Rating scale, and 52% of the participants showed 50% improvement on the Mental Health Composite Summary score of the Short Form-36 scale compared with 31.2% and 19%, respectively, in the relaxation group. The meditation group showed 43% improvement in telomerase activity compared with 3.7% in the relaxation group.

This study, described as a pilot study, found that brief daily meditation practices by family dementia caregivers can lead to improved mental and cognitive functioning and lower levels of depressive symptoms. This improvement is accompanied by an increase in telomerase activity, suggesting improvement in stress-induced cellular aging. These results need to be confirmed in a larger sample.

DIABETES

As already mentioned in the Introduction to this chapter, diabetes is a cause of considerable morbidity, especially in the aged.

Yoga as an Intervention There have been several studies investigating the usefulness of yoga in the management of diabetes. Two fairly recent studies are cited here in which the participants were seniors with diabetes.

Seventy-three healthy elderly patients with type 2 diabetes mellitus, aged 60 to 70 years, with diabetes for 5 to 10 years and with poor glycemic control (HbA(1c) > 8%) residing in Kozhikode district in southern India were recruited for the study (Beena, & Sreekumaran, 2013). The subjects were divided into three groups according to their glycemic control. Group I with HbA(1c) 8.6%–9.7%, group II with HbA(1c) 9.8%–10.7%, and group III with HbA(1c) 10.8%–12.7%. Participants did yogic practice under the supervision of an experienced yoga trainer, for 90 minutes each day for 3 months. Biochemical estimation of HbA(1c), glucose, lipid profile, cortisol, ferritin, malondialdehyde (MDA), and catalase activity were carried out on 0 day and on the 90th day.

The participants in the test group showed a statistically significant decrease in glucose, HbA(1c), lipids, cortisol, ferritin, and MDA, and a significant increase in catalase activity after yogic practice.

Another study used an exploratory randomized controlled design with in-depth process evaluation (Skoro-Kondza, Tai, Gadelrab, Drincevic, & Greenhalgh, 2009). The setting was two multi-ethnic boroughs in the United Kingdom, one with average and one with low mean socio-economic deprivation score. Participants were 59 people with type 2 diabetes not taking insulin, recruited from general practice lists or by contact with general practice staff. The intervention group was offered 12 weeks of a twice-weekly 90-minute yoga class; the control group was on a waiting list for the yoga classes. Both groups received advice and leaflets on a healthy lifestyle and were encouraged to exercise.

The primary outcome measure was HbA1c. Secondary outcome measures included attendance, weight, waist circumference, lipid levels, blood pressure, UKPDS cardiovascular risk score, diabetes-related quality of life (ADDQoL), and self-efficacy. Process measures were attendance at yoga sessions, self-reported frequency of practice between taught sessions, and qualitative data (interviews with patients and therapists, ethnographic observation of the yoga classes, and analysis of documents including minutes of meetings, correspondence, and exercise plans).

The average age of the participants was 60 ± 10 years. Attendance at yoga classes was around 50%. Yoga teachers felt that most participants were unsuitable for "standard" yoga exercises because of limited flexibility, lack of basic fitness, comorbidity, and lack of confidence. There was a small fall in HbA1c in the yoga group that was not statistically significant and that was not sustained 6 months later, and no significant change in other outcome measures.

SUMMARY

Behaviors, thinking patterns, and emotional and spiritual lifestyles in middle age—factors over which individuals have significant control—have much more impact on health and satisfaction in the seventh and eighth decade of life than was once believed possible. Successful or healthy aging is a goal within reasonable reach. Yoga has a very important role to play in healthy aging, as it influences physical, intellectual, emotional, and spiritual dimensions of life. These benefits have been summarized in Figure 15.1.

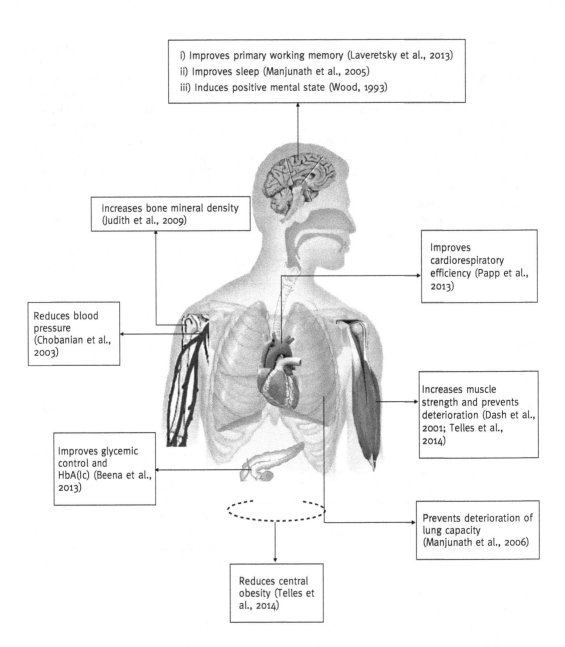

i) Improves primary working memory (Laveretsky et al., 2013)
ii) Improves sleep (Manjunath et al., 2005)
iii) Induces positive mental state (Wood, 1993)

Increases bone mineral density (Judith et al., 2009)

Improves cardiorespiratory efficiency (Papp et al., 2013)

Reduces blood pressure (Chobanian et al., 2003)

Increases muscle strength and prevents deterioration (Dash et al., 2001; Telles et al., 2014)

Improves glycemic control and HbA(1c) (Beena et al., 2013)

Prevents deterioration of lung capacity (Manjunath et al., 2006)

Reduces central obesity (Telles et al., 2014)

FIGURE 15.1   A brief summary of benefits of yoga in older persons.

DISCLOSURE STATEMENT

The authors state that there are no conflicts of interest.

REFERENCES

Alexander, C. N., Langer, E. J., Newman, R. I., Chandler, H. M., & Davies, J. L. (1989). Transcendental meditation, mindfulness, and longevity: an experimental study with the elderly. *J Pers Social Psychol, 57*(6), 950–964.

Arora, S., & Bhattacharjee, J. (2008). Modulation of immune responses in stress by Yoga. *Int J Yoga, 1*(2), 45–55.

Balkrishna, A. (2007). *Yoga in synergy with medical science.* Haridwar, India: Divya prakashan.

Bastille, J. V., & Gill-Body K. M. (2004). A yoga-based exercise program for people with chronic poststroke hemiparesis, *Physical Ther, 84*(1), 33–48.

Beena, R. K., & Sreekumaran, E. (2013). Yogic practice and diabetes mellitus in geriatric patients. *Int J Yoga, 6*(1), 47–54.

Bhasin, M. K., Dusek, J. A., Chang, B.-H., Joseph, M. G., Denninger, J. W., Fricchione, G. L., Libermann, T. A. (2013). Relaxation response induces temporal transcriptome changes in energy metabolism, insulin secretion and inflammatory pathways. *PLoS ONE, 8*(5), e62817.

Bray, G. (Ed.) (1979). *Obesity in America: Department of Health, Education, and Welfare.* Washington, DC.

Buchner, D., Larson, E., Wagner, E., Koepsell, T., & DeLateur, B. (1996). Evidence for a non-linear relationship between leg strength and gait speed. *Age Ageing, 25*(5), 386–391.

Chen K. M., Chen, M. H., Chao, H. C., Hung, H. M., Lin, H. S., & Li, C. H. (2009). Sleep quality, depression state, and health status of older adults after silver yoga exercises: Cluster randomized trial. *Int J Nurs Studies, 46*(2), 154–163.

Chen, K. M., Tseng, W. S., Ting, L. F., Huang, G. F. (2007). Development and evaluation of a yoga exercise programme for older adults. *J Adv Nurs, 57*(4), 432–441.

Chobanian, A. V., Bakris, G. L., Black, H. R., Cushman, W. C., Green, L. A., Izzo, J. L., Jr., Roccella, E. J. (2003). The seventh report of the Joint National Committee on Prevention, Detection, Evaluation, and Treatment of High Blood Pressure: the JNC 7 report. *JAMA, 289*(19), 2560–2572.

Cummings, N. A. (1998). Approaches to preventive care. In P. E. Hartman-Stein (Ed.), *Innovative behavioral healthcare for older adults: a guidebook for changing times* (pp. 1–17). San Francisco: Jossey-Bass Publishers.

Dash, M., & Telles, S. (2001). Improvement in hand grip strength in normal volunteers and rheumatoid arthritis patients following yoga training. *Indian J Physiol Pharmacol, 45*(3), 355–360.

Di Bello, V., Lattanzi, F., Picano, E., Talarico, L., Caputo, M.T., DiMuro, C., Giusti, C. (1993). Left ventricular performance and ultrasonic myocardial quantitative reflectivity in endurance senior athletes: an echocardiographic study. *Eur Heart J, 14*(3), 358–363.

Epel, E., Daubenmier, J., Moskowitz, J.T., Folkman, S., & Blackburn, E. (2009). Can meditation slow rate of cellular aging? Cognitive stress, mindfulness, and telomeres. *Ann NY Acad Sci, 1172,* 34–53.

Foley, D. J., Monjan, A. A., Brown, S. L., Simonsick, E. M., Wallace, R. B., & Blazer, D. G. (1995). Sleep complaints among elderly persons: an epidemiologic study of three communities. *Sleep, 18*(6), 425–432.

Frazer, D. W., Leicht, M. L., & Baker, M. D. (1996). Psychological manifestations of physical disease in the elderly. In L. L. Carstensen, B. A. Edelstein, & L. Dornbrand (Eds.), *The practical handbook of clinical gerontology* (pp. 217–235). Thousand Oaks, CA: Sage.

Friedland, R. P., Fritsch, T., Smyth, K.A., Koss, E., Lerner, A. J., Chen, C. H., Debanne, S. M. (2001). Patients with Alzheimer's disease have reduced activities in midlife compared with healthy control-group members. *Proc Natl Acad Sci USA, 98*(6), 3440–3445.

Frontera, W. R., Hughes, V. A., Lutz, K. J., & Evans, W. J. (1991). A cross-sectional study of muscle strength and mass in 45-to 78-yr old men and women. *J Applied Physiol, 71*(2), 644–650.

Garnero, P., Sornay-Rendu, E., Chapuy, M., & Delmas, P. (1996). Increased bone turnover in late postmenopausal women is a major determinant of osteoporosis. *J Bone Mineral Res, 11*(3), 337–349.

Hagins, M., States, R., Selfe, T., & Innes, K. (2013). Effectiveness of yoga for hypertension: systematic review and meta-analysis. *Evid-Based Compl Alt Med,* 1–13.

International Diabetes Federation. (2008, February 4). *Diabetes atlas.* Retrieved from http://www.eatlas.idf.org/Prevalence.

Judith Balk, J., Gluck, M., Bernardo, L., & Catov, J. (2009). The effect of yoga on markers of bone turnover in osteopenic women: a pilot study. *Int J Yoga Ther, 19*(1), 63–68.

Lavretsky, H., Epel, E. S., Siddarth, P., Nazarian, N., Cyr, N. S., Khalsa, D. S., Irwin, M. R. (2013). A pilot study of yogic meditation for family dementia caregivers with depressive symptoms: effects on mental health, cognition, and telomerase activity. *Int J Geriatr Psychiatry, 28*(1), 57–65.

Lazar, S. W., Kerr, C. E., Wasserman, R. H., Gray, J. R., Greve, D. N., Treadway, M. T., Fischl, B. (2005). Meditation experience is associated with increased cortical thickness. *NeuroReport, 16*(17), 1893–1897.

Lazaridou, A., Philbrook, P., & Tzika, A. A. (2013). Yoga and mindfulness as therapeutic interventions for stroke rehabilitation: a systematic review. *Evid-Based Compl Alt Med, 2013,* 1–9. 357108.

Lee, Y., Yang, M. J., Lai, T. J., Chiu, N. M., & Chau, T. T. (2000). Development of the Taiwanese depression questionnaire. *Chang Gung Med J, 23*(11), 688–694.

Luskin, F. M., Newell, K. A., Griffith, M., Holmes, M., Telles, S., DiNucci, E., Haskell, W. L. (2000). A review of mind/body therapies in the treatment of musculoskeletal disorders with implications for the elderly. *Alt Ther, 6*(2), 46–56.

Lynton, H., Kligler, B., & Shiflett, S. (2007). Yoga in stroke rehabilitation: a systematic review and results of a pilot study. *Topics Stroke Rehab, 14*(4), 1–8.

Manjunath, N. K., & Telles, S. (2004). Spatial and verbal memory test scores following yoga and fine arts camps for school children. *Indian J Physiol Pharmacol, 48*(3), 353–356.

Manjunath, N. K., & Telles, S. (2005). Influence of yoga and ayurveda on self rated sleep in a geriatric population. *Indian Journal of Medical Research, 121*(5), 683–690.

Manjunath, N. K., & Telles, S. (2006). Pulmonary functions following yoga in a community dwelling geriatric population in India. *J Indian Psychol, 24*(1), 17–25.

Mathers, C. D., Lopez, A. D., & Murray, CJ. L. (2006). The burden of disease and mortality by condition: data, methods and results for 2001. In: A. D. Lopez, C. D. Mathers, M. Ezzati, C. J. L. Murray, & D. T. Jamison (Eds.), *Global burden of disease and risk factors* (pp. 45–240). New York: Oxford University Press.

McCullough, M. E., Hoyt, W. T., Larson, D. B., Koenig, H. G., & Thoresen, C. (2000). Religious involvement and mortality: a meta-analytic review. *Health Psychol, 19*(3), 211–222.

Nidhi, R., Padmalatha, V., Nagarathna, R., & Amritanshu, R. (2013). Effects of a holistic yoga program on endocrine parameters in adolescents with polycystic ovarian syndrome: a randomized controlled trial. *J Alt Compl Med, 19*(2), 153–160.

Nolan, K. A., & Blass, J. P. (1992). Preventing cognitive decline. *Clin Geriatr Med, 8*(1), 19–34.

Ohayon, M. M. (2002). Epidemiology of insomnia: what we know and what still need to learn. *Sleep Med Rev, 6*(2), 97–111.

Pandi-Perumal, S. R., Seils, L. K., Kayumov, L., Ralph, M. R., Lowe, A., Moller, H., & Swaab, D. F. (2002). Senescence, sleep, and circadian rhythms. *Ageing Res Rev, 1*(3), 559–604.

Papp, M. E., Lindfors, P. Storck, N. & Wandell, P. E. (2013). Increased heart rate variability but no effect on blood pressure from 8 weeks of hatha yoga: a pilot study. *BMC Res Notes, 6*, 59.

Perls, T. T., Silver, M. H., & Lauerman, J. F. (1999). *Living to 100: lessons in living to your maximum potential at any age.* New York: Basic Books.

Penninx, B. W., van Tilburg, T., Kriegsman, D. M., Deeg, D. J., Boeke, A. J., & van Eijk, J. T. (1997). Effects of social support and personal coping resources on mortality in older age: the Longitudinal Aging Study Amsterdam. *Am J Epidemiol, 146*(6), 510–519.

Pilkington, K., Kirkwood, G., Rampes, H., & Richardson, J. (2005). Yoga for depression: the research evidence. *J Affect Disord, 89*(1–3), 13–24.

Pinquart, M., & Soerensen, S. (2001). How effective are psychotherapeutic and other psychosocial interventions with older adults? A meta analysis. *J Mental Health Aging, 7*, 207–243.

Reed, R. L., Pearlmutter, L., Yochum, K., Meredith, K. E., & Mooradian, A. D. (1991). The relationship between muscle mass and muscle strength in the elderly. *J Am Geriatr Soc, 39*(6), 555–561.

Reynolds, C. F., Alexopoulos, G. S., & Katz, I. R. (2002). Geriatric depression: diagnosis and treatment. *Generations, 26*(1), 28–31.

Riggs, B. L., & Melton, L. J. (1992). The prevention and treatment of osteoporosis. *New Engl J Med, 327*(9), 620–627.

Rowe J. W., & Kahn, R. L. (1998). *Successful aging.* New York: Pantheon Books.

Saltin, B. (1986). Physiological characteristics of the masters athlete. In J. R. Sutton and R. M. Brock (Eds.), *Sports medicine and the mature athlete* (pp. 59–80). Indianapolis: Benchmark Press.

Santaella, D. F., Devesa, C. R., Rojo M. R., Amato, M. B., Drager, L. F., Casali, K. R., Lorenzi-Filho, G. (2011). Yoga respiratory training improves respiratory function and cardiac sympathovagal balance in elderly subjects: a randomised controlled trial. *BMJ Open, 1*(1), Article ID e000085.

Saposnik, G., & Estol, C. J. (2011). Translational research: from observational studies to health policy: how a cohort study can help improve outcomes after stroke. *Stroke, 42*(12), 3336–3337.

Skoro-Kondza, L., Tai, S. S., Gadelrab, R., Drincevic, D., & Greenhalgh, T. (2009). Community based yoga classes for type 2 diabetes: an exploratory randomised controlled trial. *BMC Health Serv Res, 9*, 33.

Spina, R. J., Ogawa, T., Kohrt, W. M., Martin, W. H., Holloszy, J. O., & Ehsani, A. A. (1993). Differences in cardiovascular adaptations to endurance exercise training between older men and women. *J Applied Physiol, 75*(2), 849–855.

Streeter, C. C., Gerbarg, P. L., Saper, R. B., Ciraulo, D. A., & Brown, R. P. (2012). Effects of yoga on the autonomic nervous system, gamma-aminobutyric-acid, and allostasis in epilepsy, depression, and post-traumatic stress disorder. *Med Hypotheses, 78*(5), 571–579.

Telles, S., Sharma, S. K., Yadav, A., Singh, N., & Balkrishna, A. (2014). Immediate changes in muscle strength and motor speed following yoga breathing. *Indian Journal of Physiology and Pharmacology, 58*(1), 22–29.

Telles, S., Sharma, S. K., Yadav, A., Singh, N., & Balkrishna, A. (2014). A comparative controlled trial comparing the effects of yoga and walking for overweight and obese adults. *Med Sci Monitor, 20*, 894–904.

United Nations Population Division, Department for Economic and Social Information. (2008, February 4). *World population prospects: The 2006 Revision Population Database*. Retrieved from http://esa.un.org/unpp/index.asp?panel=2.

Vaillant, G. E., (2002). Adaptive mental mechanisms: their role in a positive psychology. *Am Psychol, 55*(1), 89–98.

Waelde, L. C., & Thompson, L. (2004). A pilot study of a yoga meditation intervention for dementia caregiver stress. *J Clinical Psychol, 60*(6), 677–687.

Wallace, R. K., Dillbeck, M., Jacobe, E., & Harrington B. (1982). The effects of the transcendental meditation and TM-Sidhi program on the aging process. *Int J Neurosci, 16*(1), 53–58.

Wang, H., Du, S., Zhai, F., & Popkin, B. M. (2007). Trends in the distribution of body mass index among Chinese adults, aged 20–45 years (1989–2000). *Int J Obes (Lond), 31*(2), 272–278.

Wang, L., Kong, L., Wu, F., Bai, Y., & Burton, R. (2005). Preventing chronic diseases in China. *Lancet, 366*(9499), 1821–1824.

Ware, J. E., Snow, K. K., Kosinski, M., & Gandek, B. (1993). *SF-36 Health Survey manual and interpretation guide*. Boston, MA: The Health Institute, New England Medical Center.

Weintraub, D., Furlan, P., & Katz, I. R. (2002). Depression and coexisting medical disorders in late life. *Generations, 26*, 55–58.

WHO. (2002–2003). *World Health Survey 2002–2003*. Geneva: World Health Organization.

Wilson, R. S., Bennett, D. A., & Swartzendruber, A. (1997) Age-related change in cognitive function. In P. D. Nussbaum (Ed.), *Handbook of neuropsychology and aging* (pp. 7–14). New York: Plenum Press.

Wolinsky, F., Fitzgeral, J., & Stump, T. (1997). The effect of hip fracture on mortality, hospitalization and functional status: a prospective study. *Am J Public Health, 87*(3), 398–403.

Wood, C. (1993). Mood change and perceptions of vitality: a comparison of the effect of relaxation, visualization and yoga. *J R Soc Med, 86*(5), 254–257.

Woolery, A., Myers, H., Sternlieb, B., & Zeltzer, L. (2004). A yoga intervention for young adults with elevated symptoms of depression. *Alt Ther, 10*(2), 60–63.

Wu, E., Barnes, D. E., Ackerman, S. L., Lee, J., Chesney, M., Mehling, W. E. (2015). Preventing Loss of Independence through Exercise (PLIÉ): qualitative analysis of a clinical trial in older adults with dementia. *Aging Mental Health, 19*(4), 353–362.

Zarit, S. H., & Knight, B. G. (Eds.) (1996). *A guide to psychotherapy and aging: effective clinical interventions in a life-stage context*. Washington, DC: American Psychological Association.

16

BREATHING PRACTICES FOR MENTAL HEALTH AND AGING

Patricia L. Gerbarg and Richard P. Brown

When one gives individual attention to the breath and brings it to the utmost degree of pliancy, one can become as a babe.

Lao Tsu, *Tao Teh Ching*

BREATHING PRACTICES have been used by spiritual leaders, tribal cultures, martial artists, and health practitioners throughout the world to enhance well-being into old age. Voluntarily regulated breathing practices (VRBPs) have the potential to mitigate the effects of stress on mental and physical health, enhance mechanisms of health maintenance, and, at the same time, counteract pathophysiological processes that contribute to age-related disease progression. By studying the modes of action for VRBPS, it is possible to develop specific breathing techniques to alleviate illness symptoms, support mental and physical health, and improve quality of life. Anti-aging treatments may include any preventive approach to reduce the progression of pathological processes that contribute to late-life pathology (Gems, 2014). In this sense, it is possible to consider specific breathing practices to be within the scope of anti-aging treatments.

Excess or prolonged stress has direct and indirect effects on mental health. Repeated or cumulative stressors tend to exacerbate anxiety, insomnia, depression, post-traumatic-stress disorder (PTSD), and cognitive dysfunction. Stress alters sympatho-vagal balance, hypothalamic pituitary-adrenal axis (HPA) activity, energy metabolism, and inflammation. Neuroimaging studies are finding stress-related changes in neuroanatomical structures. These changes contribute to disorders of the immune, cardiovascular, gastrointestinal, neurological, and other body systems. The ensuing illnesses and their treatments (e.g., medication or surgery) can further compound the stress. The treatment of mental illness as patients age becomes more challenging, in part because, as normal homeostatic and cellular repair systems become less robust, neurodegeneration occurs, comorbid conditions develop, and patients become less able to tolerate medications.

Voluntarily regulated breathing practices (VRBPs) include deliberate, conscious alterations in respiratory rate, phases of the respiratory cycle, forcefulness of breath, and other qualities of respiration. VRBPs are particularly suitable for addressing the challenges of aging because they are low in side effects, do not interact adversely with prescription medications, and exert positive effects on key components of the aging mind–body complex. Breath practices can be safely adapted for use in medically ill or frail patients, and they are affordable for those with limited means.

This chapter will explore aspects of VRBPs related to mental health and aging, including effects on the following: the stress response system (SRS), autonomic nervous system (ANS), heart rate variability (HRV), hypothalamic-pituitary-adrenal (HPA) axis, emotion regulatory systems, inflammation, immune response, oxidative stress, and cardiovascular and neurological systems. The use of VRBPs in the treatment of anxiety disorders, PTSD, insomnia, mood disorders, cognitive dysfunction, schizophrenia, and stress-related medical conditions will be reviewed. Most mind–body programs utilize combinations of movement, breathing, and meditative practices, rather than breathing practices alone. Therefore, this discussion will include studies of VRBPs, multi-component programs that emphasize breathing practices, and technology-guided paced breathing. We acknowledge that although better methodologies are being developed for mind–body research, many of the studies do not meet conventional standards for high quality due to small size, non-randomization, lack of an active control, inadequate description of interventions, confounding factors, and potential bias. In addition, the heterogeneity of subjects and the diversity of techniques used in the interventions complicate attempts to group the studies. Consequently, the field does not yet lend itself to meaningful meta-analysis (Boutron et al., 2008; Kinser & Robins 2013; Sherman 2012). Nevertheless, by applying current knowledge from neurophysiology, neuroanatomy, neuroimaging, and respiratory physiology, meaningful models can be constructed and beneficial treatments can be derived. Rather than a conventional research review or meta-analysis, this chapter highlights studies that contribute to our understanding of the neurophysiology and clinical benefits of mind–body practices.

VOLUNTARILY REGULATED BREATHING PRACTICES

The following VRBPs will be included in this review:

- *Paced breathing*: the number of breaths per minute is maintained at a specific respiratory rate, usually by listening to a pacing sound, watching a visual signal, or counting. Slow breathing is usually 3 to 7 breaths per minute. Advanced practitioners may breathe at 1 or 2 breaths per minute (bpm). Moderate breathing ranges from 8 to 20 bpm. Rapid breathing is faster than 20 bpm and may reach 180 or more in very rapid practices. *Kapalabhati* and *bastrika* are examples of fast or high-frequency yoga breathing (HFYB). Telles and Singh (2013) reviewed the research on voluntarily regulated yoga breathing (VRYB), including HFYB. Evidence suggests that HFYB improves performance on measures of selective attention, concentration, and visual scanning. At 120 bpm, HFYB increased sympathetic nervous system (SNS) activity, while at 60 bpm it did not (Telles, Singh, & Balkrishna, 2011).

- The relative length of each potential phase (in-breath, pause, out-breath, and pause) of the breath cycle can be set by counting. *Coherent breathing* is slow gentle breathing at 4.5–6.0 bpm with equal duration of inhalation and exhalation (3.0–4.5 bpm for individuals over 6 feet in height) (Brown & Gerbarg, 2012). *Resonant breathing* is similar to coherent breathing in that it employs slow breathing with equal duration of inhalation and exhalation, but the lips are pursed to create resistance on the out-breath in most studies. The rate of resonant breathing is the rate that produces optimal heart rate variability (HRV) for the individual: usually between 4.5 and 6 bpm. A study of cardiovascular and respiratory effects suggests that breathing at 6 bpm with equal inhalation and exhalation maximally increases baroreflex sensitivity and improves oxygenation under conditions of normoxia (Mason et al., 2013). Increasing lung tidal volume stimulates stretch receptors in the lung, which send information via vagal nerves, stimulating the Hering-Breuer reflex (Jerath et al., 2006). Slow breathing expands alveoli gradually, inducing inhibitory signals from slowly adapting stretch receptors and the stretching of connective tissue (fibroblasts), generating hyperpolarization currents (Schelegle, 2003). It has been hypothesized that these inhibitory signals synchronize rhythmic cellular activity between the cardiorespiratory and nervous system and reduce excitability in neural tissues (Jerath et al., 2013). Hypothalamic and brain-stem synchronization enhance parasympathetic nervous system (PNS) response. Greater expansion of alveoli during slow breathing also reduces anatomical dead space in the lungs and increases the alveolar surface available for oxygen exchange, thereby increasing oxygenation without increasing respiratory effort. Another common slow breath pattern is 4-4-6-2 breathing (4 counts in, 4 counts breath hold, 6 counts out, and 2 counts breath hold).

- The intensity of breathing varies from gentle to forceful. Forceful exhalation, often accompanied by a sound, such as "ha," is more stimulating and tends to increase alertness, attention, and energy. *Bhastrika* or "bellows breath," a moderate frequency, forceful breath practice, acutely increases attention (Telles & Singh, 2013).
- *Resistance breathing* creates partial obstruction to airflow using contraction of laryngeal muscles (e.g., *ujjayi*, "ocean breath," or "victorious breath") or vocal cords, pursed lips, or other methods. *Ujjayi* breathing at 7–9 bpm improved transmission of auditory evoked potentials at the level of the thalamus (Telles & Singh, 2013). *Chanting* is a form of resistance breathing in which the contraction of vocal cords partially obstructs airflow and creates sound. Bernardi observed that chanting the rosary prayer, *Ave Maria* (Hail Mary), in Latin, or a yoga mantra, paced at 6 bpm, induced powerful synchronous increases in two cardiovascular rhythms: the baroreflex sympathetic response and the vagal respiratory response (Bernardi et al., 2001). Reductions in heart rate variability and baroreflex sensitivity are predictors of increased risk after myocardial infarction or in heart failure. By synchronizing SNS and PNS outflow, breathing at 6 bpm also results in rhythmic oscillations in cerebrovascular flow (Bernardi et al., 2001). An fMRI study found that in comparison to the pronunciation of "ssss" or simple rest, the chanting of audible "om" was associated with neurohemodynamic correlates indicating bilateral deactivation of the orbitofrontal, anterior cingulate, parahippocampal gyri, thalami, and hippocampi, as well as the right amygdala. Effects were attributed to vibrational stimulation of vagal afferent branches (Kalyani et al., 2011). Thus, limbic deactivation contributes to the emotional calming effect of slow breath practices, similar to the effects of electronic vagal nerve stimulation studies.
- *Unilateral* or *alternate nostril* breathing requires the occlusion of one nostril while all air flows through the open nostril. This can be done at different rates and breath phase durations, but is usually a slow form of breathing. Unilateral right, unilateral left, or alternate nostril breathing has been shown to improve spatial memory (Joshi & Telles, 2008).
- *Breathing with movement* occurs when paced breathing is coordinated with a sequence of physical postures or movements.
- *Moving the breath* involves the imaginative movement of breath through different parts of the body (Brown & Gerbarg, 2012).

STRESS RESPONSE SYSTEMS AFFECTED BY VRBPS

Autonomic Nervous System

Autonomic nervous system dysfunction has been documented in anxiety disorders, PTSD, depression, early Alzheimer's disease, attention deficit hyperactivity disorder (ADHD), schizophrenia, autism, child behavior disorders, sociopathy, and obesity (Thayer, 2009; Porges, 2007). Heart rate variability (HRV) is derived from the fluctuations in the time intervals between consecutive R waves on an electrocardiogram (ECG). HRV, which reflects the influence of the SNS and the PNS on sinus node activity, is used to measure the activity of the SNS and the PNS.

Specific breathing techniques have been shown to increase PNS activity, improve sympatho-vagal balance, reduce inflammatory markers and cortisol release, and improve oxidative status. In addition, these practices reduce perceived stress and negative psychological states (e.g., depression, anxiety, and PTSD) (Brown, Gerbarg & Muench, 2013; Streeter, Gerbarg, Saper, et al., 2012). For most adults, breathing at 4.5–6.0 breaths per minute (bpm) induces optimal sympatho-vagal balance, as indicated by measures of HRV (Brown, Gerbarg, & Muench, 2013). Evidence supports the neurophysiological model proposed by Brown and Gerbarg (2005a, 2005b), based on polyvagal theory (Porges, 2001) and the neurovisceral integration model (Thayer & Lane, 2000; Park & Thayer, 2014), that slow gentle breathing at 4.5–6 bpm for most adults increases activity of the PNS (as indicated by increase in high frequency of heart rate variability spectra) via afferent interoceptive pathways from the respiratory receptor systems (e.g., mechanoreceptors—stretch receptors, chemoreceptors, and baroreceptors), resulting in emotional calming and cognitive enhancement (Brown & Gerberg 2005; Brown, Gerberg, & Muench 2013; Craig 2003).

An RCT of 90 healthy subjects (18–25 years old) compared fast *pranayama*(Group 1, *kapalabhati, bhastrika,* and *kukkriya*), slow *pranayama* (Groups 2, *nadishodhana, pranava,* and *savitri*), and control (Group 3, no *pranayama*). Perceived Stress Scale (PSS) scores dropped significantly in Groups 1 and 2, showing that both slow and fast *pranayama* can reduce perceived stress. Significant reductions in heart rate (HR), diastolic blood pressure (DBP), and mean arterial pressure (MAP), indicating increased PNS activity, occurred only in Group 1. These findings also suggest increased tissue perfusion with decreased workload on the heart (Sharma et al., 2013). As in this study, most young, healthy individuals (with no psychological or physical disorder) can tolerate and benefit from fast *pranayama*. However, older populations are at greater risk of adverse effects from rapid breath practices, which can seriously exacerbate symptoms of cardiovascular, cerebrovascular, or respiratory diseases.

The vagal nerves and central autonomic pathways contain the main pathways of the PNS. The PNS modulates the psycho-neuro-endocrine-immune systems, maintaining homeostasis through afferent tracts (to the hypothalamus, central ANS, limbic system, thalamus, and cortex) and efferent tracts (cholinergic anti-inflammatory pathways, CAP) to the organs and tissues of the body (Haroon, Raison, & Miller, 2012; Meregnani, Clarencon, Vivier, et al., 2011). Higher resting HRV correlates with more effective top-down (cognitive) and bottom-up (visceral afferent) regulation of emotional stimuli. Lower resting HRV is associated with hypervigilant and maladaptive cognitive responses, which may impair emotion regulation (Park & Thayer, 2014). Potential benefits of VRBPs, such as coherent breathing, alternate nostril breathing, and 4-4-6-2 breathing, include improved psycho-neuro-endocrine-immune modulation, reduced perceived stress, alleviation of negative psychological states, and enhanced executive functions. Gard and colleagues (2014) support the concept that through bidirectional feedback loops, yoga practices, such as breath regulation, can improve the regulation of cognition, emotion, behavior, and peripheral physiology. These mechanisms also support intention, motivation, executive monitoring, response inhibition, and reappraisal.

Vagal-GABA Theory and Emotion Regulation

GABA is the main inhibitory neurotransmitter in the brain. One of its functions is to reduce overactivity in the amygdala, a common feature in PTSD and anxiety disorders. Autonomic nervous system (ANS) imbalances that develop under conditions of stress are characterized by decreased PNS activity and increased SNS activity. Stress exacerbates symptoms in depression, PTSD, and chronic pain, which are characterized by low central nervous system (CNS) GABA activity, PNS underactivity (low HRV), and increased HPA axis activity (indicated by increased cortisol) (Streeter et al., 2012).

The prefrontal cortex (PFC) sends inhibitory GABAergic projections to the amygdala. Under perceived threat, the PFC may be hypoactive and may fail to inhibit overactivity of the amygdala, resulting in the emergence of limbic defensive activity, emotion dysregulation, over-reactivity, and other PTSD symptoms, such as hyper-arousal and re-experiencing. According to Vagal-GABA Theory, PFC activation associated with increased PNS activity could improve the inhibitory control over the amygdala via PFC GABA projections, decreasing amygdala overactivity and reducing PTSD symptoms (Streeter et al., 2012). Moreover, stress exacerbates depression, PTSD, chronic pain, and other stress-reactive disorders. The therapeutic effects of yoga may occur through both direct effects on the ANS and indirect effects on GABA systems.

INFLAMMATION, IMMUNE RESPONSE, AND OXIDATIVE STRESS

The autonomic nervous system, particularly the parasympathetic nervous system, modulates the immune system in chronic inflammatory disease and has anti-nociceptive effects. In vivo studies found that vagal nerve stimulation (VNS) activated the cholinergic anti-inflammatory pathway (Sun, Zhou, Wang, et al., 2013). The afferent branch of the inflammatory reflex through the vagus nerve transmits information about bodily inflammation to the CNS. The organ systems of the body are enervated by vagal efferents that release acetylcholine (Ach), which initiates an anti-inflammatory cascade. Ach modulates immune response through α7-nicotinic receptors (α7nAchRs) on human macrophages that inhibit nuclear factor kappa B (NF-κB) and cytokine

(TNF-α, IL-1) synthesis and release (Huston, 2012). The efferent arm of the inflammatory reflex, also called the cholinergic anti-inflammatory pathway, reduces peripheral inflammatory response, cytokine production, leukocyte recruitment, and NF-κB activation via α7nAchR subunit-dependent, T-lymphocyte-dependent vagus nerve signaling to the spleen (Brands, Purperhart, & Deckers-Kocken, 2011). Breath-focused yoga studies have demonstrated significant reductions of inflammatory markers: Interleukin (IL-6); TNF-a; C-reactive protein (CRP); extracellular superoxide dismutase; and malondialdehyde (MDA), protein oxidation (POX), and phospholipase A2 (PLA2) activity (Brown, Gerbarg, & Muskin, 2009; Kuttner et al., 2006; Taneja et. al., 2004). Evidence supports the concept that slow-paced VRBPs may reduce inflammation by activating vagal cholinergic anti-inflammatory pathways.

NEUROELECTROPHYSIOLOGICAL AND BRAIN-IMAGING STUDIES

Studies of the electrophysiological effects of meditative breathing have been reviewed (Brown & Gerbarg 2009, 2013; Cahn & Polich 2006). Mindful meditative breathing, non-judgmental observation of one's own breathing without engaging in thoughts, has been associated with increased alpha asymmetry (greater left-sided activation) between hemispheres in anterior frontal and temporal regions. This pattern correlates with reduced anxiety, improved mood, relaxation, and feelings of well-being (Urry et al., 2004). In contrast, concentrative meditative breathing with conscious focus of attention on the rhythm of inhalation and exhalation has been associated with enhanced attention, increased EEG intra- and inter-hemisphere theta coherence (Chan et al., 2011). In a randomized controlled study (RCT), police trainees who practiced 5 breath techniques, *pranayama*, for 1 hour daily, 4 days per week for 6 months, showed significant increases in total power, alpha and theta integrals, and significantly decreased visual auditory and discriminative auditory reaction time (RT), indicators of a more alert state, faster processing of visual input, and improved central neural processing. In addition, decreased resting EMG of frontalis muscle reflected improved muscle relaxation (Trakroo et al., 2012).

Many qi gong techniques strengthen both branches of the autonomic system by combining PNS-activating with SNS-activating breath forms within each breath cycle or by alternating periods of slow relaxed respiration with forceful stimulating breathing. Enhancements are often included, such as creating resistance to airflow, vocalizations, imagery, energy circulation, or physical movements. For example, an ancient Shaolin practice, Lao Dao Zuochan (translated as "Old Monk Taoist Breathing") from Twelve-Cycle Yang was used to heal and strengthen warriors using Guardian Chi (energy). Some of these more complex techniques have also been shown to lead to a more balanced state of alertness with calmness. For example, Shaolin Dan Tian Breathing (DTB) alternates passive and active forms of breathing. A preliminary fMRI study in experienced practitioners found that both forms activated the cingulate gyrus. Active DBT activated the bilateral amygdala and hippocampal gyri, key areas for processing emotion, attention, and memory (Chan et al., 2011). These studies of DTB excluded individuals with psychiatric disorders and CNS diseases. If the activation of the limbic structures or the SNS becomes too intense, adverse reactions could be triggered in vulnerable individuals, for example, anxiety or flashbacks in patients with panic disorder or PTSD, or hypomanic state in those with bipolar disorder. To date, we are not aware of studies demonstrating that these techniques would be feasible, safe, or effective in patients with psychological, CNS, or physical disorders.

GENOMIC STUDIES

Recent studies using gene expression profiling in circulating immune cells provide preliminary evidence that mind–body practices, including breathing techniques, may significantly affect transcriptome profiles. A review of three trials of different practices showed long-term changes in gene expression consistent with improvements in response to environmental stress. Two studies found effects on ubiquitin-related pathways and apoptosis, indicating improved survival of immune cells (Saatcioglu, 2013). The first study compared six Asian qi gong practitioners (duration of practice at least 1 year) with six healthy controls (Li et al., 2005). Gene expression profiling of neutrophils found 132 down-regulated and 118 up-regulated genes only in the qi gong practitioners. Down-regulation occurred in genes related to ubiquitin degradation pathway, genes encoding ribosomal proteins, and cellular stress response genes. Expression of two heat shock proteins increased. Up-regulation of interferon gamma-related genes was consistent with observed increased neutrophil bactericidal activity in vitro. The life span of normal neutrophils increased and the life span of inflammatory neutrophils decreased. A second genomic study compared microassays of peripheral blood lymphocytes (PBMCs) to study relaxation response (RR) in 20 healthy controls versus 19 long-term (average 9.4 years) practitioners of different mind–body practices including Vipassana, breath-focused Kripalu or Kundalini Yoga, meditation (mantra, insight, and transcendental), and repetitive prayer (Dusek et al., 2008). The characterization of these diverse practices as "relaxation response" is debatable, and the interpretation of findings from such a mixed group is challenging. Nevertheless, differential gene expression analysis indicated effects on oxidative phosphorylation, ubiquitin-dependent protein catabolism, nuclear mRNA splicing, NF-kB signaling, and apoptosis regulation. The third study compared PBMC RNA from 42 normal healthy controls with that of 42 practitioners of Sudarshan Kriya and associated practices (SK&P) (Sharma et al., 2008). Compared to controls, the SK&P group had significantly increased expression of COX-2 (antiapoptic gene), HSP-70 (stress response gene), and glutathione S-transferase mRNA. Serum assays also showed better antioxidant status, with higher levels of superoxide dismutase and glutathione. Another non-randomized study compared short-term genomic changes immediately before and after 2-hour sessions of SKY&P versus 2 hours of a nature walk and listening to relaxing music on 4 consecutive days. Microassay from PBMCs from 10 completers revealed changes in expression of 97 genes compared to 52 in the control (Qu et al., 2013). A pilot study of 35 chronic schizophrenic patients given a program of coherent breathing plus either yoga or qi gong for 1-hour sessions three times a week for 12 weeks found significant improvements in cognitive functions, attention, and memory on the Repeatable Battery for Assessment of Neuropsychological States (RBANS) and significant changes in gene expression in PBMCs: 30% decrease in Glucocorticoid receptor (GR) mRNA; 23% decrease in DNMT1mRNA (enzyme regulates DNA methylation of cytosine residues); and 22% decrease in TET1 mRNA (enzyme related to demethylation of cytosine residues) (Smith et al., 2013). Evidence of genetic effects of mind–body practices with significant breath techniques in these preliminary studies warrants further analysis

using larger samples in RCTs to elucidate the many potential implications for long-term health, stress resistance, immune defense, cognitive function, and longevity.

STRESS, ANXIETY DISORDERS, POST-TRAUMATIC STRESS DISORDER, INSOMNIA, MOOD DISORDERS, AND OBSESSIVE-COMPULSIVE DISORDER

Differences among Slow Breathing Techniques

Deep and slow breathing techniques are components of both conventional and complementary stress-reduction interventions used in the treatment of physical and psychological disorders. However, the effects of these techniques vary, depending on a variety of parameters, specific instructions given, and accompanying techniques. In order to understand the heterogeneity in research studies and to achieve optimal benefits from slow breathing, clinicians need to be aware of these differences. For example, slow breathing with eyes open is less calming than with eyes closed. Slow breathing can be effortful when accompanied by instructions to take a very deep breath, to overfill the lungs, or to maximally expel air. In contrast, it can be effortless with instructions to breathe gently and naturally. Any instructions that require effort or that engage visual or cognitive systems tend to prevent reduction of sympathetic tone and may also lessen parasympathetic activation, as the following study illustrates.

A small cross-over study ($n = 16$) of slow, deep breathing at 7 bpm with a duration ratio of 40% inhalation to 60% exhalation compared the effects of focused attention versus relaxation during the breath practice. In this study, during attentive deep slow breathing (DSB), subjects watched a monitor displaying the ideal breathing curve. They were instructed to fit their own respiration curve to the ideal curve, a task requiring constant attention and concentration. In the relaxing DSB intervention, subjects were instructed to direct awareness to the experience of breathing and to look at a spot on the wall while an instructor verbally paced their respiratory rate and depth. Both breathing interventions reduced levels of stress, negative feelings, tension, anger, and depression, as measured on the

Profile of Mood States. However, only the relaxing DSB significantly increased pain thresholds and reduced pain perception. Furthermore, only the relaxing DSB was associated with significant reduction in sympathetic activity (based on skin conductance levels, SCLs), while attentive DSB showed a non-significant increase in sympathetic activity (Busch et al., 2012). In general, prolonging the expiratory phase is more relaxing and enhances parasympathetic activity, but this effect may be lessened when it requires too much physical effort or mental work (e.g., visual tracking of physiological data on a computer monitor).

Breathing Methods to Enhance Parasympathetic Activation

Several methods can be used to augment the parasympathetic activation that occurs with slow breathing. For example, doing a movement practice, such as yoga postures, qi gong movements, or tai chi, prior to the breathing practice dispels physical tension and facilitates relaxation during VRBPs. Also, doing a very brief initial relaxation body scan for 1–2 minutes can enable anxious patients to settle into the breath practices more easily. For most adults, breathing at 4.5–6 bpm optimizes sympatho-vagal balance and induces a mental state of calm alertness, which is ideal for relaxation as well as for cognitive function, problem-solving, and stress resiliency; breathing at 3 bpm or less is more sedating and meditative.

Clinical Study of a Breathing Program for Healthcare Providers after a Mass Disaster

Clinical evidence on the effects of breathing practices used in mind–body programs for the treatment of stress, anxiety disorders, PTSD, obsessive-compulsive disorder, insomnia, and depression has been reviewed (Brown, Gerbarg, & Muench, 2013). Four randomized controlled trials (RCTs) and one open study of slow VRBPs demonstrated reductions in symptoms of stress (Brown, Gerbarg, & Muench 2013; Granath et al., 2006; Malathi & Damodaran, 1999; Nolan et al., 2005; Sakakibara & Hayano, 1996).

Healthcare providers experience work stress, particularly in areas that have suffered mass disasters. In states bordering the Gulf of Mexico, healthcare systems had not yet recovered from Hurricanes Rita and Katrina when they were further devastated by the 2010 Horizon oil spill, floods, and tornadoes. In the aftermath of disasters, mental health professionals must cope with work overload as they do their best to meet the needs of thousands of patients, including large homeless populations. Mind–body treatments have unique benefits in that they can extend services when one provider teaches stress-reducing practices to groups rather than individuals. Simultaneously, healthcare practitioners can utilize the same mind–body practices to alleviate their own stress. This concept was demonstrated in an open trial of a 3-day Breath~Body~Mind Train-the-Trainer Program in Mississippi, funded by the Mississippi Department of Mental Health. One year after the Gulf Horizon oil spill, 79 healthcare providers treating people suffering from psychological effects of the oil spill completed self-report measures before and after participating in the training. Mean scores on the Perceived Stress Scale were significantly elevated at baseline and significantly improved 6 weeks after the training. Immediately after the training program and at 6-week testing, Exercise Induced Feeling Inventory (EIFI) scores showed significant improvements in positive engagement, revitalization, tranquility, and physical exhaustion (Gerbarg, Brown, Whitfield, & Streeter, 2014). Most of the respondents reported using the breathing practices successfully in their work, including those working with groups of homeless individuals. Studies using breathing exercises have shown reductions in stress and anxiety in patients as well as in caregivers, but larger, more rigorous research is needed to validate and extend these findings.

Heart Rate Variability Biofeedback with Slow Deep Breathing

Biofeedback is being used with resonant or coherent breathing to increase HRV and to alleviate stress, anxiety, and depression. Heart-rate variability biofeedback (HRVB) utilizes instruments that measure and feed back information about physiological activity (such as HRV), enabling an individual to interpret and respond to these signals (Barragán, Loayza, et al., 2011). HRVB has shown promise in the treatment of major depressive disorder (Karavidas et al., 2007), attention deficit disorder, headaches, hypertension, and fibromyalgia (Hassett et al., 2007; Horowitz, 2006).

For example, in an RCT, 36 women who were manufacturing operators in Malaysia received five weekly sessions of biofeedback HRV training during which they were instructed to breathe slowly and deeply while receiving visual biofeedback information on a monitor displaying a respiration curve, heart rate, and HRV. The intervention group had significant reductions in scores in all three domains of the Depression, Anxiety, and Stress Scale (DASS) compared to controls (Sutarto, Wahab, & Zin, 2012).

In an inpatient perinatal psychiatry unit, HRVB therapy was administered to 15 women with prominent anxiety features of perinatal depression. Patients were trained to use deep, abdominal, or diaphragmatic breathing techniques. The use of HRVB was associated with significant improvements in the State-Trait Anxiety Inventory (STAI) ($p < 0.001$), Warwick Edinburgh Mental Well-Being Scale (WEMWBS), and Linear Analog Self Assessment (LASA) (Beckham, Greene, & Meltzer-Brody, 2013).

Breath-Focused Yoga Programs for Anxiety

Seven studies, including two RCTs, two controlled trials (CTs), and three open pilots, found significant reductions in anxiety with breath-focused yoga programs (Katzman et al., 2012; Katzman et al., 2013: Kozasa et al., 2008; Sahasi, Moha, & Kacker, 1989; Sharma, Azmi, & Settiwas, 1991; Telles, Naveen, & Dash, 2007; Telles et al., 2012). Two pilot studies evaluated breath-focused yoga programs for severe *treatment-resistant* generalized anxiety disorder (GAD) with *comorbidities*. In the first study ($n = 31$), using the 22-hour Sudarshan Kriya Yoga program of yoga postures, *ujjayi*, *bhastrika*, cyclical Sudarshan Kriya breathing, and meditation, the response rate was 73% and the remission rate was 41% (Katzman, Vermani, Gerbarg, et al., 2012). The second trial ($n = 20$) using the 12-hour Breath-Body-Mind program of breath practices, qi gong, and Open Focus attention training, resulted in significant improvements in anxiety, sleep, and depression (Katzman, Vermani, Gerbarg, et al., 2013).

Breath-Focused Yoga Programs for Post-Traumatic Stress Disorder

Autonomic dysfunction and low HRV have been associated with PTSD (Chalmers, Quintana, Abbott, & Kemp, 2014; Minassian, Geyer, Baker, et al., 2014). Studies of yoga programs emphasizing breath practices for PTSD (4 RCTs, 1 CT, and 2 open pilots) found significant improvements in PTSD, anxiety, and depression among survivors of partner abuse, mass disasters, and military service (Carter, Gerbarg, Brown, Ware, et al., 2010; Descilo, Vedamurtachar, Gerbarg, et al., 2010; Franzblau et al., 2006; Gerbarg, Streeter, & Whitfield, 2012; Seppälä, Nitschke Tudorascu, et al., 2014; Telles, Singh, Joshi, Balkrishna, et al., 2010; Brown, Gerbarg, Vermani, et al., 2010a; Brown, Gerbarg, Vermani, et al., 2010b). By improving autonomic function, VRBPs can reduce symptoms of anxiety, PTSD, and depression.

Heart Rate Variability Biofeedback for Post-Traumatic Stress Disorder

Respiratory sinus arrhythmia (RSA) is another measure of heart rate fluctuations during inhalation and exhalation. A controlled study compared RSA biofeedback to progressive muscle relaxation (PMR) as adjunctive treatments for 38 patients with PTSD in residential treatment for substance use. Significantly greater reductions in depressive symptoms and increases in HRV indices were found in the biofeedback group. Both groups significantly reduced PTSD and insomnia symptoms, and a statistical trend was observed for reduced substance craving for the biofeedback group. Increases in HRV were significantly associated with PTSD symptom reduction (Zucker, Samuelson, Muench, et al., 2009).

Breath Practices Facilitate Individual Psychotherapy

Most patients can be taught coherent breathing by their therapist, using a chime track paced at 5 bpm (Brown & Gerbarg 2012), within 20 minutes during an office visit. The integration of breath practices into individual psychotherapy can facilitate the development of trust, tolerance of painful affects, access to traumatic experiences, and resolution of symptoms, including anxiety, insomnia, nightmares, anger outbursts, disconnection, emotional numbing, sexual dysfunction, and other manifestations of trauma (Gerbarg 2008; Gerbarg& Brown 2011; Gerbarg, Gootjes, & Brown, 2014). The patient is instructed to practice coherent breathing starting with 5–10 minutes twice a day, then progressing to 20 minutes once or twice a day (depending on severity of symptoms). Most patients experience immediate improvements in anxiety and sleep if they practice regularly. Other improvements occur over time. Once patients are able to perform coherent breathing easily and comfortably, they can use it during therapy sessions, for example, to control the anxiety that arises when they try to talk about painful feelings or memories. This reduces resistance and allows the patient to better tolerate discussing painful issues that were previously avoided. Clinicians interested in offering breath practices are advised to obtain appropriate training.

MILITARY SERVICE–RELATED TRAUMA

Among military personnel and veterans, mind–body practices can help to relieve symptoms of stress, anxiety, insomnia, depression, and PTSD. As military veterans age, the physical and psychological wounds of war that have not responded to conventional treatments worsen, compounded by declining health and further losses—of family, friends, property, home, and so on. The authors (RPB and PLG) find that most active duty military personnel and veterans respond well to rounds of qi gong movements, short periods of forceful "ha" breath with brisk tapping, followed by 4-4-6-2 breathing, coherent breathing at 5 bpm, alternate nostril breathing (if time allows), breath moving, brief guided imagery, and body scan.

A 5-day multi-component, breath-focused Sudarshan Kriya Yoga program, adapted for military veterans by author Brown, was studied in a rater-blind randomized controlled trial of 30 Australian Vietnam War veterans on disability for 40 years due to severe, treatment-resistant, chronic PTSD. Their average age was 58 and they had multiple comorbid conditions, including obesity, cardiovascular disease, chronic obstructive pulmonary disease, active heavy alcohol abuse, and heavy cigarette addiction. The mean baseline score on the Clinician Admistered PTSD Scale (CAPS) was 56.3 (SD = 12.3) and dropped to 42.1 (SD = 18.2) at week 6 and 26.2 (SD = 14.8) at 24 weeks in the intervention group. Participation in the 5-day yoga course was associated with significant reductions on CAPS compared to the wait-list control at week 6 (effect size = .91) (Carter et al., 2013).

A small randomized controlled trial of Sudarshan Kriya yoga for 20 veterans of the wars in Iraq and Afghanistan found that those who participated in a 21-hour, 7-day program of Sudarshan Kriya Yoga showed significant reductions in scores on PCL-M after 1 month and 1 year, but those in the wait-list control group did not. Between-groups comparison showed moderate to large effect size for the intervention. Benefits after 1 year did not correlate significantly with the amount of at-home practice. No adverse effects were reported (Seppälä et al., 2014).

Veterans with very severe PTSD may not initially tolerate even the gentlest breath practices. In such cases, it may be necessary to begin with a quiet guided relaxation with soothing music, and gradual slowing of the breath and body scan daily. Then slow breathing can be started for a few minutes and gradually increased as tolerated over a period of weeks to 20 minutes twice a day, plus as needed for anxiety.

INSOMNIA

Elderly patients are at increased risk of cognitive impairment, syncope, and fractures due to prescription sedative-hypnotics. An RCT in geriatric subjects found that yoga techniques improved self-rated sleep safely (Manjunath & Telles 2005). Additional studies with objective sleep measures are needed to extend these promising findings.

Breath practices are particularly suited to enhancing sleep. In clinical practice, the authors (PLG and RPB) find it easy to teach patients of all ages to breathe at 5 or 6 bpm with a 1:2 ratio duration of inhalation to exhalation. Patients are instructed to use a CD soundtrack to pace their breath while lying in bed with the lights turned off. Eventually they learn to use the 1:2 slow breathing to put themselves to sleep quickly, even without the sound track to pace their respirations.

DEPRESSION

Research suggests that depression is associated with alterations in autonomic function, such as impaired baroreflex sensitivity, changes in heart rate, and reduced HRV (Karavidas, Lehrer, Vascillo, et al., 2007). Depression studies with major yoga breathing components include three RCTs and two open pilots (Brown & Gerberg, 2013). In an open study of 46 adults with dysthymia, Sudarshan Kriya Yoga (SKY) was associated with remission among those who practiced three or more times per week over 3 months (Janakiramaiah, Gangdhar, Naga Venkatesha Murthy, et al., 1998). In a one month RCT, 45 severely depressed hospitalized adults received a 1-week SKY training and practice 5 days per week for 1 month, imipramine 150 mg per day, or unipolar electroconvulsive therapy (ECT) three times a week. All three groups showed improvements in Beck Depression Inventory and Hamilton Depression Scale. The differences between group outcomes were not statistically significantly different (Janakiramaiah, Gangdhar, Naga Venkatesha Murthy, et al., 2000). A single blind RCT of 82 depressed patients found that three sessions of 30–45 minutes per week practicing relaxation and slow rhythmic breathing significantly improved depression, self-efficacy, well-being, and quality of life compared to a newspaper discussion control (Tsang. Fung, Chan, et al., 2006).

Studies of breath-based yoga programs for other psychiatric and medical conditions, which include depression measures, show significant reductions in depression in patients with fibromyalgia, inflammatory bowel disease, and in survivors of mass disasters (Abbott & Lavretsky, 2013; Brown & Gerbarg, 2013; Gerbarg, Wallace & Brown, 2011).

Breath-based mind-body programs and HRVB can improve mood, mental and physical energy, alertness, and enthusiasm in healthy individuals under stress and in people suffering from clinical depression. Further research is warranted.

STRESS-RELATED MEDICAL CONDITIONS

Inflammatory bowel disease is a prime example of a medical condition whose pathophysiology involves stress-activated inflammation.

Inflammatory Bowel Disease

Evidence suggests that stress and other negative emotional states may adversely affect the course of IBD by altering gastrointestinal motility and secretions, increasing visceral perceived pain, increasing intestinal permeability, and adversely affecting GI mucosal regeneration and blood flow. The vagus nerve-mediated cholinergic anti-inflammatory reflex is essential to prevent and repair gastrointestinal tissue damage (Thayer, 2009; van der Zanden, Boeckxsaerns, and de Jong, 2009). Mind–body practices, by increasing activity of the PNS and decreasing activity of the SNS, may counteract some of the pathophysiological effects of the sympatho-vagal imbalance associated with inflammatory bowel disease (IBD).

At the Cornell Weil Inflammatory Bowel Disease Clinic, an RCT of 29 patients with IBD (Crohn's and ulcerative colitis) found that those who participated in a 2-day 10-hour Breath-Body-Mind Workshop followed by weekly (for 6 weeks) and then monthly (for 5 months) 90-minute group Breath-Body-Mind sessions showed significantly greater improvements in measures of IBD symptoms, anxiety, depression, pain, disability, and an inflammatory biomarker (C-reactive protein) at the end of 24 weeks in comparison to a control group who participated in an educational seminar focused on management on IBD and follow-up sessions for the same number of hours (Gerbarg, Jacob, Stevens, et al., 2015). The benefits of the Breath-Body-Mind program with PNS activation may be attributed to a dual action: reduction of anxiety and stress over-reactivity and direct cholinergic anti-inflammatory effects on the bowels.

OBSESSIVE-COMPULSIVE DISORDER

Alternate nostril breathing (ANB) usually has a calming effect within 10 minutes. However, in treatment resistant disorders, such as obsessive-compulsive disorder (OCD), more extensive training and practice are often required to improve symptoms. In one small controlled trial, patients with OCD who were taught Kundalini Yoga (slow left-nostril breathing, meditation, and postures) improved significantly on the Yale-Brown Obsessive-Compulsive Scale (Y-BOCS) compared to controls given relaxation and mindfulness meditation (Shannahoff-Khalsa, 2003) (Streeter et al., 2012). Though unilateral and ANB may be intriguing adjunctive treatments for anxiety, efficacy in OCD may require 2–3 hours of daily practice. For patients who are motivated and disciplined enough to undertake this regimen, it can be beneficial.

Checking Compulsions

Compulsive behaviors, such as repeated checking, are often driven by anxiety. Patients will report that if they don't enact the compulsion, they experience increasing anxiety and that relief only occurs when they "give in" to the compulsion, for example, by rechecking a stove or door lock. In such cases, slow breath practices such as coherent breathing can be used as an adjunct to cognitive behavioral therapy (CBT), as the following case illustrates.

A Case of Rechecking Jim, a 59-year-old night watchman, sought treatment for anxiety, insomnia, and compulsive checking behaviors. His symptoms had been under good control until he was attacked by an intruder at work. After recovering from the attack, he developed severe anxiety, bordering on panic, insomnia, and exacerbation of his tendency to repeatedly check the stove and locks before leaving his house. His insomnia responded well to mirtazapine 7.5 mg at bedtime and his anxiety also diminished. Because he did not want to take additional medications, he was offered a trial of coherent breathing, *ujjayi*, and breath moving. Jim learned the practices easily during 20 minutes of his therapy session. As he practiced these breath techniques for 20 minutes in the morning and evening, his anxiety further improved, but he continued to complain of checking. He was then instructed to use coherent breathing whenever he felt the anxiety that was driving his checking compulsion and to continue the slow breathing practice while turning and walking away from the stove or lock. This provided just enough relief for him to stop the rechecking. Over the subsequent weeks, the compulsion remitted and he was pleased to report that he no longer needed to check the stove and locks more than once before leaving the house.

BRAIN AGING, COGNITIVE FUNCTION, HEART RATE VARIABILITY, AND BREATHING PRACTICES

Reduced HRV significantly correlated with lower cognitive performance in 4763 adults aged 50 years or older in the Irish longitudinal study on aging (Frewen, Finucane, Savva, et al., 2013). Orthostatic hypotension (a significant decline in blood pressure that can occur with postural changes), a sign of autonomic dysfunction, is also associated with lower cognitive performance in adults over the age of 50 who have supine hypertension (BP > 140/90 mmHg) (Frewen et al., 2013). A cross-sectional study of 80 adults aged 65 or older compared those with mild cognitive impairment (MCI) to those who had normal cognitive function. The adults with MCI were found to have greater autonomic dysfunction and orthostatic dysregulation of blood pressure (Nicolini, Ciulla, Malfatto, et al., 2014). Low HRV is associated with increased all-cause mortality, blood pressure dysregulation, and increased syncopal episodes in those with dementia. Evidence suggests that cerebral hypoperfusion

(insufficient blood flow) may lead to brain damage and progression of cognitive impairment. A study of patients with MCI found that decreased HRV was associated with increased severity of white matter lesions (Galluzzi, Nicosia, Geroldi, et. al., 2009).

Sympathetic hyperactivity and parasympathetic withdrawal may cause and sustain high blood pressure. Autonomic imbalance can reset arterial baroreflex sensitivity and chemoreflex-induced hyperventilation. Breathing at 6 bpm increases baroreflex sensitivity and reduces sympathetic activity and chemoreflex activity with potential improvement in blood pressure in hypertensives and in healthy subjects (Bernardi, Gabutti, Porta, & Spicuzza, 2001; Joseph, Porta, Casucci, et al., 2005).

A study using HRV derived from photoplethesmography (PPG) found that the strongest correlation to ECG on HRV parameters occurred during paced breathing at 6 bpm. In addition, the study found that maximum variation of heart rate had the highest negative correlation with age. Slow, deep breathing evokes the baroreflex, central to autonomic adaptive regulation. Baroreflex activity degrades with age, decreased elasticity in arterial walls, decreased lung elasticity, and reduced synaptic transmission (Russoniello, Zhirnov, Pougatchev, et. al., 2013). Breathing at 5 bpm, which improves baroreflex activity, arterial wall elasticity, and lung elasticity, may mitigate these aspects of aging.

Cognitive Function in Schizophrenia

Cognitive dysfunction, common in patients with schizophrenia, contributes to the overall difficulties functioning in daily life. Medications used to treat chronic schizophrenia contribute to the development of fatigue, inactivity, metabolic syndrome, cardiovascular disease, obesity, and other diseases of aging. These problems tend to worsen and accelerate disease progression as individuals with schizophrenia age. Yoga practices have been used to treat patients with schizophrenia, primarily in India. However, in the United States, particularly among the severe, chronic patients living in group residences, patients are often too sedentary, obese, and sedated to participate in yoga postures. An open pilot study of 35 chronic schizophrenic patients living in residences on the grounds of a hospital in the United States found that it was necessary to engage the patients in walking while performing coherent breathing at 5 bpm because if they lay down, many would fall asleep. Walking both improved their physical capacity for movement and kept them from falling asleep. Adding music to the paced breathing made the walking more enjoyable and energizing. Many of the patients could not maintain balance during yoga postures. It was easier for them to perform flowing qi gong movements. Patients participated in 1-hour sessions three times a week for 12 weeks. Sessions included 20 minutes of gentle movements (yoga or qi gong) and 20 minutes of coherent breathing. At the end of the study, mean Sum of Index Scores on Repeatable Battery for the Assessment of Neuropsychological Status (RBANS) increased significantly compared to baseline ($p = .001$), as did sub-scores for attention, delayed memory, figure copy, visual-spatial construction, semantic fluency, and language index. Analysis changes in genomic regulation from patient lymphocytes in this study are pending (Smith, Boules, Maayan, et al., 2013).

Gentle movement and breathing practices adapted for patients with schizophrenia could improve cognitive function and play a role in slowing or preventing some of the age-related and iatrogenic illnesses that add to the heavy burden of disease in these chronically ill patients. Additional research is needed in this area.

CHALLENGES IN RESEARCH AND EVALUATION OF THE EVIDENCE BASE FOR BREATHING PRACTICES

Methods developed to analyze evidence bases supporting the use of pharmaceutical agents are not readily applicable to studies of mind–body practices because of fundamental differences in the treatments, the subjects, and other confounding factors. In studies of pharmaceuticals, the identical chemical agent can be given to thousands of subjects in any number of studies. In contrast, no two mind–body programs are identical. Even if a specific breathing practice such as coherent breathing is administered, there will be variations between studies depending on the nuances of how it is taught and variations in subjects' interpretations and abilities to execute the instructions. For example, some people may breathe at 5 bpm with tension or forcefulness, while others breathe in a relaxed, gentle manner. The effects will then vary. Performing coherent breathing with tension or forcefulness introduces a greater element of sympathetic activation, rendering the parasympathetic activation less effective. Beyond individual differences in skill, there are inevitable variations between studies that use different techniques, combinations of techniques, and amounts of time devoted to each technique. There is no way to assure that the interventions are comparable among studies. Also, subjects who participate, for example, in a yoga study may already have a regular meditation practice, which will alter their neurophysiological response to the new practices. Novice subjects introduce other confounders because, being new to the practices, they may not perform them smoothly or efficiently. Nevertheless, compared to other mind–body practices, breathing is the easiest to replicate because it can be precisely timed and measured. Evaluating mind–body research using conventional scales such as the Jaded is inappropriate because it is impossible to create an identical placebo or to blind subjects to the intervention. This immediately lowers the rating on conventional scales. Attempts are being made to create more suitable evaluation methods based on better research and reporting standards, as recommended in the CONSORT (Consolidated Standards of Reporting Trials) Extension for Non-Pharmacological Interventions, developed by an international panel of 22 experts (Boutron et al., 2008a, 2008b). As researchers try to apply these standards to specific areas of mind–body research, they are being further refined (Kinser & Robbins 2013; Porcini, 2012).

FUTURE DIRECTIONS

The quality of research on breath practices will continue to improve with the use of larger groups, longer follow-up, randomization, suitable controls, clearer descriptions of the practices, standardized measures of physical and psychological symptoms, biomarkers of immune, endocrine, and metabolic response, physiological markers such as HRV, and electroencephalograms. The use of advanced technologies such as imaging studies and genomics provides new methods of exploration. Breath practices, as rapidly acting, noninvasive probes, could potentially be used to study neural networks involved in cognitive and emotion regulation. For example, a study using mass resonance spectroscopy (MRS) in depressed subjects, evaluating the effect of coherent breathing and yoga on GABA levels in the insular cortex, thalamus, and amygdala is currently in progress. However, until more funding becomes available for costly studies using advanced technologies, much can be learned from smaller high-quality studies and from careful clinical observation.

SUMMARY

Voluntarily regulated breathing practices (VRBPs) can improve mental health and mitigate the effects of aging on the stress response system (SRS), autonomic nervous system (ANS), hypothalamic-pituitary-adrenal (HPA) axis, emotion regulatory systems, inflammation, immune response, oxidative stress, and cardiovascular and neurological systems. Specific breathing techniques have been shown to increase PNS activity, improve sympatho-vagal balance, reduce inflammatory markers and cortisol release, and improve oxidative status. In addition, these practices reduce perceived stress, ameliorate negative psychological states, and may improve cognitive function. Clinical trials using breathing practices have shown reductions in symptoms of stress, anxiety, insomnia, PTSD, depression, combat stress, schizophrenia, stress-related medical conditions, and cognitive dysfunction. Larger studies are needed to validate and extend these findings.

ACKNOWLEDGMENTS AND DISCLOSURE STATEMENTS

NCCAM Award #8T007483. The Treatment of Depression with Yoga and Walking: Mass Resonance Spectroscopy Study of Brain GABA Levels in 3 ROIs. 9/1/12–6/30/17. PI: Chris Streeter. Consultants: P. L. Gerbarg and R. P. Brown.

Department of Mental Health of Mississippi, British Petroleum Grant. Breath~Body~Mind Training for Relief of stress Post-Disaster. March 1, 2011–January 30, 2012. Co-investigators: P. L. Gerbarg, R. P. Brown, C. C. Streeter.

Additional research grants from the Ratner Family Trust, Fisher Wallace Trust, Lynford Family Trust, and Humanetics.

The authors declare no other conflicts of interest.

REFERENCES

Abbott R, Lavretsky H. (2013). Tai chi and qigong for the treatment and prevention of mental disorders. *Psychiatr Clin North Am, 36*(1), 109–119. doi: 10.1016/j.psc.2013.01.011.

Antony, J., & Porcino, A. J. (2012). The greater value of the CONSORT Statement Guidelines: guideposts for designing and reporting all TMB research. *Int J Ther Massage Bodywork, 5*(4), 1–2.

Barragán Loayza, I. M/., Solà, I., & Juandó Prats, C. (2011). Biofeedback for pain management during labour. *Cochrane Database Syst Rev, 6*, CD006168. doi: 10.1002/14651858.CD006168.pub2.

Beckham, J., Greene, T. B., & Meltzer-Brody, S. (2013). A pilot study of heart rate variability biofeedback therapy in the treatment of perinatal depression on a specialized perinatal psychiatry inpatient unit. *Arch Womens Ment Health, 16*(1), 59–65. doi: 10.1007/s00737-012-0318-7

Bernardi, L., Gabutti, A., Porta, C., & Spicuzza, L. (2001). Slow breathing reduces chemoreflex response to hypoxia and hypercapnia, and increases baroreflex sensitivity. *J Hypertension, 19*, 221–229.

Bernardi, L., Sleight, P., Bandinelli, G., Cencetti, S., Fattorini, L., Wdowczyc-Szulc, J., & Lagi, A. (2001). Effect of rosary prayer and yoga mantras on autonomic cardiovascular rhythms: comparative study. *BMJ, 323*(7327), 1446–1449.

Boutron, I., Moher, D., Altman, D. G., Schulz, K. F., Ravaud, P., & CONSORT Group. (2008a). Extending the CONSORT statement to randomized trials of nonpharmacologic treatment: explanation and elaboration. *Ann Intern Med, 148*(4), 295–309.

Boutron, I., Moher, D., Altman, D. G., Schulz, K. F., Ravaud, P., & CONSORT Group. (2008b). Methods and processes of the CONSORT Group: example of an extension for trials assessing nonpharmacologic treatments. *Ann Intern Med, 148*(4), W60–66.

Brands, M. M., Purperhart, H., & Deckers-Kocken, J. M. (2011). A pilot study of yoga treatment in children with functional abdominal pain and irritable bowel syndrome. *Complement Ther Med, 19*, 109–114.

Brown, R. P., & Gerbarg, P. L. (2005a). Sudarshan Kriya yogic breathing in the treatment of stress, anxiety, and depression: Part I: neurophysiologic model. *J Alt Compl Med, 11*, 189–201.

Brown, R. P., & Gerbarg, P. L. (2005b). Sudarshan Kriya yogic breathing in the treatment of stress, anxiety, and depression: Part II: clinical applications and guidelines. *J Alt Compl Med, 11*, 711–717.

Brown, R. P., & Gerbarg, P. L. (2009).Yoga breathing, meditation, and longevity. *Ann NY Acad Sci, 1172*, 54–62.

Brown, R. P., & Gerbarg, P. L. (2012). *The healing power of the breath: simple techniques to reduce stress and anxiety, enhance concentration, and balance your emotions.* Boston: Shambhala.

Brown, R. P., Gerbarg, P. L., & Muench, F. (2013). Breathing practices for treatment of psychiatric and stress-related medical conditions. *Psychiatr Clin North Am, 36,* 121–140.

Brown, R. P., Gerbarg, P. L., & Muskin, P. R. (2009*). How to use herbs, nutrients, and yoga in mental health care.* New York: W. W. Norton.

Brown, R., Gerbarg, P., Vermani, M., et al. (2010a). *1st trial of breathing, movement and meditation for PTSD, depression, and anxiety related to September 11th New York City World Trade Center Attacks.* Presented at American Psychiatric Association, May 22, New Orleans, LA.

Brown, R., Gerbarg, P., Vermani, M., et al. (2010b). *2nd trial of breathing, movement, and meditation for PTSD, depression and anxiety related to September 11th New York City World Trade Center Attacks.* Presented at American Psychiatric Association, May 22, New Orleans, LA.

Busch, V., Magerl, W., Kern, U., Haas, J., Hajak, G., & Eichhammer, P. (2012). The effect of deep and slow breathing on pain perception, autonomic activity, and mood processing: an experimental study. *Pain Med, 13*(2), 215–228. doi: 10.1111/j.1526-4637.2011.01243.x.

Carter, J., Gerbarg, P. L., Brown, R. P., Ware, R., D'Ambrosio, C., Dirlea, M., Vermani, M., & Katzman, M. A. (2013). Multi-component yoga breath program for Vietnam veteran post traumatic stress disorder: randomized controlled trial. *J Traumat Stress Disord Treat, 2*(3), 1–10.

Chalmers, J. A., Quintana, D. S., Abbott, M. J., & Kemp, A. H. (2014). Anxiety disorders are associated with reduced heart rate variability: a meta-analysis. *Front Psychiatry, 5,* 80. doi: 10.3389/fpsyt.2014.00080.

Chan, A. S., Cheung, M. C., Sxe, S. L., Leung, W. W., & Shi, D. (2011). Shaolin dan tian breathing fosters relaxed and attentive mind: a randomized controlled neuro-electrophysiological study. *Evid Based Compl Alt Med, 2011,* 180704. doi: 10.1155/2011/180704.

Chan, B. R., & Polich, J. (2006). Meditation states and traits: EEG, ERP, and neuroimaging studies. *Psychol Bull, 132*(2), 180–211.

Craig, A. D. (2003). Interoception: the sense of the physiological condition of the body. *Curr Opin Neurobiol, 13*(4), 500–505 [Review].

Descilo, T., Vedamurtachar, A., Gerbarg, P. L., Nagaraja, D., Gangadhar, B. N., Damodaran, B., Adelson, B., Braslow, L. H., Marcus, S., & Brown, R. P. (2010). Effects of a yoga breath intervention alone and in combination with an exposure therapy for post-traumatic stress disorder and depression in survivors of the 2004 South-East Asia tsunami. *Acta Psychiatr Scand, 121*(4), 289–300.

Dusek, J. A., Otu, H. H., Wohlhueter, A. L., Bhasin, M., Zerbini, L. F., et al. (2008). Genomic counter-stress changes induced by the relaxation response. *PLoS One, 3,* e2576.

Franzblau, S. H., Smith, M., Echevarria, S., & Van Canford, T. E. (2006). Take a breath, break the silence: the effects of yogic breathing and testimony about battering on feelings of self-efficacy in battered women. *Int J Yoga Ther, 16,* 49–57.

Frewen, J., Finucane, C., Savva, G. M., Boyle, G., Coen, R. F., & Kenny, R. A. (2013). Autonomic dysfunction is a feature of mild cognitive impairment (MCI), a prodrome of dementia. *Clin Auton Res, 23*(6), 313–323.

Galluzzi, S., Nicosia, F., Geroldi, C., Alicandri, A., Bonetti, A., & Bonetti, M., et al. (2009). Cardiac autonomic dysfunction is associated with white matter lesions in patients with mild cognitive impairment. *J Gerontol A Biol Sci Med Sci 64,* 1312–1315.

Gard, T., Noggle, J. J., Park, C. L., Vago, D. R., & Wilson, A. (2014). Potential self-regulatory mechanisms of yoga for psychological health. *Front Hum Neurosci, 8,* 770. doi: 10.3389/fnhum.2014.00770.

Gems, D. (2014). What is an anti-aging treatment? *Exp Geront, Pii,* S0531-5565914 00208-3. doi: 10.1016/j.exger.2014.07.003.

Gerbarg, P. L. (2008). Yoga and neuro-psychoanalysis. In F. S. Anderson (Ed.), *Bodies in treatment: the unspoken dimension* (pp.127–150). Hillsdale, NJ: Analytic Press.

Gerbarg, P. & Brown, R. (2011). Mind-body practices for recovery from sexual trauma. In T. Bryant-Davis (Ed.), *Surviving sexual violence: a guide to recovery and empowerment* (pp. 199–216). Lanham, MD: Rowman & Littlefield.

Gerbarg, P., Gootjes, L., & Brown, R. P. (2014). Mind-body practices and the neuro-psychology of well-being. In Chu Kim-Prieto (Ed.), *Religion and spirituality across cultures.* In Antonella Delle Fave (Series Ed.), *Cross-cultural advancements in positive psychology* (vol. 9, 227–246). Milan: Springer.

Gerbarg, P. L., Jacob V. E., Stevens, L., Bosworth, B. P., Chabouni, F, DeFilippis, E. M., Warren, R., Trivellas, M. Patel, P. V., Webb, R. D., Harbus, M. D., Christos P. J., Brown R. P., Scherl E. J. The Effect of Breathing, Movement, and Meditation on Psychological and Physical Symptoms and

Inflammatory Biomarkers in Inflammatory Bowel Disease: A Randomized Controlled Trial. *J Inflammatory Bowel Disease* (in press).

Gerbarg, P. L., Jacob, V. E., Stevens, L., Bosworth, B. P., Chabouni, F., DeFilippis, E. M., Warren, R. U., Trivellas, M., Patel, P. P., Webb, C. D., Harbus, M. D., Christos, P. J., Brown, R. P., & Scherl, E. J. (2013). *The effect of breathing, movement, and meditation on psychological and physical symptoms and inflammatory biomarkers in inflammatory bowel disease: randomized controlled trial. J Inflammatory Bowel Disease* (in press).

Gerbarg, P. L., Streeter, C. C., Whitfield, T., & Brown, R. P. (2014). Breath-Body-Mind (B-B-M) training for healthcare providers post 2010 Gulf oil spill. Presented at American Psychiatric Association Annual Meeting. New York.

Gerbarg, P. L., Wallace, G., & Brown, R. P. (2011). Mass disasters and mind-body solutions: evidence and field insights. *Int J Yoga Ther, 2011,* 97–107

Granath, J., Ingvarsson, S., von Thiele, U., & Lundberg, U. (2006). Stress management: a randomized study of cognitive behavioural therapy and yoga. *Cogn Behav Ther, 35*(1), 3–10.

Haroon, E., Raison, C. L., & Miller, A. H. (2012). Psychoneuroimmunology meets neuropsychopharmacology: translational implications of the impact of inflammation on behavior. *Neuropsychopharmacology, 37*(1), 137–162. doi: 10.1038/npp.2011.205.

Hassett, A. L., Radvanski, D. C., Vaschillo, E. G., Vaschillo, B., Sigal, L. H., Karavidas, M. K., et al. (2007). A pilot study of the efficacy of heart rate variability (HRV) biofeedback in patients with fibromyalgia. *Appl Psychophysiol Biofeed, 32*(1), 1–10.

Huston, J. M. (2012). The vagus nerve and the inflammatory reflex: wandering on a new treatment paradigm for systemic inflammation and sepsis. *Surg Infect, 13,* 187–193.

Janakiramaiah, N., Gangadhar, B. N., Naga Venkatesha Murthy, P. J., Harish, M. G., Subbakrishna, D. K., & Vedamurthachar, A. (2000). Antidepressant efficacy of Sudarshan Kriya Yoga (SKY) in melancholia: a randomized comparison with electroconvulsive therapy (ECT) and imipramine. *J Affect Disord, 57*(1–3), 255–259.

Janakiramaiah, N., Gangadhar, B. N., Naga Venkatesha Murthy, P. J., Harish, M. G., Taranath Shetty, K., Subbakrishna, D. K., Meti, B. L., Raju, T. R., & Vedamurthachar, A. (1998). Therapeutic efficacy of Sudarshan Kriya Yoga (SKY) in dysthymic disorder. *NIMHANS, 17,* 21–28.

Jerath, R., Edry, J. W., Barnes, V. A., & Jerath, V. (2006). Physiology of long pranayamic breathing: neural respiratory elements may provide a mechanism that explains how slow deep breathing shifts the autonomic nervous system. *Med Hypotheses, 67*(3), 566–571.

Joseph, C. N., Porta, C., Casucci, G., Casiraghi, N., Maffeis, M., Rossi, M., & Bernardi, L. (2005). Slow breathing improves arterial baroreflex sensitivity and decreases blood pressure in essential hypertension. *Hypertension, 46,* 714–718.

Joshi, M., & Telles, S. (2008). Immediate effects of right and left nostril breathing on verbal and spatial scores. *Indian J Physiol Pharmacol, 52*(2), 197–200.

Kalyani, B. G., Venkatasubramanian, G., Arasappa, R., Rao, N. .P, Kalmady, S. V., Behere, R. V., Rao, H., Vasudev, M. K., & Gangadhar, B. N. (2011). Neurohemodynamic correlates of "OM" chanting: a pilot functional magnetic resonance imaging study. *Int J Yoga, 4*(1), 3–6. doi: 10.4103/0973-6131.78171.

Karavidas, M. K., Lehrer, P. M., Vaschillo, E., Vaschillo, B., Marin, H., Buyske, S., Malinovsky, I., Radvanski, D., & Hassett, A. (2007). Preliminary results of an open label study of heart rate variability biofeedback for the treatment of major depression. *Appl Psychophysiol Biofeed, 32*(1), 19–30.

Katzman, M., Vermani, M., Gerbarg, P. L., & Brown, R. P. (2013). *Effect of Breath Body Mind Workshop on symptoms of GAD with comorbidities.* Presented at 166th Annual Meeting of the American Psychiatric Association, May 17–22, San Francisco, CA.

Katzmann, M. A., Vermani, M., Gerbarg, P. L., Brown, R. P., Iorio, C., Davis, M., Cameron, C., Pawluk, E., & Tsirgielis, D. (2012). A multicomponent yoga-based, breath intervention program as adjunctive treatment in patients suffering from generalized anxiety disorder (GAD) with or without comorbidities. *Int J Yoga, 5*(1), 57–65.

Kinser, P. A., & Robins, J. L. (2013). Control group design: enhancing rigor in research of mind-body therapies for depression. *Evid-Based Compl Alt Med, 2013,* 140467. Article ID 140467. doi: 10.1155/2013/140467.

Kozasa, E. H., Santos, R. F., Rueda, A. D., Benedito-Silva, A. A., De Ornellas, F. L., & Leite, J. R. (2008). Evaluation of Siddha Samadhi Yoga for anxiety and depression symptoms: a preliminary study. *Psychol Rep, 103*(1), 271–274.

Kuttner, L., Chambers, C. T., Hardial, J., et al. (2006). A randomized trial of yoga for adolescents with irritable bowel syndrome. *Pain Res Manag, 11,* 217–223.

Lehrer, P. M., & Gevirtz, R. (2014). Heart rate variability biofeedback: how and why does it work? *Front Psychol, 5*, 756. doi: 10.3389/fpsyg.2014.00756.

Li, Q. Z., Li, P., Garcia, G. E., Johnson, R. J., & Feng, L. (2005) Genomic profiling of neutrophil transcripts in Asian qigong practitioners: a pilot study in gene regulation by mind-body interaction. *J Altern Complement Med, 11*, 29–39.

Malathi, A., & Damodaran, A. (1999). Stress due to exams in medical students: role of yoga. *Indian J Physiol Pharmacol, 43*(2), 218–224.

Manjunath, N. K., & Telles, S. (2005). Influence of yoga and Ayurveda on self-rated sleep in a geriatric population. *Indian J Med Res, 121*(5), 683–690.

Mason, H., Vandoni, M., Debarbieri, G., Codrons, E., Ugargol, V., & Bernardi, L. (2013). Cardiovascular and respiratory effect of yogic slow breathing in the yoga beginner: what is the best approach? *Evid Based Compl Alt Med, 2013*, 743504. doi: 10.1186/1751-0759-5-4.10.1155/2013/743504.

Meregnani, J., Clarençon, D., Vivier, M., et al. (2011). Anti-inflammatory effect of vagus nerve stimulation in a rat model of inflammatory bowel disease. *Auton Neurosci Basic Clin, 160*, 82–89.

Minassian, A., Geyer, M. A., Baker, D. G., Nievergelt, C. M., O'Connor, D. T., Risbrough, V. B., & Marine Resiliency Study Team. (2014). Heart rate variability characteristics in a large group of active-duty marines and relationship to posttraumatic stress. *Psychosom Med, 76*(4), 292–301. doi: 10.1097/PSY.0000000000000056.

Nicolini, P., Ciulla, M. M., Malfatto, G., Abbate, C., Mari, D., Rossi, P. D., Pettenuzzo, E., Magrini, F., Consonni, D., & Lombardi, F. (2014). Autonomic dysfunction in mild cognitive impairment: evidence from power spectral analysis of heart rate variability in a cross-sectional case-control study. *PLoS One, 5*, e96656. doi: 10.1371/journal.pone.0096656.

Nolan, R. P., Kamath, M. V., Floras, J. S., Stanley, J., Pang, C., & Picton, P., et al. (2005). Heart rate variability biofeedback as a behavioral neurocardiac intervention to enhance vagal heart rate control. *Am Heart J, 149*(6), 1137.

Olafsrud, S. M., Meza-Zepeda, L. A., & Saatcioglu, F. (2013). Rapid gene expression changes in peripheral blood lymphocytes upon practice of a comprehensive yoga program. *PLoS One, 8*(4), e61910. doi: 10.1371/journal.pone.0061910.

Park, G., & Thayer, J. F. (2014). From the heart to the mind: cardiac vagal tone modulates top-down and bottom-up visual perception and attention to emotional stimuli. *Front Psychol, 5*, 278. doi: 10.3389/fpsyg.2014.00278.

Porges, S. W. (2001). The polyvagal theory: phylogenetic substrates of a social nervous system. *Int J Psychophysiol, 42*(2), 123–146.

Porges, S. W. (2007). The polyvagal perspective. *Biol Psychol, 74*(2), 116–143.

Qu, S., Olafsrud, S. M., Meza-Zepeda, L. A., & Saatcioglu, F. (2013). Rapid gene expression changes in peripheral blood lymphocytes upon practice of a comprehensive yoga program. *PLoS One, 8*(4): e61910. doi: 10.1371/journal.pone.0061910.

Russoniello, C. V., Zhirnov, Y. N., Pougatchev, V. I., & Gribkov, E. (2013). Heart rate variability and biological age: implications for health and gaming. *Cyberpsychol Behav Social Networking, 17*(4), 302–308

Saatcioglu, F. (2013). Regulation of gene expression by yoga, meditation and related practices: a review of recent studies. *Asian J Psychiatr, 6*(1), 74–77. doi: 10.1016/j.ajp.2012.10.002.

Sahasi, G., Moha, D., & Kacker, C. (1989). Effectiveness of yogic techniques in the management of anxiety. *J Personal Clin Stud, 5*, 51–55.

Sakakibara, M., & Hayano, J. (1996). Effect of slowed respiration on cardiac parasympathetic response to threat. *Psychosomatic Med, 58*(1), 32–37.

Schelegle, E. S. (2003). Functional morphology and physiology of slowly adapting pulmonary stretch receptors. *Anat Rec A Discov Mol Cell Evol Biol, 270*(1), 11–16.

Seppälä, E. M., Nitschke, J. B., Tudorascu, D. L., Hayes, A., Goldstein, M. R., Nguyen, D. T., Perlman, D., & Davidson, R. J. (2014). Breathing-based meditation decreases posttraumatic stress disorder symptoms in U.S. Military veterans: a randomized controlled longitudinal study. *J Trauma Stress, 27*(4), 397–405. doi: 10.1002/jts.21936.

Shannahoff-Khalsa, D. S. (2003). Kundalini yoga meditation techniques for the treatment of obsessive-compulsive and OC spectrum disorders. *Grief Treat Crisis Intervent, 3*(3), 369–382.

Sharma, H., Datta, P., Singh, A., Sen, S., Bhardwaj, N. K., Kochupillai, V., & Singh, N. (2008). Gene expression profiling in practitioners of Sudarshan Kriya. *J Psychosom Res, 64*, 213–218.

Sharma, I., Azmi, S. A., & Settiwar, R. M. (1991). Evaluation of the effect of pranayama uin anxiety states. *Alternative Med, 3*, 227–235.

Sharma, V. K., Trakroo, M., Subramaniam, V., Rajajeyakumar, M., Bhavanani, A. B., & Sahai, A. (2013). Effect of fast and slow pranayama on perceived stress and cardiovascular parameters in young health-care students. *Int J Yoga, 6*(2), 104–110. doi: 10.4103/0973-6131.113400.

Sherman, K. J. (2012). Guidelines for developing yoga interventions for randomized trials. *Evid-Based Compl Alt Med, 2012,* 143271. Article ID 143271. doi: 10.1155/2012/143271.

Smith, R. C., Boules, S., Maayan, L., Gerbarg, P. L., Brown, R., Visceglia, E., et al. (2013). *Effects of yoga on cognition, psychiatric symptoms, and epigenetic changes in chronic schizophrenic patients.* Presented at 14th International Schizophrenia Congress, Orlando, FL, April 22.

Streeter, C. C., Gerbarg, P. L., Saper, R. B., et al. (2012). Effects of yoga on the autonomic nervous system, gamma-aminobutyric-acid, and allostasis in epilepsy, depression, and post-traumatic stress disorder. *Med Hypotheses, 78,* 571–579.

Sun P., Zhou, K., Wang S., et al. (2013). Involvement of MAPK/NF-κB signaling in the activation of the cholinergic anti-inflammatory pathway in experimental colitis by chronic vagus nerve stimulation. *PloS One, 8,* e69424.

Sutarto, A. P., Wahab, M. N., & Zin, N. M. (2012). Resonant breathing biofeedback training for stress reduction among manufacturing operators. *Int J Occup Saf Ergon, 18*(4), 549–561.

Taneja, I., Deepak, K. K., Poojary, G., et al. (2004). Yogic versus conventional treatment in diarrhea-predominant irritable bowel syndrome: a randomized control study. *Appl Psychophysiol Biofeed, 29,* 19–33.

Telles, S., Bhardwaj, A. K., Kumar, S., Kumar, N., & Balkrishna, A. (2012). Performance in a substitution task and state anxiety following yoga in army recruits. *Psychol Rep, 110*(3), 963–976.

Telles, S., Naveen, K. V., & Dash, M. (2007). Yoga reduces symptoms of distress in tsunami survivors in the andaman islands. *Evid-Based Compl Alt Med, 4*(4), 503–509.

Telles, S., & Singh, N. (2013). Science of the mind: ancient yoga texts and modern studies. *Psychiatr Clin North Am, 36,* 93–108.

Telles, S., Singh, N., & Balkrishna, A. (2011). Heart rate variability changes during high frequency

yoga breathing and breath awareness. *Biopsychosoc Med, 5,* 4.

Telles, S., Singh, N., Joshi, M., Balkrishna, A. (2010). Post traumatic stress symptoms and heart rate variability in Bihar flood survivors following yoga: a randomized controlled study. *BMC Psychiatry, 10,* 18. doi: 10.1186/1471-244X-10-18.

Thayer, J. F. (2009). Vagal tone and the inflammatory reflex. *Cleve Clin J Med, 76*(Suppl 2), S23–26.

Thayer, J. F., & Lane, R. D. (2000). A model of neurovisceral integration in emotion regulation and dysregulation. *J Affect Disord, 61*(3), 201–216.

Thayer, J. F., & Sternberg, E. M. (2009). Neural concomitants of immunity: focus on the vagus nerve. *Neuroimage, 47*(3), 908–910. doi: 10.1016/j.neuroimage.2009.05.058.

Trakroo, M., Bhavanani, A. B., Pal, G. K., Udupa, K., & Krishnamurthy, N. (2013). A comparative study of the effects of asan, pranayama and asan-pranayama training on neurological and neuromuscular functions of Pondicherry police trainees. *Int J Yoga, 6*(2), 96–103. doi: 10.4103/0973-6131.113398.

Tsang, H. W., Fung, K. M., Chan, A. S., Lee, G., & Chan, F. (2006). Effect of a qigong exercise programme on elderly with depression. *Int J Geriatr Psychiatry, 21*(9), 890–897.

Urry, H. L., Nitschke, J. B., Dolski, I., Jackson, D. C., Dalton, K. M., Mueller, C. J., et al. (2004). Making a life worth living: neural correlates of well-being. *Psychol Sci, 15*(6), 367–372.

van Der Zanden, E. P., Boeckxstaens, G. E., & de Jonge, W. J. (2009). The vagus nerve as a modulator of intestinal inflammation. *Neurogastroenterol Motil, 21,* 6–17.

Zucker, T. L., Samuelson, K. W., Muench, F., Greenberg, M. A., & Gevirtz, R. N. (2009). The effects of respiratory sinus arrhythmia biofeedback on heart rate variability and posttraumatic stress disorder symptoms: a pilot study. *Appl Psychophysiol Biofeedback, 34*(2), 135–143. doi: 10.1007/s10484-009-9085.

17

SPIRITUAL ISSUES AND INTERVENTIONS IN MENTAL HEALTH AND AGING

Sermsak Lolak, Darlinda K. Minor, Najmeh Jafari and Christina Puchalski

INTRODUCTION

Spirituality, broadly defined and inclusive of religion, is the aspect of humanity that refers to the ways in which individuals seek and express meaning and purpose, and the ways that they experience their connectedness to the moment, to self, to others, to nature, and to the significant or sacred (C. Puchalski et al., 2009). Spirituality is a dynamic dimension of human life, and is expressed through beliefs, values, traditions, and practices (C. M. Puchalski, Vitillo, Hull, & Reller, 2014). Patients use the spiritual dimension of their lives to understand and cope with their suffering (C. Puchalski & Romer, 2000). Suffering encompasses physical and emotional symptoms, and is often associated with existential or spiritual distress; therefore spirituality is a critical aspect in developing and delivering patient-centered, compassionate, whole-person care, a goal commonly emphasized by many healthcare institutions. Moreover, a focus on spirituality improves patients' health outcomes and quality of life, including in end-of-life care and care of the aging

population (Larson et al., 1986; Larson et al., 1992; C. M. Puchalski et al., 2014).

There are currently several practice guidelines available regarding how to integrate spirituality into clinical practice. A guideline from the 2009 National Consensus Project for Quality Palliative care (NCP; National Consensus Project for Quality Palliative Care, 2009; C. Puchalski et al., 2009), widely adapted in both palliative care and other clinical settings, recommends an interdisciplinary team that ideally includes spiritual care professionals to assess and address spiritual, religious, and existential dimensions of care. Building on the 2009 guidelines, international conferences were held, with the goals of reaching consensus on approaches to the integration of spirituality into healthcare structures at all levels (C. M. Puchalski et al., 2014).

Spiritual well-being offers some protection against despair in those facing illness, including those nearing the end of life (McClain, Rosenfeld, & Breitbart, 2003). In addition, spirituality may positively affect the patient's mental health and well-being in a variety of ways, such as increasing coping, facilitating social integration and support, providing meaning, and helping with self-regulation and emotional comfort (H. G. Koenig, 2013; Pargament & Lomax, 2013; Swinton, 2001). In this chapter we explore how to recognize and address spiritual issues in mental health and aging, as well as outline and critically evaluate available evidence of spiritual interventions in clinical settings, particularly in the mental health and aging population.

SPIRITUALITY IN MENTAL HEALTH AND AGING

Spiritual and Religious Coping

Religious and/or spiritual coping is very common in elderly patients and patients with persistent mental illness (H. G. Koenig et al., 1992; Tepper, Rogers, Coleman, & Malony, 2001). Spirituality may positively affect the patient's mental health and well-being in a variety of ways, such as increasing coping, facilitating social integration and support, helping with self-regulation and emotional comfort, and providing meaning (Pargament & Lomax, 2013; Swinton, 2001).

Hundreds of studies found positive associations between mental health (e.g., higher levels of psychological well-being, greater social support, less depression, less suicidal thoughts, and drug abuse) and higher levels of religious involvement (H. Koenig, King, & Carson, 2012; Lucchetti et al., 2011). This association is more robust in the elderly and in subjects with medical illness, and in general the association appears to be strong in depression, suicide, and substance abuse (Bonelli & Koenig, 2013; Dervic et al., 2011; H. G. Koenig, George, & Titus, 2004; H. G. Koenig, Zaben, & Khalifa, 2012; Moreira-Almeida, Lotufo Neto, & Koenig, 2006; Van Ness & Larson, 2002). Studies have shown that there is a high level of religion/spirituality among older adults in the United States and significant patient-reported desire to include such beliefs in healthcare settings (Phillips, Paukert, Stanley, & Kunik, 2009). However, the vast majority of these studies were focused on religious attendance and beliefs among North American Christians. Less work has been done on other religions or spiritual beliefs, especially when the subjects do not belong to or participate in an organized religion, and thus can represent selection bias (Dein, Cook, Powell, & Eagger, 2010; Jafari et al., 2013).

Negative Spiritual Coping

While positive religious coping, such as forgiveness or healthy relationship with deity, can enhance health outcomes and well-being (Tepper et al., 2001), spiritual struggle with oneself, with others, and with the divine can also damage health and well-being, particularly among psychiatric patients (Pargament & Lomax, 2013). For example, positive religious coping in bipolar patients is strongly associated with fewer depressive symptoms and higher quality of life, while negative religious coping is associated with lower quality of life (Stroppa & Moreira-Almeida, 2013). The same is true for psychotic patients; studies show that spiritual struggle (negative religious coping) is associated with greater psychotic symptoms, social isolation, depression, anxiety, and suicidal ideation, while positive coping appears to have an opposite effect (Mohr, Brandt, Borras, Gilliéron, & Huguelet, 2006; Rosmarin, Bigda-Peyton, Öngur, Pargament, & Björgvinsson, 2013). Although clinicians generally recognize the importance of spiritual and religious issues, they may not be accurately aware of a patient's religion or spiritual involvement and its impact. As such, it is important for clinicians to not only inquire about the patient's spiritual involvement but to ask about whether it is problematic for the patient, which can open the door to an exploration of religion and spirituality struggle (Pargament & Lomax, 2013).

Spiritual Suffering

The spiritual dimension of suffering can also present with physical and emotional symptoms, but is distinct from emotional and/or psychiatric causes of suffering. In addition, a patient who seems to be free of physical or psychiatric symptoms can still have significant spiritual distress, which leads to significant suffering. On the other hand, spiritual, existential, or religious distress can and often does present as a psychiatric complaint, and vice versa. Pargament categorizes the relationship between religion or spirituality and psychiatric illness as primary (a source of psychiatric illness), secondary (a byproduct of psychiatric illness), and complex (both directions) (Pargament & Lomax, 2013).

Given these complexities, a traditional psychosocial assessment may not be adequate in assessing the patient's spiritual coping and distress. The Royal College of Psychiatrists recommends that a spiritual assessment should be considered as part of every mental health assessment, as psychiatric illness can reflect a spiritual void in a person's life. In addition, the guideline also suggests that mental health professionals need to be able to distinguish between a spiritual crisis and a mental illness, particularly when these overlap (Royal College of Psychiatrists, 2013). Frequently, psychiatrists and/or mental health practitioners are called upon to address those symptoms or issues. A skilled clinician can discern the elements of existential distress and provide appropriate interventions. In the case that psychopathology is the primary source of religious distress (i.e., religious-themed hallucinations or delusions), the treatment of primary psychopathology alone may result in spiritual improvement. However, when the psychiatric symptoms are secondary to problems with spiritual or religious struggles, a focus on psychiatric treatment alone may not be sufficient (Pargament & Lomax, 2013).

In addition, an individual's spiritual beliefs, assumptions, and relationship to the significant, sacred, or divine may take shape through his or her experiences and past relationships. In some patients, spiritual views may be distorted by their past traumatic experience. For example, estranged or abusive parents may distort images of God and the patient's relationship with God (Kestenbaum & Dunn, 2014). As such, religion may be associated with restrictions and punishments, rather than with acceptance and love (H. G. Koenig, 2013). These "transferences" may also play out in the context of the therapeutic relationship between the patient and his or her mental health providers.

Psychological processes such as depression or trauma can have spiritual impacts such as anger, or a damaged relationship with God. Patients can also confuse one dimension with another, mistaking their psychopathology to be of a spiritual origin (e.g., believing that depression is a punishment from God). Balboni et al. suggest a model that differentiates among the emotional, existential, and spiritual domains of the patient's distress (Balboni, Puchalski, & Peteet, 2014). This can be accomplished by an exploration of the patient's emotions, worldview, experience, and beliefs in psychotherapy.

ASSESSING SPIRITUALITY IN THE CLINICAL SETTING

Despite recognizing the importance of the issues (Mohr et al., 2006), doctors tend to avoid or bypass the discussion of spirituality with their patients.

This may be due to professional role conflicts, having negative presumptions about spirituality, or just simply feeling uncomfortable or unprepared. Most practitioners continue to view spiritual care as something that they are unable to provide (Kalish, 2012). However, the issues of meaning, purpose, and beliefs are important to the patients, and without some signal or permission from the doctors the patients may feel that these topics are not welcome (C. Puchalski & Romer, 2000).

While the majority of patients and physicians believe in the positive impact of spiritual care, physicians hold more negative perceptions of spiritual care compared to patients (Phelps et al., 2012). Similarly, mental health professionals generally are resistant and ambivalent to discussing the issues of spirituality and religion for a complex and wide variety of reasons, including the belief that it is not scientific or not consistent with the current psychopathology model, feeling incompetent, or being concerned about imposing their beliefs on their patients (Griffith & Griffith, 2002; Swinton, 2001). Moreover, the separation of spirituality and medicine is rooted within a larger social system context that dichotomizes spiritual and non-spiritual domains (Balboni et al., 2014). However, psychiatrists and mental health practitioners may be more likely to encounter religion/spirituality issues in the clinical setting. A large survey found that psychiatrists are more open to and appreciate the importance of addressing spirituality issues with their patients (Curlin et al., 2007). Patients are unlikely to engage in a deep conversation about the deepest sides of themselves unless clinicians demonstrate a willingness to explore spiritual issues (Griffith & Griffith, 2002; Pargament & Lomax, 2013).

Approaching the Patient on the Issue of Spirituality

Spiritual care is integral in patients whose sense of meaning and worth is challenged by illness (Culliford & Eagger, 2009). It is important to recognize that for patients whose lives contain much pain and sorrow, integrating the spiritual dimension into their overall care is necessary for their treatment to progress. Spiritual issues are often central in patients suffering from demoralization or existential crises, either from physical, mental, or terminal illnesses.

There are many frameworks for understanding spirituality. A helpful approach is to start with questions that explore the issues of meaning, hope, relationship/support, and purpose (Culliford & Eagger, 2009; Griffith & Griffith, 2002). These questions, which explore the patient's existential posture, not only are helpful in getting information but also help the patient cope by mobilizing his or her inner resources, leading to resiliency (Griffith & Gaby, 2005).

Metaphors pose abstract concepts in terms of images and events drawn from daily life, which can be a valuable tool to engage the patient in the discussion of spiritual issues. By closely listening for and skillfully using metaphors, clinicians can engage at a deeper level with patients. Griffith and Griffith wrote eloquently about how to use the power of metaphor in psychotherapy with patients when exploring spiritual issues. They offer strategies for clinicians in working with metaphors, including eliciting additional metaphors, encouraging the patient to elaborate on the metaphor, or seeking alternative metaphors in order to help the patient process his or her spiritual difficulties (Griffith & Griffith, 2002).

While there is clearly a benefit in engaging the patient in exploring spiritual and/or religious issues, this has to be done in a sensitive and professional manner in order to protect vulnerable patients, such as those who suffer from mental illness, from undue influence by a clinician's personal belief system, which may not be compatible with that of the patient. Guidelines are available on how psychiatrists can sensitively and respectfully explore a patient's spiritual beliefs and history while being aware of ethical and boundary issues (Cook, 2013). Hence there is a strong need for training and the integration of spirituality education and reflection in medical education. Clinicians can draw upon their spiritual traditions and communities to help shape their professional identity and practice of medicine, while being aware of the differences between their own and their patients' beliefs or values (Balboni et al., 2014).

Obtaining a Spiritual History

The most common and most helpful method of assessing spiritual needs is getting a good spiritual history (Culliford & Eagger, 2009). Conducting a spiritual history is an important part of addressing the patient's spiritual needs. It helps the clinician to understand the roles that spirituality plays in the patient's life, illness, and coping; to identify the patient's beliefs that may affect care; and to recognize and mobilize the patient's community

of support or other interventions in order to satisfy the patient's spiritual needs. This not only can affect the patient's coping ability, compliance, and rapport, but also potentially can affect the practitioners' own spirituality and sense of "calling" and meaning, which will eventually impact both quality of care and the practitioner's own quality of life (H. G. Koenig, 2013).

Taking a spiritual history and engaging the patient in conversation about the importance of his or her spirituality in and of itself can be very therapeutic and powerful. Patients may be reluctant to bring up spiritual issues to their doctors, even though they are a very important part of their lives (C. Puchalski & Romer, 2000). By taking a spiritual history, the physician sends the message to the patient that these issues are recognized, permitted, and even encouraged to discuss. The spiritual history impacts the medical care plan, and determines decisions on spiritual interventions for a particular patient, such as referral to a chaplain (H. G. Koenig, 2013). One such approach is using one of the available spiritual assessment tools, such as FICA (Faith or beliefs, Importance and influence, Community, and Address) (Borneman, Ferrell, & Puchalski, 2010; C. Puchalski & Romer, 2000) to guide the interview. Delegating these questions to the chaplain is not sufficient, nor is it always practical. Koenig proposed using a single question, "Do you have any spiritual needs or concerns related to your health?" in a clinical situation that is rushed and does not allow more than a few moments to address the patient's spiritual needs (H. G. Koenig, 2013), with plans to follow up on the issue if it came up. This method, however, is considered a spiritual screening, not a history. A full spiritual history is recommended as part of the routine history and physical encounter, and should be done by clinicians who are responsible for developing treatment and care plans (C. Puchalski et al., 2009). Kristeller found that an inclusion of a brief (5–7 minute) semi-structured exploration of spiritual concerns to routine visit results in a positive impact on psychological well-being and perception of care (Kristeller, Rhodes, Cripe, & Sheets, 2005).

SPIRITUAL INTERVENTIONS

There is no clear consensus as to what constitutes spiritual interventions in a healthcare setting. Clearly, conducting a good spiritual history itself can accomplish a lot and could be considered a spiritual intervention in itself. In addition, it provides a better understanding of the patient's spiritual needs and type of subsequent interventions.

It has been shown that various aspects of spirituality and/or religiousness—together or alone—can decrease feelings of depression and anxiety, increase dignity and sense of purpose/meaning at the end of life, and decrease the request for hastened death. Furthermore, spiritual well-being has been cited as one of the more important factors in the lives of individuals at the end of life. Despite growth in this area of research, there have not been many efforts to translate these findings into clinical interventions. This is likely due to ethical implications given the needs of this population, as well as the fact that they may be receiving religious and spiritual interventions outside the medical setting (Candy et al., 2012).

In spite of this, there is some research available for interventions aimed at improving overall well-being and quality of life, strengthening the sense of spirituality and connectedness, increasing meaning, sense of purpose, and dignity, and improving mental health in aging populations and at the end of life. The quality of these studies, however, are varied due to methodological limitations, making interpretation challenging. In the following sections, we attempt to outline some of the widely known spiritual interventions according to the available evidence. The description of each intervention is followed by critical evaluation of the evidence of efficacy of the intervention(s). Table 17.1 shows examples of spirituality-based interventions.

Mindfulness-Based Interventions (MBIs)

MBIs have been extensively studied in a variety of populations, including mental health and aging. These interventions aim to enhance the quality of mindfulness, defined as "paying attention in a particular way: on purpose, in the present moment, and non-judgmentally" (Kabat-Zinn, 1994). While MBIs, such as mindfulness-based stress reduction (MBSR) programs, are generally classified under complementary and alternative medicine (CAM), these practices could be considered spiritual interventions given their roots in wisdom traditions, the emphasis on contemplation, and the attitude of curiosity, openness, and acceptance.

Table 17.1. Examples of Spirituality-Based Interventions

INTERVENTION	EXAMPLES OF EVIDENCE
Mindfulness-based interventions (MBIs)	Bränström et al., 2010 Kearney et al., 2013 Keng et al., 2011 Kuyken et al., 2008 Ludwig & Kabat-Zinn, 2008 Marchand, 2012 Vøllestad et al., 2011
Yoga	Chen et al., 2009 Patel et al., 2012 Smith et al., 2007
Dignity therapy	Chochinov et al., 2005 Julião at al., 2013 Chochinov et al., 2011 Houmann et al., 2014
Meaning-enhancing therapy	Ando et al., 2010 Breitbart, et al., 2007 Breitbart et al., 2012 D. K. Miller et al., 2005
Referral to chaplain or other spiritual care professionals	Culliford & Eagger, 2009 Handzo & Puchalski, 2015 Kestenbaum & Dunn, 2014 H. G. Koenig, 2013 Puchalski et al., 2009 VandeCreek & Burton, 2001

In addition, focusing on the relational and spiritual aspect, such as transcendence and the interconnectedness of mindfulness practice, may have a potential to deepen its benefits (Falb & Pargament, 2012). There is evidence suggesting the effectiveness of MBIs in a variety of medical and psychiatric disorders (Keng, Smoski, & Robins, 2011; Ludwig & Kabat-Zinn, 2008;

Marchand, 2012). In particular, a number of randomized controlled trials (RCTs) of MBSR programs show decreased self-report of various psychological symptoms, including anxiety and depression, as well as general distress, with good effect size (Keng et al., 2011; Vøllestad, Sivertsen, & Nielsen, 2011). Studies also found increased psychological well-being and sense of spirituality (Bränström, Kvillemo, Brandberg, & Moskowitz, 2010) in participants completing MBSR programs. A particular form of psychotherapy, mindfulness-based cognitive therapy (MBCT), which combines mindfulness training and elements of cognitive therapy, shows evidence for efficacy as an adjunctive treatment of both depression and anxiety, as well as reduced relapsed rate for patients with recurrent major depressive disorder (MDD), in several RCTs (Keng et al., 2011; Kuyken et al., 2008; Marchand, 2012).

While MBIs are generally found to be effective for a variety of psychological symptoms, evidence from meta-analyses are less conclusive as to the real effect size. In addition, little is known about the "minimal effective dose" of MBIs needed for different populations. In their critical review of effects of mindfulness on psychological health, Keng et al. cautioned against indiscriminate application of mindfulness as a panacea technique; rather, it should be tailored to fit the needs of specific population and target outcomes (Keng et al., 2011).

In addition to MBIs, there has been a recent growth in programs specifically addressing the cultivation of compassion informed by wisdom traditions, as well as psychological theories (Lolak, 2013). Compassion training likely works by promoting functional brain plasticity and affects the brain regions responsible for empathy, emotions, and executive function Jazaieri et al. (2013), offering a new coping strategy that fosters a positive affect even when one is confronted with the distress of others (Klimecki, Leiberg, Lamm, & Singer, 2013). Recent studies show effectiveness of interventions using loving-kindness and mindfulness meditations in veterans suffering from post-traumatic stress disorder (PTSD) (Kearney et al., 2013). However, the evidence is just beginning to accumulate, and more studies, particularly with good comparison groups and clear outcome measures, are needed.

Overall, these interventions are likely becoming more popular given their relative low cost, accessibility in a variety of settings (group, in person, or online), and lack of significant side effects,

drug interactions, and stigma compared to biological treatment. However, until we have enough high-quality comparison studies with the standard treatment that account for various methodological shortcomings and confounders, these interventions should be used to supplement traditional treatment, but not as a replacement, for those suffer from severe mental illness.

Yoga

Yoga is a popular and commonly practiced form of exercise/meditative practice that has been long practiced to enhance to the mind-body-spirit experience. It has been claimed to calm the spirit, and to help bring it into harmony with a higher being. The goal of the practice is to promote well-being in the mind, body, and spirit through meditation, various postures, and breathing techniques, and to create a sense of unity among them.

There is a plethora of evidence noting the positive effects of yoga on various measures of health (Chen et al., 2009; Patel, Newstead, & Ferrer, 2012; Smith, Hancock, Blake-Mortimer, & Eckert, 2007), including maintaining wellness, decreasing anxiety and depression scores, and increasing the sense of inner peace. Other positive aspects include that yoga is considered a self-help intervention (Smith et al., 2007), and, if successful, there is an ability to avoid poor side effect profiles in elderly patients. However, there is not much evidence for the use of yoga on the aging population (Patel et al., 2012). One can imagine that yoga presents some physical limitations due to the strenuous physical activity and stretching involved, which is usually limited in elderly individuals. There have been a few pioneers who have attempted to develop modified yoga interventions to accommodate the limited flexibility in this population. One study looked at the effects of Silver yoga against placebo in promoting mental health in elderly senior center patients in Taiwan (Chen et al., 2009). They found that after a 70-minute Silver yoga exercise three times per week for 6 months, conducted by staff and volunteers in the senior activity center who had completed a 9-hour training course, sleep quality, daytime dysfunction, physical and mental health perceptions, and depression scores had all improved at the 3-month assessment mark. These effects were maintained at 6 months as well, indicating the lasting effect of yoga on these measures.

Unfortunately, the evidence is mixed regarding yoga interventions in aging individuals. One study looked at Hatha yoga in a randomized comparative trail of 131 Australian participants with a mean age of 44 (Smith et al., 2007). The intervention was performed for 1 hour per week over the course of 10 weeks, and focused on breath awareness and internal centering, focus, sensitivity toward internal feelings, meditation, and relaxation. Compared with a progressive muscle relaxation (PMR) group, the Hatha yoga group was as effective as relaxation techniques in reducing stress and anxiety, and increasing sleep and physical and mental health. Interestingly enough, the progressive muscle relaxation group had higher long-term quality of life, and more participants had continued PMR upon follow-up than yoga.

Many of the problems with research done with yoga in aging groups are echoed in the preceding examples. However, overall, the effects of yoga are promising, and the benefits are undeniable for overall health. The key to strengthening this area is to develop a consistent, elderly-friendly intervention that can be done independently.

Jain et al. (2014) recently published a systematic review of meditation therapies for the acute and subacute phrase of depressive disorders. Of 747 abstracts screened, the authors identified 18 RCTs for the analysis. Most interventions included were MBCT and movement-based meditation therapies such as tai chi and yoga.

The data from RCTs suggest that meditative interventions may have substantial effects on depressive symptoms in patients with clinically diagnosed depressive disorders, including those currently having an acute major depressive episode (MDE) and those in partial remission (Jain 2014). The upper limit of effect sizes was larger for subjects having an acute MDE than for those with residual symptoms. Relative to the control group, most studies demonstrated moderate to large effect sizes relative to wait-list or treatment-as-usual controls. The studies using psychoeducation or pseudo-therapy control groups yielded lower upper-limit effect sizes (0.39–1.54) compared to the ones using treatment-as-usual controls (0.47–2.12). The authors note that calculation of a common effect size was not possible because of the heterogeneity of various meditation therapies included in the analysis.

Similar limitations were also echoed in the meta-analysis of yoga in older adults (Patel et al., 2012), where too many differing interventions make it difficult to have a clear understanding of what durations and interventions work regarding yoga in this population. Also, most of the studies included in his meta-analysis did not report on adverse side effects, which makes it difficult to determine if there just were no adverse effects or if they were not reported. This would be important to note in this population because of the increased potential for injury with exercise. Finally, outcomes measured vary significantly by study (Patel et al., 2012). Though there are few common variables, consistent outcome measures in well-designed, high-powered studies would certainly strengthen the results of the research. Jain et al. (2014) advocate clinical trials registration, as well as better design of control groups. The use of active control groups with a similar amount of group contact, focusing on healthy behaviors and homework time, but without the inclusion of active meditative practices, is recommended (Jain, Walsh, Eisendrath, Christensen, & Cahn, 2014). In addition, the authors suggest using the third arm of minimal treatment, such as modest psychoeducation group, in order to compare the effect of meditative therapies to minimal treatment.

Dignity Therapy

Dignity therapy was first described by Chochinov et al. (2005) as an intervention to increase a sense of meaning and purpose through increasing the sense of dignity at the end of life. It has been previously noted that patients in the end-of-life population struggle with a loss of dignity because they lose sense of their life value (Chochinov, 2007). This loss of dignity has been linked to an increase in suicides and requests for hastened deaths (Julião, Barbosa, Oliveira, Nunes, & Carneiro, 2013). Dignity therapy is one of the interventions more consistently studied, as the mechanism of performing the intervention is usually the same. Most of the providers performing dignity therapy for experimental purposes have been trained by Chochinov himself. Some of the noted advantages of this intervention include the ease of implementing it in end-of-life populations and the low costs to the participants, which means that it can be utilized across socioeconomic classes.

The intervention includes recording and transcribing information that the participant finds important to pass along to family and friends (Chochinov et al., 2005). Individuals are given a set of questions to ponder before the recording session. By sharing their personal story, which will endure beyond their death, their sense of value should increase and their level of distress decrease at the end of life. Dignity therapy provides a space for participants to share important life experiences, give advice, and settle any important issues (Julião et al., 2013). The results with this form of therapy have been promising.

In their phase 1 trial of dignity therapy with 100 end-of-life individuals, Chochinov et al. (2005) noted that a majority of the participants endorsed a higher sense of dignity, increased sense of purpose and meaning, and that this transcribed document, termed a generativity document, helped their families. A randomized trial done in a palliative care setting ($n = 326$) as a follow-up comparing dignity therapy to supportive psychotherapy and standard palliative care did not find any statistically significant differences in spiritual and psychosocial distress between the groups due to the floor effect of distress levels at baseline (Chochinov et al., 2011). However, in a follow-up survey, they found the secondary outcome measures provided the evidence for the benefit of dignity therapy. Participants in the treatment group were more likely than those in the control groups to report that dignity therapy helped them and their families, and improved their quality of life and their sense of dignity.

There is also evidence to support that dignity therapy decreases the sense of being a burden at the end of life. In a prospective evaluation study with terminal cancer patients in Denmark, participants who had some room to improve from baseline showed marked improvements in suffering, feelings of unfinished business and not being respected, depression, anxiety, and hopelessness. Even participants who reported no issues with dignity and meaningfulness at baseline found that dignity therapy made life more meaningful and strengthened their sense of dignity (Houmann, Chochinov, Kristjanson, Petersen, & Groenvold, 2014).

As with other spiritual and/or religious interventions being studied at the end of life, there are some issues with research for dignity therapy as well. Some of the limitations in the research are the same as those mentioned earlier—small sample sizes, poor attrition rates, lack of consistent outcome measures and measurement tools among available studies, and an inability to blind the groups, which could lead to better responses because of participant expectations. In dignity therapy, particularly, there have been profound floor effects, preventing the studies from showing statistically significant improvements in primary outcome measures

(Chochinov et al., 2011; Chochinov et al., 2005; Houmann et al., 2014). And although the dignity therapy treatment is consistent across studies, largely due to training by Chochinov, the study designs, including control groups and assessment timing, have been widely variable, weakening the overall body of results.

Meaning-Enhancing Therapy

Meaning-enhancing, or meaning-centered, therapy is a specific subset of psychotherapeutic interventions aimed at enhancing meaningfulness and purpose in life (Breitbart, Gibson, Poppito, & Berg, 2007). Several studies have shown the positive effects of increasing meaningfulness on depression and hopelessness, which are prevalent in the end-of-life population (Ando, Morita, Akechi, Okamoto, & Japanese Task Force for Spiritual Care, 2010; Breitbart et al., 2012; D. K. Miller, Chibnall, Videen, & Duckro, 2005). Unlike dignity therapy, there is not one specific meaning-enhancing therapy being studied in the literature. One of the biggest limitations in this intervention group is that there is no homogeneity in the interventions. Interventions range from individual to group settings; durations of the sessions and overall intervention differ, as well as the types of interventions performed.

Breitbart et al. (2010) developed a meaning-centered therapy called meaning-centered group psychotherapy (MCGP) for advanced cancer patients. It was developed as a brief, 8-week intervention to focus on lectures, discussion, and the exploration of meaning and purpose to enhance spiritual well-being. In a randomized controlled study with 90 terminally ill patients comparing MCGP to traditional supportive group therapy (D. K. Miller et al., 2005), the meaning-centered therapy group experienced significant improvements in spiritual well-being, purpose/meaning, and faith, which remained intact at a 2-month follow-up. There were no changes in depression scores in this study, but there is evidence that meaning-centered therapies help with depression.

In a study done by Ando et al. (2010), the effect of a short-term life review (STLR), in which the participant had two 30–60-minute sessions with an interviewer to review their lives and learn to accept and be satisfied with life, was studied in comparison to a control group receiving general support. STLR was an effort to enhance quality of life, acceptance, and decrease the desire for hastened death. Not only did they find improvements in sense of meaning, anxiety, and depression, but there was also improvement in elements of a good death. Participants felt like less of a burden, felt more complete, and were more prepared for death after using the technique to reflect on life and regain their sense of identity.

Some of the commonly cited limitations to this body of research include the inability to blind the treatment modality, high attrition rates in the end-of-life population, and unclear translations to clinical use—optimal numbers of sessions, duration of sessions, and treatment formats. Future research in this area is aimed at addressing these limitations to determine the feasibility of this technique in an aging population.

Other Spiritual Interventions

REFERRAL TO CHAPLAIN OR OTHER SPIRITUAL CARE PROFESSIONALS

When the patient's spiritual needs are beyond the expertise of a patient's primary healthcare or mental health professionals, a referral to a trained chaplain or other spiritual care professional, such as a pastoral counselor, is recommended. Certified professional chaplains are considered spiritual care experts in the healthcare setting. (C. Puchalski et al., 2009; H. G. Koenig, 2013; Handzo & Puchalski, 2015). Trained chaplains have gone through extensive training, followed by written and oral board exams, to meet the spiritual needs of medical or psychiatric patients, using spiritual assessments to guide the interventions (Kestenbaum & Dunn, 2014). Board-certified or board-eligible chaplains are trained to comprehensively assess and address the spiritual needs of patients from a wide range of religious traditions, as well as for those with no religious tradition or affiliation (Culliford & Eagger, 2009).

Chaplain interventions are always patient centered. Professional chaplains serve as an integral member of the patient's care team, reach across faith group boundaries, and do not proselytize (VandeCreek & Burton, 2001). Chaplains assist the patient's healing by addressing core spiritual needs such as meaning, sense of self-worth, belonging to community, and to love and be loved (reconciliation) (Kestenbaum & Dunn, 2014). This can be done through interactions with the patient, family members, the patient's other healthcare providers, and in some cases the members of the patient's spiritual communities. In addition, chaplains can make referrals to spiritual communities and classes or illness support groups, as well as leading spiritual/religious rituals or ceremony with the goal to move the patient along a path of healing (Kestenbaum & Dunn, 2014; VandeCreek & Burton, 2001).

In addition to chaplain and community clergy, a pastoral counselor may play an important and specific role in helping patients who struggle with spiritual issues, especially when unique forms of psychotherapy or counseling may be indicated, such as in outpatients with mental health issues (H. G. Koenig, 2013). According to the American Association of Pastoral Counselors (AAPC), AAPC-certified pastoral counselors are well credentialed, with postgraduate degrees from accredited universities; have experience and training in the ministry; have a current relationship with a local religious community; and have intensive, directly supervised counseling experience. They also have state licenses as social workers, marriage or family counselors, or psychologists.

OTHER INTERVENTIONS

Religious interventions have the least amount of literature available. There is minimal evidence for religious interventions, despite the ongoing evidence supporting the positive effects of religion on mental health, spiritual well-being, and overall quality of life in the end-of-life period. Religious interventions that have been studied include Bible reading, prayer, listening to religious music, and attendance at religious services and ceremonies.

In one pre-test and post-test designed trial, spirituality and ego integrity scores were examined in secular music versus spiritual music groups of 30 elderly individuals (Lowis & Hughes, 1997). There were two 30-minute tapes of secular or religious music played to the individuals weekly over a 4-week period. They found that there was no significant difference in the scores between the two groups, and there was an overall decrease in spirituality scores in both groups. Yet, in a study looking at two waves of data (2001 and 2004) from a Religion, Aging, and Health survey, it was noted that listening to religious music was significantly associated with decreased anxiety about death, and increased life satisfaction and self-control (Bradshaw, Ellison, Fang, & Mueller, 2014).

There is very little evidence on private religious practices (or non-organized religious activities) like prayer and Bible reading. In a prospective cohort study with almost 4000 elderly individuals, Helm et al. (2000) looked at how the frequency of private religious activities affected overall survival. After dividing the groups into elderly with impaired versus unimpaired activities of daily living (ADLs), they found a protective effect of religious activities on the survival of those with good ADLs. One major limitation of this study was that the private religious activities were not studied independently, making it difficult to determine the effects of each intervention alone.

The evidence for organized religious activities is also sparse. Most of the research looks at the effects of religious ceremonies on mental health and quality-of-life measures. These studies do not independently evaluate organized religious activities such as church attendance, baptisms, or festivals. Unfortunately, the religious ceremony interventions studied incorporate organized religious activities, like laying on hands, festivals, sermons, baptisms, and dancing, with private religious activities, like singing, prayer, meditation, and Bible reading. In two separate studies, patients were assessed pre- and post-ceremony to assess physical, spiritual, mental, and emotional quality of life (P. Hewson, Rowold, Sichler, & Walter, 2014; P. D. Hewson & Rowold, 2012). Though the results for spiritual (defined in religious terms) and mental quality of life have been overwhelmingly positive in these studies, the major limitation is that it is difficult to determine which elements of the ceremony have the greatest effects. In addition, it is difficult to determine if all of the elements are having any effect on these outcome measures at all. One should also consider that specific religious practices as well as personal spiritual or humanistic practices may be difficult to study using reductionist scientific methodology because that methodology does not fully capture the experience of spirituality and humanism broadly defined, or religious practices and their effect on people.

MECHANISMS

A number of explanatory mediators of the spirituality-health connection have been previously proposed in the literature. These include social support (Chatters, Taylor, Woodward, & Nicklett, 2014; Hill & Pargament, 2008), sense of coherence (Cowlishaw, Niele, Teshuva, Browning, & Kendig, 2013; George, Larson, Koenig, & McCullough, 2000), forgiveness (Toussaint, Marschall, & Williams, 2012), better coping strategies (Penley,

Tomaka, & Wiebe, 2002), emotional self-regulation (Aldwin, Park, Jeong, & Nath, 2014), and buffering the negative effects of stress on health (Nelson, 2009).

Recent studies rely on neuroimaging techniques to explore the neural mechanisms of the relationship between spirituality and mental health. In a study of 103 adults, Miller et al. (2014) examined the association between spirituality and cortical thickness in the brain regions, where a thinner cortex is a morphologic endophenotype of familial risk for MDD. They found that the high importance of spirituality or religion was associated with thicker cortices in these brain areas, suggesting the importance of spirituality or religion in protecting against MDD in people who are predisposed to developing it (L. Miller et al., 2014).

Similar studies have demonstrated that morphological changes in the regions associated with mental health are the underlying mechanism for the effects of mindfulness meditation practice on psychological well-being (Hölzel et al., 2008; Lazar et al., 2005; Luders, Toga, Lepore, & Gaser, 2009). In a controlled longitudinal study, Hölzel et al. (2008) investigated pre–post changes in brain gray matter concentration attributable to participation in an MBSR program. After an 8-week intervention, they observed increases in gray matter concentration in brain regions involved in learning and memory processes, emotion regulation, self-referential processing, and perspective taking (Hölzel et al., 2011).

Rather than the morphological changes, neurotransmitters are also involved in the interaction of spirituality or religion and mental health. Investigation of individuals with higher religiosity/spirituality scores showed lower cortisol responses to stress, resulted in buffering the negative effects of stress on health (Creswell et al., 2005; Nelson, 2009; Tartaro, Luecken, & Gunn, 2005). Increased levels of serotonin and β-endorphin release also reported during meditation and mindfulness-based practices contribute to the antidepressant effects (Mohandas, 2008).

SUMMARY

In the last two decades, empirical research on and related to spirituality has rapidly expanded in the field of mental health and medicine. However, there are still several areas of needs that should be addressed in future research in this field. The biggest challenge is the lack of consensus on a definition of spirituality in research projects and how to best conceptualize the distinct yet overlapping concepts of religion and spirituality, more broadly defined to also include humanistic, non-religious, and non-theistic beliefs. More research is needed to conceptualize not only the general concepts of spirituality and religion, but also different types of spiritual practices and spiritual outcomes (e.g., dignity, meaning, inner peace, and compassion). Also, further effort is needed to resolve uncertainties in the taxonomy of spiritual distress, an important step in the development of targeted spiritual interventions and outcome research. Another important concern is the lack of confidence and competence in assessing the spiritual needs of the elderly population among many healthcare providers. Developing evidence-based tools and guidelines and training of healthcare professionals are essential to ensure addressing elderly patients' and family members' spiritual needs in clinical practice.

Despite the significant progress in the number of studies linking spirituality and mental health, few studies have used longitudinal designs or population-based samples. Another methodological weakness is the lack of adequate control for potentially confounding variables and the short duration of interventions and outcome assessments. More longitudinal studies, especially in various clinical populations, are needed to show how and why spirituality and mental health may be functionally connected to each other. Further evidence of effectiveness and cost-effectiveness is essential before large-scale implementation.

Most research studies of the relationship of spirituality and health are conducted in the US population and in some European countries. Limited data are available in different religious groups and geographical locations, such as Asia and the Middle East (Jafari, Loghmani, & Puchalski, 2014). More research is needed to examine the association of spirituality and health in various cultural, humanistic, or religious backgrounds and to determine the cross-cultural commonalities and differences and their potential implications. Furthermore, there is still a wide gap in our knowledge on the pathways and mechanisms through which spirituality may affect psychological well-being. Previous studies mostly examined neurobiological changes due to meditation. Further exploration of mechanisms is needed for other prevalent religious, spiritual, cultural, and humanistic practices and interventions.

DISCLOSURE STATEMENTS

The Authors declare that there is no conflict of interest to disclose.

REFERENCES

Aldwin, C. M., Park, C. L., Jeong, Y., & Nath, R. (2014). Differing pathways between religiousness, spirituality, and health: a self-regulation perspective. *Psychol Relig Spiritual, 6*(1), 9.

Ando, M., Morita, T., Akechi, T., Okamoto, T., & Japanese Task Force for Spiritual Care. (2010). Efficacy of short-term life-review interviews on the spiritual well-being of terminally ill cancer patients. *J Pain Symptom Manage, 39*(6), 993–1002.

Balboni, M. J., Puchalski, C. M., & Peteet, J. R. (2014). The relationship between medicine, spirituality and religion: three models for integration. *J Religion Health, 53*(5), 1586–1598.

Bonelli, R. M., & Koenig, H. G. (2013). Mental disorders, religion and spirituality 1990 to 2010: A systematic evidence-based review. *J Religion Health, 52*(2), 657–673.

Borneman, T., Ferrell, B., & Puchalski, C. M. (2010). Evaluation of the FICA tool for spiritual assessment. *J Pain Symptom Manage, 40*(2), 163–173.

Bradshaw, M., Ellison, C. G., Fang, Q., & Mueller, C. (2014). Listening to religious music and mental health in later life. *Gerontologist, 00*(00), 1–12.

Bränström, R., Kvillemo, P., Brandberg, Y., & Moskowitz, J. T. (2010). Self-report mindfulness as a mediator of psychological well-being in a stress reduction intervention for cancer patients: a randomized study. *Ann Behav Med, 39*(2), 151–161.

Breitbart, W., Gibson, C., Poppito, S. R., & Berg, A. (2007). Psychotherapeutic interventions at the end of life: a focus on meaning and spirituality. *Focus, 5*(4), 451–458.

Breitbart, W., Poppito, S., Rosenfeld, B., Vickers, A. J., Li, Y., Abbey, J., . . . Cassileth, B. R. (2012). Pilot randomized controlled trial of individual meaning-centered psychotherapy for patients with advanced cancer. *J Clin Oncol, 30*(12), 1304–1309.

Breitbart, W., Rosenfeld, B., Gibson, C., Pessin, H., Poppito, S., Nelson, C., . . . Jacobson, C. (2010). Meaning-centered group psychotherapy for patients with advanced cancer: a pilot randomized controlled trial. *Psycho-Oncology, 19*(1), 21–28.

Candy, B., Jones, L., Varagunam, M., Speck, P., Tookman, A., & King, M. (2012). Spiritual and religious interventions for well-being of adults in the terminal phase of disease. *The Cochrane Library*, (5), 1–53.

Chatters, L. M., Taylor, R. J., Woodward, A. T., & Nicklett, E. J. (2014). Social support from church and family members and depressive symptoms among older African Americans. *American J Geriatr Psychiatry*, 23(6), 559–567.

Chen, K., Chen, M., Chao, H., Hung, H., Lin, H., & Li, C. (2009). Sleep quality, depression state, and health status of older adults after silver yoga exercises: cluster randomized trial. *Int J Nurs Studies*, 46(2), 154–163.

Chochinov, H. M. (2007). Dignity and the essence of medicine: the A, B, C, and D of dignity conserving care. *BMJ (Clinical Research Ed.)*, 335(7612), 184–187. doi: 335/7612/184.

Chochinov, H. M., Hack, T., Hassard, T., Kristjanson, L. J., McClement, S., & Harlos, M. (2005a). Dignity therapy: a novel psychotherapeutic intervention for patients near the end of life. *J Clin Oncol*, 23(24), 5520–5525.

Chochinov, H. M., Kristjanson, L. J., Breitbart, W., McClement, S., Hack, T. F., Hassard, T., & Harlos, M. (2011). Effect of dignity therapy on distress and end-of-life experience in terminally ill patients: a randomised controlled trial. *Lancet Oncol*, 12(8), 753–762.

Cook, C. (2013). How spirituality is relevant to mental healthcare and ethical concerns. Royal College of Psychiatrists. Spirituality and Mental Health Special Interest Group Publications Archive. Retrieved March 2015 from http://www.rcpsych.ac.uk/pdf/Chris%20Cook%20How%20Spirituality%20is%20Relevant%20to%20Mental%20Healthcare%20and%20Ethical%20Concerns.y.pdf.

Cowlishaw, S., Niele, S., Teshuva, K., Browning, C., & Kendig, H. (2013). Older adults' spirituality and life satisfaction: a longitudinal test of social support and sense of coherence as mediating mechanisms. *Ageing Society*, 33(07), 1243–1262.

Creswell, J. D., Welch, W. T., Taylor, S. E., Sherman, D. K., Gruenewald, T. L., & Mann, T. (2005). Affirmation of personal values buffers neuroendocrine and psychological stress responses. *Psychol Sci*, 16(11), 846–851. doi:PSCI1624 [pii]

Culliford, L., & Eagger, S. (2009). Assessing spiritual needs. In: Chris Cook, Andrew Powell and Andrew Sims (Eds.) *Spirituality and Psychiatry*, London: Royal College of Psychiatrists, 16–38.

Curlin, F. A., Lawrence, R. E., Odell, S., Chin, M. H., Lantos, J. D., Koenig, H. G., . . . Th M, M. (2007). Religion, spirituality, and medicine: psychiatrists' and other physicians' differing observations, interpretations, and clinical approaches. *Am J Psychiatry*, 164(12), 1825–1831.

Dein, S., Cook, C. C., Powell, A., & Eagger, S. (2010). Religion, spirituality and mental health. *Psychiatrist*, 34(2), 63–64.

Dervic, K., Carballo, J. J., Baca-Garcia, E., Galfalvy, H. C., Mann, J. J., Brent, D. A., & Oquendo, M. A. (2011). Moral or religious objections to suicide may protect against suicidal behavior in bipolar disorder. *J Clin Psychiatry*, 72(10), 1390–1396.

Falb, M. D., & Pargament, K. I. (2012). Relational mindfulness, spirituality, and the therapeutic bond. *Asian J Psychiatry*, 5(4), 351–354.

George, L. K., Larson, D. B., Koenig, H. G., & McCullough, M. E. (2000). Spirituality and health: what we know, what we need to know. *J Social Clin Psychology*, 19(1), 102–116.

Griffith, J. L., & Gaby, L. (2005). Brief psychotherapy at the bedside: countering demoralization from medical illness. *Psychosomatics*, 46(2), 109–116.

Griffith, J. L., & Griffith, M. E. (2002). *Encountering the sacred in psychotherapy: how to talk with people about their spiritual lives.* New York: Guilford Press.

Helm, H. M., Hays, J. C., Flint, E. P., Koenig, H. G., & Blazer, D. G. (2000). Does private religious activity prolong survival? A six-year follow-up study of 3,851 older adults. *The Journals of Gerontology Series A: Biological Sciences and Medical Sciences*, 55(7), M400–M405.

Handzo, G., & Puchalski, C. M. (2015). The role of the chaplain in palliative care. In Cherny, N., Fallon, M., Kaasa, S., Portenoy, R. K., & Currow, D. C. (Eds) *Oxford Textbook of Palliative Medicine*. Oxford: Oxford University Press.

Hewson, P. D., & Rowold, J. (2012). Do spiritual ceremonies affect participants' quality of life? A pilot study. *Compl Ther Clin Practice*, 18(3), 177–181.

Hewson, P., Rowold, J., Sichler, C., & Walter, W. (2014). Are healing ceremonies useful for enhancing quality of life? *J Alt Compl Med*, 20(9), 713–717.

Hill, P. C., & Pargament, K. I. (2008). Advances in the conceptualization and measurement of religion and spirituality: implications for physical and mental health research. *Psychology of Religion and Spirituality*, S(1), 3–17.

Hölzel, B. K., Carmody, J., Vangel, M., Congleton, C., Yerramsetti, S. M., Gard, T., & Lazar, S. W. (2011). Mindfulness practice leads to increases in regional brain gray matter density. *Psychiatry Res Neuroimaging*, 191(1), 36–43.

Hölzel, B. K., Ott, U., Gard, T., Hempel, H., Weygandt, M., Morgen, K., & Vaitl, D. (2008). Investigation of mindfulness meditation practitioners with voxel-based morphometry. *Social Cogn Affect Neurosci, 3*(1), 55–61.

Houmann, L. J., Chochinov, H. M., Kristjanson, L. J., Petersen, M. A., & Groenvold, M. (2014). A prospective evaluation of dignity therapy in advanced cancer patients admitted to palliative care. *Palliative Med, 28*(5), 448–458.

Jafari, N., Farajzadegan, Z., Zamani, A., Bahrami, F., Emami, H., & Loghmani, A. (2013). Spiritual well-being and quality of life in Iranian women with breast cancer undergoing radiation therapy. *Support Care Cancer, 21*(5), 1219–1225.

Jafari, N., Loghmani, A., & Puchalski, C. M. (2014). Spirituality and health care in Iran: time to reconsider. *J Religion Health, 53*, 1918–1922.

Jain, F. A., Walsh, R. N., Eisendrath, S. J., Christensen, S., & Cahn, B. R. (2014). Critical analysis of the efficacy of meditation therapies for acute and subacute phase treatment of depressive disorders: a systematic review. *Psychosomatics, 56*(2), 140–152.

Jazaieri, H., Jinpa, G. T., McGonigal, K., Rosenberg, E. L., Finkelstein, J., Simon-Thomas, E., . . . Goldin, P. R. (2013). Enhancing compassion: a randomized controlled trial of a compassion cultivation training program. *J Happiness Stud, 14*(4), 1113–1126.

Julião, M., Barbosa, A., Oliveira, F., Nunes, B., & Carneiro, A. V. (2013). Efficacy of dignity therapy for depression and anxiety in terminally ill patients: early results of a randomized controlled trial. *Palliat Support Care, 11*(06), 481–489.

Kabat-Zinn, J. (1994). *Wherever you go, there you are: mindfulness meditation in everyday life.* New York: Hyperion.

Kalish, N. (2012). Evidence-based spiritual care: a literature review. *Curr Opin Support Palliat Care, 6*(2), 242–246. doi: 10.1097/SPC.0b013e328353811c.

Kearney, D. J., Malte, C. A., McManus, C., Martinez, M. E., Felleman, B., & Simpson, T. L. (2013). Loving-kindness meditation for posttraumatic stress disorder: a pilot study. *J Trauma Stress, 26*(4), 426–434.

Keng, S., Smoski, M. J., & Robins, C. J. (2011). Effects of mindfulness on psychological health: a review of empirical studies. *Clin Psychol Rev, 31*(6), 1041–1056.

Kestenbaum, A., & Dunn, L. B. (2014). Spiritual AIM and the work of the chaplain: a model for assessing spiritual needs and outcomes in relationship. *Palliative and Supportive Care, 13*(01), 75–89.

Klimecki, O. M., Leiberg, S., Lamm, C., & Singer, T. (2013). Functional neural plasticity and associated changes in positive affect after compassion training. *Cereb Cortex, 23*(7), 1552–1561. doi: 10.1093/cercor/bhs142.

Koenig, H., King, D., & Carson, V. B. (2012). *Handbook of religion and health.* Oxford: Oxford University Press.

Koenig, H. G. (2013). *Spirituality in patient care: why, how, when, and what.* Philadelphia: Templeton Foundation Press.

Koenig, H. G., Cohen, H. J., Blazer, D. G., Pieper, C., Meador, K. G., Shelp, F., . . . DiPasquale, B. (1992). Religious coping and depression among elderly, hospitalized medically ill men. *Am J Psychiatry, 149*(12), 1693–1700.

Koenig, H. G., George, L. K., & Titus, P. (2004). Religion, spirituality, and health in medically ill hospitalized older patients. *J Am Geriatr Soc, 52*(4), 554–562.

Koenig, H. G., Zaben, F. A., & Khalifa, D. A. (2012). Religion, spirituality and mental health in the West and the Middle East. *Asian J Psychiatry, 5*(2), 180–182.

Kristeller, J. L., Rhodes, M., Cripe, L. D., & Sheets, V. (2005). Oncologist assisted spiritual intervention study (OASIS): patient acceptability and initial evidence of effects. *Int J Psychiatry Med, 35*(4), 329–347.

Kuyken, W., Byford, S., Taylor, R. S., Watkins, E., Holden, E., White, K., . . . Mullan, E. (2008). Mindfulness-based cognitive therapy to prevent relapse in recurrent depression. *J Consult Clin Psychol, 76*(6), 966.

Larson, D. B., Mansell, E., Pattison, M., Blazer, D. G., Omran, A. R., & Kaplan, B. H. (1986). Systematic analysis of research on religious variables. *Am J Psychiatry, 1*(43), 329.

Larson, D. B., Sherrill, K. A., Lyons, J. S., Craigie, F. C., Jr., Thielman, S. B., Greenwold, M. A., & Larson, S. S. (1992). Associations between dimensions of religious commitment and mental health reported in the American Journal of Psychiatry and Archives of General Psychiatry: 1978–1989. *Am J Psychiatry, 149*(4), 557–559.

Lazar, S. W., Kerr, C. E., Wasserman, R. H., Gray, J. R., Greve, D. N., Treadway, M. T., . . . Fischl, B. (2005). Meditation experience is associated with increased cortical thickness. *Neuroreport, 16*(17), 1893–1897.

Lolak, S. (2013). Compassion cultivation: a missing piece in medical education. *Acad Psychiatry, 37*(4), 285–285.

Lowis, M. J., & Hughes, J. (1997). A comparison of the effects of sacred and secular music on elderly people. *J Psychology, 131*(1), 45–55.

Lucchetti, G., Lucchetti, A. G. L., Badan-Neto, A. M., Peres, P. T., Peres, M. F., Moreira-Almeida, A., . . .

Koenig, H. G. (2011). Religiousness affects mental health, pain and quality of life in older people in an outpatient rehabilitation setting. *J Rehabil Med*, 43(4), 316–322.

Luders, E., Toga, A. W., Lepore, N., & Gaser, C. (2009). The underlying anatomical correlates of long-term meditation: larger hippocampal and frontal volumes of gray matter. *NeuroImage*, 45(3), 672–678.

Ludwig, D. S., & Kabat-Zinn, J. (2008). Mindfulness in medicine. *JAMA*, 300(11), 1350–1352.

Marchand, W. R. (2012). Mindfulness-based stress reduction, mindfulness-based cognitive therapy, and Zen meditation for depression, anxiety, pain, and psychological distress. *J Psychiatr Pract*, 18(4), 233–252. doi: 10.1097/01. pra.0000416014.53215.86.

McClain, C. S., Rosenfeld, B., & Breitbart, W. (2003). Effect of spiritual well-being on end-of-life despair in terminally-ill cancer patients. *Lancet*, 361(9369), 1603–1607.

Miller, D. K., Chibnall, J. T., Videen, S. D., & Duckro, P. N. (2005). Supportive-affective group experience for persons with life-threatening illness: reducing spiritual, psychological, and death-related distress in dying patients. *J Palliat Med*, 8(2), 333–343.

Miller, L., Bansal, R., Wickramaratne, P., Hao, X., Tenke, C. E., Weissman, M. M., & Peterson, B. S. (2014). Neuroanatomical correlates of religiosity and spirituality: a study in adults at high and low familial risk for depression. *JAMA Psychiatry*, 71(2), 128–135.

Mohandas, E. (2008). Neurobiology of spirituality. *Mens Sana Monographs*, 6(1), 63–80. doi: 10.4103/0973-1229.33001.

Mohr, S., Brandt, P., Borras, L., Gilliéron, C., & Huguelet, P. (2006). Toward an integration of spirituality and religiousness into the psychosocial dimension of schizophrenia. *American Journal of Psychiatry*, 163(11), 1952–1959.

Moreira-Almeida, A., Lotufo Neto, F., & Koenig, H. G. (2006). Religiousness and mental health: a review. *Rev Bras Psiquiatria*, 28(3), 242–250.

National Consensus Project for Quality Palliative Care. (2009). *Clinical practice guidelines for quality palliative care*. Third Edition, Pittsburg, PA: National Consensus Project for Quality Palliative Care.

Nelson, J. M. (2009). *Psychology, religion, and spirituality*. London: Springer Science & Business Media.

Pargament, K. I., & Lomax, J. W. (2013). Understanding and addressing religion among people with mental illness. *World Psychiatry*, 12(1), 26–32.

Patel, N. K., Newstead, A. H., & Ferrer, R. L. (2012). The effects of yoga on physical functioning and health related quality of life in older adults: a systematic review and meta-analysis. *J Alt Compl Med*, 18(10), 902–917.

Penley, J. A., Tomaka, J., & Wiebe, J. S. (2002). The association of coping to physical and psychological health outcomes: a meta-analytic review. *J Behav Med*, 25(6), 551–603.

Phelps, A. C., Lauderdale, K. E., Alcorn, S., Dillinger, J., Balboni, M. T., Van Wert, M., . . . Balboni, T. A. (2012). Addressing spirituality within the care of patients at the end of life: perspectives of patients with advanced cancer, oncologists, and oncology nurses. *J Clin Oncol*, 30(20), 2538–2544.

Phillips, L. L., Paukert, A. L., Stanley, M. A., & Kunik, M. E. (2009). Incorporating religion and spirituality to improve care for anxiety and depression in older adults. *Geriatrics*, 64(8), 15–18.

Puchalski, C. M., Vitillo, R., Hull, S. K., & Reller, N. (2014). Improving the spiritual dimension of whole person care: reaching national and international consensus. *J Palliat Med*, 642–656

Puchalski, C., Ferrell, B., Virani, R., Otis-Green, S., Baird, P., Bull, J., . . . Prince-Paul, M. (2009). Improving the quality of spiritual care as a dimension of palliative care: the report of the consensus conference. *J Palliat Med*, 12(10), 885–904.

Puchalski, C., & Romer, A. L. (2000). Taking a spiritual history allows clinicians to understand patients more fully. *J Palliat Med*, 3(1), 129–137.

Rosmarin, D. H., Bigda-Peyton, J. S., Öngur, D., Pargament, K. I., & Björgvinsson, T. (2013). Religious coping among psychotic patients: relevance to suicidality and treatment outcomes. *Psychiatry Res*, 210(1), 182–187.

Royal College of Psychiatrists. (2013). Position statement: recommendations for psychiatrists on spirituality and religion. Retrieved March 2015 from http://www.rcpsych.ac.uk/pdf/PS03_2013.pdf.

Smith, C., Hancock, H., Blake-Mortimer, J., & Eckert, K. (2007). A randomised comparative trial of yoga and relaxation to reduce stress and anxiety. *Compl Ther Med*, 15(2), 77–83.

Stroppa, A., & Moreira-Almeida, A. (2013). Religiosity, mood symptoms, and quality of life in bipolar disorder. *Bipolar Disord*, 15(4), 385–393.

Swinton, J. (2001). *Spirituality and mental health care: rediscovering a "forgotten" dimension*. London: Jessica Kingsley Publishers.

Tartaro, J., Luecken, L. J., & Gunn, H. E. (2005). Exploring heart and soul: effects of religiosity/

spirituality and gender on blood pressure and cortisol stress responses. *J Health Psychology,* 10(6), 753–766.

Tepper, L., Rogers, S. A., Coleman, E. M., & Malony, H. N. (2001). The prevalence of religious coping among persons with persistent mental illness. *Psychiatr Serv, 52*(5), 660–665.

Toussaint, L. L., Marschall, J. C., & Williams, D. R. (2012). Prospective associations between religiousness/spirituality and depression and mediating effects of forgiveness in a nationally representative sample of United States adults. *Depression Res Treat,* 1–10.

Van Ness, P. H., & Larson, D. B. (2002). Religion, senescence, and mental health: the end of life is not the end of hope. *Am J Geriatr Psychiatry,* 10(4), 386–397.

VandeCreek, L., & Burton, L. (2001). A white paper: professional chaplaincy: its role and importance in healthcare. *J Pastoral Care,* 55(1), 81–98.

Vøllestad, J., Sivertsen, B., & Nielsen, G. H. (2011). Mindfulness-based stress reduction for patients with anxiety disorders: evaluation in a randomized controlled trial. *Behav Res Ther, 49*(4), 281–288.

18

TRANCE IN LIFE TRANSITIONS

HYPNOSIS FOR BRAIN AND BODY

David Spiegel

HYPNOTIC HISTORY

Hypnosis represents the first Western conception of a psychotherapy, in that it was the first time a talking interaction between a doctor and a patient was thought to have therapeutic potential (1). Hypnosis has been used as an adjunctive tool in the treatment of traumatic experiences, pain, and anxiety for more than two centuries. Initial uses included hypnotic analgesia to help patients through traumatic surgical procedures prior to the advent of inhalation anesthesia (2). Freud, having learned hypnosis by studying with the French neurologist Charcot, began his exploration of the unconscious through the use of hypnosis (3). He abandoned its use when a patient suddenly exited a trance state and embraced him. Freud, noting that "I was modest enough not to attribute this event to my own irresistible personal attractiveness," (4) decided that hypnosis represented a mobilization of transference phenomena, and gave it up in favor of free association and psychoanalysis, though later in his career he stated that

"the pure gold of analysis might have to be alloyed with the copper of suggestion"(5). Hypnotic techniques were then used during and after World War II to treat what were then called "traumatic neuroses." They were found to be efficient and effective in helping soldiers with acute combat reactions to work through, control, or put aside the effects of traumatic experiences (6), now understood as post-traumatic stress disorder (PTSD) (7).

DEFINITION OF HYPNOSIS

Hypnosis is a state of highly focused attention, coupled with the dissociation of competing thoughts and sensations, which are relegated to the periphery of awareness, and there is enhanced response to social cues (8). Hypnosis is analogous in consciousness to what a telephoto lens does for a camera: what you see is perceived in great detail, but it is disconnected from its visual context. In the same way, hypnosis helps to focus attention and put aside distraction. It has three components: absorption, dissociation, and suggestibility. (9) Hypnosis has been referred to as "self-altering attention," the capacity to lose oneself effortlessly in the focus of one's concentration. Indeed, people who have more spontaneous experiences of losing themselves in a movie or a sunset are more hypnotizable on formal testing (10,11). This capacity to lose oneself implies dissociating, or processing potentially distracting information outside conscious awareness. The third component is suggestibility. This does not mean that hypnotized persons are unable to exert control over what they think and do, but rather that they are inclined to go along with hypnotic suggestions because they are less likely to consider alternatives and to analyze the source or context of the suggestions: Who is this person and why is he or she asking me to do this? We have all had the "it seemed like a good idea at the time" experience. In hypnosis, people focus more on "what" than "why," so compliance is more likely. This can actually be useful in getting patients to step away from old maladaptive habits and ways of thinking about problems such as somatic anxiety.

HYPNOTIZABILITY AS A TRAIT

The capacity to exert this top-down processing control called hypnosis varies considerably among adults. While most children are highly hypnotizable, substantial variation in responsiveness to hypnosis develops in early adult life and persists. Hypnotizability is a stable trait, with a test-retest correlation of 0.7 over a 25-year interval, which is greater stability than is observed for intelligence over a similar interval (12). Despite this reliability, few meaningful correlates of this trait, either psychological or neurobiological, have been identified, despite many efforts to find them (11,13–15). However, a tendency for self-altering attention, called "absorption," is moderately but significantly correlated with hypnotizability (10,11). This means that people who have hypnotic capacity tend to use it spontaneously, even without any formal training or exposure to hypnotic techniques.

One especially useful way of introducing hypnosis into the therapy is through the use of a clinical hypnotizability scale, such as the Hypnotic Induction Profile (8). This is a good way to initiate experience with hypnosis in treatment for several reasons:

1. It provides useful information about the patient's degree of hypnotizability, which provides empirical guidance for the choice of treatment. The presence and degree of a patient's hypnotizability can guide the design treatment employing hypnosis. The absence of hypnotic responsiveness, if identified, can lead to a choice of other more effective interventions, ranging from progressive muscle relaxation to medication.

2. In enables the clinician to turn the hypnotic induction into a deduction about the patient's ability to respond. This reduces performance pressure on both the patient and the clinician. Such an atmosphere can enhance the treatment alliance, defuse anxieties about loss of control, and help to demystify hypnosis.

3. All hypnosis is really self-hypnosis. Testing provides a framework for teaching patients how to use their capacity for self-hypnosis as part of their ongoing treatment and symptom management.

HYPNOTIC MODULATION OF PERCEPTION

Hypnosis is a powerful means of altering pain, anxiety, and various somatic functions, even under highly stressful circumstances such as interventional radiology procedures and surgery for breast cancer (16–20). Hypnotic alteration of perception, best studied in the somatosensory and visual systems, involves a top-down resetting of the intensity of perceptual response itself, rather than just an alteration in post-perception processing. This has been demonstrated through a reduction in early (21, p. 100) as well as late (p. 300) components of somatosensory event-related potentials (ERP) during hypnotic analgesia instructions (21). In addition, the nature of the hypnotic instruction influences the part of the brain involved in producing hypnotic analgesia. When subjects are told that the pain is there but will not bother them, the analgesia is associated with reduced activity of dorsal anterior cingulate cortex (dACC), while if they are told that they can reduce perception of the pain itself through a competing sensation such as tingling numbness, the analgesia is correlated with reduced activity in somatosensory cortex (22–24). Several studies have examined the idea that endogenous opiates account for hypnotic analgesia. However, with one partial exception (25), studies with both volunteers (26) and patients with chronic pain (27) have found that hypnotic analgesia is not blocked and is reversed by a substantial dose of naloxone, an opiate receptor blocker. In contrast, placebo analgesia is mediated by endogenous opiates (28).

Hypnosis can influence perception in other systems as well. With the use of hypnosis, believing is seeing: hypnotic alteration of color vision results in congruent changes in blood flow in the lingual and fusiform gyri (29). An instruction to drain color from a grid that looks like a Mondrian painting results in decreased blood flow in the color-processing regions, while hypnotic illusion that a black and white grid is filled with color results in both perception of the color and increased blood flow in those regions. The amount of time delay in naming a color word presented in a different color is associated with interaction between the dorsolateral prefrontal cortex (DLPFC) and the anterior cingulate cortex (ACC) (30). Hypnotic suggestion that words are written in an unknown language can reduce or eliminate the well-known Stroop color-word interference phenomenon, with concomitant reduction in activation of the dACC (14,15,31) These are examples of how hypnosis provides a model of brain control over perception and behavior. Such hypnotic effects occur more intensely when the hypnotic state is induced, so the phenomenon is more than a trait difference—it requires entry into the hypnotic state among people capable of it (32).

BRAIN REGIONS INVOLVED IN HYPNOSIS

The dorsal anterior cingulate cortex (dACC) and dorsolateral prefrontal cortex (DLPFC) contribute in important ways to both hypnotizability and sensory control. These regions are involved in the executive control network and salience, including selective attention and conflict resolution (33). The dACC and lateral PFC are also part of the mesocortical dopamine system(14), and consistent with this, hypnotizability has been found to be correlated with levels of homovanillic acid, a dopamine metabolite, in the cerebrospinal fluid (55). High-hypnotizable individuals, in contrast to low-hypnotizables, have altered activation of the dACC (15,22–24,34–39) and PFC (14,22,35,36) when they are modulating pain perception, reducing Stroop interference, and at rest (40). These findings suggest that these two

brain regions are engaged in top-down modulation of perception during hypnosis. There are detectable differences in functional connectivity between these regions among high- and low-hypnotizable individuals. (41) In a resting-state fMRI study, high- compared to low-hypnotizable individuals showed greater functional connectivity between the left DLPFC, an executive-control region of the brain, and the salience network, which is composed of the dACC, anterior insula, amygdala, and ventral striatum. This region is involved in detecting, integrating, and filtering relevant somatic, autonomic, and emotional information. These functional differences were not due to differences in brain anatomy in these regions. These results are similar to but not identical to observations that there are increases in left frontal activation during mindfulness practice (42,43). Our findings differ in emphasizing the co-activation of dACC along with DLPFC. Mindfulness is considered a practice that must be developed with considerable time and effort. Unlike hypnosis, it is not targeted at specific symptoms, but rather is a practice involving the development of a sense of open presence, scanning of the body, and compassion. Both, however, involve developing the ability to shift among mental states, which seems to provide benefit in dealing with stress and anxiety.

TEACHING SELF-HYPNOSIS

It is useful to teach patients from the beginning to experience the state of hypnosis as self-hypnosis so that they feel in control of the transition to this altered mental state. The instructions can be simple: "All hypnosis is really self-hypnosis. Now that we have demonstrated that you have a good capacity to use hypnosis, let me show you how to use it to work on a problem. While there are many ways to enter a state of self-hypnosis, one simple means is to count from one to three. On "one," do one thing: look up. On "two," do two things: slowly close your eyes and take a deep breath. On "three," do three things: let the breath out, let your eyes relax but keep them closed, and let your body float. Then, let one hand or the other float up in the air like a balloon, and that will be your signal to yourself and to me that you are ready to concentrate" (8, pp. 87–89). Once in a state of self-hypnosis, patients can be taught to produce a physical sensation of floating, lightness, or buoyancy. Their sense of physical comfort can be reinforced by having them initially imagine that they are somewhere safe and comfortable, such as floating in a bath, a lake, a hot tub, or space. This enhances their sense of control over their body.

ANXIETY: MIND AND BODY

Anxiety disorders are the most common of psychiatric problems, including in the aging population, with an overall 12-month prevalence of 18.1% and a lifetime prevalence of 28.8% (44). They are also archetypal mind–body problems, since an interaction between psychological and somatic distress is a hallmark feature of all of the anxiety disorders: generalized anxiety disorder, panic disorder, agoraphobia, and specific phobias. All of these disorders involve a reciprocating cycle of mental and physical distress. This makes techniques such as hypnosis especially salient to treatment, since it involves enhanced control by the mind over the body.

Most people with anxiety disorders are aware that, at some level, their fears are exaggerated or irrational. Yet, oddly enough, this is rarely reassuring, especially in the context of aging, since real if minor physical problems are experienced as harbingers of things to come. The very lack of definition of the source of the discomfort can exaggerate the fear, enhancing the patient's sense of helplessness and desire for avoidance. And yet the more they avoid the source of the fear, the more they consolidate an associational network that reinforces the strength of the threat. The challenge is to convert anxiety into fear, to give it a focus, so something can be done about it. In the same sense, converting depression into sadness can help such individuals work through the sources of their sadness so that the erosion of their self-worth and feelings of hopelessness and helplessness are reduced. To do this, one must offer patients tools that enable them to face their fears or sadness without a downward cycle of mental and physical distress. The ability to provide physical comfort in the face of fear is a valuable therapeutic tool.

From the point of view of therapeutic strategy, anxiety involves pathological distraction of attention from necessary day-to-day functions, and a negative feedback cycle between psychological preoccupation and somatic discomfort, a kind of "snowball effect," in which subjective anxiety and somatic tension reinforce each other. When someone notices an increase in heart rate, sweating, or tension in his or her abdomen, he or she is likely to respond with increased anxiety, reading the somatic signals as an indication of the seriousness of his or her concerns. This can in turn trigger further somatic response, in a continually reinforcing pattern. Hypnosis can be especially helpful not only because of its ability to reduce anxiety and induce relaxation (45), but because of the dissociative element of hypnosis that facilitates separation of the psychological and somatic components of anxiety.

The hypnotic technique involves having subjects imagine a sense of floating, lightness, or buoyancy, as though they were floating in a bath, a lake, a hot tub, or just floating in space. They are then taught to picture on an imaginary screen a pleasant scene to establish their ability to visualize in this manner. They are asked to picture a stressor on the left side of the screen while maintaining physical comfort, dissociating psychological from physiological stress. They are then asked to brainstorm a potential solution to the problem on the right side of the screen. This "brainstorming" is meant to help them take a more active stance toward the problem, and to widen the store of their potential responses to it.

There is evidence that hypnosis is as effective at reducing anxiety as 1 mg of alprazolam, at least among younger populations (46). Hypnosis has also been found to have as consistent anti-anxiety effects in such populations as autogenic training and quiet rest (47). It is particularly important to mobilize the dissociative capacity of patients, to help them separate their focal attention, even that devoted to anxiety-related issues, from somatic sensations of discomfort and restlessness.

INSOMNIA

Hypnosis is a state of increased concentration and awareness. From this point of view, the hypnotic state is far from sleep, although both are restful altered mental states with reduced awareness of the peripheral environment. Given the common Greek root *hypnos*, meaning "sleep," for hypnosis and hypnotic medications, there is often the mistaken assumption that hypnosis is a form of sleep. It is not that, but given the combination of focal attention and dissociation of somatic arousal, hypnosis can be helpful for inducing a state of physical relaxation that is at least compatible with sleep. As in the treatment of anxiety, a relaxing trance state may diminish the sympathetic arousal usually associated with anxious preoccupation and could facilitate entering into a restful sleep. Patients can be instructed to enter a state of self-hypnosis, then to induce a sense of floating and physical relaxation. Once this is achieved, they may use one of many different mechanisms to put worries or thoughts on hold "for tonight," knowing that they can always deal with them tomorrow. For example, patients can be taught to project those thoughts onto an imaginary screen. Then they can become a kind of "traffic director" for their thoughts, dealing with them on the screen, thereby dissociating them from the physical response to them while remaining in a quiet and relaxed state (8). This type of exercise can be used to get to sleep in the evening, and also if they wake during the night. There is limited evidence that such techniques can be effective in treating insomnia, for example among those with PTSD (48).

HYPNOTIC ANALGESIA

Hypnosis and similar techniques work through three primary mechanisms: muscle relaxation, perceptual alteration, and cognitive distraction. Pain is often accompanied by reactive muscle tension. Patients frequently splint the part of their body that hurts. Yet, because muscle tension can by itself cause pain in normal tissue and because traction on a painful part of the body can exacerbate pain, techniques that induce physical relaxation reduce pain. Therefore, having patients enter a state of hypnosis and concentrate on an image that connotes physical relaxation, such as floating or lightness, often produces physical relaxation and reduces pain.

The second major component of hypnotic analgesia is perceptual alteration. Patients can be taught to imagine that the affected body part is tingling or numb. Temperature metaphors are often especially useful, which is not surprising since pain and temperature sensations are part of the same neurosensory system, conducted through small poorly myelinated C fibers through the lateral spinothalamic tract in the spinal cord. Thus, imagining that an affected body part is cooler or warmer, using an image of dipping it in ice water or warming it in the sun, can often help patients transform pain signals. This is especially useful for extremely hypnotizable individuals who can, for example, relive an experience of dental anesthesia and reproduce the drug-induced sensations of numbness in their cheek, which they can then transfer to the painful part of their body. Rather than "fighting" the pain,

they can transform it, concentrating on competing sensations.

The third approach involves cognitive alteration, changing the context in which pain is experienced or understood. Some can also simply "switch off" perception of the pain with surprising effectiveness. Other patients prefer to imagine that the pain is a substance with dimensions that can be moved or can flow out of the body as if it were a viscous liquid. Another technique is to foster dissociation by having the patient imagine that he or she can step outside his or her body, for example, to visit another room in the house. Less hypnotizable individuals often do better with distraction techniques that help them focus on competing sensations in another part of the body. The effectiveness of the specific technique employed depends upon the degree of hypnotic ability of the subject.

It is useful to take stock both during and after the hypnotic session regarding pain ratings: "Now with your eyes closed, and remaining in this state of concentration, please describe how your body is feeling." Then ask, "On a scale of 0 to 10, please rate your level of discomfort right now." The images or metaphors used for pain control employ certain general principles:

1. *Sensory transformation*: The first is that the hypnotically controlled image may serve to "filter the hurt out of the pain." They learn to transform the pain experience. They acknowledge that the pain exists, but there is a distinction between the signal itself and the discomfort that the signal causes. The hypnotic experience, which patients create and control, helps them transform the signal into one that is less uncomfortable. So patients expand their perceptual options by having them change from an experience in which either the pain is there or it is not to an experience in which they see a third option, in which the pain is there but is transformed by the presence of such competing sensations as tingling, numbness, warmth, or coolness.

2. *Sensory accommodation*: Patients are taught not to fight the pain. Fighting pain only enhances it by focusing attention on the pain, enhancing related anxiety and depression, and increasing physical tension that can literally put traction on painful parts of the body and increase the pain signals that are generated peripherally. This is analogous to the meditation technique of "open presence," simply acknowledging feelings as they come.

SELF-HYPNOSIS FOR PAIN CONTROL

These hypnotic techniques can easily be taught to patients for self-administration (5,6). Pain patients can be taught to enter a state of self-hypnosis in a matter of seconds with some simple induction strategies, such as looking up while slowly closing their eyes, taking a deep breath and then letting the breath out, their eyes relax, and imagining that their body is floating and that one hand is so light it can float up in the air like a balloon. They are then instructed in the pain control exercise, such as coolness or warmth, tingling, or numbness, and are taught to bring themselves out by reversing the induction procedure, again looking up, letting the eyes open, and letting the raised hand float back down. Patients can use this exercise every 1–2 hours initially and any time they experience an attack of pain (8,49). It is useful to provide them with a written summary of the hypnotic induction, analgesic technique employed, and means of exiting the hypnotic state. As with any pain treatment technique, hypnosis is more effective when employed early in the pain cycle, before the pain has become so overwhelming that it impairs concentration. Patients should be encouraged to use this technique early and often because it is simple and effective and has no side effects.

MEDICAL, SURGICAL, AND DENTAL PROCEDURES

Because hypnosis can be used to induce a state of physical relaxation and to reduce anxiety, it has proved to be valuable as an adjunct to medical procedures. Once patients have been trained in the use of self-hypnosis, they can use it both in preparation for undergoing medical procedures and during them. They can use self-hypnosis to imagine themselves being somewhere else, a place that they associate with physical comfort, such as floating in a bath, a lake, a hot tub, or just floating in space, thereby dissociating their mental experience from the physical discomfort and contextual anxiety related to medical procedures. Hypnosis can also be used as a means of mastering the anxiety associated with potentially threatening diagnostic procedures (50), such as endoscopies (51,52), colonoscopies (53,54), imaging techniques (i.e., computed tomography and magnetic resonance imaging),

(55–59) bone marrow aspirations (60–62), needle insertion (63-68), liver biopsy (69), dental procedures (70), and lumbar punctures (62,67,71). Hypnosis is also helpful in helping patients through therapeutic interventions such as chemotherapy (56,72–84), external beam radiation therapy (85,86), surgery and its recovery (87,88), and interventional radiology (89–91). A randomized clinical trial involving patients undergoing percutaneous vascular and renal procedures compared training in hypnosis with the presence of a sympathetic nurse for emotional support and with routine on-demand intravenous analgesia. The subjects in the hypnosis condition used half the pain medication, and experienced significantly less pain and anxiety, fewer procedural complications, and the overall procedure time was 17 minutes shorter. The cost of the procedure was $348 less per patient in the hypnosis condition. So hypnosis made their experience less uncomfortable, less anxiety provoking, safer, and shorter.

HYPNOTIC EFFECTS ON THE BODY

There is evidence that hypnosis can facilitate a surprising amount of control over somatic functions that are not thought likely to be susceptible to mental management. For example, we examined the ability of hypnosis to both stimulate and inhibit gastric acid secretion among highly hypnotizable healthy volunteers. When subjects were hypnotized and instructed to imagine eating a series of delicious meals, gastric acid output rose from a basal mean of 3.60 ± 0.48 to a mean of 6.80 ± 0.02 mmol H+/h with hypnosis, an increase of 89% ($p = 0.0007$). In a related study, subjects underwent two sessions of gastric analysis in random order, once with no hypnosis and once with a hypnotic instruction to experience deep relaxation while not thinking about food or drink. With hypnosis there was a 39% reduction in basal acid output (4.29 ± 0.93 vs. 2.60 ± 0.44 mmol H+/h, $p < 0.05$) and an 11% reduction in peak gastric acid output stimulated by pentagastrin (28.69 ± 2.34 vs. 25.43 ± 2.98 mmol H+/h, $p < 0.05$). Thus there was bidirectional control of gastric acid output related to the type of hypnotic instruction. Hypnosis has also been used successfully in the management of such problems as pseudoepilepsy (92–94), irritable bowel syndrome (19,95–98), and contractures of the hand (99).

SUMMARY

Hypnosis is a naturally occurring state of highly focused attention. People vary in their ability to utilize it. It has special relevance to the treatment of anxiety, pain, and other problems common to the aging process, because of its ability to enhance mind–body control. The phenomena that constitute hypnosis—absorption, dissociation, and suggestibility—are mobilized spontaneously during stress, during which they may serve as a unique and adaptive defense against fear, pain, and anxiety. Thus, hypnotic phenomena underlie important aspects of the response to stress. More is being learned about brain function related to hypnosis. The hypnotic alteration of perception is accompanied by marked changes in the relevant sensory areas, as well as brain regions involving context monitoring (dorsal anterior cingulate gyrus) and executive function (dorsolateral prefrontal cortex). Hypnosis alters sensation itself, not just response to sensory input, making it a powerful tool in modulating pain as well as anxiety. Self-hypnosis is a useful skill to teach people dealing with phobias and medically related anxiety. Hypnosis is the oldest Western conception of psychotherapy, but it involves some of our newest understandings of the relationship between brain function and our ability to control pain, anxiety, and the consequences of aging and disease.

REFERENCES

1. Ellenberger HF. *The discovery of the unconscious: the history and evolution of dynamic psychiatry*. New York: Basic Books, 1970.
2. Esdaile J. *Hypnosis in medicine and surgery*. New York: Julian Press, 1846.
3. Breuer J, Freud S. Studies in Hysteria. In: Strachey J (Ed.), *The standard edition of the complete psychological works of Sigmund Freud*. London: Hogarth Press, 1893–1895 (reprinted 1995), pp. 183–251.
4. Freud S. *An autobiographical study*. London: Hogarth Press, 1959 [1925].
5. Freud S. Lines of advance in psycho-analytic therapy. *Wege der Psychoanalytischen Therapie*. 1919;5:61–68.
6. Kardiner A, Spiegel H. *War stress and neurotic illness*. New York: Hoeber, 1947.
7. APA. *Diagnostic and statistical manual of mental disorders* (5th ed., text revision). Washington, DC: American Psychiatric Association, 2013.
8. Spiegel H, Spiegel D. *Trance and treatment: clinical uses of hypnosis*. Washington, DC: American Psychiatric Publishing, 2004.
9. Elkins GR, Barabasz AF, Council JR, Spiegel D. Advancing research and practice: the revised APA Division 30 definition of hypnosis. *Int J Clin Exp Hypn*. 2015;63(1):1–9.
10. Tellegen A. Practicing the two disciplines for relaxation and enlightenment: comment on "Role of the feedback signal in electromyograph biofeedback: the relevance of attention" by Qualls and Sheehan. *J Exp Psychol Gen*. 1981;110(2):217–231.
11. Tellegen A, Atkinson G. Openness to absorbing and self-altering experiences ("absorption"), a trait related to hypnotic susceptibility. *J Abnorm Psychol*. 1974;83(3):268–277.
12. Piccione C, Hilgard ER, Zimbardo PG. On the degree of stability of measured hypnotizability over a 25-year period. *J Pers Soc Psychol*. 1989;56(2):289–295.
13. Lichtenberg P, Bachner-Melman R, Ebstein RP, Crawford HJ. Hypnotic susceptibility: multidimensional relationships with Cloninger's Tridimensional Personality Questionnaire, COMT polymorphisms, absorption, and attentional characteristics. *Int J Clin Exp Hypn*. 2004;52(1):47–72.
14. Raz A. Attention and hypnosis: neural substrates and genetic associations of two converging processes. *Int J Clin Exp Hypn*. 2005;53(3):237–258.
15. Raz A, Fan J, Posner MI. Hypnotic suggestion reduces conflict in the human brain. *Proc Natl Acad Sci U S A*. 2005;102(28):9978–9983.
16. Lang EV, Berbaum KS, Faintuch S et al. Adjunctive self-hypnotic relaxation for outpatient medical procedures: a prospective randomized trial with women undergoing large core breast biopsy. *Pain*. 2006;126(1–3):155–164.
17. Lang EV, Benotsch EG, Fick LJ et al. . Adjunctive non-pharmacological analgesia for invasive medical procedures: a randomised trial. *Lancet*. 2000;355:1486–1490.
18. Montgomery GH, Bovbjerg DH, Schnur JB et al. A randomized clinical trial of a brief hypnosis intervention to control side effects in breast surgery patients. *J Natl Cancer Inst*. 2007;99(17):1304–1312.
19. Whorwell PJ, Prior A, Faragher EB. Controlled trial of hypnotherapy in the treatment of severe refractory irritable-bowel syndrome. *Lancet*. 1984;2(8414):1232–1234.
20. Colgan SM, Faragher EB, Whorwell PJ. Controlled trial of hypnotherapy in relapse

prevention of duodenal ulceration. *Lancet.* 1988;1(8598):1299–1300.

21. Spiegel D, Bierre P, Rootenberg J. Hypnotic alteration of somatosensory perception. *Am J Psychiatry.* 1989;146(6):749–754.

22. Rainville P, Hofbauer RK, Paus T, et al. Cerebral mechanisms of hypnotic induction and suggestion. *J Cogn Neurosci.* 1999;11(1):110–125.

23. Faymonville ME, Laureys S, Degueldre C, et al. Neural mechanisms of antinociceptive effects of hypnosis. *Anesthesiology.* 2000;92(5):1257–1267.

24. Rainville P, Hofbauer RK, Bushnell MC, et al. Hypnosis modulates activity in brain structures involved in the regulation of consciousness. *J Cogn Neurosci.* 2002;14(6):887–901.

25. Frid M, Singer G. Hypnotic analgesia in conditions of stress is partially reversed by naloxone. *Psychopharmacology.* 1979;63(3):211–215.

26. Goldstein A, Hilgard ER. Failure of the opiate antagonist naloxone to modify hypnotic analgesia. *Proc Natl Acad Sci U S A.* 1975;72(6):2041–2043.

27. Spiegel D, Albert L. Naloxone fails to reverse hypnotic alleviation of chronic pain. *Psychopharmacology.* 1983;81:140–143.

28. Zubieta JK, Bueller JA, Jackson LR et al. Placebo effects mediated by endogenous opioid activity on mu-opioid receptors. *J Neurosci.* 2005;25(34):7754–7762.

29. Kosslyn SM, Thompson WL, Costantini-Ferrando MF et al. Hypnotic visual illusion alters color processing in the brain. *Am J Psychiatry.* 2000;157(8):1279–1284.

30. Morishima Y, Okuda J, Sakai K. Reactive mechanism of cognitive control system. *Cerebral Cortex.* 2010;20(11):2675–2683.

31. Raz A, Shapiro T, Fan J, Posner MI. Hypnotic suggestion and the modulation of stroop interference. *Arch Gen Psychiatry.* 2002;59(12):1155–1161.

32. Iani C, Ricci F, Baroni G, Rubichi S. Attention control and susceptibility to hypnosis. *Conscious Cogn.* 2009;18(4):856–863.

33. Pochon JB, Riis J, Sanfey AG et al. Functional imaging of decision conflict. *J Neurosci.* 2008;28(13):3468–3473.

34. Szechtman H, Woody E, Bowers KS, Nahmias C. Where the imaginal appears real: a positron emission tomography study of auditory hallucinations. *Proc Natl Acad Sci U S A.* 1998;95(4):1956–1960.

35. Maquet P, Faymonville ME, Degueldre C et al. Functional neuroanatomy of hypnotic state. *Biol Psychiatry.* 1999;45(3):327–333.

36. Derbyshire SW, Whalley MG, Stenger VA, Oakley DA. Cerebral activation during hypnotically induced and imagined pain. *Neuroimage.* 2004;23(1):392–401.

37. Schulz-Stubner S, Krings T, Meister IG et al. Clinical hypnosis modulates functional magnetic resonance imaging signal intensities and pain perception in a thermal stimulation paradigm. *Reg Anesth Pain Med.* 2004;29(6):549–556.

38. Egner T, Jamieson G, Gruzelier J. Hypnosis decouples cognitive control from conflict monitoring processes of the frontal lobe. *Neuroimage.* 2005;27(4):969–978.

39. Raij TT, Numminen J, Narvanen S et al. Brain correlates of subjective reality of physically and psychologically induced pain. *Proc Natl Acad Sci U S A.* 2005;102(6):2147–2151.

40. McGeown WJ, Mazzoni G, Venneri A, Kirsch I. Hypnotic induction decreases anterior default mode activity. *Conscious Cogn.* 2009;18(4):848–855.

41. Hoeft F, Gabrieli JDE, Whitfield-Gabrieli S et al. Functional brain basis of hypnotizability. *Arch Gen Psychiatry.* 2012;69(10):1064–1072.

42. Davidson RJ. Empirical explorations of mindfulness: conceptual and methodological conundrums. *Emotion.* 2010;10(1):8–11.

43. Davidson RJ, Kabat-Zinn J, Schumacher J et al. Alterations in brain and immune function produced by mindfulness meditation. *Psychosom Med.* 2003;65(4):564–570.

44. NIMH. *Prevalence of anxiety disorders.* http://www.nimh.nih.gov/statistics/1SPEC_ADULT.shtml 2012.

45. Spiegel D. The mind prepared: hypnosis in surgery. *J Natl Cancer Inst.* 2007;99(17):1280–1281.

46. Nishith P, Barabasz A, Barabasz M, Warner D. Brief hypnosis substitutes for alprazolam use in college students: transient experiences and quantitative EEG responses. *Am J Clin Hypn.* 1999;41(3):262–268.

47. Garvin AW, Trine MR, Morgan WP. Affective and metabolic responses to hypnosis, autogenic relaxation, and quiet rest in the supine and seated positions. *Int J Clin Exp Hypn.* 2001;49(1):5–18.

48. Abramowitz EG, Barak Y, Ben-Avi I, Knobler HY. Hypnotherapy in the treatment of chronic combat-related PTSD patients suffering from insomnia: a randomized, zolpidem-controlled clinical trial. *Int J Clin Exp Hypn.* 2008;56(3):270–280.

49. Patterson DR, Jensen MP. Hypnosis and clinical pain. *Psychol Bull.* 2003;129(4):495–521.

50. Rape RN, Bush JP. Psychological preparation for pediatric oncology patients undergoing painful procedures: a methodological critique of the research. *Child Health Care*. 1994;23(1):51–67.

51. Cavallo G, Cuomo R, Viscardi A, et al. Hypnosis for upper gastrointestinal endoscopy. *Gastrointest Endosc*. 1985;31(3):228.

52. Sutherland RJ, Knox J. Hypnosis for endoscopy. *Lancet*. 1976;2(7997):1244.

53. Cadranel JF, Benhamou Y, Zylberberg P, et al. Hypnotic relaxation: a new sedative tool for colonoscopy? *J Clin Gastroenterol*. 1994;18(2):127–129.

54. Elkins G, White J, Patel P et al. Hypnosis to manage anxiety and pain associated with colonoscopy for colorectal cancer screening: case studies and possible benefits. *Int J Clin Exp Hypn*. 2006;54(4):416–431.

55. Chandler T. Techniques for optimizing MRI relaxation and visualization. *Adm Radiol J*. 1996;15(3):16–18.

56. Covino NA, Frankel FH. Hypnosis and relaxation in the medically ill. *Psychother Psychosom*. 1993;60(2):75–90.

57. Friday PJ, Kubal WS. Magnetic resonance imaging: improved patient tolerance utilizing medical hypnosis. *Am J Clin Hypn*. 1990;33(2):80–84.

58. Simon EP. Improving tolerance of MR imaging with medical hypnosis. *AJR Am J Roentgenol*. 1999;172(6):1694–1695.

59. Simon EP. Hypnosis using a communication device to increase magnetic resonance imaging tolerance with a claustrophobic patient. *Mil Med*. 1999;164(1):71–72.

60. Ellis JA, Spanos NP. Cognitive-behavioral interventions for children's distress during bone marrow aspirations and lumbar punctures: a critical review. *J Pain Symptom Manage*. 1994;9(2):96–108.

61. Liossi C, Hatira P. Clinical hypnosis versus cognitive behavioral training for pain management with pediatric cancer patients undergoing bone marrow aspirations. *Int J Clin Exp Hypn*. 1999;47(2):104–116.

62. Hageman-Wenselaar LH. [Hypnosis for pain control during lumbar puncture and bone marrow aspirations in children with cancer]. *Tijdschr Kindergeneeskd*. 1988;56(3):120–123.

63. Bell DS, Christian ST, Clements RS, Jr. Acuphobia in a long-standing insulin-dependent diabetic patient cured by hypnosis. *Diabetes Care*. 1983;6(6):622.

64. Dash J. Rapid hypno-behavioral treatment of a needle phobia in a five-year-old cardiac patient. *J Pediatr Psychol*. 1981;6(1):37–42.

65. Morse DR, Cohen BB. Desensitization using meditation-hypnosis to control "needle" phobia in two dental patients. *Anesth Prog*. 1983;30(3):83–85.

66. Nugent WR, Carden NA, Montgomery DJ. Utilizing the creative unconscious in the treatment of hypodermic phobias and sleep disturbance. *Am J Clin Hypn*. 1984;26(3):201–205.

67. Simon EP, Canonico MM. Use of hypnosis in controlling lumbar puncture distress in an adult needle-phobic dementia patient. *Int J Clin Exp Hypn*. 2001;49(1):56–67.

68. Usberti M, Grutta d'Auria C, Borghi M et al. Usefulness of hypnosis for renal needle biopsy in children. *Kidney Int*. 1984;26(3):351–352.

69. Adams PC, Stenn PG. Liver biopsy under hypnosis. *J Clin Gastroenterol*. 1992;15(2):122–124.

70. Moore R, Abrahamsen R, Brodsgaard I. Hypnosis compared with group therapy and individual desensitization for dental anxiety. *Eur J Oral Sci*. 1996;104(5–6):612–618.

71. Kellerman J, Zeltzer L, Ellenberg L, Dash J. Adolescents with cancer: hypnosis for the reduction of the acute pain and anxiety associated with medical procedures. *J Adolesc Health Care*. 1983;4(2):85–90.

72. Hilgard JR, LeBaron S. Relief of anxiety and pain in children and adolescents with cancer: quantitative measures and clinical observations. *Int J Clin Exp Hypn*. 1982;30(4):417–442.

73. Zeltzer L, Kellerman J, Ellenberg L, Dash J. Hypnosis for reduction of vomiting associated with chemotherapy and disease in adolescents with cancer. *J Adolesc Health Care*. 1983;4(2):77–84.

74. Genuis ML. The use of hypnosis in helping cancer patients control anxiety, pain, and emesis: a review of recent empirical studies. *Am J Clin Hypn*. 1995;37(4):316–325.

75. Katz ER, Kellerman J, Ellenberg L. Hypnosis in the reduction of acute pain and distress in children with cancer. *J Pediatr Psychol*. 1987;12(3):379–394.

76. Richardson J, Smith JE, McCall G, Pilkington K. Hypnosis for procedure-related pain and distress in pediatric cancer patients: a systematic review of effectiveness and methodology related to hypnosis interventions. *J Pain Symptom Manage*. 2006;31(1):70–84.

77. Syrjala KL, Cummings C, Donaldson GW. Hypnosis or cognitive behavioral training for the reduction of pain and nausea during cancer treatment: a controlled clinical trial. *Pain*. 1992;48(2):137–146.

78. Zeltzer L, LeBaron S. Hypnosis and nonhypnotic techniques for reduction of pain and anxiety during painful procedures in children and adolescents with cancer. *J Pediatr.* 1982;101(6):1032–1035.

79. Jacknow DS, Tschann JM, Link MP, Boyce WT. Hypnosis in the prevention of chemotherapy-related nausea and vomiting in children: a prospective study. *J Dev Behav Pediatr.* 1994;15(4):258–264.

80. Renouf D. Hypnotically induced control of nausea: a preliminary report. *J Psychosom Res.* 1998;45(3):295–296.

81. Zeltzer L, LeBaron S, Zeltzer PM. The effectiveness of behavioral intervention for reduction of nausea and vomiting in children and adolescents receiving chemotherapy. *J Clin Oncol.* 1984;2(6):683–690.

82. Axelrod A, Vinciguerra V, Brennan-O'Neill E, Moore T. A preliminary report on the efficacy of hypnosis to control anticipatory nausea and vomiting caused by cancer chemotherapy. *Prog Clin Biol Res.* 1988;278:147–150.

83. Cotanch P, Hockenberry M, Herman S. Self-hypnosis as antiemetic therapy in children receiving chemotherapy. *Oncol Nurs Forum.* 1985;12(4):41–46.

84. Marchioro G, Azzarello G, Viviani F et al. Hypnosis in the treatment of anticipatory nausea and vomiting in patients receiving cancer chemotherapy. *Oncology.* 2000;59(2):100–104.

85. Steggles S. The use of cognitive-behavioral treatment including hypnosis for claustrophobia in cancer patients. *Am J Clin Hypn.* 1999;41(4):319–326.

86. Bertoni F, Bonardi A, Magno L et al. Hypnosis instead of general anaesthesia in paediatric radiotherapy: report of three cases. *Radiother Oncol.* 1999;52(2):185–190.

87. Kessler R, Dane JR. Psychological and hypnotic preparation for anesthesia and surgery: an individual differences perspective. *Int J Clin Exp Hypn.* 1996;44(3):189–207.

88. Lambert SA. The effects of hypnosis/guided imagery on the postoperative course of children. *J Dev Behav Pediatr.* 1996;17(5):307–310.

89. Lang EV, Benotsch EG, Fick LJ et al. Adjunctive non-pharmacological analgesia for invasive medical procedures: a randomised trial. *Lancet.* 2000;355(9214):1486–1490.

90. Lang EV, Joyce JS, Spiegel D et al. Self-hypnotic relaxation during interventional radiological procedures: effects on pain perception and intravenous drug use. *Int J Clin Exp Hypn.* 1996;44(2):106–119.

91. Spiegel D. Wedding hypnosis to the radiology suite. *Pain.* 2006;126(1–3):3–4.

92. Barry JJ, Atzman O, Morrell MJ. Discriminating between epileptic and nonepileptic events: the utility of hypnotic seizure induction. *Epilepsia.* 2000;41(1):81–84.

93. Devinsky O, Putnam F, Grafman J et al. Dissociative states and epilepsy. *Neurology.* 1989;39(6):835–840.

94. Levine DN. Utility of suggestion-induced spells in diagnosis of pseudoseizures. *Ann Neurol.* 1994;36(3):450.

95. Anton PA. Stress and mind-body impact on the course of inflammatory bowel diseases. *Sem Gastroint Dis.* 1999;10(1):14–19.

96. Galovsky TE, Blanchard EB. Hypnotherapy and refractory irritable bowel syndrome: a single case study. *Am J Clin Hypnos.* 2002;45(1):31–37.

97. Palsson OS, Turner MJ, Johnson DA et al. Hypnosis treatment for severe irritable bowel syndrome: investigation of mechanism and effects on symptoms. *Dig Dis Sci.* 2002;47(11):2605–2614.

98. Whorwell PJ, Prior A, Colgan SM. Hypnotherapy in severe irritable bowel syndrome: further experience. *Gut.* 1987;28:423–425.

99. Spiegel D, Chase RA. The treatment of contractures of the hand using self-hypnosis. *J Hand Surg [Am].* 1980;5(5):428–432.

19

CREATIVE ARTS THERAPIES AND OLDER ADULTS

Cathy A. Malchiodi

MOST INTERVENTIONS with older adults focus on declining physical, mental, and emotional abilities that may have been compromised by age, bereavement, or end-of-life issues. But despite what is often a negative, problem-laden view of older adulthood, medicine and mental health are also embracing what is possible during the later years of life. While twentieth-century gerontology focused on identifying and treating the inevitable changes that occur with age, practitioners in the early twenty-first century are recognizing the potential to reframe the later years of life as ones of continued growth and the capacity to learn via creative arts (Malchiodi, 2012a).

Creative arts therapies are approaches that capitalize on human potential for development that is not limited by age or by many of the physical, emotional, and even cognitive challenges that come with aging. Research indicates that even during old age the brain is still flexible in many ways and can be stimulated by engagement in purposeful and pleasurable activities; one of these activities is involvement

with the arts (Cohen, 2000, 2009; National Center for Creative Aging, 2014). The cumulative results of numerous studies on the impact of participatory art programs on the health of older adults are promising and underscore how creative expression supports wellness for many individuals in their seventies and beyond. For example, the US National Endowment for the Arts (2006) study on creativity and aging reveal strikingly positive differences in health and activities levels in older adults (65 years or older) who participate in art programs from those who do not. Gene Cohen (2000, 2006, 2009), a well-known expert on gerontology, neuroscience, and aging, cites many benefits of creativity via art in older adults, including the elimination of mood and sleep disorders, an increase in positive outlook, a boost in the immune system, and improvement of memory and other brain functions.

Just as the arts are now recognized as essential components of elder care, strategic applications of these modalities in the form of creative arts therapies are demonstrating their essential role in the health and wellness of older adults. Art, music, and dance/movement therapy and other arts-based therapies are an increasingly important part of many facilities and programs to specifically address the impact of cognitive, physical, and psychosocial challenges encountered by older adults. To this end, this chapter briefly highlights current research and practical applications of arts in therapy with older adults. The multiple roles of creative arts therapies to enhance health and well-being later in life are discussed, with an emphasis on key applications for sensory stimulation, neurorehabilitation, and psychosocial care.

WHAT ARE THE CREATIVE ARTS THERAPIES?

The creative arts therapies formally emerged in the twentieth century as distinct approaches with a variety of theoretical and methodological frameworks based on psychology, psychiatry, and behavioral medicine. These methods have been used to address a variety of emotional, behavioral, social, and physical disorders in individuals of all ages (Warren, 2004; Malchiodi, 2005, 2012b) and, in essence, are defined as action-oriented, sensory-based interventions. Art expression, music making and singing, dance and movement, and drama enactment and imaginative play involve action and include multiple sensory experiences. For example, art making, even in its simplest sense, can involve arranging, touching, gluing, constructing, painting, forming, and many other active experiences; music involves not only sound, but also may include participation in playing a musical instrument or singing with others. All creative arts therapies encourage clients to become empowered participants in the therapeutic process and stimulate and energize the senses, focus and redirect attention, and influence emotions and behavior.

The creative arts therapies are most commonly defined as follows (summarized in Malchiodi, 2005, 2012b):

- *Art therapy* is the purposeful use of visual art materials and media in intervention, counseling, psychotherapy, and rehabilitation; it is used with individuals of all ages, families, and groups (Malchiodi, 2006).
- *Music therapy* uses music to effect positive changes in the psychological, physical, cognitive, or social functioning of individuals with health,

behavioral, social, emotional, or educational challenges (American Music Therapy Association, 2014; Wheeler, 2015).
- *Drama therapy* is defined as an active, experiential approach to facilitating change through storytelling, projective play, purposeful improvisation, and performance (Johnson, 2009; National Drama Therapy Association, 2014).
- *Dance/movement therapy* is based on the assumption that body and mind are interrelated and is defined as the psychotherapeutic use of movement as a process that furthers the emotional, cognitive, and physical integration of the individual and influences changes in feelings, cognition, physical functioning, and behavior (Goodill, 2005; National Dance Therapy Association, 2014; Payne, 2013).
- *Poetry therapy and bibliotherapy* are terms used synonymously to describe the intentional use of poetry and other forms of literature for healing and personal growth (Micozzi, 2010).

The terms *expressive therapies* and *expressive arts therapies* are sometimes used interchangeably with the term *creative arts therapies*. However, the term *expressive therapies* is more correctly used to describe the application of two or more of the creative arts involving, but not limited to, all the arts therapies and various forms of play therapy (props, games, and sand play). An *integrated arts approach*, or *intermodal therapy*, involves two or more expressive therapies in an individual or group session. Integrated arts and intermodal or multimodal therapy are distinguished from their closely allied domains of art therapy, music therapy, dance/movement therapy, and drama therapy by focusing on the interrelatedness of the arts. They are based on a variety of orientations, including arts as therapy, art psychotherapy, and the use of arts for traditional healing (Knill, Barba, & Fuchs, 2004).

In recent years, two major influences have promoted greater recognition of the value of creative arts therapies as complementary interventions with older adults. One is the 2009 documentary, *I Remember Better When I Paint* (Ellena & Heubner, 2009), which highlights the film directors' mother, who painted prolifically before dying of Alzheimer's disease. It also spotlights programs around the world that engage people with dementia in art, whether by making art within assisted-living facilities, bringing people to museums, or immersing them in other creative experiences. But perhaps the greatest influences are the seminal contributions of Gene Cohen (2000, 2006, 2009), which are central to the growing understanding of how the arts and arts therapies benefit older adults. Cohen's research and writings underscore the multiple positive health outcomes that result from engagement in the arts later in life. His work not only continues to be an enduring influence on clinical applications and research on the creative arts therapies with older adults, but also has a wide-ranging impact on the development of art-based activities programs for individuals in independent living, assisted care, Alzheimer's disease settings, and elder care in general.

CREATIVE ARTS AND BRAIN PLASTICITY

Possibly the most significant influence on the understanding of how the arts therapies complement health and wellness in old age is the concept of neuroplasticity—the brain's ability to learn new concepts and activities throughout the life span. Cozolino (2008) observes that greater amounts of gray matter in the specific parts of the brain later in life set the stage for self-transcendence, a quality related to more mature creativity and an openness to novel thinking that is key to imagination. Additionally, there are numerous examples that point to the fact that "it's never too late for art," no matter what one's age or challenges (Mental Health Foundation, 2011). "Grandma" Elizabeth Layton, an octogenarian, overcame lifelong depression at the age of 68 years, in part by making contour drawings, a technique she learned in an art class. Her drawings went on to be displayed at the Smithsonian Museum in Washington, D.C., and her story was told at a US Congressional hearing on aging in 1991 (Cohen, 2006). Similarly, older individuals like Layton who did not become involved in art until after the age 65 predominantly create what is commonly known as "folk art" (Cohen, 2000, 2006).

Well-known author and neurologist Oliver Sacks (2008) underscores the impact of the arts on higher brain functions, observing that dementia patients recognize and react to works of art and enjoy painting even when unresponsive to words, unable to communicate, and disoriented under other circumstances. Reports on the arts' impact on people with dementia document through multiple case studies that artistic ability is preserved in people with dementia (Cohen, 2006; Fornazzari, 2005; Fornazzari et al., 2006; Fornazzari et al., 2013). The creative arts therapies also capitalize on examples from the art world that demonstrate the impact of visual art making on memory disorders. For example, Willem de Kooning, a well-known modern abstract artist, became more productive as his Alzheimer's disease progressed; some forms of dementia cause many people with no previously identified skill in art to begin to develop remarkable artistic talent and interest in art making (Ramachandran, 1998, 2011). In people with frontotemporal dementia (FTD), new artistic abilities are reported to emerge as the disease progresses (Schott, 2012). This underscores that there is still potential for experiences, such as artistic expression, that give dementia patients pleasure because new avenues of expression may develop as other faculties are lost.

Finally, Cohen (2000, 2006) believes that being active in the arts capitalizes on the opportunity for the left and right brain to interact, a function known as *bilaterization*. In part, this may account for the fact that older people find that the arts become more important as they age and why some people who never created art earlier in life do so in their later years. Similarly, the creative arts therapies are essentially "right-brain dominant" interventions (Malchiodi, 2014); while engagement in art making, music, or dance/movement are essentially whole-brain activities, they are also sensory-based experiences that tap regions of the brain that are more right-brain dominant. Overall, the value of creative arts therapies in work with older adults with memory disorders, stroke, traumatic brain injury, or other challenges is essentially based on the idea that one part of the brain often takes on activities that are usually accomplished by another part.

CREATIVE ARTS THERAPIES AND OLDER ADULTS: OVERALL CONSIDERATIONS

With any population, there are practical considerations in the specific application of expressive arts for the purpose of therapy, including complementary medicine and integrative health care. In applying creative arts therapies with older adults who may have cognitive and/or physical challenges, these considerations include, but are not limited to, the following:

1. *Physical aspects*: Aging inevitably affects vision, hearing, perception of size and color, mobility, vestibular and proprioceptive changes, and coordination. Tactile senses may be altered, potentially reducing the abilities to compare objects and surfaces and to handle materials easily.

2. *Cognitive functioning*: During the course of the life span, cognitive changes may occur that impact memory and other executive functions. Adaptations may be necessary to negotiate a variety of cognitive challenges in providing art, music, or dance/movement therapy in order to accommodate memory, language, and comprehension.

3. *Psychosocial changes*: Age may be viewed with fear and trepidation and with concern about changing social status and negative stereotypes of the elderly that still permeate many cultures. Views of the self also gradually change during aging, as roles shift with retirement and within families and communities; there may be experiences of loss and grief or illness that alter self-concept. Creative arts therapies strategies may specifically address these changes while supporting the dignity and self-efficacy of the individual faced with intrapersonal and interpersonal changes and challenges.

Weiss (1984), an early pioneer in creative arts therapy with older adults, summarizes practical objectives and goals in work with this population as follows:

1. To rediscover interpersonal and intrapersonal meaning in life;

2. To enhance interaction and communication with others;

3. To develop and enhance self-worth and self-esteem;

4. To stimulate intellectual, physical, and emotional functioning;

5. To review life events, come to terms with oneself, and see value in one's life;

6. To experience a "wholeness in one's being" through fulfilling one's potential and meaning of one's life (adapted from Weiss, 1984, p. 27).

While published several decades ago, these objectives and goals are still relevant to contemporary creative arts therapies with older adult populations and are achievable through sensitive and knowledgeable

application of various media and approaches with older adults.

For the remainder of this chapter, two key concepts in applying the creative arts therapies to work with older adults are described: (1) sensory stimulation and neurorehabilitation; and (2) psychosocial care. Current research and examples of applications of art therapy, music therapy, and dance/movement therapy are provided to help readers understand best practices in creative arts therapies programming in elder care.

SENSORY STIMULATION AND NEUROREHABILITATION

Each of the creative arts therapies provides specific opportunities for *sensory stimulation*. In brief, sensory stimulation refers to the impact the environment has on our minds and bodies as we receive information through our senses—tactile, visual, auditory, olfactory, gustatory, vestibular, and proprioceptive. In most programs that include creative intervention for elderly clients, individuals receive stimulation through arts-based activities and related recreational experiences to enhance sensory stimulation in various ways. Some of these activities may encourage active participation, such as making art, moving, or singing, while others may involve stimulation through exposure to films, listening to music, or other passive, viewer-oriented experiences. In general, art therapy, music therapy, and dance/movement therapy include a variety of specific applications with the purpose of sensory stimulation to address a variety of issues and complement medical and psychosocial interventions.

Neurorehabilitation is closely related to the concept of sensory stimulation; in the creative arts therapies, it is defined as specific forms of sensory stimulation that are intended to increase or enhance functional skills after neurological impairment due to stroke, brain injury, or other conditions. Creative arts therapies often are used to complement occupational, physical, and other therapies or are used as primary methods to address functional skills in older adults challenged by stroke, dementias, neurological diseases, and loss of function due to normal aging.

Art Therapy

Art therapy is frequently cited as an approach to sensory stimulation for all individuals of all ages, but particularly with older adults (Elkis-Abuhoff et al., 2008; Levine-Madori, 2009). For example, Levine-Madori (2009) provides a comprehensive, creative arts therapies approach to address the retention of skills and abilities in aging populations. The Therapeutic Thematic Arts Programming (TTAP Method®) is a series of nine structured arts activities presented in a sequential way to provide neurological stimulation, encourage brain wellness and neural regeneration, maximize interaction among participants, and address social/emotional needs. The goal is to provide a viable means for enhancing cognitive functioning through a variety of sensory activities, including art making. For individuals who have lost some or all of their verbal capabilities due to stroke or other illness, art is a well-recognized alternative modality that uses sensory means to stimulate nonverbal expression (Johnson & Sullivan-Marx, 2004). For example, an art therapy session may focus on experimentation and choice of materials or paint colors, allowing an individual to be recognized and understood through creative abilities (sensory channels) rather than language.

Sensory stimulation via art making can have a powerful effect on emotions in older adults, even those with challenging disabilities. For example, the activity of viewing art in a museum has powerful affects on those individuals in assisted care. Programs like "Meet Me at MOMA" (Museum of Modern Art, 2011) are demonstrating that regular attendance at art museums for people with dementia or Alzheimer's disease improves mood and memory by stimulating the senses in a number of ways. Intellectual stimulation derived from experiencing art provides opportunities for new learning; the shared experiences with family and friends promote social engagement through relaxed and normalizing situations, including gallery tours and docent-led discussions in an accepting environment. Coupled with facilitators who are empathetic and interactive with participants, engagement with others and a renewed interest in life are stimulated through the sensory experiences of viewing art.

In the area of neurorehabilitation, art therapy is being successfully applied to work with those challenged by stroke, traumatic brain injury, and various diseases that cause memory and motor difficulties (Malchiodi, 2013). For example, Elkis-Abuhoff et al. (2008) encourage individuals diagnosed with Parkinson's disease (PD) to manipulate and be creative with modeling clay and monitored changes in their emotional and symptomatic reactions. Since many individuals with PD experience hand tremors and/or a deficit in fine motor abilities, modeling clay is used as the art medium because it is easily controllable, is applicable to all skill levels, and encourages fine and gross motor skills. The researchers evaluated behavior pre- and post-intervention and found that obsessive-compulsive thinking, phobia, and depression were not only significantly decreased, but also were reduced to within normal adult range. These three emotional symptoms are particularly important in individuals with PD because they often ruminate about their symptoms, develop fears, and, as a result, may experience depression. In brief, the sensory use of an art therapy via clay manipulation encouraged PD patients to use their fine and gross motor skills to experience a sense of control within their environment and created a tactile "connection" to the world, thus giving them the sensation of regaining a "grip on the world."

Music Therapy

Music not only stimulates auditory senses, but also is a kinesthetic experience that involves rhythm and movement; music listening, for example, not only recruits auditory areas in the brain but also involves larger neural networks including the limbic and cortical systems (Levitin, 2006). Specific patterns of rhythm and melody can help to stimulate movement, resulting in a type of memory in the central nervous system called motor memory. A simple example of motor memory is the ability of a musician to play several notes in a few seconds without having to recall every individual note. With older adults, music can be a sensory experience that stimulates the recall of coordination and even complex series of movements. These types of sensory experiences have been applied in neurologic music therapy (NMT), particularly through a technique termed *rhythmic auditory stimulation* (RAS), in which rhythm is used strategically as an external timekeeper to help individuals organize and sequence complex movements. Specific applications of RAS have been shown to improve motor function in people who have had strokes (Thaut, McIntosh, Prassas, & Rice, 1993) or traumatic brain injury due to accidents or other events (Hurt, Rice, McIntosh, & Thaut, 1998), and in individuals with Parkinson's disease (Thaut, McIntosh, McIntosh, & Hoemberg, 2001). Music also serves as a form of entrainment and stress reduction; that is, music can impact mood and physiology, including blood pressure, respiration, and heart rate. Walt and Duffy

(2010) reviewed 13 articles on music therapy and dementia and found that the majority of the data indicated that the application of various forms of music therapy significantly reduced agitation and improved mood.

Tamplin (2015) notes that the body of clinical research on music therapy treatment in neurore-habilitation is steadily increasing. For example, a Cochrane review on music therapy for acquired brain injury found evidence to indicate that rhythmic auditory stimulation may improve gait in stroke patients (Bradt et al., 2010); other positive outcomes have resulted from single studies that demonstrate improved upper extremity function and improved speech for people with aphasia. In general, active participation from the individual is used to stimulate the senses and encourage neurorehabilitation involving physical, speech and language, cognitive, and psychosocial skills.

Tamplin (2015) offers several reasons that music therapy approaches are beneficial in neurorehabilitation, including (1) rhythm as a cue for movement coordination; (2) music as stimulation for unconscious physiological responses (e.g., foot tapping); (3) motivation through music to increase engagement and extend participation length by energizing patients; and (4) playing a musical instrument as visual, kinesthetic, and aural feedback. Music therapy also has a key role in the neurorehabilitation of speech and language difficulties (Hurkmans et al., 2012); research demonstrates improvement in word and phrase production, rate of speech, voice volume, and speech naturalness, among other benefits, following music therapy intervention (Tamplin, 2008; Tamplin et al., 2013; Tomaino, 2012). Additionally, singing familiar song lyrics may help with word retrieval, particularly with patients with verbal fluency disorders (Tamplin, 2015).

Dance/Movement Therapy

People of all ages may encounter challenges in organizing sensory experiences; in particular, older adults may experience reduced abilities to move effectively, lose vestibular and proprioceptive capacities, and/or experience decreased adaptive responses in terms of movement. Dance/movement therapy has a variety of applications with older adults in terms of sensory stimulation. These include locomotion (the movement of the body through space) and motor planning, vestibular capacity, proprioception (sensations from muscles and joints),

body image (the perception of one's own body), and adaptive response (responding to an environmental demand). In particular, sensory integration, the combination of many neural networks related to movement, is a key concept and goal in dance/movement therapy.

The kinesthetic sense, or internal muscle sense, is an essential component of dance/movement therapy with older adults. It may include assisting individuals in proper breathing, improving sitting and standing postures, and how to move with greater ease (Hoban, 2000; Wickstrom, 2004). While dance/movement therapy can address psychosocial aspects of aging, this aspect of physical activity and kinesthetic experience is a sensory foundation necessary to improving cognitive and emotional functioning in older adults (American Dance Therapy Association, 2014).

In terms of neurorehabilitation, there are several studies that support the use of dance/movement therapy with Parkinson's disease (PD), a progressive disorder of the nervous system that develops gradually, starting with a barely noticeable tremor in an extremity, and also causes stiffness or slowing of movement. The four main signs of PD include tremors, slowness of movements, rigidity in gait, and loss of postural reflexes. McKinley et al. (2008) were among the first to report the benefits of Argentine tango with older adults, noting that it significantly improved functional balance and confidence in this population. Dance/movement therapy currently is a widely accepted approach to address several areas of neurorehabilitation of gait, movement, balance, and tremor in PD through the specific use of music, movement strategies, balance exercises, and strength and flexibility (Earhart, 2009; Hackney & Bennett, 2014). For example, engaging individuals in movements from the Argentine tango involves walking backward, practicing posture, and keeping one's balance, all to the rhythm of tango music.

Finally, dance and movement as therapy are also applied to the rehabilitation of people with various forms of dementia. In general, preliminary dance/movement studies support the use of specific strategies to improve individuals' concentration and communication with others (Hamill, Smith, & Rohricht, 2011; Newman-Bluestein & Hill, 2010). While more studies are needed, current research and best practices in dance/movement therapy demonstrate that unresponsive individuals with dementia disorders who are relatively unresponsive pre–dance interventions can find significant benefits through specific movement strategies and connection with others via dance/movement therapy strategies.

PSYCHOSOCIAL CARE

Rather than viewing old age as a series of endings, the creative arts therapies embrace the idea that psychosocial growth continues and can be enhanced and even celebrated during the natural process of aging. Cohen (2000) provides a template for understanding psychosocial potential in four distinct phases:

1. The midlife re-evaluation phase, from the early forties to the late fifties (realization of mortality increases the desire to explore one's untapped potential);
2. The liberation phase, from the mid-fifties to the mid-seventies (freedom to explore new options in retirement);
3. The summing-up phase, from the late sixties to the eighties (re-examination of life in an attempt to make sense);
4. The encore phase, from the late seventies to the end of life (reaffirmation and acceptance of the major themes or lessons from life).

These phases provide a structure for adapting creative arts therapies to older adults because they emphasize the possibility for creative potential, as opposed to inevitable decline. For example, the liberation phase implies increased freedom and confidence to develop new interests and try new things, such as artistic self-expression, that might not have been feasible during work life. The summing up phase lends itself to life review via visual expression and social interactions, which become opportunities to share one's experiences and wisdom with others. In the following sections, the ways in which art therapy, music therapy, and dance/movement therapy are applied to psychosocial care are briefly explained, with an emphasis on how these approaches enhance self-expression, insight, personal narrative, and social connection.

Art Therapy

Art therapy has traditionally been used a method for helping individuals of all ages explore and express psychological challenges and concerns throughout the life span. Psychosocial issues and self-perception change during the aging process,

and art expression is one way to help older adults examine these changes, make adjustments, and reflect on the aging process. Art therapy may focus on current interests of participants, increasing quality of life, assisting with adjustment to life changes, distress, grief or loss, and enhancing socialization through group art activities. While intervention may be insight oriented, it is also predicated on the functional level of the individual in terms of cognition and physical capacities. Additionally, the use of art as a form of communication takes on a slightly different role by providing opportunities for older adults to share wisdom and life experiences through creative expression, while also offering the possibility to revisit unresolved issues (Malchiodi, 2012a).

Current research indicates that art therapy is particularly valuable in promoting a psychological sense of well-being and increased quality of life in older adults. For example, Kim (2012) conducted a study of older adults that underscores the psychological benefits of increased self-esteem, reduced negative emotions, and decreased anxiety. Additionally, small group art therapy experiences can help to decrease social isolation and can enhance connection and mutual support through working together, sharing art materials and projects, and assisting one another (Weisberg & Wilder, 2001).

Creating a drawing, painting, sculpture, or craft item is often a way of sharing something of oneself with others in a group or community through storytelling about an art expression. Similarly, life review using art as a means of communication is a commonly used approach in art therapy with older adults. Johnson and Sullivan-Marx (2004) note that reminiscence-oriented art therapy groups are particularly effective for life review. Drucker (1995) additionally observes that art therapy may provide an outlet for missed opportunities and to make sense of past events. In all cases, sharing narratives through personal art expression is a way to convey life wisdom and to instill hope, despite functional challenges (Waller, 2002).

Music Therapy

Music therapy provides multiple benefits that support psychosocial aspects of patients' lives. For example, singing in a choir or participating in group singing activities may improve the perception of health and well-being in older adults; research indicates that choir singing leads to positive physiological changes and develops social relationships through participation in choirs (Clift, 2012). These influences on health and well-being are derived from the motivational and emotional role of music (Ridder & Wheeler, 2015); in brief, the positive health effects from music are initiated through both music experiences and positive social interactions that stimulate the brain to release dopamine, the body's "feel-good" hormone and neurotransmitter. Older adults who enjoy music and social engagement can benefit from both active music making and music listening with social engagement. Other practitioners note that receptive music therapy interventions, such as song-based discussion and music-assisted relaxation, can also be used to support psychosocial goals (Steele, 2005). This becomes particularly important in work with individuals who have degenerative neurological conditions and who may only be able to engage in receptive approaches when the disease process is progressive and voluntary motor movement is too difficult or painful.

Many music therapy methods address emotional needs and encourage mood states that support psychosocial aspects of treatment. For example, writing a song, singing, or play music can be non-confrontational ways to express emotions for some older individuals. Music-assisted counseling can help individuals to address issues of grief, pain, anger, and anxiety; the use of song discussion may encourage a person to identify with concepts and emotions presented in song lyrics, comparing them to personal feelings or experiences. The effect of music therapy on mood may also have a positive influence on older adults' social interaction and motivation to participate in rehabilitation and therapy (Nayak et al., 2000).

One of the most compelling aspects of music therapy is the capacity for music therapists to use music and psychosocial intervention to enhance communication and literally "bring out" responses from older adults who are withdrawn, depressed, or challenged by dementia and other disorders. Ridder and Wheeler (2015) provide a compelling example of how therapeutic singing helped one individual (Mrs. Wilson) communicate with the therapist (Feil) in the following excerpt:

Mrs. Wilson is sitting with closed eyes in a chair, with Feil in front of her. Feil explains that when people are old and deteriorated and no one enters their world, they withdraw inwards more and more. Still, *inside there is a desperate need for connection and a longing for closeness. Feil shows that she is attentive to these needs of Mrs. Wilson. Mrs. Wilson expresses her needs through her movements, and Feil puts into words what she sees, for example, that Mrs. Wilson is crying and that there is a tear on her cheek. Feil asks if there is a pain, if she is sad or afraid. The pace is slow, and she waits for Mrs. Wilson to answer. She touches Mrs. Wilson's cheek, like a mother would touch her child, and afterwards explains that this opens up communication. Mrs. Wilson relates to religious songs, as church music is tied to emotion and safety for her. Feil sings "Jesus Loves Me," and, almost immediately, Mrs. Wilson follows the rhythm of the song by tapping her hand at her armrest. She opens her eyes and looks directly at Feil. Mrs. Wilson's hand tapping increases in tempo and dynamic, and Feil follows her in the song. She matches the intensity of her voice with the intensity of Mrs. Wilson's movements and describes that, for a split second, when they share the music, they become one person. After this Mrs. Wilson appears peaceful and her breathing slows down. She gently grabs Feil and pulls her close. Their foreheads touch . . . Feil sings one more song, and Mrs. Wilson joins in singing . . . Finally, Feil asks if she feels safe, and Mrs. Wilson whispers, "Yes." (p. 374)*

This excerpt illustrates how the therapist uses voice, tempo, and intensity of singing to mirror what the individual is expressing. In brief, music therapy as a psychosocial intervention may best be summarized by Sacks (2008), who notes, "at least at these times, (illness) is no bar to emotional depth. Once one has seen such responses, one knows that there is still a self to be called upon, even if music, and only music, can do the calling" (p. 385).

Dance/Movement Therapy

While dance/movement therapy may be perceived to be mainly a physical experience, the experience of dance or movement is also essentially a social experience. In a systematic review of existing literature on dancing as a psychosocial intervention, Guzman-Garcia et al. (2012a) concluded that it decreased problematic behaviors and improved mood, cognition, communication, and socializing. In particular, studies report that dancing induces social interaction and decreases isolation (Guzmán-Garcia et al., 2012b; Hackney & Bennett, 2014). In brief, dance/movement intervention not only increases physical function and control, it includes extensive social interaction that improves the perception of quality of life.

Additionally, body movement is one way to tell life stories without words to others; postures or movements are verbally acknowledged and often mirrored by the therapist to validate expression (American Dance Therapy Association, 2014). In addition, an environment of playfulness via movement is a fundamental experience of "aliveness" and the here-and-now. In this sense, dance/movement therapy recapitulates experiences of positive attachment and attunement via the therapist and the group that may be compromised by physical disorders or emotional losses in later years.

SUMMARY

Edna Eckert, an octogenarian artist, notes, "I think creative people are often long-lived because we are always re-inventing life; what we did yesterday, we create anew tomorrow. Inherent in this process is hope" (in Weiss, 1984, p. 25). In essence, Eckert underscores the core of creativity arts therapies and aging; they provide experiences of hope that demonstrate that life is not over as long as individuals can create through images, sound, and/or movement. As research on applications of creative arts therapy with older adults continues, there undoubtedly will be a greater understanding of how it facilitates sensory stimulation, enhances cognitive and physical abilities and social connection, and maintains psychological growth into old age. As Eckert implies, it also may have an impact not only on the quality of life, but also on the life span, by keeping older adults engaged through creativity and self-expression.

Creative arts therapies do not change the course of disease, but they do positively influence individuals' experiences of the challenges of aging, illness, and loss. Art, music, and dance/movement therapies not only emphasize the application of creative methods of intervention for specific disorders and conditions of old age, they also underscore what is possible via creative expression despite age. In brief, these action-oriented, sensory-based forms of treatment demonstrate the importance of encouraging older adults' fullest potential in later life while providing the multiple physical, cognitive, emotional, and interpersonal benefits of creative expression.

DISCLOSURE STATEMENT

Cathy Malchiodi has received royalties from McGraw-Hill, Guilford Press, and Routledge.

REFERENCES

American Dance Therapy Association. (2014). About dance/movement therapy. Retrieved on October 1, 2014, from http://www.adta.org/about_dmt.

American Music Therapy Association. (2014). *What is music therapy?* Retrieved on October 1, 2014, from http://www.musictherapy.org/about/musictherapy/.

Bradt, J., Magee, W. L., Dileo, C., Wheeler, B. L., & McGilloway, E. (2010). Music therapy for acquired brain injury. *Cochrane Database Syst Rev, 7*, CD006787.

Clift, S. (2012). Singing, wellbeing, and health. In R. MacDonald, G. Kreutz, & L. Mitchell (Eds.), *Music, health, & wellbeing* (pp. 113–124). New York: Oxford University Press.

Cohen, G. (2000). *The creative age: awakening human potential in the second half of life.* New York: Quill.

Cohen, G. (2006). *The mature mind: the positive power of the aging brain.* New York: Basic Books.

Cohen, G. (2009). New theories and research findings on the positive influence of music and art on health with aging. *Art Health, 1*(1), 48–63.

Cozolino, L. (2008). *The healthy aging brain: sustaining attachment, attaining wisdom.* New York: Norton.

Drucker, K. (1995). Swimming upstream: Art therapy with the psychogeriatric population in one health district. In M. Liebmann (Ed.), *Art Therapy in Practice.* London: Jessica Kingsley.

Earhart, G. M. (2009). Dance as therapy for individuals with Parkinson's disease. *Eur J Phys Rehabil Med, 45* (2), 231–238.

Elkis-Abuhoff, D., Goldblatt, R., Gaydos, M., Coratto, S. (2008). The effects of clay manipulation on somatic dysfunction and emotional distress in patients diagnosed with Parkinson's disease. *Art Therapy, 25*(3), 122–128.

Ellena, E., & Huebner, B. (2009). *I remember better when I paint.* Paris: French Connections Films.

Fornazzari, L. (2005). Preserved painting creativity in an artist with Alzheimer's disease. *Eur J Neurol, 12*(6), 419–424.

Fornazzari, L., Castle, T., Nadkarni, S., Ambrose, M., Miranda, D., Apanasiewicz, N., & Phillips, F. (2006). Preservation of episodic musical memory in a pianist with Alzheimer disease. *Neurology, 66*(4), 610–611.

Fornazzari, L., Ringer, T., Ringer, L., & Fischer, C.E. (2013). Preserved drawing in a sculptor with dementia. *Can J Neurol Sci, 40*(5), 736–737.

Goodill, S. (2005). *Introduction to medical dance/movement therapy.* London: Jessica Kingsley.

Guzman-Garcia, A., Hughes, J., James, I., & Rochester, L. (2012a). Dancing as a psychosocial intervention in care homes: a systematic review of the literature. *Int J Geriatr Psychiatry*, doi: 10.1002/gps.3913.

Guzmán-García A., Mukaetova-Ladinska, E., & James, I. (2012b). Introducing a lesson of Latin ballroom dance class to people with dementia living in care homes, benefits and concerns: a pilot study. *Dementia, 1*, 1–13.

Hackney, M., & Bennett, C. (2014). Dance therapy for individuals with Parkinson's disease: Improving quality of life. *J Parkinsonism RLS, 20* (4), 17–25.

Hamill, M., Smith, L., & Rohricht, F. (2011). Dancing down memory lane: circle dancing as a psychotherapeutic intervention in dementia. *Dementia*, 1–16. doi: 10.1177/1471301211420509.

Hoban, S. (2000). Motion and emotion: The dance/movement therapy experience. *Nursing Homes, 49*(11), 33–34.

Hurkmans, J., de Bruijn, M., Boonstra, A. M, Jonkers, R., Bastiaanse, R., Arendzen, H., & Reinders-Messelink, H. A. (2012). Music in the treatment of neurological language and speech disorders: a systematic review. *Aphasiology, 26*(1), 1–19.

Hurt, C. P., Rice, R. R., McIntosh, G. C., & Thaut, M. H. (1998). Rhythmic auditory stimulation in gait training for patients with traumatic brain injury. *J Music Ther, 35*, 228–291.

Johnson, C., & Sullivan-Marx, E. (2004). Art therapy: using the creative process for healing and hope among African American older adults. *Geriatric Nurs, 27*(5), 309–316.

Johnson, D. R. (2009). *Current approaches in drama therapy.* Springfield, IL: Charles C. Thomas.

Kim, S. K. (2012). A randomized, controlled study of the effects of art therapy on older Korean-Americans' healthy aging. *Arts Psychother, 40* (1), 158–164.

Knill, P., Barba, & Fuchs, M. (2004). *Minstrels of the soul: intermodal expressive therapy.* Toronto, ON: EGS Press.

Levine-Madori, L. (2009). Uses of therapeutic thematic arts programming (TTAP Method©) for enhanced cognitive and psychosocial functioning in the geriatric population. *Am J Recreation Ther, 8* (1), 25–31.

Levitin, D. (2006). *This is your brain on music.* New York: Dutton.

Malchiodi, C. A. (2005). *Expressive therapies.* New York: Guilford Publications.

Malchiodi, C. A. (2006). *The art therapy sourcebook* (2nd ed.). New York: McMillan.

Malchiodi, C. A. (2012a). Creativity and aging: An art therapy perspective. In C. Malchiodi (Ed.), *Handbook of art therapy* (pp. 275–287). New York: Guilford Publications.

Malchiodi, C. A. (2012b). *Handbook of art therapy* (2nd ed.). New York: Guilford Publications.

Malchiodi, C. A. (2013). *Art therapy and healthcare.* New York: Guilford Publications.

Malchiodi, C. A. (2014). Creative arts therapy approaches to attachment issues. In C. Malchiodi & D. Crenshaw (Eds.), *Creative arts and play therapy for attachment problems* (pp. 3–18). New York: Guilford Publications.

McKinley, P., Jacobson, A., Bednarczyk, V., Leroux, A., Rossignol, M., & Fung, J. (2008). Effect of a community-based Argentine tango dance program on functional balance and confidence in older adults. *J Aging Phys Activity, 16*(4):435–453.

Mental Health Foundation. (2011). *An evidence review of the impact of participatory arts on older adults.* Edinburgh, UK: Mental Health Foundation.

Micozzi, (2010). *Fundamentals of complementary and alternative medicine* (4th ed.). St. Louis, MO: Saunders/Elsevier.

Museum of Modern Art. (2011). *Meet me at MoMA.* Retrieved on October 1, 2014, from http://www.moma.org/meetme/.

National Center for Creative Aging. (2014). *Why creative people age better.* Retrieved on October 1, 2014, from http://www.creativeaging.org/news-blog/news/why-creative-people-age-better.

National Drama Therapy Association. (2014). What is drama therapy? Retrieved on October 1, 2014, from http://www.nadta.org/what-is-drama-therapy.html.

National Endowment for the Arts. (2006). *The creativity and aging study: Final report.* Washington, DC: NEA.

Nayak, S., Wheeler, B. L., Shiflett, S. C., & Agostinelli, S. (2000). Effect of music therapy on mood and social interaction among individuals with acute traumatic brain injury and stroke. *Rehabil Psychology, 45*(3), 274–283.

Newman-Bluestein, D., & Hill, H. (2010). Movement as the medium for connection, empathy, playfulness. *J Dementia Care, 18*, 24–27.

Payne, H. (2013). *Dance movement therapy: theory, research and practice*. New York: Routledge.

Ramachandran, V. (2011). *The tell-tale brain: a neuroscientist's quest for what makes us human*. New York: Norton.

Ramachandran, V. S. (1998). *Phantoms in the brain*. New York: Quill.

Richardson, H., & Glass, J. (2002). A comparison of scoring protocols on the clock drawing test in relation to ease of use, diagnostic group, and correlations with Mini-Mental State Examination. *J Am Geriatr Soc, 50*, 169–173.

Ridder, H. M., & Wheeler, B. (2015). Music therapy and older adults. In B. Wheeler (Ed.), *Handbook of music therapy* (pp. ////). New York: Guilford Publications.

Sacks, O. (2008). *Musicophilia: tales of music and the brain*. New York: Random House.

Schott, G. (2012). Pictures as neurological tools: lessons from enhanced and emergent artistry in brain disease. *Brain, 135* (6), 1947–1963.

Steele, M. (2005). Coping with multiple sclerosis: a music therapy viewpoint. *Aust J Music Ther, 16*, 70–87.

Stewart, E. (2004). Art therapy and neuroscience blend: working with patients who have dementia. *Art Therapy, 21*(3), 148–155.

Understanding clinical benefits of modeling clay exploration with patients diagnosed with Parkinson's disease. *Arts in Health*.

Tamplin, J. (2008). A pilot study into the effect of vocal exercises and singing on dysarthric speech. *Neurorehabilitation, 23*(3), 207–216.

Tamplin, J. (2015). Music therapy for adults with traumatic brain injury and other neurological disorders. In B. Wheeler (Ed.), *Handbook of music therapy*. New York: Guilford Publications.

Tamplin, J., Baker, F., Grocke, D., Brazzale, D., Pretto, J. J., Ruehland, W. R., . . . Berlowitz, D. J. (2013). The effect of singing on respiratory function, voice, and mood following quadriplegia: a randomized controlled trial. *Arch Phys Med Rehabil, 94*(3), 426–434.

Thaut, M. H., McIntosh, K. W., McIntosh, G. C., & Hoemberg, V. (2001). Auditory rhythmicity enhances movement and speech motor control in patients with Parkinson's disease. *Funct Neurol, 16*(2), 163–172.

Thaut, M. H., McIntosh, G. C., Prassas, S. G., & Rice, R. R. (1993). Effect of rhythmic auditory cuing on temporal stride parameters and EMG patterns in hemiparetic gait of stroke patients. *J Neurol Rehabil, 7*, 9–16.

Tomaino, C. M. (2012). Effective music therapy techniques in the treatment of nonfluent aphasia. *Ann NY Acad Sci, 1252*(1), 312–317.

Wall, M., & Duff, A. (2010). The effects of music therapy for older people with dementia. *Br J Nursing, 19* (2), 108–113.

Waller, D. (2002). *Art therapies and progressive illness: nameless dread*. New York: Brunner-Routledge.

Warren, B. (2004). *Using the creative arts in therapy: a practical introduction* (2nd ed.). New York: Routledge.

Weisberg, N., & Wilder, R. (2001). *Expressive arts with elders: a resource*. London: Jessica Kingsley.

Weiss, J. (1984). *Expressive therapies with elders and the disabled: touching the heart of life*. New York: The Haworth Press.

Wheeler, B. A. (2015). *Music therapy handbook*. New York: Guilford Publications.

Wikstrom, B. M. (2004). Older adults and the arts: the importance of aesthetic forms of expression later in life. *J Gerontol Nurs, 30*(9), 30–36.

Woolhiser, J. S. (2010). Collage as a therapeutic modality for reminiscence in patients with dementia. *Art Therapy, 27*(3), 136–140.

20

USING THE INTERNET TO FIND CAIM RESOURCES FOR MENTAL HEALTH PROFESSIONALS AND THEIR OLDER PATIENTS

Ellen Gay Detlefsen

WHEN CONSIDERING the prospect of identifying Internet and web-based or digital (1) resources on complementary, alternative, and integrative medicine that are appropriate to use with older patients and their families, three questions often come to mind:

- Do elders really use the Internet to find information in the first place?
- Do their clinicians have the time and evaluation expertise to locate appropriate information?
- Is there actually reliable and appropriate Internet-based information on the topic anyway?

In 2015, the answer to all three questions is "yes."

First, researchers at the highly regarded Pew Research Center noted in 2014 that "[o]verall, technology adoption among seniors has been increasing slowly but surely. Today, three quarters of seniors have a cell phone, six in ten use the internet, and almost half have broadband at home. Those still trail the national average, but they have been steadily increasing since we began tracking these metrics way back in 2000" (2). These scholars go on to posit that "[y]ounger, higher-income, and more highly educated seniors use the internet and broadband at rates approaching—or even exceeding—the general population; internet use and broadband adoption each drop off dramatically around age 75" (3). Recent research has also shown that while some seniors seek training for accessing digital information, and they trust what they find, others find that "[i]nformation seeking on the Internet is especially complex because it requires a general knowledge of the topic of interest, basic knowledge of hardware and software operations, information seeking skills (e.g., knowledge of how the Internet or a Web page is organized and how links, search boxes, and search histories work), and the ability to judge whether information sources are credible . . . " (4).

Second, a number of studies have also shown that physician–patient communication about complementary, alternative, and integrative medicine, even in older populations, occurs successfully (5).

Physician discomfort with discussions of CAIM (complementary, alternative, and integrative medicine) topics is diminishing (6). Specifically, investigators who looked at a population of older patients and their physicians noted that "[r]egardless of a physician's stance or knowledge about CAM, she or he can help patients negotiate CAM treatment decisions . . . [and] providers do not have to possess extensive knowledge about specific CAM treatments to have meaningful discussions with patients and to give patients a framework for evaluating CAM treatment use" (7). Recent work indicates that CAIM services have even begun to be offered in the hospice setting, with benefits for older individuals at the end of life (8).

Finally, the Internet and the World Wide Web do have excellent sources of information for seniors and their clinicians on the topic of complementary, alternative, and integrative medicine in general, as well as specific information on mental health concerns. Caution is needed, however, when looking for, or choosing to use, the information that is dispensed widely via the Internet.

When looking for or using Internet-accessible materials with older people, there are helpful guidelines from major public health institutions. For instance, the World Health Organization (in a planning document for designing information for elders who are at risk in emergency and disaster situations), recommends that web-based information for elders should

- provide information about . . . resources in formats and communication channels that are accessible to older persons so they can make informed personal decisions; and
- provide information and public education to prepare for to meet health needs . . . in formats that are accessible to persons with less education and low literacy (9).

Other sources suggest that good websites for older users should

- avoid Internet or subject-specific jargon;
- have a reading level no higher than eighth grade;
- have pages that load quickly, even with a slow Internet connection;
- have pages that are accessible from both PCs and Macintosh/Apple computers;
- use formats that work on at least three common platforms (computers, tablets, cell phones); and

- create the feeling of a "trusted, knowledgeable friend" (10).

Furthermore, ideally, web-based information for the special population of older people needs to be

- specifically prepared for elders;
- culturally fluent for differing communities whether identified by race/ethnicity, faith tradition, disability status, or even generation; and
- easily printed.

Experts from the National Library of Medicine, working together with colleagues from the National Institute on Aging, created an excellent guide for designing "senior-friendly" websites. This tool is helpful as both a design aid and an evaluation guide for measuring the accessibility of web-based information for older people. Websites should also be created using the "plain language" guidelines familiar to health professionals who write and administer informed consent documents (11) (see Figure 20.1).

Other useful tools for assessing the quality of health-related sites are available through the MedlinePlus® portal, including two web pages with patient-friendly language, entitled a "MedlinePlus Guide to Healthy Web Surfing, and Evaluating Health Information"; the NLM has also created a helpful web-based instructional tool for people who may experience low literacy or low health literacy, entitled "Evaluating Internet Health Information: A Tutorial" (12).

Several other NIH institutes have also created excellent guides for assessing the quality of Internet-accessible and web-based information. Two useful examples come from the National Cancer Institute and the newly renamed National Center for Complementary and Integrative Health (NCCIH). The NCI's web page, entitled "Evaluating Online Sources of Health Information: How can you be careful about cancer information on websites, Twitter, YouTube, blogs, Facebook, and e-mail?" is particularly timely in that it advises health consumers about a variety of approaches to evaluating health information, including social media (13). The NCCIH site, entitled "Finding and Evaluating Online Resources on Complementary Health Approaches," is one of the few NIH sites that specifically address consumer and health professional concerns about web-based and Internet-accessible information in the realm of CAIM (14) (see Figure 20.2).

■ ◆ ✖ ✴
NATIONAL INSTITUTE ON AGING

NATIONAL LIBRARY
OF MEDICINE

NATIONAL INSTITUTES OF HEALTH
Department of Health and Human Services

Making Your Website Senior Friendly
Tips from the National Institute on Aging and the National Library of Medicine

This tip sheet offers research-based guidelines that can help you create websites that work well for older adults, the fastest-growing group of Internet users. Besides sending and receiving email, older adults search the web for health, financial, and religious or spiritual information. They also use the Internet to shop, play games, perform genealogy searches, and book travel. As the baby boomers age, the number of older adults using the Internet will continue to grow, and web designers will increasingly be called on to tailor websites to this population.

This tip sheet is organized into the following sections:

■ Basing Web Design on Research
■ Organizing Web Information for Older Adults
■ Writing Online Text for Older Adults
■ Designing Readable Online Text for Older Adults
■ Making Web Information Easy for Older Adults to Find
■ Including Other Media
■ Making Sure That Older Adults Can Use Your Website

Key Tips for Making Your Website Senior Friendly

■ Break information into short sections.
■ Give instructions clearly and number each step.
■ Minimize the use of jargon and technical terms.
■ Use single mouse clicks.
■ Allow additional space around clickable targets.
■ Use 12- or 14-point type size, and make it easy for users to enlarge text.
■ Use high-contrast color combinations, such as black type against a white background.
■ Provide a speech function to hear text read aloud.
■ Provide text-only versions of multimedia content.
■ Minimize scrolling.
■ Choose a search engine that uses keywords and doesn't require special characters or knowledge of Boolean terms.

Visit www.NIHSeniorHealth.gov for an example of a website that incorporates these senior-friendly guidelines.

FIGURE 20.1   Making your website senior friendly.

Source: http://www.nlm.nih.gov/pubs/checklist.pdf

When specifically looking for tools and materials that focus on the needs and concerns of older individuals, the National Institute on Aging plays a leading role. The Institute includes a helpful guide to "Online Health Information: Can You Trust It?" as one of its long-standing *AgePage* series; the material is freely available as a print brochure or as an online tool (15) (see Figure 20.3).

In the NIA's major web tool, known as *NIH SeniorHealth: Built with You in Mind,* and created cooperatively with the National Library of Medicine, there is a very full section entitled "Complementary

Finding and Evaluating Online Resources on Complementary Health Approaches

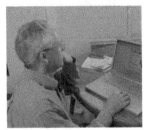

© Matthew Lester

The number of Web sites offering health-related resources—including information about complementary health approaches (often called complementary and alternative medicine)—grows every day. Social media sites have also become an important source of online health information for some people. Many online health resources are useful, but others may present information that is inaccurate or misleading, so it's important to find sources you can trust and to know how to evaluate their content. This guide provides help for finding reliable Web sites and outlines things to consider in evaluating health information from Web sites and social media sources.

Checking Out a Health Web Site: Five Quick Questions

If you're visiting a health Web site for the first time, these five quick questions can help you decide whether the site is a helpful resource.

Who? Who runs the Web site? Can you trust them?

What? What does the site say? Do its claims seem too good to be true?

When? When was the information posted or reviewed? Is it up-to-date?

Where? Where did the information come from? Is it based on scientific research?

Why? Why does the site exist? Is it selling something?

Key Facts

Not all online health information is accurate. Be cautious when you evaluate health information on the Internet, especially if the site

- Is selling something
- Includes outdated information
- Makes excessive claims for what a product can do
- Is sponsored by an organization whose goals differ from yours.

U.S. DEPARTMENT OF HEALTH AND HUMAN SERVICES

National Institutes of Health
National Center for Complementary and Alternative Medicine

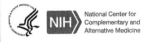

National Center for Complementary and Alternative Medicine

FIGURE 20.2   Finding and evaluating online resources on complementary health approaches.

Source: https://nccih.nih.gov/health/webresources

Health Approaches" with content covering clinical and research issues, and tips for being an informed consumer and on communicating with the health-care team (16). This site is particularly useful, as it offers the capability to resize the type, can be seen in a high-contrast mode, and can be printed as a handout—all features that are specifically targeted to older users. The NIH Senior Health materials

National Institute on Aging

AgePage

Online Health Information: Can You Trust It?

A group of older adults are gathered for their weekly computer class. They are learning to use the Internet to find health information. Maria's husband, who is 75, had a stroke the month before so she's searching the web for some basic facts about stroke rehabilitation. Walter, who is 68, has questions about what causes Alzheimer's disease because he thinks that's what his mother had. Shirley and Howard, married for 48 years, are trying to find out if the cataract surgery their eye doctor suggests really is as safe as he says. The whole group has one big worry—"How can we trust the health information we get on the Internet?"

There are thousands of health-related websites on the Internet.

Some of the information on these websites is reliable and can be trusted. Some of it is not. Some of the information is current. Some of it is not. Choosing which website to trust is worth thinking about.

How do I find reliable health information online?

As a rule, health websites sponsored by Federal government agencies are good sources of health information. You can reach all Federal websites by visiting *www.usa.gov*. Large professional organizations and well-known medical schools may also be good sources of health information.

The main page of a website is called the home page. The home page shows you the features on the website. You should be able to spot the name of the sponsor of the website right away.

What questions should I ask?

As you search online, you are likely to find websites for many health agencies and organizations that are not well-known. By answering the following questions you should be able to find more information about these websites. A lot of these details

2

FIGURE 20.3   Online health information: Can you trust it?

Source: http://www.nia.nih.gov/sites/default/files/online_health_information_can_you_trust_it_1.pdf

can also be readily shared via a single click to many social media tools, which makes the information widely available for family members who may be at a distance from their elders (see Figure 20.4).

If the need is to locate focused mental health information in an Internet-accessible or web-based format, the materials from the National Institute of Mental Health and several national associations for mental health professionals who care for older adults are key. The NIMH web-based resources found at their page on "Older Adults and Mental Health" are targeted to depression and Alzheimer's disease (17). More specific information on a wider range of topics is available from the Geriatric Mental Health Foundation (associated with the American Association for Geriatric Psychiatry), which has a large array of consumer- and

family-focussed materials at their website; their Internet-accessible brochures are listed under the tab entitled "Consumer/Patient Information," and include web-accessible and printable brochures on alcohol/drug abuse/misuse, substance abuse and misuse, alcohol and aging, Alzheimer's disease, anxiety, caregiving, dementia, depression, disaster preparedness, healthy aging, and sleep (18). The Health in Aging Foundation, created by the American Geriatrics Society, also offers materials on a variety of general mental health issues experienced by elders with their A-to-Z section and their "tip sheets," including one short entry in the A-to-Z section for "Alternative Remedies" (19). None of these sites, however, offers much information about CAIM-specific approaches for geriatric mental health.

(b)

Places To Start

There are a few good places to start if you are looking for online health information. An excellent source of reliable information is the National Institutes of Health (*www.nih.gov*). You can start here to find information on almost every health topic, including:

✦ managing heart disease (*www.nhlbi.nih.gov*)

✦ dealing with deafness (*www.nidcd.nih.gov*)

✦ taking care of dentures (*www.nidcr.nih.gov*)

✦ caring for a loved one with Alzheimer's disease (*www.alzheimers.nia.nih.gov*)

In addition, you can visit the National Library of Medicine's Medline Plus (*www.medlineplus.gov*) for dependable information on more than 700 health-related topics.

You can also visit NIHSeniorHealth.gov (*www.nihseniorhealth.gov*)—a website with health information designed specifically for older people.

can be found under the heading, "About Us" or "Contact Us."

1. *Who sponsors the website? Can you easily identify the sponsor?*

Websites cost money—is the funding source readily apparent? Sometimes the website address itself may help— for example:

✦ .gov identifies a government agency

✦ .edu identifies an educational institution

✦ .org identifies professional organi- zations (e.g., scientific or research societies, advocacy groups)

✦ .com identifies commercial websites (e.g., businesses, pharmaceutical companies, sometimes hospitals)

2. *Is it obvious how you can reach the sponsor?*

Trustworthy websites will have contact information for you to use. They often have a toll-free telephone number. The website home page should list an e-mail address, phone number, or a mailing address where the sponsor and/or the authors of the information can be reached.

3

4

FIGURE 20.3   Continued

However, the National Center for Complementary and Integrative Health (NCCIH; the NIH Institute formerly known as NCCAM) clearly focuses on CAIM-oriented web-based infor- mation, with one page specifically entitled "Aging," and another page entitled "Seniors or Older Adults or Elderly Information" (20). Those seeking addi- tional NCCIH information specifically on geriatric mental health will have to find it by searching the NCCIH website for topics, diagnoses, and con- cerns typically found in an older population. For example, there are full entries and patient education "tip sheets" for CAIM materials on subjects such as Alzheimer's disease, arthritis, cognitive func- tion, dementia, depression, hospice care, insom- nia, menopausal symptoms, neurodegenerative

diseases, osteoarthritis, pain, Parkinson's disease, sleep disorders, and stroke—all areas of inter- est for older people and their family and profes- sional caregivers. Health professionals can also use the NCCIH tools to access continuously updated PubMed MEDLINE searches, with active links that identify and, in many cases, provide full-text access to current systematic reviews, meta-analyses, and reports of randomized controlled trials on CAIM and aging, and CAIM and Alzheimer's disease (21). Health professionals—clinicians and research- ers alike—will also find that the NCCIH page on CAIM research entitled "Spotlighted Research Results—Aging" includes information useful for older populations; a recent issue of the NCCIH *Clinical Digest*, a monthly e-newsletter for health

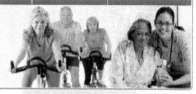

NIHSeniorHealth

Built with You in Mind

Resize Text: A A A   Change Contrast ◑   Print 🖨 Sign Up ✉ Share ➕

In This Topic

→ **What Are Complementary Health Approaches?**

Natural Products

Safety Of Natural Products

Mind And Body Practices

Safety Of Mind And Body Practices

Other Complementary Approaches

Safety Of Other Complementary Approaches

Research On Diseases Affecting Older Adults

Research On Pain Management

Be An Informed Consumer

Tell Your Health Care Providers

Frequently Asked Questions

Learn More

Complementary Health Approaches Videos

Quiz Yourself

MedlinePlus For More Information

National Institute On Aging

Related Topics

Eating Well As You Get Older

The information in this topic was provided by the National Center for Complementary and Integrative Health

Topic Last Reviewed: September 2013

Complementary Health Approaches

What Are Complementary Health Approaches?

Today, many people use complementary health approaches for a variety of diseases or conditions. But what exactly are these approaches, and how do they differ from standard medical care?

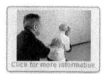

Complementary health approaches are medical and health care systems, practices, and products that originated outside of mainstream medicine. They include techniques performed by a practitioner (such as acupuncture, spinal manipulation, and massage therapy) and natural products (such as herbs, probiotics, and fish oil). Some approaches, including acupuncture and yoga, originated in Eastern countries such as China or India but are now used in Western countries as well.

Little research has been done on many complementary health approaches. Therefore, in many instances, it's uncertain whether they are safe or effective. The National Institutes of Health (NIH) is sponsoring research to learn more about the safety and effectiveness of complementary approaches.

Complementary vs. Alternative

When people talk about health care practices with non-mainstream origins, they often use the words "alternative" and "complementary" as though they mean the same thing, but the two words usually refer to different concepts.

- "Complementary" refers to use of a non-mainstream approach together with conventional medicine.
- "Alternative" refers to use of a non-mainstream approach in place of conventional medicine.

True "alternative" medicine is not common. Most people who use non-mainstream approaches use them along with conventional treatments.

Integrative Medicine

Non-mainstream health care approaches may also be considered part of integrative medicine or integrative health care. For example, cancer treatment centers with integrative health care programs may offer services such as acupuncture and massage to patients who are receiving conventional cancer treatments such as chemotherapy. These approaches may help patients manage some of the symptoms and side effects of treatment.

Integrative health care is a growing trend in the United States, but research on its potential value is in its early stages. Therefore, it's hard for people to make informed decisions about whether to try this kind of care.

FIGURE 20.4   What are complementary health approaches?.

Source: http://nihseniorhealth.gov/complementaryhealthapproaches/whatarecomplementaryhealthapproaches/01.html

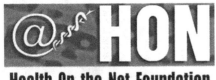

Health On the Net Foundation

Non Governmental Organization

www.HealthOnNet.org

FIGURE 20.5   HON Code.

Source: http://www.hon.ch/web.html

professionals, offered evidence-based information on CAIM approaches on the use of dietary supplements and cognitive function and dementia (22).

Similarly, major websites from well-known clinical providers often provide information about complementary and integrative modalities, but they rarely mention specific mental health or geriatric topics. Typical examples come from the Mayo Clinic (23), the Cleveland Clinic (24), and Stanford HealthCare (25), all of which contain positive information about a wide range of CAIM approaches, but none of which focuses specifically on the needs or concerns of an older population. The UPMC Center for Integrative Health in Pittsburgh includes information about a number of mental health conditions for which integrative treatment is offered, but none is specifically or uniquely geriatric (26). The International Network of Integrative Mental Health, a "global organization dedicated to advancing an integrative whole person approach to mental health," with a website rich with links to web-based and Internet-accessible mental health resources, does not have a specific section for older persons' mental health (27).

The clinician or consumer seeking web-based, Internet-accessible, digital information about complementary, integrative, and/or alternative approaches to dealing with mental health issues and older patients or family members is left with sifting the information from various, sometimes dubious, sites. Beginning with a Google® or Yahoo® or a Wikipedia® search is not recommended, as the first stops on the information journey should be the NIH SeniorHealth site or the NCCIH site.

If, however, web surfing or "googling" is undertaken, then using the tools for assessing quality from the NCCIH, MedlinePlus, and the National Institute on Aging will arm the searcher with skills to filter and choose wisely from the flood of material that is dumped out by the search engines. Learning a simple rubric or mnemonic for measuring quality is useful; the *Trust It or Trash It* model (28), developed by the genetic disease community as a tool for consumers searching for digital information on complex medical problems, is helpful. Additionally, looking for the HON Code symbol prominently displayed on a health website is also useful; this mark, assigned by the long-standing and highly regarded Health On the Net Foundation only to those sites that have been vetted and approved by their expert staff, is an international quality marker (29) (see Figure 20.5).

If there is web-accessible, Internet-accessible CAIM information that is available from websites other than those associated with NIH institutes, professional associations, and/or major medical centers, there are several points to remember when assessing the quality of these materials. As one physician blogger put it in 2014, there are five questions to ask:

1. Does the website claim to cure everything?
2. Are they trying to sell you something?
3. Has this treatment already worked for thousands of anonymous people?
4. Is this the "medical secret" doctors don't want you to know about?
5. Are there any peer-reviewed medical studies that can support their claims?

If the answer to any two of these questions is "yes," then one should be very skeptical of those web resources (30).

Finally, seeking out the services of a trained consumer health information specialist may also be an option. Hospital and medical center libraries, and some larger public libraries, may have personnel who are especially trained in consumer health information services; each of the eight Regional Medical Libraries of the National Network of Libraries of Medicine has a staff member with responsibility for consumer health materials as well (31). These colleagues may be helpful in identifying consumer health materials that are locally produced or distributed.

DISCLOSURE STATEMENT

Ellen Gay Detlefsen DLS has no conflicts to disclose as of January 2015.

REFERENCES

1. A note of clarification: The terms *Internet* and *Web* are often used interchangeably, but in fact the two terms are not synonymous. The "Internet" is a massive network of networks, which connects millions of computers so that any computer can communicate with any other computer as long as they are both connected to the network known as the Internet. The "World Wide Web," or the "Web," is a way of accessing information over the Internet that uses common protocols for communication in order to share information. You may want to think of the Internet as the way the content moves around, and the Web as the software that lets you use the content. It is probably more accurate to use terms like "web-accessible information" and "Internet-delivered information." Digital information is a newer term used to describe the information that is shared via the Web, and across the Internet. In practice, however, most laypeople simply use the words *Internet, web,* and even *digital,* to mean the same thing—the information that is obtained by a search with a computer that is connected to the worldwide network known as the Internet. There is a very friendly explanation of these terms and concepts on the website of the Computer History Museum, in Mountain View, CA, at http://www.computerhistory.org/revolution/networking/19.

2. Pew Research Center. *Older adults and technology use*, 2014. http://www.pewinternet.org/2014/04/03/older-adults-and-technology-use/.

3. Pew Research Center Internet Project. *Seniors continue to lag in tech adoption*, 2014. http://pewinternet.tumblr.com/post/81584916842/technology-adoption-among-seniors-has-been.

4. Xie B. Improving older adults' e-health literacy through computer training using NIH online resources. *Library Information Sci Res* 2012;34:63–74 (2012); Zulman DM, Kirch M, Zheng K, An LC. Trust in the Internet as a health resource among older adults: analysis of data from a nationally representative survey. *J Med Internet Res* 2011 Feb 16;13(1):e19, http://www.jmir.org/2011/1/e19/; Czaja SJ. Aging, e-health tools, and health literacy, in Centers for Disease Control and Prevention, *Improving health literacy for older adults: expert panel report 2009.* Atlanta: US Department of Health and Human Services; 2009.

5. AARP [and] National Center for Complementary and Integrative Health. *Complementary and alternative medicine: what people aged 50 and older discuss with their health care providers.* Consumer Survey Report. https://nccih.nih.gov/news/camstats/2010.

6. Shelley BM, Sussman AL, Williams RL, Segal AR, Crabtree BF. "They don't ask me so I don't tell them": patient-clinician communication about traditional, complementary, and alternative medicine. *Ann Fam Med.* 2009 Mar–Apr;7(2):139–147; Corbin Winslow L, Shapiro H. Physicians want education about complementary and alternative medicine to enhance communication with their patients. *Arch Intern Med.* 2002 May 27;162(10):1176–1181.

7. Koenig CJ, Ho EY, Yadegar V, Tarn DM. Negotiating complementary and alternative medicine use in primary care visits with older patients. *Patient Educ Couns.* 2012 Dec;89(3):368–373; Sleath B, Rubin RH, Campbell W, Gwyther L, Clark T. Ethnicity and physician-older patient communication about alternative therapies. *J Altern Complement Med.* 2001 Aug;7(4):329–335.

8. Helwick C. Few hospices providing CAM services to patients. *Medscape Medical News.* May 23, 2014. http://www.medscape.com/viewarticle/825676#vp_2.

9. *Older persons in emergencies: an active ageing perspective.* Geneva: World Health Organization, 2008. http://www.who.int/ageing/publications/EmergenciesEnglish13August.pdf.

10. Devlin M. Network librarians conclude outreach projects. Part III: Health information for elders. *Dragonfly* 2003;34(4). http://nnlm.gov/pnr/news/200310/devlin.html.

11. National Library of Medicine & National Institute on Aging. *Making your website senior friendly.* http://www.nia.nih.gov/health/publication/making-your-website-senior-friendly; http://www.nlm.nih.gov/pubs/staffpubs/od/ocpl/agingchecklist.html; Hart TA, Chaparro BS, Halcomb CG. Evaluating websites for older adults: adherence to "senior-friendly" guidelines and end-user performance. *Behav Inform Technol* 2008 May;27(3):191–199; Plain Language Action and Information Network. *Federal plain language guidelines.* http://www.plainlanguage.gov/howto/guidelines/FederalPLGuidelines/TOC.cfm.

12. National Library of Medicine. *MedlinePlus guide to healthy web surfing.* http://www.nlm.nih.gov/medlineplus/healthywebsurfing.html; National Library of Medicine. *Evaluating health information.* http://www.nlm.nih.gov/

medlineplus/evaluatinghealthinformation.html; National Library of Medicine. *Evaluating Internet health information: a tutorial from the National Library of Medicine*. http://www.nlm.nih.gov/medlineplus/webeval/webeval.html.

13. National Cancer Institute. *Evaluating online sources of health information: how can you be careful about cancer information on websites, Twitter, YouTube, blogs, Facebook, and e-mail?* http://www.cancer.gov/cancertopics/cancerlibrary/health-info-online.

14. National Center for Complementary and Integrative Health. *Finding and evaluating online resources on complementary health approaches*. https://nccih.nih.gov/health/webresources.

15. National Institute on Aging. *Online health information: can you trust it?* http://www.nia.nih.gov/sites/default/files/online_health_information_can_you_trust_it_1.pdf.

16. National Library of Medicine & National Institute on Aging. *Complementary health approaches*. http://nihseniorhealth.gov/complementaryhealthapproaches/whatarecomplementaryhealthapproaches/01.html.

17. National Institute of Mental Health. *Older adults and mental health*. http://www.nimh.nih.gov/health/topics/older-adults-and-mental-health/index.shtml.

18. Geriatric Mental Health Foundation. *Consumer/patient materials*. http://www.gmhfonline.org/.

19. Health in Aging Foundation. *Aging and health A-to-Z* [and] *tip sheets*. http://www.healthinaging.org/aging-and-health-a-to-z/; http://www.healthinaging.org/news/tip-sheets/; http://www.healthinaging.org/aging-and-health-a-to-z/topic:alternative-remedies/.

20. National Center for Complementary and Integrative Health. *Aging* https://nccih.nih.gov/health/aging; *Seniors or older adults or elderly information* https://nccih.nih.gov/taxonomy/term/506; *Time to talk tips*. https://nccih.nih.gov/health/tips.

21. National Center for Complementary and Integrative Health. *Evidence-based medicine: literature reviews*. https://nccih.nih.gov/health/providers/litreviews.htm.

22. National Center for Complementary and Integrative Health. *Spotlighted research results—aging*. https://nccih.nih.gov/health/50/research; NCCIH Clinical Digest. *Dietary supplements and cognitive function, dementia, and Alzheimer's disease*. https://nccih.nih.gov/health/providers/digest/alzheimers.htm.

23. Mayo Clinic. *Complementary and integrative medicine*. http://www.mayoclinic.org/departments-centers/general-internal-medicine/minnesota/overview/specialty-groups/complementary-integrative-medicine; http://www.mayo.edu/research/centers-programs/complementary-integrative-medicine/complementary-integrative-medicine-program/overview.

24. Cleveland Clinic. *About integrative and lifestyle medicine*. http://my.clevelandclinic.org/services/wellness/integrative-medicine/about; http://my.clevelandclinic.org/services/wellness/integrative-medicine/treatments-services/brainhealthandwellness.

25. Stanford Health Care. *Integrative medicine center*. https://stanfordhealthcare.org/medical-clinics/integrative-medicine-center/conditions.html.

26. UPMC Center for Integrative Medicine. *Conditions we treat*. http://upmc.com/Services/integrative-medicine/Pages/conditions.aspx.

27. The International Network of Integrative Mental Health. http://www.inimh.org/index.asp.

28. *Trust it or trash it*. http://www.trustortrash.org/; Genetic Alliance. *Trust it or trash it? creating & assessing genetic health information*. Washington, DC: Genetic Alliance; 2010. *Trust it or trash it? a tool to help evaluate and create genetics health information*. http://www.ncbi.nlm.nih.gov/books/NBK115530/.

29. Health On the Net Foundation. http://www.hon.ch/Global/HON_mission.html.

30. Baum N. *Health information on the Internet: 5 questions to ask*. http://www.kevinmd.com/blog/2014/10/health-information-internet-5-questions-ask.html.

31. National Network of Libraries of Medicine. *Health information on the Web*. http://nnlm.gov/hip//

21

RESILIENCE-BUILDING INTERVENTIONS FOR SUCCESSFUL AND POSITIVE AGING

Alexandrea L. Harmell, Rujvi Kamat, Dilip V. Jeste and Barton W. Palmer

INTRODUCTION

The United States continues to be a rapidly aging society, with the number of adults aged 65 and older expected to more than double between 2010 and 2050 (Vincent & Velkoff, 2010) and the number of adults aged 85 and older projected to increase by 350% (Wiener & Tilly, 2002). Advancing age is often associated with increased vulnerability to a unique set of stressors, including retirement, medical comorbidity, loss of loved ones, and the threat of reduced independence. As such, there has been a recent surge in both public and research interest in exploring factors that contribute to aging more successfully. One such aspect of successful aging is the concept of resilience (Vaillant, 2015).

Positive constructs such as resilience may be thought of as being complements to traditional medicine in that they emphasize personal strength rather than disease or deficits (Jeste & Palmer, 2015; Jeste, Palmer, Rettew, & Boardman, 2015). In other words, whereas the standard medical model typically addresses how to treat diseases or symptoms, complementary/alternative medicine does this while also focusing on positive attributes in an effort to help older individuals not only live longer, but also live better. The study of resilience coincides with the rising trend toward a strengths-based approach to aging, which is slowly starting to replace, or at least complement, the traditional negative deficits view of aging. One of the goals of positive aging is for individuals to evolve, adapt, and find meaning and purpose, despite whatever particular circumstances may arise.

The critical role of resilience in successful aging has been well documented (Lamond et al., 2008; Montross et al., 2006; Moore et al., 2015). For example, in a recent study by our group, Jeste and colleagues (2013) found significant associations between resilience and self-rated successful aging in a sample of over 1000 community-dwelling older adults. The magnitude of these effects were comparable in size to that of physical health, suggesting that increasing resilience may have as strong an effect in successful aging as reducing physical disability. This finding was further corroborated by Manning, Carr, & Kail (2014), who reported that high levels of resilience protect against the deleterious impact of chronic new conditions in older adults. Some research has suggested that, in addition to protecting against possible declines in physical health, high levels of resilience significantly contribute to longevity and become even more profound at very advanced ages, with centenarians being more resilient than any other age group (Zeng & Shen, 2010).

Given the emerging importance of resilience in health outcomes, the purpose of the present chapter is to examine the concept of resilience, specifically within the context of positive aging. We review various definitions that have been proposed and discuss how resilience can be construed within a hierarchical individual- and systems-based approach. In addition, we discuss how to measure resilience by reviewing the currently available scales. Further, we consider interventions that promote resilience. Finally, we provide suggestions for future research and give recommendations for further development of resilience interventions for older adults.

DEFINING RESILIENCE

Although at face value, resilience may appear to be a relatively simple construct to define, it is actually quite complex and multifaceted. Developing a universally accepted definition has posed a significant challenge. Initially, resilience was studied primarily within the framework of developmental psychology. Specifically, children at risk of developing later psychopathology (due to environmental adversities or genetic vulnerabilities) were followed longitudinally, which led to the discovery that there was great variability in outcomes, with some children appearing to be more impervious to adverse circumstances than others (Masten & Tellegen, 2012). This observation prompted interest in the topic of resilience, which was used as a proxy to describe successful adaptation to adversity. Following the early developmental studies, the empirical literature employing the construct of resilience has expanded considerably to describe diverse sets of groups across the life span who seem to be able to adapt and to overcome a wide range of stressful circumstances.

The term *resilience* was originally derived from the mid-seventeenth century Latin word *resilire*, which means "to jump back or recoil." However, more recent groups, such as the American Psychological Association (APA), do not define *resilience* in terms of one's ability to bounce back to a current level of functioning but merely as "the *process* of adapting well in the face of adversity, trauma, tragedy, threats, or even significant sources of stress" (APA, 2015). In the field of developmental psychology, APA's definition is commonly expanded even further to include not only the process of, but also the capacity for, or outcome of, successful adaptation despite challenging or threatening circumstances (Masten & Tellegen, 2012). These nuanced definitions lead to one of the main controversies in resilience research, which is whether resilience should be best conceptualized as a fixed trait, an outcome, or a dynamic and fluid developmental process. In the field of aging, perhaps it is most appropriate for resilience to not simply be reduced to binary terms (i.e., whereby a person is or is not resilient), but rather to reflect a continuum of differing degrees of resilience across different contexts. Aging adults often encounter numerous acute and chronic stressors, and the psychological and physiological responses to these stressors likely depend not only on the individual's inherent ability to adapt to stress in general, but perhaps more specifically on the individual's ability to adapt to the stressors within a particular context and at a particular time in his or her life.

Recently, some researchers have identified a constellation of unique characteristics that have been associated with resilience. This approach tends to be person focused by grouping together individuals who seem better equipped to manage adversity and studying the commonalities between them. One study found that older adults who were more resilient tended to report fewer multiple adversities and were more likely to use adaptive, solution-driven coping, rather than avoidant coping strategies, when faced with challenges (Hildon, Montgomery, Blane, Wiggins, & Netuveli, 2010). Additional individual characteristics that have been viewed as being important contributors to resilience include commitment, dynamism, humor in the face of adversity, optimism, faith, altruism, and perceiving adversity as an opportunity to learn and grow (Lavretsky, 2014).

Investigators have also suggested that resilience may not just be an isolated quality inherent in an aging individual, but also something that can be derived from external systems, such as social support from the family. A family-perspective approach to resilience tends to focus on the entire family system and how the family responds as a unit or system when confronted with various stressors. In contrast to focusing on individually based traits, researchers interested in family resilience emphasize the critical role of close relationships on personal outcomes. Three key concepts that have been cited as being important to successful aging from a family-resilience stance include flexibility, social support, and spirituality/religiosity (Martin, Distelberg, & Elahad, 2015). Flexibility corresponds to a family's ability to adapt to a challenge by brainstorming potential solutions, setting positive expectations, and learning to accept major life fluctuations. Social support is based on the theory that feelings of connectedness and belonging buffer the impact of deleterious outcomes. This especially holds true for older adults who are at increased risk for isolation due to factors such as retirement, loss of friends and peers, and decreased mobility. Several reports indicate that older adults with better personal connections live longer and report improved physical and cognitive functioning (Chodosh, Kado, Seeman, & Karlamangla, 2007; Stewart & Yuen, 2011). Spirituality has also been viewed through the lens of family resilience, as families with a shared spirituality have been shown to have a more optimistic outlook on adverse events as they can use their faith to help find inspiration, meaning, and purpose in a particular adverse event (Black & Lobo, 2008). Since older adults more frequently experience loss of loved ones, turning to family and spirituality/religion in times of grieving can act as an important coping mechanism.

In addition to individual and family resilience, the concept of community-based resilience is also gaining recognition. Among some of the community resources that have been shown to foster resilience are social connectedness and cohesion (Langdon, 1997). Communities are variable in their ability to influence individual health and well-being outcomes in terms of community characteristics such as walkability, air quality, crime rates, and educational quality. For older adults, being included in and having access to community activities, social clubs, or volunteering may act as a protective factor against stressful circumstances. Despite its importance, one of the main limitations in studying community resilience is that the complexity of communities makes measuring resilient outcomes a formidable challenge. Compounding this difficulty even further is trying to tease out the nature of the relationship between individual, family, and community contributions of resilience. Likely, one's response to stressful experiences is best captured by

how these various hierarchical levels interact with one another.

In defining resilience, it is also important to note that resilience may change as a function of development and life tasks. For example, in accord with Erikson's stages of psychosocial development, different ages pose different challenges. For example, the common challenges and stresses of an 18-year-old, which may include successful identity formation, are very different from the common challenges and stresses of an 80-year-old, which may include developing integrity and seeing him- or herself as having led a meaningful life. For this reason, it is important for researchers and clinicians to look at resilience from a life-span perspective. For older adults, specifically, old age can be typified as a period of gains, losses, and accompanied by the need to maintain stability and find meaning. The challenge of old age and how old age is viewed continues to evolve. Therefore, careful attention needs to be paid to understanding the unique stressors faced by older adults and the remarkable ability for some individuals to reduce or somehow adapt to the long-term consequences of stressors. The more we can learn about the underpinnings of resilience and all of the intricacies involved in helping to define it, the more potential there is to develop interventions to promote successful aging.

RESILIENCE SCALES

With increasing attention on resilience over the past few decades, different approaches to measuring this construct have been developed. Most of the scales used to measure resilience have not been widely adopted; thus there is little evidence to inform the selection of specific instruments in research and clinical settings. Furthermore, the wide range of measures used across studies has led to inconsistencies relating to the characterization of potential risk factors, protective processes, and prevalence estimates of resilience (Windle, Bennett, & Noyes, 2011).

Windle et al. (2011) identified 15 validated measures of resilience. These instruments targeted groups across the life span; we focus on three instruments that have been used to measure resilience specifically in older adults. The Resilience Scale (Wagnild & Young, 1993) was developed using a sample of 810 community-dwelling older adults and assesses the degree of individual competence and acceptance of self and life events. The measure consists of items that were derived verbatim from interviews with participants; unfortunately, data regarding the comprehensive nature or generalizability of the items are not available. Scores greater than 145 indicate moderately high to high resilience, scores of 125–145 reflect moderately low to moderate levels of resilience, and scores of 120 and below indicate low resilience. In one study, this scale was examined in a sample of 125 Swedish people over the age of 85 years; this group reported higher resilience compared to a comparison sample of younger adults (Nygren et al., 2005). These data suggest that this measure may be appropriate for use in older adults.

The Psychological Resilience scale (Windle, Markland, & Woods, 2008) is a self-report measure that was derived in part from the Resilience Scale, using a cohort of 50–90-year-old adults in Britain. Via factor analysis, items relating to self-esteem, personal competence, and interpersonal control were selected. These three aspects are theorized to serve as protective factors against risks and adversities. In a follow-up report by the same group (Windle, Woods, & Markland, 2010) resilience, as measured by this scale, appeared to moderate the negative effects of illness on perceptions of well-being in individuals, particularly among those in the 60–90-year-age groups. This measure has received limited use in the empirical study of resilience. Additional factors, such as self-acceptance and spirituality/religion, which appear to be important elements of resilience, were not included in this measure, which is another potential limitation of the instrument.

Another commonly used measure of resilience is the Connor-Davidson Resilience Scale (CD-RISC) (Connor & Davidson, 2003). This 25-item instrument was developed as a measure of coping in stressful situations and targets five factors: personal competence, trust/tolerance/strengthening effects of stress, acceptance of change and secure relationships, control, spiritual influences. A study from our research group (Lamond et al., 2008) showed the CD-RISC is an internally consistent scale (Cronbach's alpha = .92) for assessing resilience among community-dwelling older women ($n = 1395$). It yielded four factors that reflected personal control/goal orientation, adaptation and tolerance for negative affect, leadership and trust in instincts, and spiritual coping. These factors were somewhat different from those previously reported among younger adults, which could suggest that resilience in older adults reflects a different process

than among younger adults. In older cohorts, acceptance and tolerance of negative affect versus tenacity (which appears to be important in younger individuals) may contribute to resilience. This study raises an important issue regarding the measurement of resilience: aging may be associated with alterations in the underlying factor structure of instruments. The skills, qualities, or processes of a resilient response may change with different challenges associated with different times in one's life span. This possibility has important implications for the assessment of resilience in clinical and research settings within the context of aging.

There is also a 10-item abbreviated Connor Davidson Scale that has been developed for use in research (Campbell-Sills & Stein, 2007). This abridged version contains items that reflect the ability to tolerate experiences such as change, personal problems, illness, pressure, failure, and painful feelings. This 10-item measure of resilience was the scale employed in the study from our research group described earlier, finding significant associations between resilience and self-rated successful aging among community-dwelling older adults (Jeste et al., 2013). Nonetheless, most of the studies employing this measure have focused on younger adults; additional research would be helpful in determining the relative merits of the 25-item versus 10-item version for use with older adults.

As noted by Windle et al. (2011), currently available measures of resilience insufficiently address cultural variability and its effect on resilience. Importantly, different cultures may place different values on what constitutes "successful outcomes." Extant measures of resilience also typically ignore or greatly minimize the role of communities in shaping individual resilience. This is especially true in the few measures that are applied to older adults. Another limitation of current resilience measures is that, thus far, there is no general consensus on what measure is most appropriate to use in older adults, which often leads to inconsistent results across studies. Additionally, greater efforts are needed to examine the psychometric properties of measures, including their reliability and validity. There is also a paucity of studies exploring resilience in more diverse samples of older adults, such as institutionalized older adults, which is a major growing segment of the American population. Future efforts to develop more comprehensive scales would benefit from addressing these issues.

INTERVENTIONS

To our knowledge, there are no published interventions specifically targeting resilience in older adults, but data from intervention studies to enhance resilience in adults more generally provide interesting avenues for potential therapeutic strategies for older adults (see Table 21.1). One example is well-being therapy to boost resilience (Fava & Tomba, 2009). This validated and empirically supported intervention promotes resilience by targeting dimensions of psychological well-being, such as environmental mastery (e.g., the individual has difficulty managing everyday affairs or improving surrounding context), personal growth (e.g., the individual has a sense of personal stagnation), purpose in life (e.g., the individual lacks beliefs that give life meaning), autonomy (e.g., the individual relies on the judgment of others to make important decisions), self-acceptance (e.g., the individual feels dissatisfied with self), and positive relations with others (e.g., the individual has difficulty forming and sustaining close relationships). Functioning in these domains is improved by training individuals to monitor instances of well-being, to identify thoughts and beliefs associated with premature interruption of well-being, to challenge these automatic thoughts, and to pursue activities that promote well-being. This intervention has been validated in samples with mood and anxiety disorders (Fava, Rafanelli, Cazzaro, Conti, & Grandi, 1998). Aspects of this intervention may be adapted to boost well-being and resilience in older adults; for example, individuals may be encouraged to observe when they have positive interactions with friends or family members, to facilitate acceptance of changing cognitive and health status, to improve environmental mastery by education regarding community resources, and to assist with reflecting on their life to discover and appreciate their accomplishments.

Padesky and Mooney (2012) describe a four-step Strengths-Based Cognitive Behavioral Therapy Model designed to strengthen resilience. The four steps to resilience include (1) a search for strengths, (2) construction of a personal model of resilience, (3) applying the personal model of resilience to areas of life difficulties, and (4) practicing resilience. Specifically, in this treatment approach, therapists help teach individuals how to search for areas of competence, such as good health, positive relationships with others, self-efficacy, emotion-regulation skills, and the belief that one's life has meaning. The purpose of this search is based on the notion that individuals are already resilient in some areas of their lives, yet often are unaware of their strengths. Using the individual's own strengths, a personal model of resilience is created, which may then be used by the individual in a variety of situations, including challenging settings. This intervention also appears to be amenable for use with older adults, although it has not yet been validated with this population.

There is also growing interest in positive interventions that increase happiness and other positive psychosocial factors through pleasure, engagement, and/or meaning (Parks et al., 2015). These are salient to resilience, and many of these interventions may have some benefit in the efforts to boost resilience in a range of populations, including older adults. These positive interventions often target a variety of skills, such as maintaining a present focus and attending to the positive aspects of an experience. Individuals may also be trained in loving-kindness meditation and gratitude as a way to promote social support and life satisfaction. Goal setting, reminiscing about positive experiences, and increasing engagement in rewarding activities also appear to promote happiness. Although the utility of these interventions in strengthening resilience in older adults is unknown, they may provide potentially useful avenues to explore.

That resilience skills can be taught, sustained, and enhanced is highlighted by the US Army's Master Resilience Trainer (MRT) course (Reivich, Seligman, & McBride, 2011). Through a 10-day course, army officers are taught to build resilience by improving self-awareness of one's thoughts, emotions, and behaviors, regulating impulses, thoughts, or behaviors to attain goals, practicing optimism, identifying strengths in oneself and others, and promoting strong interpersonal relationships through effective communication and willingness to ask for and offer help. Participants are taught to identify when others are experiencing challenges to their resilience and how the MRT skills may be adapted across challenging settings, thus facilitating the maintenance of these skills over time. Additional techniques, such as goal setting, confidence building, and energy management, are used to enhance these skills and promote mastery. An interesting aspect of this program is that it was designed for delivery in a large-group setting with breakout-group training. This suggests the possibility of adapting such a group-based program for civilian community settings to promote individual and group resilience.

Table 21.1. Descriptions of Interventions Designed to Enhance Resilience

NAME OF INTERVENTION	AUTHORS AND YEAR	POPULATION TARGETED	BRIEF DESCRIPTION	SESSIONS	GOAL OF INTERVENTION
Well-Being Therapy	Fava & Tomba (2009)	Patients with mood and anxiety disorders	This is a structured, directive, individualized short-term therapy that extends over 8–12 sessions.	*Initial sessions:* Focus on identifying positive experiences through the use of a diary. *Intermediate sessions:* Encourage the patient to identify thoughts and beliefs leading to premature interruption of well-being. *Final sessions:* Patient is expected to be able to identify moments of well-being, to be aware of interruptions to well-being feelings, and to pursue optimal experiences.	The promotion of resilience and psychological well-being
Strengths-Based Cognitive Behavioral Therapy	Padesky & Mooney (2012)	Can be applied to a wide range of populations, including patients with depression and anxiety disorders, chronic pain, and sleep disorders	Highly collaborative and empirical therapy. The therapist engages the patient so that each step of therapy is a mutual construction and exploration. Patients rely on their own observations of their experience and test their personal resilience model by setting up real-world behavioral experiments.	Four steps to resilience: (1) Search for hidden strengths within everyday experiences; (2) use existing strengths to construct a personal model of resilience which includes metaphors and images; (3) apply the personal model of resilience to areas of life difficulty; (4) practice by designing behavioral experiments and making resilience predictions.	Designed to help patients build positive qualities and strengthen personal resilience

Program	Citation	Population	Description	Goal
Army's Master Resilience Trainer Course	Reivich, Seligman, & McBride (2011)	Sergeants and soldiers	10-day course to teach non-commissioned officers a set of skills and techniques that build resilience so that they, in turn, can teach other soldiers.	The course teaches three components: (1) *Preparation*: Focuses on defining resilience, building mental toughness (through concepts such as problem-solving and minimizing catastrophic thinking), identifying top character strengths, and strengthening relationships among and between soldiers and their family members; (2) *Sustainment*: Focuses on familiarizing soldiers with what to expect in terms of psychological demands and reactions at various points of the deployment cycle; (3) *Enhancement*: Teaches mental skills foundations, how to build confidence, goal setting, attention control, energy management, and mental imagery.	Increase resilience to enhance soldiers' ability to handle adversity, prevent depression and anxiety, prevent PTSD, and enhance overall well-being and performance
Stress Management and Resiliency Training (SMART)	Loprinzi, Prasad, Schroeder, & Sood (2011)	Women diagnosed with breast cancer	Adapted from Attention and Interpretation Therapy. Program consists of two 90-minute group training sessions, an optional brief individual session, and three follow-up telephone calls.	*Group sessions*: Patients learn structured relaxation (diaphragmatic breathing) and how to delay judgment and direct their attention away from fixed prejudices toward more flexible thinking. In addition, patients cultivate skills such as gratitude, compassion, acceptance, forgiveness, and higher meaning and purpose. *Individual sessions*: Optional one-on-one 30–60-minute follow-up session with a physician to review learned information. *Telephone Calls*: Follow-up calls from the investigator at 4-week intervals to remind the patients to practice and to answer any questions the patients have regarding the intervention.	Designed to improve resilience and quality of life, and reduce perceived stress and anxiety

In a cohort of middle-aged and older women with breast cancer, Loprinzi et al. (2011) demonstrated the possible efficacy of the Stress Management and Resiliency Training (SMART) program in increasing resiliency and overall quality of life. In this intervention, participants attended two 90-minute group sessions in which they were taught relaxation skills, as well as techniques to delay judgment and attend to novel aspects of the environment rather than one's thoughts. Participants also learned to adopt a flexible disposition and to practice gratitude, compassion, and acceptance. The authors found that relative to the wait-list control group, women who received the SMART intervention reported improved resilience as well as quality of life, and reductions in anxiety, stress, and fatigue. The evidence of the feasibility of such a brief intervention is promising in the context of adapting a resilience-training program for older adults.

SUGGESTIONS FOR FUTURE RESEARCH

Although there have been multiple efforts to characterize resilience and develop interventions to boost resilience, there are notable limitations that may be targeted by future research. At present, there is no independent gold standard of resilience, which is required when developing and testing new measures of this construct. The available measures of resilience rely on self-report, which may be susceptible to social desirability bias.

Future work with resilience in older adults will benefit from better understanding of the underlying neurobiologic parameters. For example, in their review of relevant literature, Charney et al. (2004) suggested that severe recurrent mood disorders may be associated with decreased neuroplasticity and cellular resilience, and that development of medications to attenuate maladaptive stress responses may prove helpful in enhancing plasticity and cellular resilience. Another aspect of resilience that appears to improve with age is the construct of wisdom, which neurobiologically appears to be related to functioning in the prefrontal cortex and limbic striatum (Jeste & Harris, 2010; Meeks & Jeste, 2009). Yet another potential component of resilience in late life may be the maintenance of intact cognitive functioning. In part, such maintenance may reflect what has been labeled "brain reserve" or "cognitive reserve" (e.g., Satz, Cole, Hardy, & Rassovsky, 2011; Steffener & Stern, 2012). For example, in a 9-year follow-up study of healthy septuagenarians in the Health, Aging, and Body Composition (Health ABC) study, Rosano et al. (2012) found that maintenance of cognitive functioning was associated with greater medial temporal gray matter volume, and lower microstructure diffusivity in the cingulate cortex. In another recent report of data from the Health ABC study, Kaup et al. (2015) examined cognitive resilience over 1 to 11 years among 670 participants with the apolipoprotein ε4 allele (APOE ε4). Within this sample, cognitive resilience was found to be significantly associated with older age, higher education and literacy, more reading time, absence of diabetes mellitus and/or obesity, and absence of negative life events in the preceding year. Such findings are important in demonstrating that even among those genetically at risk for cognitive decline, cognitive resilience and/or neuroplasticity may be fostered by some potentially modifiable health and lifestyle factors.

In older adults, resilience appears to share variance with personality traits such as optimism (Lamond, et al., 2008). However, data from younger age groups suggest that resilience may be associated with adaptive coping mechanisms in response to particular stressors. Within older cohorts the characterization of the construct of resilience (i.e., whether it is related to positive attitudes or specific coping methods) warrants empirical attention. Furthermore, longitudinal research methods will be needed to examine whether the nature of resilience changes as older adults age. Similarly, the association of this construct with long-term health outcomes also remains to be fully examined.

Also related to the issue of neurocognitive resilience among the elderly, there is some emerging evidence that physical exercise may be associated with later onset or reduced age-related cognitive decline or neurodegenerative disorders (Ahlskog, Geda, Graff-Radford, & Petersen, 2011; Meeusen, 2014), but further prospective research is needed to determine the degree to which exercise has clinically significant neuroprotective effects at the individual patient level (Kirk-Sanchez & McGough, 2014), as well as the precise neurobiological mechanisms of such protective effects (Phillips, Baktir, Srivatsan, & Salehi, 2014; Zigmond & Smeyne, 2014). Related avenues for future research include the potential neuroprotective value of good sleep hygiene (Sexton, Storsve, Walhovd, Johansen-Berg, & Fjell, 2014). There is also some reason to think that antidepressant medications could have neuroprotective benefits among older adults with depression (Castren, 2004; Young, 2002), but the latter is also a possibility warranting further prospective research before firm conclusions for clinical practice can be drawn.

There is some evidence suggesting gene–environment interactions and their impact on behavioral outcomes in animals (Francis, Mellem, & Maricq, 2003) and humans (Rutter, Moffitt, & Caspi, 2006). These data indicate that a particular set of genes may have a beneficial effect by protecting the individual from "bad" environments; another possible interpretation is that "good" environments mitigate the effect of "bad" genes. There is need to examine these gene–environment interactions in the context of resilience. Few studies have examined the relationship between genes and resilience in older adults (Moore et al., 2015). Data from our research group suggests that positive psychological traits such as optimism and resilience may be associated with selected single-nucleotide polymorphisms in *MAOA*, *IL-10*, and *FGG* genes (Rana et al., 2014). These preliminary findings warrant replication with larger sample sizes and additional methods such as pathway-based analyses, sequence-based association studies, and copy number variation analyses, as this would provide a better understanding of the complex relationship between genes and positive psychological traits.

As efforts to better characterize and assess the construct of resilience in older adults evolve, attention to intervention approaches is also necessary. As noted earlier, there are no empirically supported interventions specifically designed to increase resilience in older adults. Evidence from resilience interventions in younger cohorts and interventions to reduce loneliness in older adults (Winningham & Pike, 2007) suggest important targets for future research. For example, it is likely that concepts such as identifying areas of competence and planning how to use these strengths during challenging situations may be useful for older adults. However, the application of these methods may need modification based on the cognitive and health status of the individual. Furthermore, the nature of challenging situations and available competencies may dramatically change as the individual ages, necessitating revision of the individual's personal resilience model (Padesky & Mooney, 2012). In their study of an intervention to target loneliness in older adults

living in an assisted-living facility, Winningham and Pike (2007) found that loneliness may dramatically increase and social support decrease without intervention. It is possible that this decline may apply to resilience as well, and future interventions may develop methods to maintain positive psychological traits in older adults living in retirement or assisted-living facilities.

Efforts to build future interventions for resilience should consider longitudinal change in the cognitive and health status of older adults and the effect of these factors on learning and executing skills to promote resilience. For example, the development of autonomy, which is often central to some resilience interventions, may or may not generalize across diverse groups of older adults.

Future interventions may also strive to promote the enhancement of both internal resources (e.g., effective coping strategies, enhanced self-efficacy) and external resources (e.g., increased social support) that may help offset stress exposure. Internal resources may be enhanced via coaching, modeling of positive responses, or group therapy support. External resources may be increased through interventions that reduce loneliness and social isolation and help to build social skills. Interventions used to foster volunteering or helping also hold promise in enhancing resilience as the value of helpful engagement has been tied to successful aging (Kahana & Force, 2008) and enhanced quality of life and well-being (Carr & Moorman, 2011; Cornwell, 2011). Additional strategies found on the APA website to help foster resilience include, but are not limited to, accepting that change is a part of living, developing and moving toward realistic goals, looking for opportunities for self-discovery, participating in activities that bring enjoyment and relaxation, and engaging in meditation and spiritual practices (APA, 2015).

In addition, future interventions should account for the fact that there are different types of interacting resilience systems. In other words, individuals comprise families, and families comprise communities. These three hierarchical levels are not mutually exclusive, and interventions that target any one of these domains will inevitably impact resilience functioning at the other levels. Therefore, experts working together from a broad range of disciplines may be the most effective at deciding what specific level would be most appropriate for intervention in order to produce the greatest amount of change.

SUMMARY

In sum, with the advancement of modern medicine, people are living longer than ever before. With advancing age comes more opportunity to be exposed to various types of stressors. Despite this increase in frequency to stressors, however, some older adults are astonishingly successful at being able to adapt, respond to, and recover from stressful experiences. One of the main goals of a positive psychiatry of aging should be to try to help elucidate some of the mechanisms that help distinguish older individuals who seem to demonstrate higher levels of resilience from those who do not (Jeste & Palmer, 2013).

This chapter was written in an effort to help shed light on the critical role of resilience on successful aging. To this effect, we have provided various proposed definitions of resilience and have reviewed the difficulty surrounding the creation of a universally accepted model. Further refinement of a universal definition is a necessary step in order to make significant progress in the area of resilience research. Researchers should be confident that they are speaking the same language and that the results from one study of resilience are generalizable and can be used to help inform the results of a separate study of resilience. We also have discussed individual, familial, and community aspects of resilience and have noted the importance of acknowledging how these three dynamic systems interact with one another. We further have highlighted how older adults face very different challenges from those of younger adults and have provided a rationale for the importance of evaluating resilience across the life span.

In our review of resilience measures commonly used in older adults, we found several inherent limitations. Such limitations included lack of cultural sensitivity, insufficiently reported psychometric properties, and failure to use these measures in more diverse samples of older adults (e.g., older adults living in assisted-living facilities). Figuring out ways to circumvent some of these limitations by either strengthening existing measures or developing new reliable and valid measures to assess resilience in older adults should be a priority for researchers interested in this area.

A main focus of this chapter was also to review interventions that target ways to enhance resilience, as well as to provide suggestions for future research. Although there were several interventions that were shown to be effective in enhancing resilience, none of them primarily focused on older adults. This major gap in resilience research provides an important opportunity for further investigation. New innovative interventions can play a very important role in facilitating successful aging by reducing the impact of stress exposure in late life. We expect that, over time, resilience definitions, measures, and interventions will continue to improve, providing a welcome addition to the field as well as a great benefit to older adults.

DISCLOSURE STATEMENT

The authors have no conflicts of interest to declare.

REFERENCES

Ahlskog, J. E., Geda, Y. E., Graff-Radford, N. R., & Petersen, R. C. (2011). Physical exercise as a preventive or disease-modifying treatment of dementia and brain aging. *Mayo Clin Proc, 86*(9), 876–884.

American Psychological Association. (2015). The road to resilience. Retrieved April 3, 2015, from http://www.apa.org/helpcenter/road-resilience.aspx.

Black, K., & Lobo, M. (2008). A conceptual review of family resilience factors. *J Fam Nurs, 14*(1), 33–55.

Campbell-Sills, L., & Stein, M. B. (2007). Psychometric analysis and refinement of the Connor-Davidson Resilience Scale (CD-RISC): Validation of a 10-item measure of resilience. *J Trauma Stress, 20*(6), 1019–1028.

Carr, D. C., & Moorman, S. M. (2011). Social relations and aging. In R. A. Settersten & J. L. Angel (Eds.), *Handbook of sociology of aging* (pp. 145–160). New York: Springer.

Castren, E. (2004). Neurotrophic effects of antidepressant drugs. *Curr Opin Pharmacol, 4*(1), 58–64.

Charney, D. S., Dejesus, G., & Manji, H. K. (2004). Cellular plasticity and resilience and the pathophysiology of severe mood disorders. *Dialogues Clin Neurosci, 6*(2), 217–225.

Chodosh, J., Kado, D. M., Seeman, T. E., & Karlamangla, A. S. (2007). Depressive symptoms as a predictor of cognitive decline: MacArthur studies of successful aging. *Am J Geriatr Psychiatry, 15*(5), 406–415.

Connor, K. M., & Davidson, J. R. (2003). Development of a new resilience scale: The Connor-Davidson Resilience Scale (CD-RISC). *Depress Anxiety, 18*(2), 76–82.

Cornwell, B. (2011). Independence through social networks: bridging potential among older women and men. *J Gerontol B, 66B*(6), 782–794.

Fava, G. A., Rafanelli, C., Cazzaro, M., Conti, S., & Grandi, S. (1998). Well-being therapy: a novel psychotherapeutic approach for residual symptoms of affective disorders. *Psychol Med, 28*(2), 475–480.

Fava, G. A., & Tomba, E. (2009). Increasing psychological well-being and resilience by psychotherapeutic methods. *J Pers, 77*(6), 1903–1934.

Francis, M. M., Mellem, J. E., & Maricq, A. V. (2003). Bridging the gap between genes and behavior: recent advances in the electrophysiological analysis of neural function in caenorhabditis elegans. *Trends Neurosci, 26*(2), 90–99.

Hildon, Z., Montgomery, S. M., Blane, D., Wiggins, R. D., & Netuveli, G. (2010). Examining resilience of quality of life in the face of health-related and psychosocial adversity at older ages: what is "right" about the way we age? *Gerontologist, 50*(1), 36–47.

Jeste, D. V., & Harris, J. C. (2010). Wisdom: a neuroscience perspective. *JAMA, 304*(14), 1602–1603.

Jeste, D. V., & Palmer, B. W. (2013). A call for a new positive psychiatry of ageing. *Br J Psychiatry, 202*(2), 81–83.

Jeste, D. V., & Palmer, B. W. (2015). Introduction: what is positive psychiatry? In D. V. Jeste & B. W. Palmer (Eds.), *Positive psychiatry: a clinical handbook* (pp. 1–16). Arlington, VA: American Psychiatric Press.

Jeste, D. V., Palmer, B. W., Rettew, D. C., & Boardman, S. (2015). Positive psychiatry: its time has come. *J Clin Psychiatry, 76*(6) 675–683.

Jeste, D. V., Savla, G. N., Thompson, W. K., Vahia, I. V., Glorioso, D. K., Martin, A. S., . . . Depp, C. A. (2013). Association between older age and more successful aging: critical role of resilience and depression. *Am J Psychiatry, 170*(2), 188–196.

Kahana, J., & Force, L. T. (2008). Toward inclusion: a public-centered approach to promote civic engagement by the elderly. *Public Policy Aging Rep, 18*(3), 30–35.

Kaup, A. R., Nettiksimmons, J., Harris, T. B., Sink, K. M., Satterfield, S., Metti, A. L., . . . Yaffe, K. (2015). Cognitive resilience to apolipoprotein e epsilon4: Contributing factors in black and white older adults. *JAMA Neurol., 72*(3), 340–348.

Kirk-Sanchez, N. J., & McGough, E. L. (2014). Physical exercise and cognitive performance in the elderly: current perspectives. *Clin Interv Aging, 9*, 51–62.

Lamond, A. J., Depp, C. A., Allison, M., Langer, R., Reichstadt, J., Moore, D. J., . . . Jeste, D. V. (2008). Measurement and predictors of resilience among community-dwelling older women. *J Psychiatr Res, 43*(2), 148–154.

Langdon, P. (1997). *A better place to live: reshaping the american suburb.* Amherst: University of Massachusetts Press.

Lavretsky, H. (2014). *Resilience and aging: research and practice.* Balitmore, MD: Johns Hopkins University Press.

Loprinzi, C. E., Prasad, K., Schroeder, D. R., & Sood, A. (2011). Stress management and resilience training (smart) program to decrease stress and enhance resilience among breast cancer survivors: a pilot randomized clinical trial. *Clin Breast Cancer, 11*(6), 364–368.

Manning, L. K., Carr, D. C., & Kail, B. L. (2014). Do higher levels of resilience buffer the deleterious impact of chronic illness on disability in later life? *The Gerontologist, 00*, 1–12.

Martin, A. S., Distelberg, B. J., & Elahad, J. A. (2015). The relationship between family resilience and aging successfully. *Am J Fam Ther, 43*(2), 163–179.

Masten, A. S., & Tellegen, A. (2012). Resilience in developmental psychopathology: Contributions of the project competence longitudinal study. *Dev Psychopathol., 24*(02), 345–361.

Meeks, T. W., & Jeste, D. V. (2009). Neurobiology of wisdom: a literature overview. *Arch Gen Psychiatry, 66*(4), 355–365.

Meeusen, R. (2014). Exercise, nutrition and the brain. *Sports Med, 44*(Suppl 1), S47–S56.

Montross, L. P., Depp, C. A., Daly, J., Reichstadt, J., Golshan, S., Moore, D. J., . . . Jeste, D. V. (2006). Correlates of self-rated successful aging among community-dwelling older adults. *Am J Geriatr Psychiatry, 14*(1), 43–51.

Moore, R. C., Eyler, L. T., Mills, P. J., O'Hara, R. M., Wachman, K., & Lavretsky, H. (2015). Biology of positive psychiatry. In D. V. Jeste & B. W. Palmer (Eds.), *Positive psychiatry: a clinical handbook* (pp. 261-283). Arlington, VA: American Psychiatric Press.

Moore, R. C., Martin, A. S., Kaup, A. R., Thompson, W. K., Peters, M. E., Jeste, D. V., . . . Eyler, L. T. (2015). From suffering to caring: a model of differences among older adults in levels of compassion. *Int J Geriatr Psychiatry, 30*(2), 185–191.

Nygren, B., Alex, L., Jonsen, E., Gustafson, Y., Norberg, A., & Lundman, B. (2005). Resilience, sense of coherence, purpose in life and self-transcendence in relation to perceived physical and mental health among the oldest old. *Aging Ment Health, 9*(4), 354–362.

Padesky, C. A., & Mooney, K. A. (2012). Strengths-based cognitive-behavioural therapy: a four-step model to build resilience. *Clin Psychol Psychother, 19*(4), 283–290.

Parks, A. C., Kleiman, E. M., Kashdan, T. B., Hausmann, L. R. M., Meyer, P. S., Day, A. M., . . . Kahler, C. W. (2015). Positive psychotherapeutic and behavioral interventions. In D. V. Jeste & B. W. Palmer (Eds.), *Positive psychiatry: a clinical handbook* (pp. 147–165). Arlington, VA: American Psychiatric Press.

Phillips, C., Baktir, M. A., Srivatsan, M., & Salehi, A. (2014). Neuroprotective effects of physical activity on the brain: a closer look at trophic factor signaling. *Front Cell Neurosci, 8*, 170.

Rana, B. K., Darst, B. F., Bloss, C., Shih, P. A., Depp, C., Nievergelt, C. M., . . . Jeste, D. V. (2014). Candidate SNP associations of optimism and resilience in older adults: exploratory study of 935 community-dwelling adults. *Am J Geriatr Psychiatry, 22*(10), 997–1006.

Reivich, K. J., Seligman, M. E., & McBride, S. (2011). Master resilience training in the U.S. Army. *Am Psychol, 66*(1), 25–34.

Rosano, C., Aizenstein, H. J., Newman, A. B., Venkatraman, V., Harris, T., Ding, J., . . . Yaffe, K. (2012). Neuroimaging differences between older adults with maintained versus declining cognition over a 10-year period. *Neuroimage, 62*(1), 307–313.

Rutter, M., Moffitt, T. E., & Caspi, A. (2006). Gene-environment interplay and psychopathology: Multiple varieties but real effects. *J Child Psychol Psychiatry, 47*(3–4), 226–261.

Satz, P., Cole, M. A., Hardy, D. J., & Rassovsky, Y. (2011). Brain and cognitive reserve: Mediator(s) and construct validity, a critique. *J Clin Exp Neuropsychol, 33*(1), 121–130.

Sexton, C. E., Storsve, A. B., Walhovd, K. B., Johansen-Berg, H., & Fjell, A. M. (2014). Poor sleep quality is associated with increased cortical atrophy in community-dwelling adults. *Neurology, 83*(11), 967–973.

Steffener, J., & Stern, Y. (2012). Exploring the neural basis of cognitive reserve in aging. *Biochim Biophys Acta, 1822*(3), 467–473.

Stewart, D. E., & Yuen, T. (2011). A systematic review of resilience in the physically ill. *Psychosomatics, 52*(3), 199–209.

Vaillant, G. E. (2015). Resilience and post-traumatic growth. In D. V. Jeste & B. W. Palmer (Eds.), *Positive psychiatry: a clinical handbook* (pp. 45–70). Arlington, VA: American Psychiatric Press.

Vincent, G. K., & Velkoff, V. A. (2010). The next four decades the older population in the United States: 2010 to 2050. *Current Population Reports* (May 2010), 1–14. Retrieved from http://www.census.gov/prod/2010pubs/p25-1138.pdf.

Wagnild, G. M., & Young, H. M. (1993). Development and psychometric evaluation of the resilience scale. *J Nurs Meas, 1*(2), 165–178.

Wiener, J. M., & Tilly, J. (2002). Population ageing in the United States of America: implications for public programmes. *Int J Epidemiol, 31*(4), 776–781.

Windle, G., Bennett, K. M., & Noyes, J. (2011). A methodological review of resilience measurement scales. *Health Qual Life Outcomes, 9*(8), 1–18.

Windle, G., Markland, D. A., & Woods, R. T. (2008). Examination of a theoretical model of psychological resilience in older age. *Aging Ment Health, 12*(3), 285–292.

Windle, G., Woods, R. T., & Markland, D. A. (2010). Living with ill-health in older age: the role of a resilient personality. *J Happiness Stud, 11*, 763–777.

Winningham, R., & Pike, N. (2007). A cognitive intervention to enhance institutionalized older adults' social support networks and decrease loneliness. *Aging Ment Health, 11*(6), 716–721.

Young, L. T. (2002). Neuroprotective effects of antidepressant and mood stabilizing drugs. *J Psychiatry Neurosci, 27*(1), 8–9.

Zeng, Y., & Shen, K. (2010). Resilience significantly contributes to exceptional longevity. *Curr Gerontol Geriatr Res, 2010*, 525693. Retrieved from doi:10.1155/2010/525693.

Zigmond, M. J., & Smeyne, R. J. (2014). Exercise: is it a neuroprotective and if so, how does it work? *Parkinsonism Relat Disord, 20*(Suppl 1), S123–S127.

PART IV

INTEGRATIVE INTERVENTIONS OF COGNITIVE AGING AND LATER LIFE MENTAL DISORDERS

SECTION A

COGNITIVE AGING, DEMENTIA PREVENTION, AND INTEGRATIVE THERAPIES

22

MEMORY TRAINING AND AGING

Karen J. Miller, John Geirland, Megan E. Gomez, Richelin V. Dye and Linda M. Ercoli

AGING HAS been associated with cognitive decline, including changes in executive functioning, processing speed, and memory (Park et al., 2002; Salthouse, 2009). Early neuronal studies of the brain appeared to show that aging is also correlated with widespread neuronal loss, leading researchers to believe that there was no neurogenesis in the aging brain, and that nothing could be done to reverse or slow cognitive decline associated with age. However, with better techniques and methodologies, and converging evidence from animal and human studies, we began to learn that neurogenesis can indeed occur in the brain throughout the life span (Fuchs & Flugge, 2014), and that although regional neuronal loss occurs with age, large-scale and severe neuronal loss is not a feature of normal aging (Epp, Barker, & Galea, 2009; Myczek, Yeung, Castello, Baglietto-Vargas, & LaFerla, 2014; Yeung et al., 2014). The apparently enduring neuroplasticity of the brain suggests the potential for older adults to continue to benefit from training and learning experiences. Thus, the impact of cognitive

exercises as a means of mitigating cognitive decline in the aging brain has become a topic of great interest to both consumers and researchers.

In this chapter we will present an overview of cognitive training, including classroom-based programs, peer-led courses, computerized brain fitness tools, and applications (apps) for smartphones. We will also discuss the relevance of these programs for various populations, including normal aging, mild cognitive impairment (MCI), and persons with dementia (e.g., Alzheimer's disease [AD]), along with the transferability and long-term impact of these training modalities.

TYPES OF COGNITIVE INTERVENTIONS

Interventions aimed at improving cognitive abilities can generally be organized into three approaches: *cognitive or mental stimulation, cognitive rehabilitation,* and *cognitive training* (Clare & Woods, 2009). Cognitive stimulation engages the individual in activities that are enlivening in order to arouse general brain activity for individuals with dementia, and may be used as a control condition in cognitive training research studies. Cognitive stimulation may include activities such as listening to music, having a discussion, learning something new, playing video or word games or chess, or doing crossword puzzles or Sudoku.

Cognitive rehabilitation is designed for patients with a specific neurological disorder (e.g., stroke, brain injury). Cognitive rehabilitation is an individualized intervention that first identifies personally relevant functional goals in day-to-day living, and then develops strategies that enhance those functional tasks and activities of daily living (Clare & Woods, 2009; Wilson, 2002). Cognitive rehabilitation may entail the use of computerized attention training, behaviorally based techniques to promote self-monitoring and task completion (e.g., checklists, self-instructional training), and strategies to promote new learning and retrieval by minimizing errors while learning (errorless learning) and increasing retention intervals (spaced retrieval).

In this chapter, we focus on cognitive training, which involves learning and practicing strategies to improve specific cognitive functions, such as memory, attention, or problem-solving. These programs are often referred to as "memory training" or "brain fitness." Broadly speaking, cognitive training has been administered to both the young and old, and to cognitively intact as well as impaired populations. The target populations are typically those with cognitive changes or complaints related to normal aging. Given the efficacy of cognitive training in healthy older adults (Martin, Clare, Altgassen, Cameron, & Zehnder, 2011; Verhaeghen, Marcoen, & Goossens, 1992), more recent studies have included individuals with mild cognitive impairment (MCI). Although some studies have explored the use of cognitive training for individuals with dementia (Bahar-Fuchs, Clare, & Woods, 2013), for the most part cognitive training has limited benefits for dementia patients. Later in this chapter we will discuss the efficacy of cognitive training for individuals with various degrees of cognitive decline.

The goal of cognitive training is to maintain or improve cognition by teaching skills and strategies in a standardized and structured format to individuals or small groups (Belleville, Chertkow, & Gauthier, 2007). More recently, computerized training approaches have been developed (Clare & Woods, 2009).

Memory Training in Classroom Instruction with Small Groups

Cognitive training in a classroom instruction setting, which is often referred to as memory training programs (MTPs), have existed decades before the advent of the digital industry boom. Presently, MTP instruction is still an efficient and convenient way to offer memory training, particularly for older adults, many of whom enjoy the social aspects of a classroom setting and may not be computer savvy. A trained professional (e.g., a psychologist or social worker) usually leads MTPs at a clinic or community center. MTPs are typically delivered in small group formats, based on the assumption that objective and subjective memory might be improved by training in a group versus individual format (Kelly et al., 2014a). MTPs typically vary in duration and frequency of sessions, and at times might comprise as little as one hour of instruction (Mahncke, Connor, & Appelman, 2006; Verhaeghen et al., 1992; Zarit, Zarit, & Reever, 1982). MTPs are often multifactorial in design (Stigsdotter, 2000), meaning that they address both cognitive (memory, attention, problem-solving, reasoning) and non-cognitive factors (self-efficacy, expectations, anxiety, and general education about memory) that contribute to overall memory functioning (Floyd & Scogin, 1997; Verhaeghen et al., 1992; West, Bagwell, & Dark-Freudeman, 2008). MTPs usually target functions that are primarily subserved by the declarative memory system, which involves the conscious recollection of information, such as facts (semantic memory), and experienced events linked to time and place (episodic memory; Tulving, 1983). Daily life examples of declarative memory include autobiographical information and remembering people, object placements (e.g., keys, glasses), appointments, errands, shopping lists, and more. MTPs teach techniques, usually called *mnemonics*, that have been specifically developed to improve the encoding or learning of new information and to facilitate recall (Gross & Rebok, 2011; Verhaeghen et al., 1992) through the use of imagery and association. These techniques vary with respect to complexity, structure, and application (Gross, Manly, & Pa, 2012). *Mnemonic strategies* are usually part of the core curriculum in MTPs (DeVreese, Mirco, Fioravanti, Belloi, & Zanetti, 2001; Logan & Balota, 2008).

Mnemonic strategies facilitate encoding and aid retrieval by enhancing the meaningfulness or personal relevance of information (Yesavage, 1983). Specific strategies include (1) *verbal organization* (e.g., forming acronyms), (2) *semantic clustering* (grouping a list of to-be-remembered items into clusters or subgroups of items that share something in common), (3) *elaboration* (creating a story linking all target words on a list), and (4) *visual imagery* (creating a mental picture of what is to be remembered) (Kessels & DeHaan, 2003; McCarty, 1980; Sohlberg & Mateer, 2001; Yesavage, 1983). Two well-researched and common mnemonic strategies include the method of loci and the face–name association method. The *method of loci* (aka "memory palace," "Roman room," or "journey method") was first used by Roman orators to remember long speeches (Foer, 2011). The method of loci (Yesavage, Sheikh, Friedman, & Tanke, 1990) is used to remember items in a specific order. The technique involves visualizing a familiar path and identifying unique landmarks along the path. For instance, the familiar path can be a mental walk through one's home, and the landmarks can be articles of furniture or other objects in each room. Next, the to-be-remembered items, such as items on a shopping list, are associated with each of the landmarks along the path using visual imagery. To recall the items on the list, one needs only to take a mental "walk" along the familiar path and recall each image associated with each landmark, which then cues recall of each item. The path should always be remembered in the same order, since this will facilitate recalling items in order. Another mnemonic strategy is the *face–name association* technique (McCarty, 1980), which is a visual associative strategy used to learn and recall a person's face and name. The strategy involves three steps: (1) looking at a person's face and identifying a prominent feature, (2) transforming the person's name into something meaningful, and (3) developing a visual image associating the prominent facial feature with the transformed name. For instance, Mr. Coly may have prominent dark eyes, therefore, his name can be transformed to "coal" and he can be imagined as having two large coal briquettes for eyes.

Peer-Led MTPs and Other Exportable Memory Training Programs

Although many MTPs have been tested in the laboratory, few programs have led to widespread and affordable cognitive training applications in the community until recently. Within the last decade,

MTPs have become more exportable and available due to standardizing curriculums and training allied healthcare professionals or community peers to implement such programs. Specifically, peer-led educational programs are MTPs that are taught to community-residing adults by their peers. These programs can be more affordable to administer and can reach a broader audience. Often, peers have good credibility, and can be role models that people can relate to for changing lifestyles. Thus, many peer-led programs have been created to address health behaviors and promote wellness. These programs have addressed alcohol consumption, breast cancer awareness, and diabetes self-management. The same strategies for peer-led programs directed at improving health behaviors can be applied to promoting memory health.

Our group at UCLA developed a unique 5-week, peer-led community education/intervention program to improve memory functioning in older adults with age-related memory changes. The impetus for this program was recognition of the need to bring cognitive training to a wider audience and into the community. The peer-led MTP involves training community volunteers to use a scripted, standardized curriculum to teach memory strategies to community-residing older adults, thus increasing its portability and access to a larger number of older adults. The peer-led MTP is paced comfortably for individuals 60 and older and addresses normal aging memory complaints, and is not aimed at individuals with more significant memory difficulties, such as dementia (Ercoli, Cernin, & Small, 2011). Peer-trainers present the curriculum, model the memory-enhancement techniques, help with in-class exercises, and praise both effort and excellence. Each of the five sessions includes two or three mnemonic techniques (e.g., verbal associations, visual imagery, and organizational strategies), pair-wise and group classroom exercises, and home practice exercises (see Table 22.1 for a list of exercises).

This program led to other exportable memory education programs, both peer-led and individualized. For instance, our group developed a 14-day healthy lifestyle program that involved a schedule of memory-training exercises, healthy diet suggestions, relaxation exercises, and light cardiovascular exercise. Individuals (middle-aged and older adults) who were randomly assigned to the healthy lifestyle program showed immediate benefits on recall, as

Table 22.1. Specific Mnemonic Techniques

TECHNIQUE	DESCRIPTION
Categorization	Breaking down or "chunking" of items into smaller subgroups
Look-Snap-Connect	Attention, visualization, and association techniques (Small, 2003)
Sentence and Link Methods	Creating sentences to remember short lists and creating stories to remember longer lists
Faces and Names	3-step method that requires (1) paying attention to a face, (2) forming an association with the face and name, and (3) linking the face and name using an image (McCarty, 1980)
Numbers and Months	Participants learn associations for remembering numbers and months.
Organizational Strategies	Tips/Discussion on practical memory aids (e.g., written and auditory reminders, "memory places")
Memory-Impacting Factors	Lifestyle, health-related variables, distraction, multitasking, stress, and anxiety

well as a change in brain metabolism, compared to the "usual lifestyle" group (Small, Silverman, Siddarth, Ercoli, Miller, Wright, Bookheimer, Barrio, & Phelps, 2006). Based on these findings, we developed a 6-week (12 sessions) curriculum for older adults living in assisted-living communities. We tested the program in a sample of 115 older adults who were randomly assigned to a treatment (classroom instruction in memory enhancement, stress reduction, tips for improving nutrition) or a wait-list control group (Miller, Siddarth, Gaines, Parrish, Marx, Ronch, Pilgram, Burke, Barczak, Bacock, and Small, 2011). The treatment group exhibited improvement in both subjective and objective memory, including fewer memory concerns and better performance on immediate and delayed recall measures compared to controls.

Given the many older adults experiencing age-related memory decline and the potential benefits of the intervention, the impact of peer-led and exportable memory training programs can be considerable. To date, the UCLA Longevity Center (www.semel.ucla.edu/longevity) has facilitated the implementation of these memory-training programs in a variety of venues (e.g., senior centers, hospitals, assisted-living homes, academic institutions) across 14 states, with more than 4,000 individuals completing at least one course. Currently,

the Alzheimer's Association offers other peer-led programs.

Computerized Brain Fitness

The digital age has changed the landscape of health care, and now the military, governments, and educators are using the modern approach of computer-based games. This electronic format offers a personalized approach to cognitive training based on the functionality of the gamer or patient. Computer-based games can be organized by the platform or delivery system of the game (i.e., video console, personal computer, online game, virtual worlds, and alternate reality games) and tailored for specific behavioral and learning outcomes, such as knowledge acquisition, perceptual and cognitive skills, motor skills, physiological or social outcomes (Connolly, Boyle, MacArthur, Hainey, & Boyle, 2012). Like other health-related studies, game-based interventions are categorized as preventive, therapeutic, assessment, educational, and informatics (Sawyer, 2008).

Computer-based programs not only need to be engaging, they also need to be interactive, with valid and reliable measures of outcomes (Baranowski, Buday, Thompson, & Baranowski, 2008). Other factors, such as the capabilities and limitations of platforms (e.g., full computer screen, handheld game, or smartphone) impact the participants' experience. Age-related preferences must also be considered in developing computer-based cognitive training/gaming. One study assessed the specific preferences and potential barriers of older adults regarding a web-based platform for cognitive testing. Results from qualitative interviews with a sample of older adults, half of whom had MCI, revealed a desire for cognitive exercises to have interesting topics and to have communication features to increase motivation (Haesner, O'Sullivan, Govercin, & Steinhagen-Thiessen, 2014).

Research on computer-based cognitive programs has been mixed. On the one hand, some evidence supports their effectiveness and public appeal (Anguera et al., 2013; Nacke, Nacke, & Lindley, 2009; Nouchi et al., 2012); on the other hand, other studies argue that although computer-based brain training is a lucrative industry, there is no scientific evidence to support the notion that improved cognitive performance in game tasks transfers to untrained tasks (Owen et al., 2010). Some studies (Baranowski et al., 2008; Primack et al., 2012), suggest that computer-based games are associated with improved perceptual, cognitive, behavioral, affective, and motivational outcomes (Connolly et al., 2012). Studies have also demonstrated that computer-based cognitive training has improved learning efficiency in healthy older adults (Hickman, Rogers, & Fisk, 2007) in the areas of learning/memory, working memory, and information processing (Mate-Kole et al., 2007). For patients with dementia, the benefits may be concentrated in select areas of cognition, such as short-term memory, behavioral and social improvements, and higher global cognitive functioning (Mate-Kole et al., 2007).

Computer-based cognitive programs whose efficacy has empirical support include Lumosity, CogniFit Personal Coach, Posit Science, Dakim Brain Fitness Program, Brain Age, Megame, and Super Nogin. There are a number of other programs that have little or no research support for their use (SAIDO Learning, MasterQuiz, etc.). We will explore the efficacy of computer-based cognitive programs for people with dementia later in the chapter.

One question is how much training—and with what frequency and intensity—is required to obtain measurable improvements in cognitive performance? Some computer-based programs have been shown to improve cognitive functions in older adults in as little as 4 weeks, with 15-minute sessions 5 days a week (Nouchi et al., 2012), whereas other programs were administered in a minimum of 40 hours of instruction spaced over a 6-month period (Miller et al., 2013). Interestingly, beneficial effects from computer-based programs have been found even with individuals who do not regularly use this type of technology, including improvement in executive-based skills, after just 23.5 hours of playing time (Basak, Boot, Voss, & Kramer, 2008). There is some evidence suggesting that more intensive training may result in greater benefits. For instance, the recent study of the Dakim Brain Fitness computerized program, which provided cognitive training and stimulation in language, visual processing, and memory domains, showed promising results for individuals with mild memory difficulties (both normal aging and those with MCI) who could participate in the higher levels of the program, with specific improvement for memory and language (Miller et al., 2013). Cognitive training programs from Posit Science, which contain challenging tasks, have also shown cognitive gains for intact older adults (Mahncke et al., 2006; Smith, Housen, & Yaffe, 2009). Finally, Lumosity's games have been found to increase performance in MCI participants who completed 30 sessions of cognitive training when compared to a wait-list control group, although the generalizability of training was limited to a visual sustained-attention task (Finn & McDonald, 2011).

As to whether computer-based cognitive interventions provide greater benefits than simply playing conventional computer games (e.g., Tetris, snake, puzzles, Memory Simon, memory pairs) was a question that was addressed in a systematic review of 151 research studies (Kueider, Parisi, Gross, & Rebok, 2012). These authors reported that the effect sizes (ES) ranged from 0.06 to 6.32 for *traditional training programs* (like the MTPs described earlier), 0.19 to 7.14 for *neuropsychological software interventions* (e.g., CogniFit, Einstein Memory Trainer, Posit Science), and 0.09 to 1.70 for *video game interventions* (e.g., SuperTetris, Wii Big Brain Academy, Pac Man). Outcome measures often included formal tests of memory, processing speed, attention, or executive functioning. The authors concluded that computerized training was as effective as traditional cognitive training programs.

The importance of computer programs for cognitive training is likely to increase with the aging of the Baby Boom generation, who are more likely than previous cohorts of older adults to be technologically savvy. As with any intervention, these computer-based training interventions have both strengths and limitations. The strengths include engaging interfaces, flexibility, incorporating simulations of real-life environments, integration of goal-directed behaviors, immediate feedback, and greater ecological validity (Gunther, Schafer, Holzner, & Kemmler, 2003; Schreiber, Schweizer, Lutz, Kalveram, & Jancke, 1999). However, there is evidence that the efficacy and efficiency of training may be stronger using pen and paper (Nacke, et al., 2009), calling into question the ecological validity of certain tasks included in these computerized programs. Comfort level and previous exposure to technology are also issues, particularly for persons who find using these products anxiety provoking, although learning a new computer-based skill in itself can result in positive brain changes (Small, Moody, Siddarth, & Bookheimer, 2009). Technology-based devices may be more appropriate for individuals with less impairment, considering the burden the caregiver may experience in supporting the use of such programs in terms of instruction (Nygard, 2008). Given these strengths and limitations, future research should continue to investigate whether computerized cognitive training programs for older adults can combat cognitive decline, improve abilities, and translate to everyday functioning, including essential activities of daily living (e.g., remembering to take medication, driving safely, paying bills on time).

Cognitive Training and Smartphone Apps

As of 2012, 85% of people between the ages of 68 and 88 own a mobile phone, while only 16% of these individuals have a smartphone, according to research from Forrester. Among individuals aged 65 and older, 13% reported that they have not upgraded to a smartphone because it was too complicated or hard to use. Despite the low number of older adults who own a smartphone, the market for cognitive training apps will likely grow, particularly as the younger Baby Boomers (aged 47–56) reach the age of 65 in the next decade. In the same survey, 92% of younger Baby Boomers own a mobile phone, and 39% own a smartphone. Interestingly, there is already increasing interest in the use of smartphones as a memory aid among rehabilitative patients (Migo et al., 2014; Ramsberger & Messamer, 2014).

Currently, there are a handful of smartphone apps that are marketed as "brain games," which might be of interest for older adults. These include Lumosity, CogniFit Brain Fitness, Brain Trainer Special, Brain Fitness Pro, Fit Brains Trainer, and Eidetic. These apps vary in subscription price (free to $15/month), and have been developed to improve cognitive abilities, such as memory, attention, problem-solving, and processing speed, through varied and challenging games. Further research regarding the long-term outcomes of brain game apps will be useful, particularly as the use of these apps gains interest and popularity among aging adults.

EFFICACY OF COGNITIVE TRAINING FOR DIFFERENT POPULATIONS OF OLDER ADULTS

Normal Aging

Numerous individual studies have been performed over the past 40 years assessing the efficacy of a variety of mnemonic techniques (see Table 22.2 for a representative sample of recent studies). In general, these studies indicate that cognitive training is beneficial and results in improvement on measures of memory, reasoning, processing speed, and problem-solving compared to active control or wait-list groups (Ball, Berch, & Helmers, 2002; Brooks, Friedman, Pearman, Gray, & Yesavage, 1999; Gross et al., 2012; Kelly et al., 2014a; Kelly et al., 2014b; Verhaeghen et al., 1992; Willis et al., 2006; Yesavage et al., 1990; Zehnder, Martin, Altgassen, & Clare, 2009). In some cases, improved cognitive performance has been found after just one or two sessions (Rebok & Balcerak, 1989). MTPs as short as 4 or 6 weeks can be as effective as longer programs, including those 4–12 months long (Becker, Jr., Douglas, & Arheart, 2008; Miller et al., 2011; Rozzini et al., 2007).

A seminal study of the effects of cognitive training in older adults is the Advanced Cognitive Training for Independent and Vital Elderly (ACTIVE) study (Ball et al., 2002). This randomized, controlled, single-blind trial was conducted from March 1998 to October 1999, with 2-, 5-, and 10-year follow-ups (Rebok et al., 2014; Willis et al., 2006). The initial ACTIVE intervention consisted of 10 hour-long sessions held over a 5–6-week period. The 2832 participants were randomly assigned to one of three treatment conditions or

Table 22.2. Representative Studies Providing Evidence of Benefit from Cognitive Training in Healthy Older Adults

AUTHOR	INTERVENTION	N	OUTCOME
Bailey, West, & Anderson (2010)	Training older adults to employ metacognitive skills at home	Treatment $n = 29$ Control $n = 27$	Significant gains in self-testing, study allocation for learning new information. Metacognition training at home (ES = 0.63).
Cheng et al. (2012)	Single vs. multi-domain cognitive training	$n = 270$; cognitive training	Improved memory, visual reasoning, visuospatial construction, attention, and neuropsychological status. Multi-domain Visual Reasoning (ES = 0.53); Multi-domain RBANS Immediate Memory, ES = 0.53; Multi-domain RBANS Delayed Memory (ES = 0.51).
Vranić, Španić, Carretti, & Borella (2013)	Training in metamemory strategies and motivation	$n = 51$; cognitive training	Significant gains in immediate list recall task (criterion measure). Immediate list recall (ES = 0.85).
Youn, Lee, Kim, & Ryu (2011)	Multistrategic memory training	Treatment $n = 20$ Control $n = 20$	Improvements in Word List Short-term, Delayed Free (ES = 0.68), and Cued Recall (ES = 0.66); Word-list Long-term, Delayed Free (ES = 0.88), and Cued Recall (ES = 0.92); Visuospatial span forwards (ES = 0.42); and Categorical Fluency Test (ES = 0.15).
Zinke et al. (2014)	Visuospatial, verbal, executive working memory tasks	$n = 80$; cognitive training	Improvement in all training tasks; near transfer to verbal working memory task (ES = 0.80) and far transfer to a fluid intelligence task (ES = 0.29).

a no-contact control group. The three treatment groups focused solely on the training of memory using mnemonics, inductive reasoning, or processing speed (computerized training). The training interventions resulted in improved cognitive performance for 87% of individuals in the speed training group, 74% of those in the reasoning training group, and 26% of the memory training group (Ball, Berch, Helmers, et al., 2002). Booster sessions were provided to random subsamples within each intervention group. Five of the 10 booster sessions focused on strategic instruction, and the remaining five sessions focused on the practice of these strategies.

While most studies of cognitive training involve far fewer participants than the ACTIVE project (typically fewer than 50 subjects), several meta-analyses conducted over the past 20 years have attempted to pool findings from dozens of studies to examine not only the efficacy of cognitive interventions, but also the effects on outcomes of different forms of training, the length and intensity of training, the range of techniques employed, and other program facets.

Verhaeghen et al. (1992) examined pre- to post-performance gains on episodic memory tasks for older adults. Inclusion criteria for studies included healthy normal subjects (absence of cognitive problems due to organic pathology) age 60 and older, and use of pre- and post-treatment measures (studies of long-term effects were excluded), yielding 33 studies with a total sample of 1539 persons, with mean ages ranging from 61.35 to 78. Thirteen of the 31 studies employed a control group, placebo group, or both (no description of control/placebo group activities). Study participants attended a mean of 5.76 training sessions (range of 1 to 20 sessions) with a mean duration of 1.49 hours (range of 0.33 to 2.50 hours). These studies produced 49 effect sizes (ES) among the memory training groups with a mean ES of 0.73, compared to ES = 0.38 for the control groups and ES = 0.37 for placebo groups. Among memory-training groups, the ES ranged from 0.14 in the earliest cited study (DeLeon, 1974) to 1.82 (Yesavage & Rose, 1983). The authors found no significant differences in ESs for different forms of memory training (e.g., method of loci, name–face), though most methods (except for organization) involved the element of imagery. Training effects were greater for subjects who were younger, who had received pre-training, had attended group sessions, and had participated in shorter sessions. These findings provide evidence that cognitive training generally benefited the individuals in these studies, and that participants performed better when training sessions were shorter as opposed to longer, suggesting that fatigue may be a factor in overly long sessions.

Recently, Kelly et al. (2014) performed a meta-analysis of cognitive training studies published from 2005 to 2012. Like Verhaeghen et al. (1992), the researchers only included studies involving older adults with no known cognitive impairments. Their inclusion criteria differed somewhat in that studies with slightly younger participants (> 50 years of age) were included, as well as studies that employed either cognitive training or "general mental stimulation" as interventions. A distinction was made between "no intervention" and "active" control groups, the latter participating in activities such as watching DVD-based lectures, trivia learning, or playing conventional computer games. Kelly and associates obtained 31 eligible studies with 1806 participants in cognitive training groups, 386 receiving general mental stimulation, 1541 having no intervention (controls), and 822 in active control groups. Subjects' ages ranged from 50 to 99, with most being above age 65. Interventions were heterogeneous, both in the length and depth of training and in the training programs employed. The number of sessions ranged from as few as 3 sessions to 180 sessions, with the sessions occurring over a period of any where from a couple of weeks to a 2-year time period.

The ESs were reported as standardized mean difference (SMD) and were indicated by the outcome (e.g., face–name recall, paired associates, etc.). Compared to active controls, the largest statistically significant ES was seen for processing speed (SMD = 0.82), followed by recognition (0.47), working memory (0.47), and cognitive functioning (0.23). A somewhat different set of statistically significant ESs were found for studies of cognitive training groups compared to "no intervention" control groups: paired associates (0.65), recognition (0.44), face–name recall (0.44), and subjective memory (0.36). The six mental stimulation RCTs were too few to permit the pooling of data, though significant intervention effects were observed in half the measures of memory and executive function. Kelly and associates included two studies that compared individual and group training formats and found, like Verhaeghen et al. (1992), that cognitive interventions are maximized in group settings.

Another key meta-analysis was conducted by Martin et al. (2011). Unlike Verhaeghen et al. (1992) and Kelly et al. (2014), Martin and colleagues included studies with MCI participants (dementia patients were excluded) and attempted to analyze all RCT cognitive interventions from 1970 to 2007. Thirty-six RCTs were included in their analysis, involving 2229 participants with an estimated mean age of 69 years. These researchers found significant improvement in some outcome variables in studies with no treatment control groups, including immediate recall (ES = 1.03) and delayed verbal recall (ES = 3.40). However, when studies with active control groups were analyzed, training gains were not significantly larger than those obtained from active controls. When studies involving MCI participants were separately analyzed, a similar pattern of results was obtained. Martin and colleagues concluded that there is insufficient evidence to attribute performance gains to cognitive training, either for healthy adults or for persons with MCI. The researchers speculate on several reasons for the weak evidence for training effects in their meta-analysis, including the heterogeneity of "procedures, durations, intensities, methods of dealing with absent training participants, use

Table 22.3. Representative Studies Providing Evidence of Benefit from Cognitive Training in Older Adults with MCI

AUTHOR	INTERVENTION	N	OUTCOME
Barnes, Yaffe, & Belfor (2009)	Computer-based cognitive training in auditory processing speed and accuracy vs. passive computer activities	$n = 47$; cognitive training	Except RBANS score (ES = 0.33), no significant differences between the intervention and control groups. Trend for domain-specific effect (e.g., intervention group—verbal learning and memory measures tended to favor the intervention group).
Belleville et al. (2006)	Training in episodic memory strategies	Treatment $n = 21$ Control $n = 16$	Improvement in delay list recall (Pre: 7.39 / Post: 9.06), face–name association (Pre: 5.78 / Post: 7.56), subjective memory (personal events; Pre: 2.76 / Post: 2.38) and well-being (Pre: 66.00 / Post: 68.90)
Cipriani, Bianchetti, & Trabucchi (2006)	Computer based neuropsychological training	AD $n = 10$ MCI $n = 10$ MSA $n = 3$	The AD group showed a significant improvement on MMSE scores (Pre: 23.9 / Post: 26.0) and in the areas of verbal production (Phonemic fluency z score; Pre: −0.8 / Post: −0.5) and executive functions (Trail Making Test B, # of errors; Pre: 11.8 / Post: 7.3). MCI patients significantly improved in behavioral memory (RBMT z score; Pre: −0.4 / Post: 0.6).
Banningh et al. (2010)	CBT group therapy for patients with MCI & their significant others	$n = 23$ patient-significant others dyads	Patients showed a significant increased level of acceptance (ES = 0.34) and a trend for an increased marital satisfaction. The significant others reported an increased awareness of memory and behavioral problems.
Kinsella et al. (2009)	Prospective memory tasks	$n = 52$; cognitive training	Enhanced prospective memory (prospective memory at 2-week follow-up: ES = 0.41), knowledge and use of memory (strategy knowledge at 2-week follow-up: ES = 0.38), subjective memory
Rapp, Brenes, & Marsh (2002)	Mnemonics instruction	Treatment $n = 9$ Control $n = 10$	Treated group had significantly better memory appraisals than controls at the end of treatment (5.36 vs. 3.98) and at 6-month follow-up (4.86 vs. 3.81).
Rozzini et al. (2007)	Cognitive training in language, attention, reasoning, visual spatial skills	Treatment $n = 15$ Control $n = 22$	Enhanced memory (Short Story; Baseline: 7.5 / 12-month follow-up: 11.0), abstract reasoning (Raven's Coloured Matrices; Baseline: 24.2 / 12-month follow-up: 26.6), depression (GDS; Baseline: 2.1 / 12-month follow-up: 1.3)
Unverzagt et al. (2007)	Memory, reasoning, speed of processing training	Memory impaired $n = 193$ Normal = 2580	Normal gains for MCI participants in processing speed (ES = −1.420) and reasoning (ES = 0.573)

of a variety of training contents, content combinations, and matching of evaluation instruments to training contents" (Martin et al., 2011).

Gross et al. (2012) addressed the issue of control group condition in their meta-analysis involving 35 cognitive training studies and 3797 participants. They reported strong results for memory training (ES = 0.43) as compared to controls (ES = 0.06). The authors performed a meta-regression analysis of ESs on selected predictors and found no significant effect for type of control condition (Beta = −0.10). Zehnder et al. (2009) also found significant findings for studies with both no intervention/contact controls and active control groups, though the pattern of findings was different for the two control conditions. For instance, studies with no contact controls exhibited significant training effects for paired associates learning (ES = 2.71) and delayed verbal recall (ES = 0.88), while participants in studies with active controls performed significantly better at face recall (ES = 0.93) but more poorly on visuospatial memory (ES = −0.94).

When comparing the various meta-analytical studies, it appears that there is a heterogeneous pattern of outcomes. For example, Verhaeghen et al. (1992) obtained strong ESs for memory-training groups when compared to control groups and placebo groups. Similarly, Zehnder et al. (2009) also found significant findings for studies with both no intervention/contact controls and active control groups. In contrast, some researchers (Martin et al., 2011) reported that when active control groups were analyzed, the gains of the intervention groups were not significantly larger than those obtained from active controls. The issues of methodological weaknesses and heterogeneity of methods will be revisited in the "Future Directions" section of this chapter.

Mild Cognitive Impairment

Given that 80% of those with MCI will likely go on to develop dementia (Petersen, Smith, & Waring, 1999), and because medication may provide only temporary improvements, there has been much interest in the use of cognitive training as a non-pharmacological treatment for MCI. Older studies of cognitive training employing MCI participants have been small, typically fewer than 20 subjects. Recent studies have employed larger samples and have focused on improving memory for daily tasks and maintaining a level of functional

independence (Talassi et al., 2007). For instance, a 4-week multi-component rehabilitation program resulted in improvement in activities of daily living, memory functioning, and mood compared to a wait-list control group (Requena, Maestu, Campo, Fernandez, & Ortiz, 2006). Hwang et al. (2012) found significant enhancement in delayed recall in amnestic MCI subjects following a multi-component cognitive training program and observed persisting improvements in episodic memory 3 months after the end of training. Additional representative studies involving MCI participants can be found in Table 22.3.

Meta-analytic studies involving MCI participants are beginning to appear, such as that of Li et al. (2011). These researchers included 17 studies in their meta-analysis, 11 of which employed cognitive training/stimulation and 6 involving cognitive rehabilitation, with a total of 345 participants (mean age ranged from 62 to 78 years). As in previous meta-analyses, intervention types were heterogeneous (e.g., "memory training with Memory Support System," "auditory processing speed, auditory processing speed, auditory working memory," "memory, organizational, and attention skills"). The frequency and duration of training sessions were similarly diverse, ranging from daily to weekly sessions that could be as short as 13 minutes or as long as 2 hours. About two-thirds of the studies had a control group as part of the study design, some of which involved activities and others wait-list controls.

In order to study whether there was a common population effect in the meta-analytical studies, the researchers utilized Q tests (a homogeneity statistic) (Li et al., 2011). The Q tests performed by the authors showed that MCI participants in the cognitive intervention groups performed better than those in MCI control groups for overall cognition ($Q = 16.21$, $p < .001$), overall self-ratings ($Q = 6.92$, $p = .009$), episodic memory ($Q = 13.96$, $p < .001$), and executive function/working memory ($Q = 5.40$, $p = 0.02$). Effect sizes ranging from moderate to small were obtained for several outcomes, such as self-rated functional ability (ES = 0.55), episodic memory (ES = 0.45), and attention/processing speed (ES = 0.35); however, all failed to reach statistical significance. These authors noted that studies without an MCI control group had larger ESs in overall cognition and self-ratings. Li and colleagues (2011) concluded that persons with MCI could benefit from cognitive interventions, although the small number of studies made it impossible to make meaningful comparisons between cognitive training, stimulation, and rehabilitation approaches. It should be noted that the MCI studies described by Li and associates vary widely in quality of design, and not all are RCTs. Overall, the meta-analysis and individual studies cited earlier suggest that people with MCI can benefit from cognitive interventions, but more and higher quality research is needed to ascertain the degree of benefit that can be obtained, to identify which techniques hold the most promise, and how they might best be delivered.

Dementia

In a recent review of the literature, Bahar-Fuchs, Clare, and Woods (2013) concluded that evidence of cognitive training benefiting dementia patients "remains limited," and that the "quality of the evidence needs to improve." Rather than specific lesson-based interventions, as seen with the MTPs, studies focused on the dementia population have often employed a cognitive stimulation, often because individuals with dementia find training in mnemonic strategies too challenging. Several studies did find that cognitive stimulation resulted in some benefit in patients with dementia. Orrell and colleagues (2014) conducted a large study with a single-blind, pragmatic randomized controlled trial. All subjects participated in a 7-week, 14-session cognitive stimulation training (CST) program and then were assigned to intervention and control groups. At 6 months, improvements were observed for the treatment group in terms of self-rated quality of life (Orrell et al., 2014). Similarly, Mapelli and associates (2013) provided structured cognitive stimulation to an experimental group, occupational therapy to a placebo group, and a continuation of usual activities for a control group; after 8 weeks, the experimental group improved for cognitive tests and exhibited a decrease in behavior symptoms (Mapelli, Rosa, Nocita, & Sava, 2013). Cheng and colleagues (2006) studied the effect of mahjong (a popular game) on cognitive functioning in 62 persons with dementia; participants were randomly assigned either to a twice weekly or four times weekly condition over a 16-week period; all improved in select aspects of memory (S. Cheng, Chan, & Yu, 2006). They later created an intervention that combined Mahjong with tai chi exercises in a study of 110 nursing home residents with dementia. Participants were assigned to mahjong,

tai chi, and control groups (simple handcrafts). The researchers observed that while control group participants deteriorated, participants in the experimental groups "maintained their abilities over time," including higher MMSE scores 9 months later (Y. Cheng et al., 2012).

Transfer of Training and Generalizability

The ultimate goal of cognitive training for older adults is to enhance cognitive functioning in a variety of daily activities (e.g., planning a trip, remembering the name of an acquaintance, or finding a flight number on a display screen in a bustling airport). Ideally, the cognitive skills that older adults acquire from MTPs, computerized games, or smartphone apps can be applied in a variety of real-life situations, which is referred to in the literature as "transfer of training."

"Transfer of training" comes out of the early work of Thorndike and Woodworth (1901) and the concept of transfer of learning, that is, how persons employ learning from one situation in another, perhaps different, situation (Ellis, 1965). Transfer of training can be "near," "medium," or "far," depending on the extent to which there is overlap in situations and contexts from the training experience to a new situation in which the acquired skill can be used. Near transfer, where there is a great deal of overlap, implies that the cognitive training can improve a skill within the same cognitive domain (e.g., learn a memory technique to improve performance on a memory test or the ability to recall something specific), whereas far transfer, that with little or no overlap, suggests that cognitive training (e.g., memory exercises) could also improve a different cognitive domain (e.g., language or executive skills).

Verhaeghen and colleagues (1992) observed limited far transfer effects, noting that if the mnemonic skill could be applied (e.g., method of loci for the memorization of a word list) the outcome was better than if it was not applicable (e.g., method of loci for memorizing face–names). Kelly and associates (2014) found in their meta-analytic study of healthy older adults that 21 studies demonstrated that cognitive training produces near transfer effects, mostly to tasks "within the same cognitive domain," while seven studies also showed that training transferred to "untrained cognitive domains." These authors found that studies employing adaptive and repetitive training sessions, or training over longer periods of time, were more likely to produce far transfer effects.

There are certain individual studies that have reported specific examples of transfer effects, including (1) near transfer of working memory training to a verbal working memory task, as well as far transfer to a task of fluid intelligence (Zinke et al., 2014); (2) far transfer of a verbal working memory training program for fluid intelligence and processing-speed tasks (Borella, Carretti, Riboldi, & Beni, 2010); (3) far transfer effects from computerized training on spatial and verbal working memory tasks to sustained attention and subjective daily cognitive functioning (Brehmer, Westerberg, & Bäckman, 2012).

As valuable as these studies are for illustrating transfer effects to various outcome measures, limited research has been conducted on the application of training to daily life (Kelly et al., 2014). One possible explanation for the failure to find transfer effects in everyday activities may be that individuals need to be taught how to transfer training beyond the classroom or laboratory. One approach is to give training participants "homework assignments" that involve applying learned techniques to new situations (Cavallini et al., 2010). Another approach involves teaching participants how to perform task analysis in order to modify or adapt techniques to new situations and tasks (Bottiroli, Cavallini, & Vecchi, 2008). Clearly, additional research is needed to facilitate the transfer of training in order to make cognitive training relevant and useful in the lives of training participants.

Neuroplasticity and Ancillary Benefits of Cognitive Training

The question of the neuroplasticity for both normal aging and MCI undergoing cognitive training has been addressed in some studies that used brain imaging to examine changes in brain functioning following a training intervention. Engvig and colleagues used diffusion tension imaging (DTI) to examine the effects of cognitive training in those with MMSE > 26. The intervention group received 1 hour of classroom training on the method of loci and participated in 4 days of homework exercises. Participants exhibited an increase in anterior fractional anisotropy compared with controls, in addition to improved memory. Overall, the authors concluded that cognitive interventions were related to specific changes in white matter, and that these changes were associated with improved memory performances among participants in the intervention group (Engvig et al., 2012). Another group reported evidence of neuroplasticity in MCI subjects participating in a cognitive stimulation group; the researchers employed fMRI brain scans to measure increased activation of the frontal, temporal, and parietal areas (Belleville et al., 2011). In another fMRI study, Rosen and colleagues had MCI participants perform exercises known to improve verbal memory as part of a 2-month training program; individuals in the experimental group exhibited significantly improved memory scores relative to controls and significantly increased left hippocampal activation, suggesting that those with MCI "may retain sufficient neuroplasticity to benefit from cognitive training" (Rosen, Suguira, Kramer, Whitfield-Gabrieli, & Gabrieli, 2011, p. 349). Hosseini and associates (2014) found that compared to healthy older adults who also underwent cognitive training, individuals at risk of AD exhibited increased brain activity in medial temporal, prefrontal, and posterior default mode networks. Based on careful analysis of these imaging data, the researchers believe that for persons at risk of AD, cognitive training "mainly improves compensatory mechanisms and partly restores the affected functions" (Hosseini, Kramer, & Kesler, 2014). As mentioned earlier, our group examined a 14-day healthy lifestyle program addressing memory, nutrition, exercise, and stress reduction (Small et al., 2006). Along with improved word fluency, participants had a 5% decrease in left dorsolateral prefrontal cortex activity as measured by FDG-PET scans. These results were interpreted as greater cognitive efficiency for the brain region related to working memory.

There are also a small number of studies focused on the ancillary benefits from cognitive training, including (1) slowed degradation of balance and improved gait (Smith-Ray et al., 2013) after 10 weeks of cognitive training; (2) improved sleep after 8 weeks of computerized cognitive training (Haimov & Shatil, 2013); and (3) improved cognitive functioning, with and without the treatment of lithium, in MCI adults after 8 sessions of cognitive training (Brum, Forlenza, & Yassuda, 2009).

LONG-TERM OUTCOMES OF COGNITIVE TRAINING

There is controversy as to the long-term benefits of cognitive training and whether training effects transfer to daily tasks (Owen et al., 2010) or extend to other domains beyond the training (Harrison et al., 2013). In this section we will examine the longitudinal data on both classroom and computerized cognitive training, including the potential impact on instrumental activities of daily living (IADLs). Examples of specific cognitive training techniques employed in representative studies are shown in Table 22.4.

A number of studies show that longitudinal benefits from formal classroom instruction interventions are robust, and may last from 3 months to 10 years (Anschutz, Camp, Markley, & Kramer, 1987; O'Hara et al., 2007; Rebok et al., 2014; Scogin & Bienias, 1998; Stigsdotter & Backman, 1993; Willis et al., 2006; Wolinsky, Weg, Howren, Jones, & Dotson, 2013). Most notable are the

10-year results from the ACTIVE study, which examined the long-term effects of the durability of training on cognitive abilities and the transferability of cognitive training to IADLs (i.e., medication management, financial management, and driving), examined at 2 years, 5 years, and 10 years (Rebok, et al., 2014). Longitudinal results at 2 years and 5 years revealed that participants in each cognitive intervention group (memory, inductive reasoning, processing speed) demonstrated improved performances on objective measures of cognitive ability for which they were trained (Ball, Berch, Helmers, et al., 2002; Willis et al., 2006). At 10 years, the reasoning and speed of processing effects were maintained on the targeted abilities, and booster sessions

Table 22.4. Representative Cognitive Training Techniques Employed in Studies of Healthy Older Adults and Older Adults with MCI

STUDY	COGNITIVE TRAINING TECHNIQUES
Cheng et al. (2012)	Loci memory training; face–name memory training
Vranic et al. (2013)	Training and hands-on experiences with memory systems, impact of aging, role of psychological well-being, beliefs about memory.
Youn et al. (2011)	Techniques relating to memory process, structure, attention, brain, environment, and perception.
Zinke et al. (2014)	Working memory training: visuospatial (picture grid task), verbal (subtract-2-span task). Executive control: Tower of London task.
Ball et al. (2002)	Memory: Categorizing, visual imagery, mental association. Speed-of-processing: Visual search skill training. Reasoning: Strategies for identifying patterns.
Barnes et al. (2009)	Computer-based program (Posit Science) for speed of processing and auditory primary and working memory (e.g.: identify target syllable, distinguish between two sounds, match sounds on a spatial grid).
Kinsella et al. (2009)	Strategies for improving organizational and attention skills, face–name recall training, verbal categorization and elaboration, visual imagery, spaced-retrieval.
Banningh et al. (2010)	CBT principles combined with psychoeducation and memory rehabilitation techniques, strategies for memory improvement (e.g., note taking), relaxation techniques.
Bailey et al. (2010)	Training in use of a self-testing technique applied to memorizing paired associates.
Rapp et al. (2002)	Relaxation (systematic breathing), general discussion of memory problems, cueing, categorization, chunking, method of loci.

resulted in additional improvement for these interventions; however, memory training effects were no longer maintained for memory performance (Rebok et al., 2014). Additionally, intervention groups reported less difficulty performing IADLs than the control group (Rebok et al., 2014), with modest ES for all three groups (0.48 for memory, 0.38 for reasoning, 0.36 for speed). A subsample of participants in the ACTIVE study (n = 908; mean age: 73.1), who received speed of processing and reasoning training, demonstrated an approximately 50% lower rate of at-fault motor vehicle collisions than controls, based on state motor collision reports (Ball, Edwards, Ross, & McGwin, 2010); no significant differences were found for participants in the memory training group. These findings suggest that cognitive interventions may help to maintain safety and independence in older adults, and that these benefits last several years after the intervention.

While the ACTIVE program examined the effect of single-domain cognitive training, Cheng and colleagues (2012) examined the effect of multi-domain versus single-domain cognitive training. A sample of Chinese healthy older adults (aged 65–75) in small groups met twice a week for 12 weeks (total of 24 sessions), receiving either multi-domain or single-domain cognitive training. Multi-domain cognitive training involved memory, reasoning, problem-solving, visual spatial map reading, and physical exercise; single-domain focused specifically on reasoning. At 6 months, 60% of the initial training participants received three booster sessions. Longitudinal results at 12 months demonstrated that participants who received multi-domain cognitive training improved in delayed memory and visual reasoning tasks, while those who received single-domain cognitive training improved on a word interference task. Participants who received booster sessions improved on visual reasoning, visual spatial abilities, and processing speed (Y. Cheng et al., 2012). Authors concluded that multi-domain cognitive training resulted in greater benefit than single-domain cognitive training, and similar to the ACTIVE study and the 5-year follow-up study with O'Hara et al. (2007), booster sessions extend long-term outcomes.

Similar results have been noted by researchers regarding computerized cognitive training, including sustained improvement for attention at 3-month follow-up (Mahncke, et al., 2006) and improved memory at 6 months (Miller et al.,

2013). Additionally, a large randomized controlled trial (Iowa Healthy and Active Minds Study; n = 681) examined whether 10 hours of visual speed of processing training would prevent age-related declines and potentially improve cognitive processing speed (Wolinsky et al., 2013). Participants completed computerized visual speed of processing (either 10 hours onsite; 14 hours onsite: 10 hours + 4 hours of booster sessions; or 10 hours at home), or were placed in a control group (computerized crossword puzzles for 10 hours). Outcomes were assessed at baseline and at 1 year; all three visual speed of processing training groups demonstrated improvements, including divided attention, processing speed, and executive skills. Another study found that participants who had 10 hours of computerized speed and accuracy of visual processing training actually improved on tasks of timed IADLs (Edwards, Ruva, O'Brian, Haley, & Lister, 2013). Notably, the effect of training on timed IADLs was fully mediated by improved speed of processing for a divided attention task.

Taken together, these studies suggest that the benefits of cognitive training can be maintained for several years after the intervention, even with as little as 10 intervention sessions. Booster sessions appear to extend long-term outcomes. Outcomes include not only improved performances on memory tasks, but reduced self-reported decline in daily activities (managing finances or medications) and reduced auto collisions, thus indicating the important potential of cognitive interventions in maintaining safety and independence in older adults for several years after the intervention.

FUTURE DIRECTIONS

Research on cognitive training has been criticized for methodological weaknesses, including heterogeneity in methodology and content, making it difficult to draw strong conclusions about the efficacy of cognitive training, particularly for populations with memory impairment (e.g., Martin et al., 2011). Progress in terms of understanding how cognitive training benefits individuals with MCI and dementia is underway, but additional research is still needed to address the transferability and generalizability of gains to everyday activities. There is a need to better understand how we can increase motivation to keep utilizing memory techniques on a regular basis (shift in lifestyle) in hopes of continuing to benefit from the cognitive strategies within everyday interactions (beyond the classroom or computer). Can this be achieved with booster sessions, or perhaps within a coaching or therapy context, particularly for individuals with MCI? Additionally, computer or online-based cognitive training, the use of apps for smartphones, and the ability to measure improvement via brain imaging are important endeavors for the future of cognitive training research. Also, with the increased interest in E-health self-care interventions, including the management of chronic conditions (Glueckauf et al., 2009), it is crucial to focus on the development of web-based cognitive training programs that can reach a wider audience for little to no cost. Finally, future directions of cognitive training may include examining the combined effects of cognitive training with meditation, productive engagement, or healthy behaviors like exercise (Gard, Hölzel, & Lazar, 2014; Nascimento et al., 2014; Park et al., 2014; Small et al., 2013).

SUMMARY

In sum, cognitive training is beneficial for individuals during the aging process, but may be mediated by age, cognitive reserve, neuroplasticity (including level of memory impairment), breadth/depth of training (i.e., multi-factorial), and the duration or intensity of training. Peer-led training, computerized brain fitness programs, and apps for smartphones have expanded the reach of cognitive training to a larger audience of individuals. Future research, including brain imaging, may offer more insight into the impact of cognitive training on the brain. Further, more studies are needed that incorporate measurement of IADLs to better understand how training transfers to real world needs, such as independence with driving, finances, and medication management. Finally, some researchers propose that an international meeting of clinicians and researchers be convened to establish guidelines for the development and implementation of effective cognitive training programs based on the latest science (Walton, Mowszowski, Lewis, & Nasmith, 2014). Advances in our understanding of the plasticity of the brain are making possible new, non-pharmaceutical interventions for preserving and enhancing the cognitive functioning of older adults.

REFERENCES

Anguera, J., Boccanfuso, J., Rintoul, J., Al-Hashimi, O., Faraji, F., Janowich, J., . . . Gazzaley, A. (2013). Video game training enhances cognitive control in older adults. *Nature, 501*, 97–101. doi: 10.1038/nature12486.

Anschutz, L., Camp, C., Markley, R., & Kramer, J. (1987). Remembering mnemonics: a three-year follow-up on the effects of mnemonics training in elderly adults. *Exper Aging Res, 13*(3), 141–143.

Bahar-Fuchs, A., Clare, L., & Woods, B. (2013). Cognitive training and cognitive rehabilitation for persons with mild to moderate dementia of the Alzheimer's or vascular type: a review. *Alzheimers Res Ther, 5*(4). doi: 10.1186/alzrt189.

Bailey, K., West, R., & Anderson, C. (2010). A negative association between video game experience and proactive cognitive control. *Psychophysiology, 47*, 34–42. doi: 10.1111/j.1469-8986.2009.00925.x.

Ball, K., Berch, D., & Helmers, K. (2002). Effects of cognitive training interventions with older adults. *JAMA, 348*(23), 2508–2516.

Ball, K., Berch, D., Helmers, K., Jobe, J., Leveck, M., Marsiske, M., et al. (2002). Effects of cognitive training interventions with older adults: a randomized controlled trial. *JAMA, 288*(18), 2271–2281.

Ball, K., Edwards, J. D., Ross, L., & McGwin, G. (2010). Cognitive training decreases motor vehicle collision involvement of older drivers. *J Am Geriatr Soc, 58*(11), 2107–2113.

Banningh, L. J.-W., Prins, J., Vernooij-Dassen, M., Wijnen, H., Rikkert, M. O., & Kessels, R. (2010). Group therapy for patients with mild cognitive impairment and their significant others: results of a waiting-list controlled trial. *Gerontologist, 57*(5), 444–454. doi: 10.1159/000315933

Baranowski, T., Buday, R., Thompson, D., & Baranowski, J. (2008). Playing for real: video games and stories for health-related behavior change. *Am J Prev Med, 34*(1), 74–82.

Barnes, D., Yaffe, K., & Belfor, N. (2009). Computer-based cognitive training for mild cognitive impairment: results from a pilot randomized, controlled trial. *Alzheimer Dis Assoc Disord, 23*(3), 205–210.

Basak, C., Boot, W., Voss, M., & Kramer, A. (2008). Can training in a real-time strategy video game attenuate cognitive decline in older adults? *Psychol Aging, 23*(4), 765–777.

Becker, H., Jr., G. M., Douglas, N., & Arheart, K. (2008). Comparing the efficiency of eight-session versus four-session memory intervention for older adults. *Arch Psychiatr Nurs*, 22(2), 87–94.

Belleville, S., Gilbert, B., Fontaine, F., Gagnon, L., Menard, E., Gauthier, S. (2006). Cognitive training for persons with mild cognitive impairment. *Dementia Geriatr Cogn Disord*, 22, 486–499.

Belleville, S., Chertkow, H., & Gauthier, S. (2007). Working memory and control of attention in persons with Alzheimer's disease and mild cognitive impairment. *Neuropsychology*, 21, 458–469.

Belleville, S., Clement, F., Mellah, S., Gilbert, B., Fontaine, F., & Gauthier, S. (2011). Training-related brain plasticity in subjects at risk of developing Alzheimer's disease. *Brain*, 134(6), 1623–1634.

Borella, E., Carretti, B., Riboldi, R., & Beni, R. (2010). Working memory training in older adults: evidence of transfer and maintenance effects. *Psychol Aging*, 23(4), 767–778.

Bottiroli, S., Cavallini, E., & Vecchi, T. (2008). Long-term effects of memory training in the elderly: a longitudinal study. *Arch Gerontol Geriatrics*, 47, 277–289.

Brehmer, Y., Westerberg, H., & Bäckman, L. (2012). Working-memory training in younger and older adults: training gains, transfer, and maintenance. *Front Human Neurosci*, 6, 1–7.

Brooks, J., Friedman, L., Pearman, A., Gray, C., & Yesavage, J. (1999). Mnemonic training in older adults: effects of age, length of training, and type of cognitive pretraining. *Int Psychogeriatric*, 11(1), 75–84.

Brum, P., Forlenza, O., & Yassuda, M. (2009). Cognitive training in older adults with Mild Cognitive Impairment: Impact on cognitive and functional performance. *Dementa Neuropsychologia*, 3(2), 124–131.

Cavallini, E., Dunlosky, J., Bottiroli, S., Vecchi, T. (2010). Promoting transfer in memory training for older adults. *Aging Clin Exper Res*, 22(4), 314–323.

Cheng, S., Chan, A., & Yu, E. (2006). An exploratory study of the effect of mahjong on the cognitive functioning of persons with dementia. *Int J Geriatr Psychiatry*, 21(7), 611–617.

Cheng, Y., Wu, W., Feng, W., Wang, J., Chen, Y., Shen, Y., . . . Li, C. (2012). The effects of multi-domain versus single-domain cognitive training in non-demented older people: a randomized controlled trial. *BMC Med*, 10(30). doi: 10.1186/1741-7015-10-30.

Cipriani, G., Bianchetti, A., & Trabucchi, M. (2006). Outcomes of a computer-based cognitive rehabilitation program on Alzheimer's disease

patients compared with those on patients affected by mild cognitive impairment. *Arch Gerontology Geriatrics*, 43, 327–335.

Clare, L., & Woods, B. (2009). Cognitive rehabilitation and cognitive training for early-stage Alzheimer's disease and vascular dementia (Review). *Cochrane Database Syst Rev [serial online]* 4. Retrieved from http://www.cochrane.org/reviews/en/ab003260.html.

Connolly, T., Boyle, E., MacArthur, E., Hainey, T., & Boyle, J. (2012). A systematic literature review of empirical evidence on computer games and serious games. *Computers Education*, 59(2), 661–686.

DeLeon, J. (1974). Effects of training in repetition and mediation on paired-associate learning and practical memory in the aged. *Dissertation Abstracts International*, 1–79.

DeVreese, L., Mirco, N., Fioravanti, M., Belloi, L., & Zanetti, O. (2001). Memory rehabilitation in Alzheimer's disease: a review of progress. *Int J Geriatr Psychiatry* (8) 794–809.

Edwards, J., Ruva, C., O'Brian, J., Haley, C., & Lister, J. (2013). An examination of mediators of the transfer of cognitive speed of processing training to everyday functional performance. *Psychol Aging*, 28(2), 314–321.

Ellis, H. (1965). *The transfer of learning.* New York: MacMillan.

Engvig, A., Fjell, A., Westlye, L., Moberget, T., Sundseth, O., Larsen, V., & Walhovd, K. (2012). Memory training impacts short-term changes in aging white matter: A longitudinal diffusion tensor imaging study. *Human Brain Mapp*, 33, 2390–2406.

Epp, J., Barker, J., & Galea, L. (2009). Running wild: neurogenesis in the hippocampus across the lifespan in wild and laboratory-bred Norway rats. *Hippocampus*, 19, 1043–1043.

Ercoli, L., Cernin, P., & Small, G. (2011). Peer-led memory training programs to support brain fitness. In P. Hartman-Stein & A. LaRue (Eds.), *Enhancing cognitive fitness in adults: a guide to the use and development of community-based programs* (pp. 213–229). New York: Springer.

Finn, M., & McDonald, S. (2011). Computerised cognitive training for older persons with mild cognitive impairment: a pilot study using a randomised controlled trial design. *Brain Impairment*, 12(3), 187–199.

Floyd, M., & Scogin, F. (1997). Effects of memory training on the subjective memory functioning and mental health of older adults: a meta-analysis. *Psychol Aging*, 12, 150–161.

Foer, J. (2011). *Moonwalking with Einstein: the art and science of remembering everything.* New York: Penguin Press.

Fuchs, E., & Flugge, G. (2014). Adult neuroplasticity: more than 40 years of research. *Neural Plasticity, 2014,* 1–10.

Gard, T., Hölzel, B., & Lazar, S. (2014). The potential effects of meditation on age-related cognitive decline: a systematic review. *Ann NY Acad Sci, 1307,* 89–103.

Glueckauf, R., Davis, W., Allen, K., Chipi, P., Schettini, G., Tegen, L., . . . Ramirez, C. (2009). Integrative cognitive-behavioral and spiritual counseling for rural dementia caregivers with depression. *Rehabil Psychology, 54*(4), 449–461.

Gross, A., Manly, J., & Pa, J. (2012). Cortical signatures of cognition and their relationship to Alzheimer's disease. *Brain Imaging Behav,*(4), 584–598. doi: 10.1007/s11682-012-9180-5.

Gross, A., Paris, J., Spira, A., Kueider A., Ko, J., Saczynski J., Samus Q., & Rebok, G. (2012). Memory training interventions for older adults: a meta-analysis. *Aging Mental Health, 16*(6), 722–234.

Gross, A., & Rebok, G. (2011). Memory training and strategy use in older adults: Results from the ACTIVE study. *Psychol Aging, 26*(3), 503–517. doi: 10.1037/a0022687

Gunther, V., Schafer, P., Holzner, B., & Kemmler, G. (2003). Long-term improvements in cognitive performance through computer-assisted cognitive training: a pilot study in a residential home for older people. *Aging Mental Health, 7*(3), 200–206.

Haesner, M., O'Sullivan, J., Govercin, M., & Steinhagen-Thiessen, E. (2014). Requirements of older adults for a daily use of an internet-based cognitive training platform. *Inform Health Soc Care.* (2), 139–153. doi: 10.3109/17538157.2013.879149.

Haimov, I., & Shatil, E. (2013). Cognitive training improves sleep quality and cognitive function among adults with insomnia. *PloS Medicine, 8*(4), 1–17. doi: 10.1371/journal.pone.0061390

Harrison, T., Shipstead, Z., Hicks, K., Hambrick, D., Redick, T., & Engle, R. (2013). Working memory training may increase working memory capacity but not fluid intelligence. *Psychol Sci, 12,* 2409–2419.

Hickman, J., Rogers, W., & Fisk, A. (2007). Training older adults to use new technology. *J Gerontol Behav Psychol Sci Soc Sci, 62B,* 77–84.

Hosseini, S., Kramer, J., & Kesler, S. (2014). Neural correlates of cognitive intervention in persons at risk of developing Alzheimer's disease. *Front Aging Neurosci, 6*(231), 1–9.

Hwang, H., Choi, S., Yoon, S., Yoon, B., Suh, Y., Lee D., Han I., Hong C. (2012). The effect of cognitive training in patients with mild cognitive impairment and early Alzheimer's disease: a preliminary study. *J Clin Neurol, 8*(3), 190–197.

Kelly, M. E., Loughrey, D., Lawlor, B., Robertson, I., Walsh, C., & Brennan, S. (2014). The impact of cognitive training and mental stimulation on cognitive and everyday functioning of healthy older adults: a systematic review and meta-analysis. *Ageing Res Rev, 15,* 28–43.

Kessels, R., & DeHaan, E. (2003). Mnemonic strategies in older people: a comparison of errorless and errorful learning. *Age Ageing, 32*(5), 529–533.

Kinsella, G., Mullaly, E., Rand, E., Ong, B., Burton, C., Price, S., . . . Storey, E. (2009). Early intervention for mild cognitive impairment: a randomised controlled trial. *J Neurol Neurosurg Psychiatry, 80,* 730–736. doi: 10.1136/jnnp.2008.148346.

Kueider, A., Parisi, J., Gross, A., & Rebok, G. (2012). Computerized cognitive training with older adults: a systematic review. *PloS Med, 7*(7), 1–13. doi: 10.1371/journal.pone.0040588.

Li, H., Li, J., Li, N., Li, B., Wang, P., & Zhou, T. (2011). Cognitive intervention for persons with mild cognitive impairment: a meta-analysis. *Ageing Res Rev, 10*(2), 285–296.

Logan, J., & Balota, D. (2008). Expanded vs. equal interval spaced retrieval practice: exploring different schedules of spacing and retention interval in younger and older adults. *Neuropsychol Devel Cogn Aging, 15,* 257–280.

Mahncke, H., Connor, B., & Appelman, J. (2006). Memory enhancement in healthy older adults using a brain plasticity-based training program: a randomized, controlled study. *Proc Natl Acad Sci, 103*(33), 12523–12528.

Mapelli, D., Rosa, D., Nocita, R., & Sava, D. (2013). Cognitive stimulation in patients with dementia: randomized controlled trial. *Dementia Geriatr Cogn Disord, 3*(1), 263–271.

Martin, M., Clare, L., Altgassen, A., Cameron, M., & Zehnder, F. (2011). Cognition-based interventions for healthy older people and people with mild cognitive impairment. *Cochrane Database Syst Rev, 1*(1), 1–49.

Mate-Kole, C., Fellows, R., Said, P., McDougal, J., Catayong, K., Dang, V., & Gianesini, J. (2007). Use of computer assisted and interactive cognitive training programmes with moderate to severely demented individuals: a preliminary study. *Aging and Mental Health, 11*(5), 485–495.

McCarty, D. (1980). Investigation of a visual imagery mnemonic device for acquiring face-name associations. *J Exper Psychology, 6*, 145–155.

Migo, E., Haynes, B., Harris, L., Friedner, K., Humphreys, K., & Kopelman, M. (2014). Health and memory aids: levels of smartphone ownership in patients. *J Mental Health*, Sep. 4: 1–5.

Miller, K., Dye, R., Kim, J., Jennings, J., O'Toole, E., Wong, J., & Siddarth, P. (2013). Effect of a computerized brain exercise program on cognitive performance in older adults. *Am J Geriatr Psychiatry, 21*(7), 655–663.

Miller, K., Ercoli, L., Kim, J., & Small, G. (2011). Memory training for older adults. In M. Abou-Saleh, C. Katona, & A. Kumar (Eds.), *Principles and practices of geriatric psychiatry* (3rd ed., pp. 397–402). Hoboken, NJ: Wiley-Blackwell.

Miller, K., Siddarth, P., Gaines, J., Parrish, J., Marx, K., Ronch, J., ... Small, G. (2011). The memory fitness program: cognitive effects of a healthy aging intervention. *Am J Geriatr Psychiatry*. doi: 10.1097//JGP.0b013e318227f821

Myczek, K., Yeung, S., Castello, N., Baglietto-Vargas, D., & LaFerla, F. (2014). Hippocampal adaptive response following extensive neuronal loss in an inducible transgenic mouse model. *PloS Med, 9*(9), 1–12. doi: 10.1371/journal.pone.0106009

Nacke, L., Nacke, A., & Lindley, C. (2009). Brain training for silver gamers: effects of age and game form on effectiveness, efficiency, self-assessment, and gameplay experience. *CyberPsychol Behav, 12*(5), 493–399. doi: 10.1089/cpb.2009.0013.

Nascimento, C., Pereira, J., deAndrade, L., Garuffi, M., Talib, L., Forlenza, O., ... Stella, F. (2014). Physical exercise in MCI elderly promotes reduction of pro-inflammatory cytokines and improvements on cognition and BDNF peripheral levels. *Curr Alzheimer Res, 11*(8), 799–805.

Nouchi, R., Taki, Y., HTakeuchi, Hashizume, H., Akitsuki, Y., Shigemune, Y., ... Kawashima, R. (2012). Brain training game improves executive functions and processing speed in the elderly: a randomized controlled trial. *PloS Med, 7*(1), e29676.

Nygard, L. (2008). The meaning of everyday technology as experienced by people with dementia who live alone. *Dementia, 7*(4), 481–502.

O'Hara, R., 3rd, J. B., Friedman, L., Schröder, C., Morgan, K., & Kraemer, H. (2007). Long-term effects of mnemonic training in community-dwelling older adults. *J Psychiatr Res, 41*(7), 585–590.

Orrell, M., Aguirre, E., Spector, A., Hoare, Z., Woods, R., Streater, A., ... Russel, I. (2014). Maintenance cognitive stimulation therapy for dementia: single-blind, multicentre, pragmatic randomised controlled trial. *Br J Psychiatry, 204*(6), 454–461. doi: 10.1192/bjp.bp.113.137414.

Owen, A., Hampshire, A., Grahn, J., Stenton, R., Dajani, S., Burns, A., ... Ballard, C. (2010). Putting brain training to the test. *Nature, 465*(7299), 775–778.

Park, D., Lautenschlager, G., Hedden, T., Davidson, N., Smith, A., & Smith, P. (2002). Models of visuospatial and verbal memory across the adult lifespan. *Psychol Aging, 17*(2), 229–320.

Park, D., Lodi-Smith, J., Drew, L., Haber, S., Hebrank, A., Bischof, G., & Aamodt, W. (2014). The impact of sustained engagement on cognitive function in older adults the synapse project. *Psychol Sci, 25*(1), 103–112.

Petersen, R., Smith, G., & Waring, S. (1999). Mild cognitive impairment: Clinical characterization and outcome. *Arch Neurol, 56*, 303–308.

Primack, B., Carroll, M., McNamara, M., Klem, M., King, B., Rich, M., ... Nayak, S. (2012). Role of video games in improving health-related outcomes: A systematic review. *Am J Prevent Med, 42*(6), 630–638.

Ramsberger, G., & Messamer, P. (2014). Best practices for incorporating non-aphasia specific apps into therapy. *Seminars Speech Language, 35*(1), 17–24. doi: 10.1055/s-0033-1362992.

Rapp, S., Brenes, G., & Marsh, A. (2002). Memory enhancement training for older adults with mild cognitive impairment: a preliminary study. *Aging Mental Health, 6*(1), 5–11.

Rebok, G., & Balcerak, L. (1989). Memory self-efficacy and performance differences in young and old adults: the effect of mnemonic training. *Dev Psychol, 25*(5), 714–721.

Rebok, G., Ball, K., Guey, L., Jones, R., Kim, H., King, J., ... Willis, S. (2014). Ten-year effects of the advanced cognitive training for independent and vital elderly cognitive training trial on cognition and everyday functioning in older adults. *J Am Geriatr Soc, 62*(1), 16–24.

Requena, C., Maestu, F., Campo, P., Fernandez, A., & Ortiz, T. (2006). Effects of cholinergic drugs and cognitive training on dementia: 2-year follow-up. *Dementia Geriatr Cogn Disord, 22*, 339–345.

Rosen, A., Suguira, L., Kramer, J., Whitfield-Gabrieli, S., & Gabrieli, J. (2011). Cognitive training changes hippocampal function in mild cognitive impairment: A pilot study. *J Alzheimers Dis, 26*(Suppl 3), 349–357.

Rozzini, L., Costardi, D., Chilovi, B., Franzoni, S., Trabucchi, M., & Padovani, A. (2007).

Efficacy of cognitive rehabilitation in patients with mild cognitive impairment treated with cholinesterase inhibitors. *Int J Geriatr Psychiatry, 22*(356–360).

Salthouse, T. (2009). When does age-related cognitive decline begin? *Neurobiol Aging, 30,* 507–514.

Sawyer, B. (2008). From cells to cell processors: Tte integration of health and video games. *IEEE Comput Graph Applic, 28*(6), 83–85.

Schreiber, M., Schweizer, A., Lutz, K., Kalveram, K., & Jancke, L. (1999). Potential of an interactive computer-based training in the rehabilitation of dementia: an initial study. *Neuropsychol Rehabil, 9*(2), 155–167.

Scogin, F., & Bienias, J. (1998). A three-year follow-up of older adult participants in a memory-skills training program. *Psychol Aging, 3*(4), 334–337.

Small, G. (2003). *The memory bible: An innovative strategy for keeping your brain young. Hyperion.*

Small, G., Moody, T., Siddarth, P., & Bookheimer, S. (2009). Your brain on Google: patterns of cerebral activation during Internet searching. *Am J Geriatr Psychiatry, 17*(2), 116–126.

Small, G., Siddarth, P., Ercoli, L., Chen, S., Merrill, D., & Torres-Gil, F. (2013). Healthy behavior and memory self-reports in young, middle-aged, and older adults. *Int Psychogeriatrics, 25*(6), 981–989. doi: 0.1017/S1041610213000082.

Small, G., Silverman, D., Siddarth, P., Ercoli, L., Miller, K., Wright, B., . . . Phelps, M. (2006). Effects of a 14-day healthy longevity lifestyle program on cognitive and brain functioning. *Am J Geriatr Psychiatry, 14,* 538–545.

Smith, G., Housen, P., & Yaffe, K. (2009). A cognitive training program based on principles of brain plasticity: results from the Improvement with Plasticity-based Adaptive Cognitive Training (IMPACT) study. *J Am Geriatr Soc, 57*(4), 594–603.

Smith-Ray, R., Hughes, S., Prohaska, T., Little, D., Jurivich, D., & Hedeker, D. (2013). Impact of cognitive training on balance and gait in older adults. *J Gerontol B. 70*(3), 357–366. doi: 10.1093/geronb/gbt097.

Sohlberg, M., & Mateer, C. (2001). *Cognitive rehabilitation: an integrative neuropsychological approach.* New York: Guilford Press.

Stigsdotter, N. (2000). Multifactorial memory training in normal aging: in search of memory improvement beyond the ordinary. In R. Hill, L. Backman, & A. Stigsdotter-Neely (Eds.), *Cognitive rehabilitation in old age* (pp. 63–80). New York: Oxford University Press.

Stigsdotter, N., & Backman, L. (1993). Long-term aintenance of gains from memory training in older

adults: two 3/12 years follow-up studies. *J Gerontol Psychol Sci, 48*(5), 233–237.

Talassi, E., Guerreschi, M., Feriani, M., Fedi, V., Bianchetti, A., & Trabucci, M. M. (2007). Effectiveness of a cognitive rehabilitation program in mild dementia (MD) and mild cognitive impairment (MCI): a case control study. *Arch Gerontol Geriatrics, 44*(Suppl 1), 391–399.

Thorndike, E., & Woodworth, R. (1901). The influence of improvement in one mental function upon the efficiency of other functions. *Psychol Rev, 8,* 247–261.

Tulving, E. (1983). *Elements of episodic memory.* Cambridge: Oxford University Press.

Unverzagt, F., Kasten, L., Johnson, K., Rebok, G., Marsiske, M., & Koepke, K. (2007). Effect of memory impairment on training outcomes in ACTIVE. *J Neuropsychol, 13,* 953–960.

Verhaeghen, P., Marcoen, A., & Goossens, L. (1992). Improving memory performance in the aged through mnemonic training: a meta-analytic study. *Psychol Aging, 7,* 242–251.

Vranić, A., Španić, A., Carretti, B., & Borella, E. (2013). The efficacy of a multifactorial memory training in older adults living in residential care settings. *Int Psychogeriatrics, 25*(11), 1885–1897.

Walton, C., Mowszowski, L., Lewis, S., & Nasmith, S. (2014). Stuck in the mud: time for change in the implementation of cognitive training research in ageing? *Front Aging Neurosci, 6*(43). doi: 10.3389/fnagi.2014.00043.

West, R., Bagwell, D., & Dark-Freudeman, A. (2008). Self-efficacy and memory aging; the impact of a memory intervention based on self efficacy. *Neuropsychol Devel Cogn Aging, 15*(3), 302–329.

Willis, S., Tennstet, S., Marsiske, M., Ball, K., Elias, J., & Koepke, K. (2006). Long-term effects of cognitive training on everyday functional outcomes in older adults. *JAMA, 296*(23), 2805–2814.

Wilson, B. (2002). Towards a comprehensive model of cognitive rehabilitation. *Neuropsychol Rehabil, 12*(2), 97–110.

Wolinsky, F., Weg, M. V., Howren, M., Jones, M., & Dotson, M. (2013). A randomized controlled trial of cognitive training using a visual speed of processing intervention in middle aged and older adults. *PloS One, 8*(5), e61624.

Yesavage, J. (1983). Imagery pretraining and memory training in the elderly. *Gerontology, 29*(4), 271–275.

Yesavage, J., & Rose, T. (1983). Concentration and mnemonic training in elderly subjects with memory complaints: a study of combined therapy and order effects. *Psychiatr Res, 9*(2), 157–167.

Yesavage, J., Sheikh, J., Friedman, L., & Tanke, E. (1990). Learning mnemonics: roles of aging and subtle cognitive impairment. *Psychol Aging, 51*(1), 133–137.

Yeung, S., Myczek, K., Kang, A., Chabrier, M., Baglietto-Vargas, D., & Laferla, F. (2014). Impact of hippocampal neuronal ablation on neurogenesis and cognition in the aged brain. *Neuroscience, 259*, 214–222.

Youn, J., Lee, J., Kim, S., & Ryu, S. (2011). Multistrategic memory training with the metamemory concept in healthy older adults. *Psychiatry Invest, 8*(4), 354–361. doi: 10.4306.

Zarit, S., Zarit, J., & Reever, K. (1982). Memory training for severe memory loss: effects on senile dementia patients and their families. *Gerontologist, 4*, 373–377.

Zehnder, F., Martin, M., Altgassen, M., & Clare, L. (2009). Memory training effects in old age as markers of plasticity: a meta-analysis. *Restor Neurol Neurosci, 27*(5), 507–520.

Zinke, K., Zeinti, M., Rose, N., Putzmann, J., Pydde, A., & Kilegel, M. (2014). Working memory training and transfer in older adults: effects of age, baseline performance, and training gains. *Dev Neuropsychol, 50*(1), 304–315. doi: 10.1037/a0032982.

23

COMPLEMENTARY AND ALTERNATIVE MEDICINE AGENTS IN THE PREVENTION OF LATE-LIFE DEPRESSION AND COGNITIVE DECLINE

Ankura Singh and Olivia I. Okereke

INTRODUCTION
Importance of Prevention

As the population of adults aged over 65 years continues to grow in the United States and other developed countries, the prevalence of late-life depression and age-related cognitive decline in these countries will increase (Djernes, 2006; Mathers and Loncar, 2006). Unipolar depressive disorders are projected to become the second leading cause of global disease burden by the year 2030, and are currently the leading cause of disease burden in middle- and high-income countries (Mathers and Loncar, 2006; Mihalopoulos, Vos, et al., 2011). It has been estimated that 2%–4% of community-dwelling older adults are affected by major depression, while an additional 7%–10% have clinically relevant depressive symptoms (Beekman, Copeland, et al., 1999; Chen, Chong, et al., 2007; Djernes, 2006). Depression has a strong negative impact on the well-being and daily functioning of older adults; furthermore,

this impact appears independent of other chronic illnesses and is associated with higher healthcare costs (Beekman, Penninx, et al., 2002; Katon, Lin, et al., 2003). Finally, although the incidence of depression and clinically significant depressive symptoms among older adults is not quite as high as that observed among younger persons, the rate (estimated at approximately 20–25 cases/1,000 person-years) (Luijendijk, van den Berg, et al., 2008; Norton, Skoog, et al., 2006; Pálsson, Ostling, et al., 2001) is as high as reported later-life incidence rates for several major diseases—including cardiovascular disease (Ridker, Cook, et al., 2005) and breast cancer (Cook, Lee, et al., 2005). Thus, the need for a heightened focus on the prevention of late-life depression, in conjunction with ongoing efforts concerned with treatment, is increasingly recognized by the field (Okereke, Lyness, et al., 2013; Reynolds, 2008; Reynolds, Cuijpers, et al., 2012; Smit, Beekman, et al., 2004).

The identification of risk factors and prevention strategies for age-related cognitive decline is also necessary, as studies have estimated that more than half of adults diagnosed with mild cognitive impairment will go on to develop dementia within 5 years (Gauthier, Reisberg, et al., 2006). This high rate of progression to dementia is concerning, as mild cognitive impairment is a common condition among older individuals; it is estimated to affect 14%–18% of elderly adults (Petersen, Roberts, et al., 2009). There are now over 5 million cases of Alzheimer's disease in the United States alone (Alzheimer's Association 2013), and more than 36 million dementia cases worldwide (Barnett, Hachinski, et al., 2013). Current treatments for Alzheimer's disease and vascular dementia are largely ineffective, as they fail to slow disease progression (Alzheimer's Association 2013). The current lack of treatment options makes the prevention of late-life cognitive decline a major public health priority.

Increasing Role of CAM Strategies

Complementary and alternative medicine (CAM) use has increased worldwide over the past two decades, and recent surveys have estimated that 36% of adults over 18 and 33% of elderly persons in the United States now use at least one CAM treatment (Lavretsky, 2009). Medical practices that do not fall under the category of conventional medicine, such as herbal medicine and nutritional interventions, are considered to be CAM techniques (Mahadevan & Park, 2008). Older adults are increasingly turning to CAM strategies to prevent and manage late-life cognitive and mood disorders; since these strategies have been associated with fewer side effects and drug interactions than conventional treatments, they tend to be well tolerated by older patients taking multiple prescription medications (Lavretsky, 2009; Sarris, Panossian, et al., 2011). As CAM encompasses a wide range of practices, including cognitive training, relaxation therapies, and dietary interventions, the efficacy of these treatments also greatly varies (Lavretsky, 2009). More high-quality randomized controlled trials evaluating the effectiveness of CAM in preventing depression or cognitive decline in older adults are needed, as there is currently a limited amount of evidence regarding the benefits of CAM interventions in this population.

CAM AND LATE-LIFE DEPRESSION

Observational Evidence for CAM Strategies

While it remains unclear whether some of the aforementioned categories of CAM treatments may benefit older adults who are at risk for late-life depression, recent data from numerous large-scale observational cohort studies have highlighted possible dietary risk factors, such as low intakes and serum levels of certain vitamins and minerals. In a cohort of Korean adults (Kim, Stewart, et al., 2008), aged $\geq$ 65 years and free of depression at the start of the study, baseline serum folate and vitamin B_{12} levels were both found to be inversely related to development of depression after an average of 2.4 years of follow-up ($p = 0.010$ and $p = 0.012$, respectively). Inverse associations between B vitamins and incident depression were also found in the Chicago Health and Aging Project (CHAP) (Skarupski, Tangney, et al., 2010), another observational study of adults aged over 65 years; the associations were significant for total intakes of vitamin B_6 ($p = 0.04$) and vitamin B_{12} ($p = 0.01$). In the Women's Health Initiative Observational Study (Bertone-Johnson, Powers, et al., 2011), a cohort of postmenopausal women between the ages of 50 and 79, participants with at least 400 IU vitamin D intake from food sources per day had a 20% lower risk of developing depressive symptoms over a 3-year follow-up period compared to those with daily intakes of less than 100 IU (OR: 0.80; 95% CI: 0.67, 0.95; p trend < 0.001); the results from this study suggested that low consumption of vitamin D from food sources alone may be a risk factor for depression.

Regarding mineral intakes, the relation of dietary zinc to later-life depression has also been studied. Low dietary zinc intakes were related to incident depression in middle-aged and elderly adults in the Australian Longitudinal Study on Women's Health (ALSWH) and the Hunter Community Study (HCS) (Vashum, McEvoy, et al., 2014). Although no dose-response relationship between dietary zinc and incident depressive symptoms was observed in either study, ALSWH participants who had zinc intakes within quintiles 2–5 had a 30% lower odds of developing depressive symptoms during the 6-year follow-up period than those in quintile 1 (lowest quintile). HCS participants who were in quintiles

2–4 of zinc intake had ~50% lower odds of developing depressive symptoms over 5 years compared to those in quintile 1, even though participants in quintile 5 had only a statistically non-significant reduction in odds versus the lowest quintile (Vashum, McEvoy, et al., 2014). By contrast, no association between dietary zinc and 20-year risk of depression was seen among middle-aged Finnish men in the Kuopio Ischemic Heart Disease Risk Factor Study (Lehto, Ruusunen, et al., 2013), in which the outcome of hospital discharge diagnosis of depression was not related to baseline zinc intake.

Increasingly, attention has turned toward examining dietary patterns, as these incorporate intakes of a variety of foods and may be more readily translatable to dietary recommendations (Willett, 1998; Jacobs & Tapsell, 2007). The ALSWH and CHAP studies both examined the relation of the Mediterranean dietary pattern to depressive symptoms. The Mediterranean diet is typically characterized based on adherence to a pattern of intakes of specific foods: higher intakes of whole grains, fruit, vegetables, legumes, nuts, olive oil (monounsaturated fat), and fish, moderate intake of alcohol/wine, and low intakes of red meat and saturated fat (Samieri, Sun, et al., 2013). Both the ALSWH (Rienks, Dobson, et al., 2013) and CHAP (Skarupski, Tangney, et al., 2013) studies found a linear trend association between higher adherence to the Mediterranean diet pattern and lower relative likelihood of depression: participants with the highest adherence to this dietary pattern were significantly less likely to develop depressive symptoms than those with the lowest adherence (p trend < 0.001 for both studies). Similarly, an inverse association was found between baseline Mediterranean diet score and psychological distress after 12 years of follow-up in the Melbourne Collaborative Cohort Study (Hodge, Almeida, et al., 2013) (OR : 0.86; 95% CI: 0.75, 0.98).

Finally, some studies have addressed specific nutrient components of key foods with regard to late-life depression risk. For example, the relation of intake of omega-3 fatty acids (nuts and fatty fish are particularly good sources of omega-3 fatty acids) to late-life depression risk has been examined. Intake of omega-3 fatty acids from plant sources (α-linolenic acid), but not marine sources, was inversely associated with relative risk of depression over 10 years of follow-up among middle-aged and elderly Nurses' Health Study participants (RR for 0.5 g/day increment = 0.82; 95% CI: 0.71, 0.94) (Lucas, Mirzaei, et al., 2011). Recent data from other observational cohorts—albeit with somewhat younger and middle-aged participants on average—are consistent with what Lucas and colleagues observed among the older participants of the Nurses' Health Study (who were on average older than 60 years at the start of follow-up). For example, in the SUN cohort (Sanchez-Villegas, Verberne, et al., 2011), participants classified as being in the highest quintile of polyunsaturated fatty acid (PUFA) intake had a significantly lower risk of developing depression compared with those in the lowest quintile after a median of 6.1 years of follow-up (p trend = 0.03); a dose-response relation was observed. Results from the CARDIA study (Colangelo, He, et al., 2009) showed that increasing quintiles of omega-3 fatty acid intake corresponded with a reduced risk of depressive symptoms after 3 years in women but not men (p trend = 0.008).

Overall, the data from the above-reviewed observational studies suggest that mid-life and older adults with either low nutrient levels or low dietary intakes of specific foods and nutrients might particularly benefit from dietary CAM nutritional interventions to prevent depression.

Clinical Trial Evidence for CAM Strategies

The availability and tolerability of dietary supplements and many other CAM interventions (Table 23.1) have made them desirable treatment alternatives and adjuncts among older adults with depression or depressive symptoms (Sarris, Panossian, et al., 2011). Although many of the aforementioned observational studies indicated that poor nutritional status is a risk factor for depressive disorders, limited evidence exists to support the use of dietary supplements to prevent late-life depression (Lavretsky, 2009). Low levels of serum folate and B vitamins have been linked to depression in cross-sectional studies, and so several clinical trials have been conducted to investigate the potentially protective effect of these vitamins on major depression in older adults (Andreeva, Galan, et al., 2012). Two RCTs (Ford, Flicker, et al., 2008; Okereke, Cook, et al., 2014) that had enrolled elderly subjects without clinically significant depression both found that daily folate, vitamin B_6, and vitamin B_{12} supplementation did not reduce the incidence of late-life

Table 23.1. Clinical Trials: CAM and Depression

AUTHOR	STUDY POPULATION	N	INTERVENTION	DURATION	OUTCOME MEASURE	RESULTS
Kasper et al. (2006)	Adult outpatients having an episode of mild or moderate major depression	332	600 mg/day or 1200 mg/day of St. John's wort extract WS 5570	6 weeks	HAM-D	A significantly greater decrease in HAM-D score occurred in each of the treatment groups than in the placebo group over the 6-week period ($p < 0.001$). Mean decreases in HAM-D scores in the 600 mg/day, 1200 mg/day and placebo groups were 11.6 ± 6.4, 10.8 ± 7.3 and 6.0 ± 8.1, respectively.
Kalb et al. (2001)	Adult outpatients with mild or moderate MDD	72	900 mg/day St. John's wort (Hypericum) extract	6 weeks	HAM-D	The average HAM-D score of the treatment group had decreased a significantly greater amount than that of the control group (10.8 ± 5.0 vs. 5.7 ± 6.4, $p < 0.001$).
Randløv et al. (2006)	Adults aged 25–70 with minor depression (HAM-D score > 7) or dysthymia	150	270 mg St. John's wort extract (either 0.12% hypericine or 0.18% hypericine) daily	6 weeks	HAM-D, BDI	Within the subgroup of participants without dysthymia, the group that received Hypericum had a significantly greater number of subjects with HAM-D scores of less than 7 at the end of the study period than the placebo group ($p = 0.03$).
Walker et al. (2010)	Community-dwelling adults aged 60–74	909	400 µg/day folic acid & 100 µg/day vitamin B12	24 months	PHQ-9	The change in PHQ-9 scores over the study period in the supplement group was not significantly different from that of the placebo group ($p = 0.476$).

Study	Population	N	Intervention	Duration	Measure	Results
Ford et al. (2008)	Men ≥ 75 w/o clinically significant depression	299	2 mg folic acid, 25 mg vitamin B_6 and 400 µg vitamin B_{12}/day	24 months	BDI	Although participants who received the intervention had a 24% lower risk of developing depression than those in the placebo group, the difference was not significant (95% CI: 0.68, 2.28). B-vitamin treatment did not prevent or reduce depressive symptoms compared with placebo ($p = 0.284$).
Okereke et al. (2014)	Women without depression (mean age = 63.6) in WAFACS	4331	2.5 mg folic acid, 50 mg vitamin B_6 and 1 mg vitamin B_{12}/day	7 years	Self-reported clinician diagnosis of depression or clinically significant depressive symptoms	There was no difference in risk of incident depression between the B vitamin and placebo groups (RR: 1.02; 95% CI: 0.86, 1.21, $p = 0.81$).
Andreeva et al. (2012)	Adults aged 45–80 in the SU.FOL.OM3 trial	2000	0.56 mg 5-methyl-tetrahydrofolate, 3 mg vitamin B_6 and 0.02 mg vitamin B_{12}/day, 600 mg EPA + DHA/day, or both	5 years	GDS	B vitamin supplementation did not have a significant effect on depressive symptoms (OR: 0.91; 95% CI: 0.75, 1.11). N-3 PUFA supplementation was associated with a greater risk of depressive symptoms compared to placebo in men only (OR: 1.28; 95% CI: 1.03, 1.61).
Gariballa et al. (2007)	Hospitalized patients ≥ 65	225	Daily multivitamin supplement	6 weeks	GDS-15, AMT	The mean GDS score of the supplement group significantly decreased compared to that of the placebo group ($p = 0.021$).

(continued)

Table 23.1. Continued

AUTHOR	STUDY POPULATION	N	INTERVENTION	DURATION	OUTCOME MEASURE	RESULTS
Bertone-Johnson et al. (2012)	Postmenopausal women (aged 50–79) in the Women's Health Initiative Calcium and Vitamin D (CaD) Trial	2263	1000 mg elemental calcium and 400 IU vitamin D_3/day	2 years	Burnam scale, antidepressant use	The mean change in Burnam scale score in the treatment group was not significantly different from that of the placebo group. Women receiving the supplements were not significantly less or more likely to have depressive symptoms at follow-up than women who received placebo (OR: 1.16; 95% CI: 0.86, 1.56).
Dumville et al. (2006)	Female primary care patients ≥ 70	2117	800 IU vitamin D/day	6 months	Mental Component Score of SF-12	The average MCS scores of the supplement and placebo groups were not significantly different after 6 months of follow-up, adjusting for baseline scores ($p = 0.262$).
Sánchez-Villegas et al. (2013)	Adults aged 55–80 in the PREDIMED trial with CVD risk factors	3923	Mediterranean diet supplemented with nuts or olive oil, or low-fat diet	3+ years	Self-reported depression diagnosis or antidepressant use	Participants in the Mediterranean diet + nuts group had a lower risk of developing depression than those in the low-fat/control group, though the association was not significant (HR: 0.78; 95% CI: 0.55, 1.10). When only including participants with type II diabetes in the analysis, the inverse association between Mediterranean diet + nuts and incident depression was significant (HR: 0.59; 95% CI: 0.36, 0.98).

Study	Population	N	Intervention/Dose	Duration	Measures	Results
Van de Rest et al. (2008)	Community-dwelling adults ≥ 65 without depression	302	1800 mg EPA + DHA/day or 400 mg EPA + DHA/day	26 weeks	CES-D, MADRS, GDS-15, HADS-A	There were no significant differences between the mean changes in CES-D, MADRS, HADS-A or GDS-15 scores of the placebo group and those of the fish oil groups after 26 weeks.
Haberka et al. (2013)	Patients who were hospitalized for acute MI	52	1 g n-3 PUFA/day	1 month	BDI	After one month, BDI scores in the intervention group had decreased significantly more than BDI scores in the control/standard therapy group ($p = 0.04$).
Sinn et al. (2012)	Adults ≥ 65 with mild cognitive impairment	50	EPA-rich supplement (1.67 g EPA + 0.16 g DHA/day) or DHA-rich supplement (1.55 g DHA + 0.40 g EPA/day)	6 months	GDS-15	Mean GDS-15 scores in the EPA and DHA groups significantly decreased over the study period compared to that of the control group ($p = 0.04$ and $p = 0.01$, respectively).
Gitlay et al. (2011)	Hospital patients aged 60–80 who had experienced an MI	4116	400 mg EPA + DHA/day, 2 g ALA/day, or both	40 months	GDS-15, Life Orientation Test-Revised	No significant differences were found between any of the 3 groups and placebo regarding levels of depressive symptoms after 40 months (p for EPA-DHA vs. placebo = 0.41; mean difference = −0.048 ± 0.044).
Wang et al. (2013)	Young, middle aged and elderly adult participants of 15 RCTs	1154	Qi gong intervention (mostly Eight Section Brocade Exercise)	70 minutes–4 months	Diabetes Specific Quality of Life Scale, SCL-90, GDS, SF-36	3 RCTs of patients with type II diabetes were included in a meta-analysis, which found that qi gong reduced depressive symptoms compared to the control interventions (effect size: −0.29; 95% CI: −0.58, 0.00).

(continued)

Table 23.1. Continued

AUTHOR	STUDY POPULATION	N	INTERVENTION	DURATION	OUTCOME MEASURE	RESULTS
Hui et al. (2006)	Hospital outpatients aged 42–76 with cardiac diseases	59	8 20-minute sessions of qi gong or progressive relaxation	8 sessions	Chinese version of SF-36	The qi gong group had a greater improvement on one of the psychologic measures of the SF-36 than the progressive relaxation group ($p = 0.027$). 7 of the 8 SF-36 measures had significantly improved in the qi gong group over the study period, compared to 1 out of 8 in the relaxation group.
Sephton et al. (2007)	Adult women with fibromyalgia	91	Mindfulness-based stress reduction (MBSR) intervention consisting of weekly sessions led by a clinical psychologist	8 weeks	BDI	The MBSR group had a greater reduction in depressive symptoms than the control group ($p = 0.001$). The effect of treatment on depressive symptoms was still significant 2 months after the intervention period had ended.
Würtzen et al. (2013)	Women aged 18–75 who had recently received treatment for breast cancer	336	Weekly sessions of a mindfulness-based stress reduction program	8 weeks	SCL-90, CES-D	A significantly greater reduction in depressive symptoms occurred in the MBSR group vs. the control group, according to both the SCL-90 ($p < 0.0001$) and the CES-D ($p = 0.04$).
Wang et al. (2009)	Adults with knee osteoarthritis (mean age = 65)	40	60 minute session of Tai Chi 2x/week	12 weeks	CES-D	The tai chi group had a significantly lower mean CES-D score after 12 and 48 weeks of follow-up than the control group (mean difference: −8.90; 95% CI: −13.83, −3.97; $p = 0.0006$).

depression compared with placebo. The study by Ford et al. (Ford, Flicker, et al., 2008) involved 299 men aged 75 and older who received 2 mg folic acid, 25 mg vitamin B_6, and 400 µg vitamin B_{12} daily for 24 months. The study by Okereke and colleagues involved a large sample ($n = 4331$) of older women who were administered daily a high-dose folic acid/B-vitamin combination pill (2.5 mg folic acid, 50 mg vitamin B_6, and 1 mg vitamin B_{12}/day) over a lengthy treatment period (mean treatment duration = 7 years). Results from the SU.FOL.OM3 trial (Andreeva, Galan, et al., 2012), which involved adults aged 45–80 receiving daily supplements of folate and vitamins B_6 and B_{12} for 5 years, also showed no association between supplementation and depressive symptoms. Finally, in a 24-month RCT (Walker, Mackinnon, et al., 2010) that included community-dwelling adults aged 60–74, subjects who took daily supplements of folic acid and vitamin B_{12} did not experience a greater reduction in depressive symptoms than those in the control group.

Overall, the existing randomized trial data do not provide support for use of B-vitamin supplementation to prevent incident depression or reduce depressive symptoms among community-dwelling older adults who are generally healthy and adequately nourished. However, it cannot be inferred from these trial data whether there are subsets of individuals at risk (e.g., due to biochemical nutrient deficiency, genetic polymorphism, or other predisposing factors) who may benefit from preventive treatment with B-vitamin supplements.

There are few clinical trials that examine the effects of other vitamin supplements on the psychological well-being of elderly persons, compared with the number of studies that focus on B vitamins. A sub-study (Bertone-Johnson, Powers, et al., 2012) conducted within the Women's Health Initiative Calcium and Vitamin D (CaD) Trial found that postmenopausal women who received supplements of 1000 mg elemental calcium and 400 IU vitamin D_3 per day for 2 years were not less likely to experience depressive symptoms at follow-up than women who were taking placebo. Results from another RCT (Dumville, Miles, et al., 2006) showed no difference between the SF-12 Mental Component scores of elderly women receiving 800 IU vitamin D daily and those of the placebo group after 6 months of treatment. Garibella and colleague (Garibella & Forster,

2007) observed that geriatric inpatients who were administered a daily multivitamin supplement for 6 weeks had a significant reduction in depressive symptoms relative to control group participants ($p = 0.021$); these differences were apparent at a 6-month follow-up assessment. Overall, results from the above-mentioned studies illustrate that the trial literature is limited regarding contributions of vitamin D and multivitamins to depression risk in older adults—particularly with regard to the benefits and/or risks of long-term supplementation with these agents at high doses.

Since the data from numerous cohort studies suggested that omega-3 fatty acid and/or Mediterranean diet intake may play a role in preventing depression in older adults, a number of clinical trials have recently been carried out to better examine these associations. A statistically nonsignificant inverse relationship was found between a Mediterranean diet intervention and incident depression in the PREDIMED trial (Sanchez-Villegas, Martinez-Gonzalez, et al., 2013) (HR: 0.78; 95% CI: 0.55, 1.10), an RCT that included adults aged 55–80 with cardiovascular disease risk factors. When only participants with type II diabetes were included in the analysis, however, the inverse association between randomization to the trial arm of Mediterranean diet supplemented with nuts for at least 3 years and incident depression was significant (HR: 0.59; 95% CI: 0.36, 0.98).

Two RCTs (Sinn, Milte, et al., 2012; Haberka, Mizia-Stec, et al., 2013) that involved adults with medical comorbidities provided evidence that omega-3 fatty acid supplementation may reduce depressive symptoms. Participants who took daily omega-3 fatty acid supplements for the duration of the study, which was either 1 month (Haberka, Mizia-Stec, et al., 2013) or 6 months (Sinn, Milte, et al., 2012), had a greater decrease in depressive symptoms than those receiving placebo ($p < 0.05$ for both). Two other clinical trials (Giltay, Geleijnse, et al., 2011; van de Rest, Geleijnse, et al., 2008) that included only adults over age 60 did not show an association between omega-3 supplementation and Center for Epidemiologic Studies Depression Scale (CES-D) or Geriatric Depression Scale-15 (GDS-15) scores, however, and the SU.FOL.OM3 trial (Andreeva, Galan, et al., 2012) found that taking a 600 mg EPA (eicosapentaenoic acid) + DHA (docosahexaenoic acid) supplement daily for 5 years was associated with a greater risk of depressive symptoms compared to placebo in men (OR: 1.28; 95% CI: 1.03, 1.61). The available data on the effect of omega-3 fatty acids on depressive symptoms in older adults are therefore inconclusive, and intervention studies that evaluate the role of omega-3s in preventing depression in this population are needed.

CAM interventions other than vitamins, minerals, food, and nutrients have also been examined in trials; these have included, for example, herbal medicines, physical exercise, and meditation/mindfulness-based interventions. Among CAM treatments for depression, St. John's wort has been particularly popular. St. John's wort extract, or *Hypericum perforatum*, is an herbal supplement that has been found to alleviate mild to moderate depressive symptoms in numerous clinical trials (Varteresian & Lavretsky, 2014). Although studies that focus specifically on the treatment of older adults with St. John's wort are rare, two RCTs (Randlov, Mehlsen, et al., 2006; Mannel, Kuhn, et al., 2010) that included adults up to age 70 demonstrated that both 270 mg and 600 mg daily doses of St. John's wort were more effective at reducing depressive symptoms than placebo. In studies of interventions that involved higher doses of St. John's wort, and which were administered to adult outpatients experiencing a mild to moderate depressive episode, it was found that daily doses of 900 mg (Kalb, Trautmann-Sponsel, et al., 2001) or 1200 mg (Kasper, Anghelescu, et al., 2006) for 6 weeks significantly reduced scores on the Hamilton Rating Scale for Depression compared with placebo; however, while these higher doses appeared to be well tolerated by participants, neither of these studies included individuals over 65. Furthermore, none of the aforementioned RCTs examined the use of St. John's wort as a possible prevention strategy. Thus, there is clearly a need for more trials evaluating the safety and efficacy of St. John's wort, at a broader range of possible doses, for use among older adults.

Although higher levels of participation in physical activities have generally been observed to be inversely related to late-life depression, the potential preventive effects of CAM physical and cognitive therapies such as tai chi, qi gong and meditation have not been extensively studied in elderly populations (Lavretsky, 2009). Recent studies suggest that these interventions have positive effects on the mental health and well-being of medically ill adults—thus providing evidence of their usefulness specifically in selective prevention of depression. In a review of several RCTs with young, middle-aged, and elderly participants, Wang and colleagues (Wang, Man, et al., 2013) found that qi gong reduced depressive symptoms in type II diabetes patients compared to the control interventions (effect size: −0.29; 95% CI: −0.58, 0.00). A qi gong intervention that was provided to middle-aged and elderly hospital outpatients was also associated with improved psychological well-being, according to the SF-36 (Hui, Wan, et al., 2006). Another clinical trial (Wang, Schmid, et al., 2009) examined the effect of tai chi on the mood of older adults with knee osteoarthritis; results showed that subjects who participated in the 12 weeks of tai chi sessions had significantly lower CES-D scores after the intervention and at the 48-week follow-up assessment than those in the control group ($p = 0.009$ and $p = 0.0006$, respectively). In two RCTs (Sephton, Salmon, et al., 2007; Wurtzen, Dalton, et al., 2013), mindfulness meditation was found to lessen depressive symptoms in adult women with medical comorbidities; the 8-week mindfulness-based stress reduction treatment was more effective at reducing depression scores than the control intervention in each study. Though these outcomes appear to support the use of alternative therapies, additional studies involving meditation, tai chi, and qi gong must be conducted in older populations free of depression at baseline before their efficacy in preventing late-life depression can be confirmed.

CAM AND LATE-LIFE COGNITIVE DECLINE

Observational Evidence for CAM Strategies

Some of the same CAM treatments that were administered with the hope of preventing depression or reducing depressive symptoms among older adults have also been used in studies where cognitive function is the outcome of interest. Indeed, CAM intervention studies involving dietary supplements have been inspired in large part by the numerous observational studies linking dietary exposures to improved cognitive outcomes. In the Veterans Affairs Normative Aging Study (Tucker, Qiao, et al., 2005), positive associations were found between spatial copying score after 3 years and baseline levels of plasma folate, vitamin B_6, and vitamin B_{12} ($p < 0.0001$, $p < 0.01$, and $p < 0.05$, respectively). The associations were also statistically significant when focusing on dietary intake of these vitamins and spatial copying score, and dietary folate was also positively correlated with verbal fluency score ($p < 0.05$). Serum concentrations of folate, but not vitamin B_{12}, were inversely related to incident dementia in another cohort of older adults (Ravaglia, Forti, et al., 2005): subjects with folate concentrations of less than 11.8 nmol/L had a higher risk of dementia (HR: 1.87; 95% CI: 1.21, 2.89; $p = 0.005$) and Alzheimer's disease (HR: 1.98; 95% CI: 1.15, 3.40; $p = 0.014$) over an average of 4 years, compared to those without low folate. Consistent with this finding, Luchsinger and colleagues (Luchsinger, Tang, et al., 2007) found that in a cohort of adults over age 65 without dementia at baseline, participants with total folate intakes in the highest quartile had a 50% reduced risk of developing Alzheimer's disease (AD) compared with those categorized in the lowest quartile (95% CI: 0.3, 0.9; p trend = 0.02), but total intakes of vitamins B_6 and B_{12} were not significantly related to the outcome. Finally, in the Chicago Health and Aging Project (Morris, Evans, et al., 2004), an inverse dose-response relationship was observed for niacin intake and 4-year risk of AD (p trend = 0.04). Thus, these observational studies indicate that low folate consumption or biochemical levels appear related to poor cognitive outcomes; however, the association between other B vitamins and long-term cognitive change is less consistent.

There has also been investigation into whether other types of vitamin intakes (i.e., non-B vitamins) are associated with late-life cognitive change. Higher dietary levels of vitamin D appeared to protect against incident AD among females over age 75 in the EPIDOS Toulouse study (Annweiler, Rolland, et al., 2012), as those who had the highest intakes of vitamin D from food sources were significantly less likely to develop AD over the 7-year study period than subjects in the lower quintiles of intake (OR Q5 vs. Q1–4: 0.23; 95% CI: 0.08, 0.67). In the Canadian Study of Health and Aging (Maxwell, Hicks, et al., 2005), the use of a combination of vitamin C and vitamin E supplements was inversely related to cognitive decline; however, this association was not seen for vitamin C or E supplementation alone (Maxwell, Hicks, et al., 2005). Being in the highest tertile of dietary vitamin E intake versus the bottom tertile corresponded to a reduced 5-year risk of dementia in the Rotterdam Study (Devore, Grodstein, et al., 2010) (HR: 0.75; 95% CI: 0.59, 0.95); however, no difference in dementia risk was found between the highest and lowest tertiles of vitamin C, beta carotene, or flavonoid intake. In two additional cohort studies that also featured older adults (Fillenbaum, Kuchibhatla, et al., 2005; Luchsinger, Tang, et al., 2003), no significant associations were observed between dietary, supplemental, or total intakes of vitamins C or E and incident dementia or AD.

The evidence linking the consumption of omega-3 fatty acids and a Mediterranean-style diet to cognitive function late in life appears to be stronger, and suggests a beneficial effect of dietary intake of fish and/or Mediterranean diet-related foods. In three large cohorts of community-dwelling older adults (Feart, Samieri, et al., 2009; Tangney, Kwasny, et al., 2011; Wengreen, Munger, et al., 2013), Mediterranean diet score was associated with reduced decline in cognitive test scores over follow-up periods lasting between 4 and 11 years ($p = 0.03, 0.0004,$ and 0.001, respectively). Another study (Koyama, Houston, et al., 2014) found that Mediterranean diet score was related to a significantly better trajectory of scores on the Modified Mini-Mental State Examination over the course of 8 years among black, but not white, participants. Samieri and colleagues (Samieri, Grodstein, et al., 2013) did not find an association between the Mediterranean diet and any of the cognitive measures in the Women's Health Study, although a high monounsaturated-to-saturated fat ratio was associated with better trajectories of mean cognitive scores in elderly women over time ($p = 0.03$ for global cognition and $p = 0.05$ for verbal memory). Stricter adherence to a Mediterranean-style dietary pattern was related to a decreased 4-year risk of incident AD, however, in two analyses involving populations of older adults in New York (p trend = 0.01 and 0.007) (Gu, Nieves, et al., 2010; Scarmeas, Stern, et al., 2006).

Associations between fish and/or omega-3 fatty acid intake and measures of late-life cognitive change were also observed in some of the cohort studies mentioned earlier. In the Chicago Health and Aging Project (Morris, Evans, et al., 2005), the annual rate of cognitive decline over 6 years was 13% lower among participants who consumed fish two or more times per week than among those with infrequent fish intake ($p = 0.04$). Women's Health Study participants over age 65 who had one or more servings of dark-flesh finfish per week had significantly higher verbal memory scores after a 4-year follow-up period than those who consumed less than one serving (difference = 0.079 SU; $p <$

0.01); no association was found between light-flesh finfish and cognitive test scores (Kim, Grodstein, et al., 2013). The difference in results for dark-flesh versus light-flesh finfish in the work by Kim and colleagues is particularly relevant to the omega-3 hypothesis, as dark-meat fish and tuna have substantially higher levels of long-chain omega-3 fatty acids than light-meat fish. Finally, in a study examining biochemical levels of intakes, plasma levels of long-chain omega-3 fatty acids (DHA and EPA) were associated with a reduced decline in verbal fluency over 6 years in a cohort of middle-aged and older adults (Beydoun, Kaufman, et al., 2007) (OR: 0.74; 95% CI: 0.57-0.97). In contrast with findings from all the above-mentioned studies, neither omega-3 intake nor fish consumption was related to incident dementia in the Rotterdam Study (Devore, Grodstein, et al., 2009) over an average follow-up period of 9.6 years. Overall, while most of the existing data from elderly cohorts seem to indicate that higher intakes of fish, folate, and Mediterranean diet–related foods (and the relevant biochemical nutrient levels) are related favorably to cognitive aging, the associations for other dietary factors on late-life cognitive outcomes are less clear.

Clinical Trial Evidence for CAM Strategies

The efficacy of vitamin supplements in preventing cognitive decline has been the focus of a number of clinical trials involving older adults. Intervention studies that assess the impact of B vitamins on late-life cognitive decline (Table 23.2) have had mixed results. In the VITACOG trial (de Jager, Oulhaj, et al., 2012; Smith, Smith, et al., 2010), adults over age 70 with mild cognitive impairment were given daily supplements of 0.8 mg folic acid, 0.5 mg vitamin B_{12}, and 20 mg vitamin B_6 for 24 months. Subjects receiving the intervention had higher executive function scores ($p = 0.015$) (de Jager, Oulhaj, et al., 2012) and lower yearly rates of brain atrophy ($p = 0.001$) (Smith, Smith, et al., 2010) than control group participants at the end of the study period. Similarly, in another clinical trial (Walker, Batterham, et al., 2012), study investigators found that 24 months of daily supplementation with 400 μg folic acid and 100 μg vitamin B_{12} improved the cognitive status of elderly adults with elevated psychological distress compared to those receiving placebo ($p = 0.032$). However, results from the much larger Women's Antioxidant and Folic Acid

Cardiovascular Study (WAFACS) (Kang, Cook, et al., 2008) did not show any differences on the outcome of cognitive decline in the active B-vitamin versus control groups. Another important element of the WAFACS trial was that the intervention was well-dosed—providing participants with 2.5 mg folic acid, 50 mg vitamin B_6, and 1 mg vitamin B_{12} per day versus matching inert placebo—and was conducted over a lengthy duration of approximately 6.6 years.

Data from existing RCTs in which older adults were treated with other vitamin supplements do not indicate a protective effect of these vitamins on incident cognitive decline. When evaluating results from the Women's Health Initiative Calcium and Vitamin D trial, Rossom and colleagues (Rossom, Espeland, et al., 2012) found that the risk of developing dementia in the supplement group was not significantly different from that of the placebo group. They also did not observe an association between the treatment and development of mild cognitive impairment over an average of 7.8 years of follow-up. A cognitive substudy within the Women's Health Study (Kang, Cook, et al., 2006) showed no difference in the global cognition scores of women who received 600 IU of vitamin E on alternate days for an average of 9.6 years and women who were given placebo. Similarly, long-term vitamin E supplementation did not differ from placebo with regard to effects on cognitive change in the Women's Antioxidant Cardiovascular Study (Kang, Cook, et al., 2009), an RCT of women over age 65 taking vitamin E, vitamin C, beta carotene supplements, or placebo. Beta carotene and vitamin C supplementation also failed to produce differences in cognitive change overall in this sample compared with placebo, although participants receiving vitamin C had higher cognitive test scores at the final cognitive assessment ($p = 0.0005$) (Kang, Cook, et al., 2009). A comparably conducted trial examined the effects of different vitamin treatments on cognitive decline among male physicians over age 65 in the Physicians' Health Study II (PHSII; Grodstein, Kang, et al., 2007). The PHSII included both short-term and long-term beta carotene treatment groups, in addition to a separate trial arm involving daily multivitamin supplements. While beta carotene supplementation did not affect cognitive change in the short-term treatment group, men who received the supplements for an average of 18 years (beginning when the men were, on average, in their early 50s) had significantly higher

Table 23.2. Clinical Trials: CAM and Cognitive Decline

AUTHOR	STUDY POPULATION	n	INTERVENTION	DURATION	OUTCOME MEASURE	RESULTS
Cockle et al. (2000)	Community dwelling elderly volunteers (mean age = 68.8)	5028	120 mg/day Ginkgo biloba extract	4 months	Line analogue rating scale (LARS), B-ADL scale, and self-rated activities of daily living scale (SR-ADL)	The mean change in B-ADL score in the intevention group was significantly different than that of the control group ($p < 0.001$). A greater increase in B-ADL score occurred in the control group, indicating a greater decline in daily activity performance among those who were not receiving treatment. SR-ADL scores in the intervention group significantly declined compared to those in the control group over the 4-month period ($p < 0.001$), which indicates an improvement in self-rated abilities.
Vellas et al. (2012)	Adults ≥ 70 who reported memory problems to their PCP	2854	120 mg Ginkgo biloba extract 2x/day	5 years	DSM-IV diagnosis of Alzheimer's disease	The incidence rate of AD in the intervention group (1.2/100 person-years) was not significantly different from that of the placebo group (1.4/100 person-years; HR: 0.84; 95% CI: 0.60, 1.18; $p = 0.306$).
Mix et al. (2002)	Cognitively intact adults ≥ 60	262	180 mg/day Ginkgo biloba extract	6 weeks	Selective Reminding Test, WAIS-III BD, WAIS-III DS, WMS-III FI and FII	The EGb 761 group had a significantly greater mean increase in scores on the delayed free recall ($p < 0.04$) and delayed recognition ($p < 0.01$) tasks of the Selective Reminding Test than the placebo group. Mean scores on the delayed recognition task of the WMS-III Faces II also improved more in the EGb 761 group compared to the control group over the 6-week period ($p < 0.025$).

(continued)

Table 23.2. Continued

AUTHOR	STUDY POPULATION	n	INTERVENTION	DURATION	OUTCOME MEASURE	RESULTS
DeKosky et al. (2008)	Adults ≥ 75 with either normal cognition or mild cognitive impairment, but without dementia	3069	120 mg Ginkgo biloba extract 2x/day	Median of 6.1 years	DSM-IV diagnosis of dementia, AD, Modified Mini-Mental State Examination	There was no significant difference in the incidence rate of dementia in the treatment vs. placebo groups (HR: 1.2; 95% CI: 0.94, 1.33; $p = 0.21$). The incidence rate of AD among those receiving Ginkgo was also not significantly different from that of the placebo group (HR: 1.16; 95% CI: 0.97, 1.39; $p = 0.11$).
De Jager et al. (2012)	Adults ≥ 70 with mild cognitive impairment	266	0.8 mg/day folic acid, 0.5 mg/day vitamin B_{12}, 20 mg/day vitamin B_6	2 years	MMSE, Hopkins Verbal Learning Test (HVLT DR), executive function (CLOX), category fluency, homocysteine levels	Executive function (CLOX) scores were significantly higher among participants receiving B vitamins vs. placebo ($p = 0.015$). When only including participants with high baseline homocysteine (≥ 11.3 μmol/L) in the analysis, there was a significant protective effect of treatment on MMSE score ($p < 0.001$), HVLT DR ($p = 0.001$), and category fluency ($p = 0.037$), indicating that B vitamin supplementation reduced cognitive decline among those with elevated homocysteine.
Smith et al. (2010)	Adults ≥ 70 with mild cognitive impairment	187	0.8 mg/day folic acid, 0.5 mg/day vitamin B_{12}, 20 mg/day vitamin B_6	2 years	Rate of brain atrophy/year	At the end of the 24-month period, MRI scans had shown that the mean rate of brain atrophy per year in the treatment group was significantly lower than that of the placebo group (0.76% vs. 1.08%; $p = 0.001$).

Study	Population	N	Intervention	Duration	Outcome measure	Results
Walker et al. (2012)	Adults aged 60–74 with elevated psychological distress	900	400 μg folic acid and 100 μg B_{12}/day	2 years	Telephone Interview for Cognitive Status-Modified (TICS-M)	The TICS-M total scores of participants in the supplement group had significantly increased compared with the scores of the control group ($p = 0.032$; effect size = 0.17). There was a significantly greater increase in average TICS-M immediate score ($p = 0.046$; effect size = 0.15) and TICS-M delayed recall score ($p = 0.013$; effect size = 0.18) in the supplement group vs. the placebo group.
Kang et al. (2008)	Women ≥ 65 in the Women's Antioxidant and Folic Acid Cardiovascular Study with either CVD or CVD risk factors	2009	2.5 mg folic acid, 50 mg vitamin B_6 and 1 mg vitamin B_{12}/day	6.6 years	Global composite cognition score averaging 5 tests of general cognition, verbal memory, and category fluency	The mean change in global cognitive score per year in the B vitamin group was not different from that of the placebo group (mean difference in cognitive decline/year = 0.03 SU; 95% CI: −0.03, 0.08). No significant association was found between B vitamin supplementation and any of the individual cognitive measures. Supplementation reduced cognitive decline according to the TICS among women with low dietary intakes of B vitamins (mean difference in cognitive change = 0.74; 95% CI: 0.23, 1.25), but not among those with adequate intakes.
Rossom et al. (2012)	Women ≥ 65 in the Women's Health Initiative Calcium and Vitamin D trial	4143	1,000 mg calcium carbonate and 400 IU vitamin D_3 per day	7.8 years on average	Diagnosis of dementia or mild cognitive impairment	No significant difference in risk of developing dementia was observed between the 2 groups (HR: 1.11; 95% CI: 0.71, 1.74; $p = 0.64$). There was also no significant association found between supplementation and development of MCI (HR: 0.95; 95% CI: 0.72, 1.25; $p = 0.72$).

(continued)

Table 23.2. Continued

AUTHOR	STUDY POPULATION	n	INTERVENTION	DURATION	OUTCOME MEASURE	RESULTS
Kang et al. (2009)	Women ≥ 65 in the Women's Antioxidant and Cardiovascular Study	2824	402 mg (600 IU) of vitamin E or 50 mg of beta carotene every other day, or 500 mg of vitamin C/day, for an average	8.9 years on average	Global composite cognition score averaging 5 tests of general cognition, verbal memory, and category fluency	There was no difference in the average rates of cognitive change in the vitamin E vs. placebo groups (mean difference = −0.01; 95% CI: −0.05, 0.04; $p = 0.78$). Beta carotene and vitamin C supplementation were also not associated with rate of cognitive change (mean difference = 0.03 and 0.02, and $p = 0.28$ and 0.39, respectively). Participants receiving vitamin C supplements had higher cognitive scores at the last cognitive assessment than those receiving placebo (mean difference = 0.13; 95% CI: 0.06, 0.20; $p = 0.0005$).
Kang et al. (2006)	Women ≥ 65 in the Women's Health Study	6377	600 IU of vitamin E on alternate days	9.6 years on average	Global composite cognition score averaging 5 tests of general cognition, verbal memory, and category fluency	The average global cognition score in the vitamin E group was not different than that of the placebo group (mean difference = 0.00; 95% CI: −0.04, 0.04). The vitamin E group also did not experience less cognitive decline between the initial and final cognitive assessments (4 yrs) than the placebo group (mean difference = 0.02; 95% CI: −0.01, 0.05).

Author (year)	Population	N	Intervention	Duration	Outcome measure	Results
Grodstein et al. (2007)	Males ≥ 65 in the Physicians' Health Study II	5956	Short-term or long-term supplementation of 50 mg beta carotene every other day	Either 1 year or 18 years	Global composite cognition score averaging 5 tests of general cognition, verbal memory, and category fluency	No association was found between treatment group and global cognition score among the men who received short-term beta carotene supplementation. Among those in the long-term supplementation group, men receiving the supplements had significantly higher global cognition scores than those who received placebo (mean difference = 0.047 SU; $p = 0.03$). Men in the long-term beta carotene group also had significantly greater verbal memory scores than those in the long-term placebo group (mean difference = 0.063; $p = 0.007$).
Grodstein et al. (2013)	Males ≥ 65 in the Physicians' Health Study II	5947	Daily multivitamin	12 years	Global composite cognition score averaging 5 tests of global cognition, verbal memory, and category fluency	The average difference in cognitive change between the multivitamin and placebo groups was not significant (difference = −0.01 SU; 95% CI: −0.04, 0.02). There was also no significant difference in change in verbal memory between the two groups (difference = −0.005 SU; 95% CI: −0.04, 0.03).
McNeill et al. (2007)	Community dwelling adults ≥ 65	910	Daily multivitamin tablet with 16 vitamins/minerals	12 months	Digit span forward and verbal fluency tests to assess cognitive function	There was no difference between the mean change in test scores over time of the multivitamin and placebo groups. In a subgroup analysis including only participants aged 75 and older, a weak positive effect of supplementation on verbal fluency was observed (mean difference = 2.8; 95% CI: −0.6, 6.2). A similar effect on verbal fluency was observed among participants who were at increased risk of nutritional deficiency (mean difference = 2.5; 95% CI: −1.0, 6.1).

(continued)

Table 23.2. Continued

AUTHOR	STUDY POPULATION	n	INTERVENTION	DURATION	OUTCOME MEASURE	RESULTS
Martinez-Lapiscina et al. (2013)	Adults aged 55–80 in the PREDIMED trial	522	Mediterranean diet supplemented with nuts or olive oil, or low-fat diet for a mean follow-up of 6.5 years	6.5 years on average	MMSE, Clock Drawing Test	Participants in both the Mediterranean diet + EVOO group and the Mediterranean diet + nuts group had significantly higher MMSE and CDT scores than those in the control group after an average of 6.5 years (EVOO: $p = 0.005$ and 0.001; nuts: $p = 0.015$ and 0.048).
Sydenham et al. (2012)	Adults ≥ 60 without dementia or cognitive impairment	4080	Omega-3 PUFAs via gel capsules or margarine spread	6, 24 or 40 months	MMSE, word learning, digit span, verbal fluency	In two of the studies, no significant difference in MMSE score was found between the omega-3 and placebo groups at the end of the study periods (mean difference = -0.07; 95% CI: -0.25, 0.10). In the third study, no difference was found between the omega-3 group and placebo group on any of the other cognitive measures.
Desideri et al. (2012)	Elderly patients of the Alzheimer unit of the University of L'Aquila Geriatric Division who had mild cognitive impairment	90	Cocoa drink with either 45 mg, 520 mg, or 990 mg of flavanol/day	8 weeks	MMSE, Trail Making Test, verbal fluency test, blood pressure, insulin resistance, lipid peroxidation	Some improvement in cognitive function was observed in the high and medium flavanol groups, compared to the low flavanol group. Trail making tests A & B were completed in significantly shorter periods of time by participants in both treatment groups vs. those in the control group ($p < 0.05$), and subjects in the high flavanol group experienced a significantly greater improvement in verbal fluency test scores than those who consumed low flavanol ($p < 0.05$).

| Rebok et al. (2014) | Community-dwelling adults ≥ 65 in the ACTIVE study | 2832 | 10 cognitive training sessions over 5–6 weeks followed by 4 sessions of booster training for a subset of participants | 10 years | Memory, reasoning, speed of processing and IADL function measures | Participants who received the reasoning and speed processing interventions had improved cognitive outcomes in those areas compared with the control group (reasoning effect size = 0.23; 99% CI: 0.09, 0.38; speed of processing effect size = 0.66; 99% CI: 0.43, 0.88). Those receiving the memory intervention did not have significantly greater memory performance than controls at follow-up. |

late-life global cognition scores ($p = 0.03$) and verbal memory scores ($p = 0.007$) than those who were given placebo during that time period (Grodstein, Kang, et al., 2007). In the multivitamin arm of the PHSII, long-term (12 years on average) multivitamin treatment did not have a significantly different impact on late-life global or verbal cognitive change compared to placebo (Grodstein, O'Brien, et al., 2013). Similarly, another RCT (McNeill, Avenell, et al. 2007) that involved providing daily multivitamins to elderly persons reported null associations. However, when restricting the analyses in the latter study to include only participants over age 75, or only those with possible micronutrient deficiencies, a weak positive association between multivitamin treatment and verbal fluency score was observed. Overall, while the above-mentioned vitamin trials reported null findings for broad preventive benefits of these agents on late-life cognitive decline, they also provide important hints for future research directions. The findings by Grodstein et al. regarding significant benefits of long-term, but not short-term, treatment with beta carotene speak to the notion that preventive interventions for cognitive decline must be implemented at much earlier ages than has generally been the case in the extant trial literature. Finally, the suggestive findings by McNeill and colleagues among the subset of persons at high risk due to nutrient deficiency, while requiring a cautious interpretation as with any subgroup analysis, highlight the importance of targeted, or selective, prevention. Other dietary interventions to improve cognitive measures have had more promising results, even though the available data on these treatments are still limited and/or inconclusive. In the PREDIMED trial (Martinez-Lapiscina, Clavero, et al., 2013), adults aged 55–80 were assigned to a Mediterranean diet supplemented with either nuts or extra-virgin olive oil (EVOO), or a low-fat diet. Participants in both of the Mediterranean diet groups had significantly higher MMSE (EVOO: $p = 0.005$; nuts: $p = 0.015$) and Clock Drawing Test (EVOO: $p = 0.001$; nuts: $p = 0.048$) scores than those in the low-fat group after an average follow-up period of 6.5 years. The specific effects of omega-3 fatty acid supplementation on late-life cognitive outcomes, however, have been inconsistent. In a meta-analysis of 10 RCTs (Mazereeuw, Lanctot, et al., 2012), omega-3 supplements were found to improve immediate recall and processing speed in the subgroup of elderly subjects with mild cognitive impairment, but not in healthy subjects or those

with Alzheimer's disease. Another meta-analysis by Sydenham and colleagues (Sydenham, Dangour, et al., 2012) included three RCTs with older adults who were free of dementia or cognitive impairment at baseline; however, this review did not find any effect of 6, 24, or 40 months of omega-3 supplementation on MMSE score or other cognitive measures.

The herbal product Ginkgo biloba is also commonly taken as a supplement for the prevention and treatment of cognitive problems (Mahadevan & Park, 2008), even though the available literature does not consistently support its use for this purpose. In two studies that had populations of community-dwelling elderly subjects and lasted for 6 weeks (Mix & Crews, 2002) and 4 months (Cockle, Kimber, et al., 2000), respectively, participants who received daily supplements of Ginkgo biloba extract had improved performance on several cognitive tests compared with those who were taking placebo. Also, the activities of daily living (ADL) scores at the follow-up assessment in the 4-month study indicated that the treatment group had experienced significantly less decline in daily activity performance than the control group ($p < 0.001$) (Cockle, Kimber, et al., 2000). In the 6-week study, Ginkgo biloba supplementation was associated with a greater improvement in scores on the delayed free recall ($p < 0.04$) and delayed recognition ($p < 0.01$) tasks of the Selective Reminding Test (Mix and Crews 2002). Promising results from these short-term studies involving Ginkgo biloba stand in contrast, however, with those from longer-term trials. Long-term use of Ginkgo biloba extract was not found to prevent Alzheimer's disease or all-cause dementia in two large RCTs (DeKosky, Williamson, et al., 2008; Vellas, Coley, et al., 2012) that involved adults over age 70 years. Vellas and colleagues (Vellas, Coley, et al., 2012) observed that participants taking 120 mg supplements twice daily for 5 years did not have a significantly lower risk of developing Alzheimer's disease than those who received placebo, and results from the second study (DeKosky, Williamson, et al., 2008) showed that the incidence rates of dementia in the Ginkgo biloba and placebo groups were not different after a median of 6.1 years of follow-up. Thus, while Ginkgo biloba supplementation may lead to some short-term improvement in some cognitive functions among older persons, there is a lack of evidence supporting its use for the prevention of cognitive decline and dementia.

The use of CAM interventions other than dietary supplements and herbal medicines to prevent late-life cognitive decline and dementia has not been extensively tested. However, a few well-designed RCTs provide preliminary indication that certain other treatments may be beneficial for improving late-life cognitive function. Cocoa flavanol supplementation was observed to improve certain measures of cognitive function in the 8-week-long CoCoA study (Desideri, Kwik-Uribe, et al., 2012). Elderly adults with mild cognitive impairment who consumed a beverage containing either 520 mg or 990 mg of flavanols each day performed better on the Trail Making Tests A & B than did those who received a 45 mg flavanol drink ($p < 0.05$). Regarding non-herbal or non-nutritional interventions, some promising evidence was recently reported for cognitive exercise. Rebok and colleagues (Rebok, Ball, et al., 2014) investigated the 10-year outcome of cognitive training sessions in the ACTIVE trial, and concluded that the reasoning and speed-processing interventions were associated with improved outcomes in those areas (effect sizes = 0.23 and 0.66, respectively), though the memory intervention did not affect memory performance at follow-up. More studies examining these types of CAM therapies are needed to determine whether they are effective at improving late-life cognitive performance or reducing the risk of late-life cognitive decline.

CAM GUIDELINES AND SAFETY INFORMATION

Current Recommendations and Guidelines

CAM techniques such as herbal medicines and dietary supplements are generally considered to be safer than common pharmacological treatments, but the tolerability of these alternative treatments in aging populations must be evaluated (Table 23.3). Although results from RCTs have shown that doses of 240 mg/day of Ginkgo biloba (DeKosky, Williamson, et al., 2008) and 900 mg/day of St. John's wort (Kalb, Trautmann-Sponsel, et al., 2001) are both well tolerated by study participants, these herbal supplements are associated with certain side effects and drug interactions. In a study (Brattstrom, 2009) in which subjects received 500 mg of St. John's wort extract per day for 1 year, the most common treatment-related adverse events were gastrointestinal distress and skin problems due to sun sensitivity. St. John's wort is also known to induce the cytochrome P450 enzyme system, altering the effectiveness of medications metabolized via this pathway (Mannel, 2004; Varteresian & Lavretsky, 2014). The Food and Drug Administration (FDA) has issued a Public Health Advisory regarding this potential for interaction, and has advised against the concurrent use of St. John's wort and HIV protease inhibitors in particular (FDA, 2000).

High doses of Ginkgo leaf extract may lead to gastrointestinal discomfort and headaches, and in some cases excessive bleeding or hemorrhage, though the existing literature suggests that Ginkgo biloba appears generally to be a safe product for older adults (Carlson, Farquhar, et al., 2007; Koch, 2005; Varteresian & Lavretsky, 2014). Elderly patients who are at an elevated risk of bleeding, including those being treated with warfarin or other anticoagulant drugs, should be monitored with caution when taking these supplements (Lavretsky, 2009). Ginkgo biloba can interact with anticoagulant, antidiabetic, and anti-epileptic medications, NSAIDs (non-steroidal anti-inflammatory drugs), and the antidepressant trazodone due to selective inhibition of certain liver enzymes, such as cytochrome P450 (Mahadevan & Park, 2008).

The FDA considers all vitamins, in addition to herbal medicines such as Ginkgo biloba and St. John's wort, to fall under the category of dietary supplements; they are therefore subject to different regulations than food or drug products (FDA, 2014). According to the FDA, ensuring the safety and accurate labeling of dietary supplements before they go on the market is the responsibility of manufacturers (FDA, 2014). The Institute of Medicine, however, has released information on the recommended daily upper intake levels and possible overdose effects of certain vitamins and minerals. While high doses of vitamin C, vitamin B_{12}, and beta carotene are not associated with serious adverse effects (Food and Nutrition Board, 1998, 2000), consuming excessive amounts of vitamin D may lead to hypercalcemia and decreased renal function (Food and Nutrition Board, 1997). High folic acid intake has been known to mask vitamin B_{12} deficiency (Food and Nutrition Board, 1998), and niacin and vitamin B_6 toxicity are associated with skin flushing/rashes and sensory neuropathy (Food and Nutrition Board, 1998), respectively. Long-term daily vitamin E supplementation has been related to an increased risk of hemorrhagic stroke in some RCTs (Food and Nutrition Board, 2000; Sesso, Buring, et al., 2008), and one

Table 23.3. Dose Ranges and Possible Side Effects of Select CAM Agents

TREATMENT	TYPE	DOSE RANGES STUDIED	NOAEL (NO OBSERVED ADVERSE EFFECT LEVEL)	POSSIBLE SIDE EFFECTS OR INTERACTIONS
Ginkgo biloba	Herbal supplement	120–240 mg/day	Not available	Nausea, headaches, GI discomfort, excessive bleeding Possible interactions: warfarin/anticoagulants, aspirin, trazodone, NSAIDs, antidiabetic and antiepileptic medications
St. John's wort	Herbal supplement	270 mg–1200 mg/day	Not available	GI discomfort, photosensitivity, headache, induces the cytochrome P450 enzymes and P-glycoprotein drug transporter (causing interactions) Possible interactions: hormonal contraceptives, HIV protease and non-nucleoside reverse transcriptase inhibitors, immunosuppressants, warfarin, other antidepressants (serotonin syndrome)
Folate/Folic acid	Dietary supplement	400 µg/day–5 mg/day	1 mg/day; LOAEL (lowest observed adverse effect level), 5 mg/day	Possible neurological complications in vitamin B_{12}-deficient individuals, masks vitamin B_{12} deficiency
Vitamin B_6	Dietary supplement	3 mg–50 mg/day	200 mg/day	Sensory neuropathy, photosensitivity/rashes
Vitamin B_{12}	Dietary supplement	100 µg/day–1 mg/day	Not available. No adverse effects known for vitamin B_{12} from foods or supplements in amounts far in excess of needs	

Supplement	Form	Dose	Upper limit / notes	Adverse effects / interactions
Vitamin C	Dietary supplement	500 mg/day	Not available; UL (tolerable upper intake level), 2 g/day	GI discomfort, nausea
Vitamin D	Dietary supplement	400 IU–800 IU/day	Not available; UL for vitamin D_3, 2000 IU/day	Hypercalcemia, reduced renal function, urinary tract stones, GI discomfort
Vitamin E	Dietary supplement	400 IU–600 IU every other day	540 mg/day (800 IU/day); UL, 270 mg/day (400 IU/day)	Impaired blood clotting, risk of hemorrhagic stroke
Beta carotene	Dietary supplement	15 mg–50 mg every other day	Not available. 20 mg/day or more is contraindicated for current, heavy smokers	Carotenodermia (yellowing of the skin), carcinogenesis in heavy smokers. Possible interactions: alcohol
Zinc	Dietary supplement	5 mg–50 mg/day	50 mg/day; UL, 25 mg/day	GI discomfort, nausea, vomiting. Possible interactions: reduced absorption when taken with iron
Omega-3 (ω-3) fatty acids	Dietary supplement	400 mg–1800 mg/day	Not available. FDA: marine omega-3 fatty acid (as total intake of eicosapentaenoic acid or docosahexaenoic acid) not exceeding 3 g/d is "Generally Recognized as Safe."	GI discomfort, internal bleeding

meta-analysis (Miller et al., 2005), albeit debated, of trials involving high-dose vitamin E supplementation (≥ 400 IU/d) reported that use at such levels may be related to increased risk of all-cause mortality. Finally, omega-3 fatty acids have been found to inhibit platelet aggregation, raising concerns about an elevated risk of excessive bleeding during supplement use (Bays, 2007); the only side effect of omega-3 fatty acid intake that has been observed in clinical trials, however, is gastrointestinal discomfort (Bays, 2007; Sydenham, Dangour, et al., 2012). Although the occurrence of treatment-related adverse events during vitamin or omega-3 supplementation is rare, the benefits and risks of long-term use of these CAM strategies in older adults should be assessed before they are recommended as treatment options.

FUTURE CONSIDERATIONS

Current CAM Trials Underway

In order to determine whether or not vitamins, dietary supplements, and other CAM treatments are safe and effective prevention strategies for late-life depression and cognitive decline, additional CAM intervention studies involving older adult participants must be carried out (Table 23.4). Though results from previous clinical trials do not consistently indicate that omega-3 fatty acid supplementation improves mental health outcomes in older persons, several ongoing RCTs that are currently investigating these potential associations will provide more insight into the effects of daily omega-3 use. Several interventions that consist of administering vitamin D supplements to elderly subjects are also in progress, and multiple other studies will test the impact of other vitamins on incident cognitive decline or depression. While most of the data from existing studies do not provide definitive support for the use of these supplements as preventive measures, the results have been inconclusive, and the new RCTs should help clarify the benefits.

SUMMARY

The rising popularity of complementary and alternative medicines among older adults underscores a need to investigate the impact of each CAM treatment on cognitive status and mood. The limited data from existing clinical trials that involve CAM interventions and older populations have indicated that taking supplements of Ginkgo biloba or vitamins C, D, or E does not affect one's risk of incident cognitive impairment, dementia, and/or depression. Analyses from observational studies, however, seem to suggest that vitamin treatments might prevent these outcomes in elderly persons with nutrient deficiencies. There is some evidence that long-term use of B-vitamin, beta carotene, or omega-3 fatty acid supplements may protect against poor mental health outcomes; nevertheless, several well-designed RCTs found that these treatments had no effect. A Mediterranean-style diet appeared to be inversely associated with the development of cognitive decline and depression in both cohort studies and clinical trials, and the herbal medicine St. John's wort was consistently found to reduce depressive symptoms, although not in a prevention design framework. Finally, RCTs that involved using alternative physical and mental therapies to prevent and/or reduce depression have had promising results, but additional trials involving such interventions (e.g., tai chi, qi gong and meditation) need to be carried out among older adults in order to determine the broader benefits of these strategies.

DISCLOSURE STATEMENT

Ms. Singh has no conflicts to disclose.

Dr. Okereke is Editor of a book title with Springer Publishing on the prevention of late-life depression. Dr. Okereke currently receives funding from the National Institutes of Health/National Institute of Mental Health (R01 MH091448; R01 MH096776) for research on risk factors and/or prevention of late-life depression. In the past 3 years, Dr. Okereke has received grant funding from the NIH/National Institute on Aging (K08 AG029813), Harvard Medical School Diversity Inclusion and Community Partnership Fellowship, Harvard University Milton Fund, and the Alzheimer's Association (NIRG-09-13383) for research related to risk factors and/or prevention of late-life depression and/or cognitive decline. In the past 3 years, Dr. Okereke has been a Member of the Board of Directors of the Massachusetts/New Hampshire Chapter of the Alzheimer's Disease and Related Disorders Association, Inc., a nonprofit agency focused on matters related to prevention,

Table 23.4. Current CAM Trials in Late-life Depression and/or Cognitive Decline

INSTITUTION/ SPONSOR	YEARS	AGE RANGE	ESTIMATED N	INTERVENTION	DURATION	OUTCOME MEASURES
Clinica Universidad de Navarra	2012–2014	≥ 75	170	Omega-3 fatty acid supplementation	1 year	MMSE, verbal fluency test
University of Cincinnati	2010–2014	62–80	140	2.4 g omega-3 fatty acids and a blueberry powder supplement/ day	6 months	Working memory, GDS
University Hospital, Toulouse	2008–2014	≥ 70	1680	Omega-3 fatty acid supplementation (800 mg DHA)	36 months	Memory function
Brigham and Women's Hospital	2010–2017	≥ 50	25875	2000 IU vitamin D_3 and 840 mg omega 3 fatty acids/day	5 years	Clinical Depressive Syndrome; Mood score
Brigham and Women's Hospital	2010–2017	≥ 60	3226	2000 IU vitamin D_3 and 840 mg omega 3 fatty acids/day	5 years	Global composite cognitive score
University Hospital, Angers	2012–2014	≥ 60	160	200 IU/day of vitamin D	12 weeks	Trail Making Test
VU University Medical Center	2014–2017	≥ 40	240	16800 IU/week vitamin D	1 year	CESD, SF-12
University of Miami	2014–2015	≥ 55	130	4000 IU/day of vitamin D	6 months	BDI
University of Kentucky	2002–2014	60–90	10400	400 IU vitamin E and/or 200 μg selenium/day	7–12 years	Alzheimer's disease
University of Georgia	2012–2015	18–95	120	Carotenoids (10 mg lutein + 2 mg zeaxanthin)	1 year	Executive function, reaction time, and short-term memory
University of California Los Angeles	2013–2014	55–90	66	Kundalini yoga and meditation for 60 minutes/week	12 weeks	Memory function, GDS

treatment, advocacy, and/or care in Alzheimer's disease and related cognitive disorders.

REFERENCES

Andreeva, V. A., Galan, P., et al. (2012). Supplementation with B vitamins or n-3 fatty acids and depressive symptoms in cardiovascular disease survivors: ancillary findings from the SUpplementation with FOLate, vitamins B-6 and B-12 and/or OMega-3 fatty acids (SU.FOL.OM3) randomized trial. *Am J Clin Nutr, 96*(1), 208–214.

Annweiler, C., Rolland, Y., et al. (2012). Higher vitamin D dietary intake is associated with lower risk of alzheimer's disease: a 7-year follow-up. *J Gerontol A Biol Sci Med Sci, 67*(11), 1205–1211.

Alzheimer's Association. (2013). 2013 Alzheimer's disease facts and figures. *Alzheimers & Dementia, 9*(2), 208–245.

Barnett, J. H., Hachinski, V., et al. (2013). Cognitive health begins at conception: addressing dementia as a lifelong and preventable condition. *BMC Med, 11*, 246.

Bays, H. E. (2007). Safety considerations with omega-3 fatty acid therapy. *Am J Cardiol, 99*(6A), 35C–43C.

Beekman, A. T., Copeland, J. R., et al. (1999). Review of community prevalence of depression in later life. *Br J Psychiatry, 174*, 307–311.

Beekman, A. T., Penninx, B. W., et al. (2002). The impact of depression on the well-being, disability and use of services in older adults: a longitudinal perspective. *Acta Psychiatr Scand, 105*(1), 20–27.

Bertone-Johnson, E. R., Powers, S. I., et al. (2011). Vitamin D intake from foods and supplements and depressive symptoms in a diverse population of older women. *Am J Clin Nutr* 94(4): 1104–1112.

Bertone-Johnson, E. R., Powers, S. I., et al. (2012). Vitamin D supplementation and depression in the women's health initiative calcium and vitamin D trial. *Am J Epidemiol, 176*(1), 1–13.

Beydoun, M. A., Kaufman, J. S., et al. (2007). Plasma n-3 fatty acids and the risk of cognitive decline in older adults: the Atherosclerosis Risk in Communities Study. *Am J Clin Nutr, 85*(4), 1103–1111.

Brattstrom, A. (2009). Long-term effects of St. John's wort (Hypericum perforatum) treatment: a 1-year safety study in mild to moderate depression. *Phytomedicine, 16*(4), 277–283.

Carlson, J. J., Farquhar, J. W., et al. (2007). Safety and efficacy of a ginkgo biloba-containing dietary supplement on cognitive function, quality of life, and platelet function in healthy, cognitively intact older adults. *J Am Diet Assoc, 107*(3), 422–432.

Chen, C. S., Chong, M. Y., et al. (2007). Clinically significant non-major depression in a community-dwelling elderly population: epidemiological findings. *Int J Geriatr Psychiatry, 22*(6), 557–562.

Cockle, S. M., Kimber, S., et al. (2000). The effects of Ginkgo biloba extract (LI 1370) supplementation on activities of daily living in free living older volunteers: a questionnaire survey. *Hum Psychopharmacol, 15*(4), 227–235.

Colangelo, L. A., He, K., et al. (2009). Higher dietary intake of long-chain omega-3 polyunsaturated fatty acids is inversely associated with depressive symptoms in women. *Nutrition, 25*(10), 1011–1019.

Cook, N. R., Lee, I. M., et al. (2005). Low-dose aspirin in the primary prevention of cancer: the Women's Health Study: a randomized controlled trial. *JAMA, 294*(1), 47–55.

de Jager, C. A., Oulhaj, A., et al. (2012). Cognitive and clinical outcomes of homocysteine-lowering B-vitamin treatment in mild cognitive impairment: a randomized controlled trial. *Int J Geriatr Psychiatry, 27*(6), 592–600.

DeKosky, S. T., Williamson, J. D., et al. (2008). Ginkgo biloba for prevention of dementia: a randomized controlled trial. *JAMA, 300*(19), 2253–2262.

Desideri, G., Kwik-Uribe, C., et al. (2012). Benefits in cognitive function, blood pressure, and insulin resistance through cocoa flavanol consumption in elderly subjects with mild cognitive impairment: the Cocoa, Cognition, and Aging (CoCoA) study. *Hypertension, 60*(3), 794–801.

Devore, E. E., Grodstein, F., et al. (2009). Dietary intake of fish and omega-3 fatty acids in relation to long-term dementia risk. *Am J Clin Nutr, 90*(1), 170–176.

Devore, E. E., Grodstein, F., et al. (2010). Dietary antioxidants and long-term risk of dementia. *Arch Neurol, 67*(7), 819–825.

Djernes, J. K. (2006). Prevalence and predictors of depression in populations of elderly: a review. *Acta Psychiatr Scand, 113*(5), 372–387.

Dumville, J. C., Miles, J. N., et al. (2006). Can vitamin D supplementation prevent winter-time blues? A randomised trial among older women. *J Nutr Health Aging, 10*(2), 151–153.

FDA. (2000). *Risk of drug interactions with St. John's wort and Indinavir and other drugs.* Retrieved from http://www.fda.gov/ Drugs/DrugSafety/ PostmarketDrug SafetyInformationfor PatientsandProviders/ ucm052238.htm.

FDA. (2014). *Dietary supplements.* Retrieved from http://www.fda.gov/Food/DietarySupplements/ default.htm.

Feart, C., Samieri, C., et al. (2009). Adherence to a Mediterranean diet, cognitive decline, and risk of dementia. *JAMA, 302*(6), 638–648.

Fillenbaum, G. G., Kuchibhatla, M. N., et al. (2005). Dementia and Alzheimer's disease in community-dwelling elders taking vitamin C and/or vitamin E. *Ann Pharmacother, 39*(12), 2009–2014.

Food and Nutrition Board, Institute of Medicine. (1997). *Dietary reference intakes for calcium, phosphorus, magnesium, vitamin D, and fluoride.* Washington, DC: National Academy of Sciences.

Food and Nutrition Board, Institute of Medicine. (1998). *Dietary reference intakes for thiamin, riboflavin, niacin, vitamin B6, folate, vitamin B12, pantothenic acid, biotin, and choline.* Washington, DC: The National Academies Press.

Food and Nutrition Board, Institute of Medicine. (2000). *Dietary reference intakes for vitamin C, vitamin E, selenium, and carotenoids.* Washington, DC: National Academy of Sciences.

Ford, A. H., Flicker, L., et al. (2008). Vitamins B12, B6, and folic acid for onset of depressive symptoms in older men: results from a 2-year placebo-controlled randomized trial. *J Clin Psychiatry, 69*(8), 1203–1209.

Gariballa, S., & Forster, S. (2007). Effects of dietary supplements on depressive symptoms in older patients: a randomised double-blind placebo-controlled trial. *Clin Nutr, 26*(5), 545–551.

Gauthier, S., Reisberg, B., et al. (2006). Mild cognitive impairment. *Lancet, 367*(9518), 1262–1270.

Giltay, E. J., Geleijnse, J. M., et al. (2011). Effects of n-3 fatty acids on depressive symptoms and dispositional optimism after myocardial infarction. *Am J Clin Nutr, 94*(6), 1442–1450.

Grodstein, F., Kang, J. H., et al. (2007). A randomized trial of beta carotene supplementation and cognitive function in men: the Physicians' Health Study II. *Arch Intern Med, 167*(20), 2184–2190.

Grodstein, F., O'Brien, J., et al. (2013). Long-term multivitamin supplementation and cognitive function in men: a randomized trial. *Ann Intern Med, 159*(12), 806–814.

Gu, Y., Nieves, J. W., et al. (2010). Food combination and Alzheimer disease risk: a protective diet. *Arch Neurol, 67*(6), 699–706.

Haberka, M., Mizia-Stec, K., et al. (2013). Effects of n-3 polyunsaturated fatty acids on depressive symptoms, anxiety and emotional state in patients with acute myocardial infarction. *Pharmacol Rep, 65*(1), 59–68.

Hodge, A., Almeida, O. P., et al. (2013). Patterns of dietary intake and psychological distress in older Australians: benefits not just from a Mediterranean diet. *Int Psychogeriatr, 25*(3), 456–466.

Hui, P. N., Wan, M., et al. (2006). An evaluation of two behavioral rehabilitation programs, qigong versus progressive relaxation, in improving the quality of life in cardiac patients. *J Altern Complement Med, 12*(4), 373–378.

Jacobs, D. R., Jr., & Tapsell, L. C. (2007). Food, not nutrients, is the fundamental unit in nutrition. *Nutr Rev, 65*, 439–450.

Kalb, R., Trautmann-Sponsel, R. D., et al. (2001). Efficacy and tolerability of hypericum extract WS 5572 versus placebo in mildly to moderately depressed patients. A randomized double-blind multicenter clinical trial. *Pharmacopsychiatry, 34*(3), 96–103.

Kang, J. H., Cook, N., et al. (2006). A randomized trial of vitamin E supplementation and cognitive function in women. *Arch Intern Med, 166*(22), 2462–2468.

Kang, J. H., Cook, N., et al. (2008). A trial of B vitamins and cognitive function among women at high risk of cardiovascular disease. *Am J Clin Nutr, 88*(6), 1602–1610.

Kang, J. H., Cook, N. R., et al. (2009). Vitamin E, vitamin C, beta carotene, and cognitive function among women with or at risk of cardiovascular disease: The Women's Antioxidant and Cardiovascular Study. *Circulation, 119*(21), 2772–2780.

Kasper, S., Anghelescu, I. G., et al. (2006). Superior efficacy of St John's wort extract WS 5570 compared to placebo in patients with major depression: a randomized, double-blind, placebo-controlled, multi-center trial [ISRCTN77277298]. *BMC Med, 4*, 14.

Katon, W. J., Lin, E., et al. (2003). Increased medical costs of a population-based sample of depressed elderly patients. *Arch Gen Psychiatry, 60*(9), 897–903.

Kim, D. H., Grodstein, F., et al. (2013). Seafood types and age-related cognitive decline in the Women's Health Study. *J Gerontol A Biol Sci Med Sci, 68*(10), 1255–1262.

Kim, J. M., Stewart, R., et al. (2008). Predictive value of folate, vitamin B12 and homocysteine levels in late-life depression. *Br J Psychiatry, 192*(4), 268–274.

Koch, E. (2005). Inhibition of platelet activating factor (PAF)-induced aggregation of human thrombocytes by ginkgolides: considerations on possible bleeding complications after oral intake of Ginkgo biloba extracts. *Phytomedicine, 12*(1–2), 10–16.

Koyama, A., Houston, D. K., et al. (2014). Association between the Mediterranean diet and cognitive decline in a biracial population. *J Gerontol A Biol Sci Med Sci*, 70(3), 354–359.

Lavretsky, H. (2009). Complementary and alternative medicine use for treatment and prevention of late-life mood and cognitive disorders. *Aging Health*, 5(1), 61–78.

Lehto, S. M., Ruusunen, A., et al. (2013). Dietary zinc intake and the risk of depression in middle-aged men: a 20-year prospective follow-up study. *J Affect Disord*, 150(2), 682–685.

Lucas, M., Mirzaei, F., et al. (2011). Dietary intake of n-3 and n-6 fatty acids and the risk of clinical depression in women: a 10-y prospective follow-up study. *Am J Clin Nutr*, 93(6), 1337–1343.

Luchsinger, J. A., Tang, M. X., et al. (2003). Antioxidant vitamin intake and risk of Alzheimer disease. *Arch Neurol*, 60(2), 203–208

Luchsinger, J. A., Tang, M. X., et al. (2007). Relation of higher folate intake to lower risk of Alzheimer disease in the elderly. *Arch Neurol*, 64(1), 86–92.

Luijendijk, H. J., van den Berg, J. F., et al. (2008). Incidence and recurrence of late-life depression. *Arch Gen Psychiatry*, 65(12), 1394–1401.

Mahadevan, S., & Park, Y. (2008). Multifaceted therapeutic benefits of Ginkgo biloba L.: chemistry, efficacy, safety, and uses. *J Food Sci*, 73(1), R14–19.

Mannel, M. (2004). Drug interactions with St John's wort: mechanisms and clinical implications. *Drug Saf*, 27(11), 773–797.

Mannel, M., Kuhn, U., et al. (2010). St. John's wort extract LI160 for the treatment of depression with atypical features: a double-blind, randomized, and placebo-controlled trial. *J Psychiatr Res*, 44(12), 760–767.

Martinez-Lapiscina, E. H., Clavero, P., et al. (2013). Mediterranean diet improves cognition: the PREDIMED-NAVARRA randomised trial. *J Neurol Neurosurg Psychiatry*, 84(12), 1318–1325.

Mathers, C. D., & Loncar, D. (2006). Projections of global mortality and burden of disease from 2002 to 2030. *PLoS Med*, 3(11), e442.

Maxwell, C. J., Hicks, M. S., et al. (2005). Supplemental use of antioxidant vitamins and subsequent risk of cognitive decline and dementia. *Dement Geriatr Cogn Disord*, 20(1), 45–51.

Mazereeuw, G., Lanctot, K. L., et al. (2012). Effects of omega-3 fatty acids on cognitive performance: a meta-analysis. *Neurobiol Aging*, 33(7), 1482. e17–1482.e29.

McNeill, G., Avenell A., et al. (2007). Effect of multivitamin and multimineral supplementation on cognitive function in men and women aged 65 years and over: a randomised controlled trial. *Nutr J*, 6, 10.

Mihalopoulos, C., Vos, T., et al. (2011). The economic analysis of prevention in mental health programs. *Annu Rev Clin Psychol*, 7, 169–201.

Miller, E. R., 3rd, Pastor-Barriuso, R., Dalal, D., Riemersma, R. A., Appel, L. J., & Guallar, E. (2005). Meta-analysis: high-dosage vitamin E supplementation may increase all-cause mortality. *Ann Intern Med*, 142(1), 37–46.

Mix, J. A., & Crews, W. D., Jr. (2002). A double-blind, placebo-controlled, randomized trial of Ginkgo biloba extract EGb 761 in a sample of cognitively intact older adults: neuropsychological findings. *Hum Psychopharmacol*, 17(6), 267–277.

Morris, M. C., Evans, D. A., et al. (2004). Dietary niacin and the risk of incident Alzheimer's disease and of cognitive decline. *J Neurol Neurosurg Psychiatry*, 75(8), 1093–1099.

Morris, M. C., Evans, D. A., et al. (2005). Fish consumption and cognitive decline with age in a large community study. *Arch Neurol*, 62(12), 1849–1853.

Norton, M. C., Skoog, I., et al. (2006). Three-year incidence of first-onset depressive syndrome in a population sample of older adults: the Cache County study. *Am J Geriatr Psychiatry* 14(3): 237–245.

Okereke, O. I., Cook, N. R., et al. (2015). Effect of long-term supplementation with folic acid and B-vitamins on risk of depression in older women. *Br J Psychiatry*, 206(4), 324–331.

Okereke, O. I., Lyness, J. M., et al. (2013). Depression in late-life: a focus on prevention. *Focus*, 11(1), 22–31.

Pálsson, S. P., Ostling, S., et al. (2001). The incidence of first-onset depression in a population followed from the age of 70 to 85. *Psychol Med*, 31(7), 1159–1168.

Petersen, R. C., Roberts, R. O., et al. (2009). Mild cognitive impairment: ten years later. *Arch Neurol*, 66(12), 1447–1455.

Randlov, C., Mehlsen, J., et al. (2006). The efficacy of St. John's Wort in patients with minor depressive symptoms or dysthymia: a double-blind placebo-controlled study." *Phytomedicine*, 13(4), 215–221.

Ravaglia, G., Forti, P., et al. (2005). Homocysteine and folate as risk factors for dementia and Alzheimer disease. *Am J Clin Nutr*, 82(3), 636–643.

Rebok, G. W., Ball, K., et al. (2014). Ten-year effects of the advanced cognitive training for independent and vital elderly cognitive training trial on cognition and everyday functioning in older adults. *J Am Geriatr Soc*, 62(1), 16–24.

Reynolds, C. F., 3rd (2008). Preventing depression in old age: it's time. *Am J Geriatr Psychiatry*, *16*(6): 433–434.

Reynolds, C. F., 3rd, Cuijpers, P., et al. (2012). Early intervention to reduce the global health and economic burden of major depression in older adults. *Annu Rev Public Health*, *33*, 123–135.

Ridker, P. M., Cook, N. R., et al. (2005). A randomized trial of low-dose aspirin in the primary prevention of cardiovascular disease in women. *N Engl J Med*, *352*(13), 1293–1304.

Rienks, J., Dobson, A. J., et al. (2013). Mediterranean dietary pattern and prevalence and incidence of depressive symptoms in mid-aged women: results from a large community-based prospective study. *Eur J Clin Nutr*, *67*(1), 75–82.

Rossom, R. C., Espeland, M. A., et al. (2012). Calcium and vitamin D supplementation and cognitive impairment in the women's health initiative. *J Am Geriatr Soc*, *60*(12), 2197–2205.

Samieri, C., Grodstein, F., et al. (2013). Mediterranean diet and cognitive function in older age. *Epidemiology*, *24*(4), 490–499.

Samieri, C., Sun, Q., et al. (2013). The association between dietary patterns at midlife and health in aging: an observational study. *Ann Intern Med*, *159*(9), 584–591.

Sanchez-Villegas, A., Martinez-Gonzalez, M. A., et al. (2013). Mediterranean dietary pattern and depression: the PREDIMED randomized trial. *BMC Med*, *11*, 208.

Sanchez-Villegas, A., Verberne, L., et al. (2011). Dietary fat intake and the risk of depression: the SUN Project. *PLoS One*, *6*(1), e16268.

Sarris, J., Panossian, A., et al. (2011). Herbal medicine for depression, anxiety and insomnia: a review of psychopharmacology and clinical evidence. *Eur Neuropsychopharmacol*, *21*(12), 841–860.

Scarmeas, N., Stern, Y., et al. (2006). Mediterranean diet and risk for Alzheimer's disease. *Ann Neurol*, *59*(6), 912–921.

Sephton, S. E., Salmon, P., et al. (2007). Mindfulness meditation alleviates depressive symptoms in women with fibromyalgia: results of a randomized clinical trial. *Arthritis Rheum*, *57*(1), 77–85.

Sesso, H. D., Buring, J. E., et al. (2008). Vitamins E and C in the prevention of cardiovascular disease in men: the Physicians' Health Study II randomized controlled trial. *JAMA*, *300*(18), 2123–2133.

Sinn, N., Milte, C. M., et al. (2012). Effects of n-3 fatty acids, EPA v. DHA, on depressive symptoms, quality of life, memory and executive function in older adults with mild cognitive impairment: a 6-month randomised controlled trial. *Br J Nutr*, *107*(11), 1682–1693.

Skarupski, K. A., Tangney, C., et al. (2010). Longitudinal association of vitamin B-6, folate, and vitamin B-12 with depressive symptoms among older adults over time. *Am J Clin Nutr*, *92*(2), 330–335.

Skarupski, K. A., Tangney, C. C., et al. (2013). Mediterranean diet and depressive symptoms among older adults over time. *J Nutr Health Aging*, *17*(5), 441–445.

Smit, F., Beekman, A., et al. (2004). Selecting key variables for depression prevention: results from a population-based prospective epidemiological study. *J Affect Disord*, *81*(3), 241–249.

Smith, A. D., Smith, S. M., et al. (2010). Homocysteine-lowering by B vitamins slows the rate of accelerated brain atrophy in mild cognitive impairment: a randomized controlled trial. *PLoS One*, *5*(9), e12244.

Sydenham, E., Dangour, A. D., et al. (2012). Omega 3 fatty acid for the prevention of cognitive decline and dementia. *Cochrane Database Syst Rev*, *6*, CD005379.

Tangney, C. C., Kwasny, M. J., et al. (2011). Adherence to a Mediterranean-type dietary pattern and cognitive decline in a community population. *Am J Clin Nutr*, *93*(3), 601–607.

Tucker, K. L., Qiao, N., et al. (2005). High homocysteine and low B vitamins predict cognitive decline in aging men: the Veterans Affairs Normative Aging Study. *Am J Clin Nutr*, *82*(3), 627–635.

van de Rest, O., Geleijnse, J. M., et al. (2008). Effect of fish-oil supplementation on mental well-being in older subjects: a randomized, double-blind, placebo-controlled trial. *Am J Clin Nutr*, *88*(3), 706–713.

Varteresian, T., & Lavretsky, H. (2014). Natural products and supplements for geriatric depression and cognitive disorders: an evaluation of the research. *Curr Psychiatry Rep*, *16*(8), 456.

Vashum, K. P., McEvoy, M., et al. (2014). Dietary zinc is associated with a lower incidence of depression: findings from two Australian cohorts. *J Affect Disord*, *166*, 249–257.

Vellas, B., Coley, N., et al. (2012). Long-term use of standardised Ginkgo biloba extract for the prevention of Alzheimer's disease (GuidAge): a randomised placebo-controlled trial. *Lancet Neurol*, *11*(10), 851–859.

Walker, J. G., Batterham, P. J., et al. (2012). Oral folic acid and vitamin B-12 supplementation to prevent cognitive decline in community-dwelling older adults with depressive symptoms: the Beyond Ageing Project: a randomized controlled trial. *Am J Clin Nutr*, *95*(1), 194–203.

Walker, J. G., Mackinnon, A. J., et al. (2010). Mental health literacy, folic acid and vitamin B12, and physical activity for the prevention of depression in older adults: randomised controlled trial. *Br J Psychiatry, 197*(1), 45–54.

Wang, C., Schmid, C. H., et al. (2009). Tai Chi is effective in treating knee osteoarthritis: a randomized controlled trial. *Arthritis Rheum, 61*(11), 1545–1553.

Wang, F., Man, J. K., et al. (2013). The effects of qigong on anxiety, depression, and psychological well-being: a systematic review and meta-analysis. *Evid Based Complement Alternat Med, 2013,* 152738.

Wengreen, H., Munger, R. G., et al. (2013). Prospective study of Dietary Approaches to Stop Hypertension- and Mediterranean-style dietary patterns and age-related cognitive change: the Cache County Study on Memory, Health and Aging. *Am J Clin Nutr, 98*(5), 1263–1271.

Willett, W. (1998). *Nutritional epidemiology.* New York: Oxford University Press.

Wurtzen, H., Dalton, S. O., et al. (2013). Mindfulness significantly reduces self-reported levels of anxiety and depression: results of a randomised controlled trial among 336 Danish women treated for stage I-III breast cancer. *Eur J Cancer, 49*(6), 1365–1373.

24

LIFESTYLE INTERVENTIONS, INCLUDING NUTRITION AND EXERCISE, FOR COGNITIVE AND BIOLOGICAL AGING

David A. Merrill

INTRODUCTION

Lifestyle Medicine and Cognitive Aging

Lifestyle medicine is an evolving field promoting the prevention, treatment, and management of chronic modern health problems with predominantly lifestyle-based etiologies. Lifestyle interventions include, but are not limited to, diet (nutrition), conventional and mindful physical exercise, stress reduction and management, smoking cessation, and pharmacology. Lifestyle medicine has been applied to most common chronic diseases, including vascular disease, heart disease, hypertension, type-2 diabetes, obesity, osteoporosis, and many types of cancer. In this chapter, we review and consider novel applications of lifestyle medicine approaches to conditions impacting cognitive and biological aging.

The greatest risk factor for cognitive decline is age, with age-related memory change increasing by approximately 10% per decade after the age of 60 and affecting half of all adults age 65 and older (Bassett and Folstein, 1993, Larrabee and Crook, 1994). Cognitive change with aging begins in midlife and includes declines in processing speed, frontal executive function, and spontaneous recall of facts and events (including names) (Christensen, 2001). Such "subjective memory impairment" (SMI) is considered clinically normal, conferring an approximately 1% per year risk of developing more serious memory loss over time. Mild cognitive impairment (MCI), an elevated risk-state of memory decline present in 10%–20% of older adults, involves subjective memory complaints plus deficits on neuropsychological testing (e.g., scoring greater than one standard deviation below average on two or more age- and education-matched evaluations with intact performance on tasks of daily function) (Petersen et al., 1999). MCI can further be classified as involving only memory (amnestic), other cognitive domains (non-amnestic), or both (multiple domains). MCI is associated with a 10%–15%

risk per year of conversion to functionally impairing dementia syndromes, the most common of which is Alzheimer's disease (AD), which accounts for and/or contributes to about 70% of all dementia cases (e.g., mixed vascular and AD dementia) (Hanninen et al., 2002; Lopez et al., 2003; Mitchell and Shiri-Feshki, 2009).

Once memory and cognitive decline causes significant impairment in daily function, a diagnosis of dementia is warranted (Small et al., 1997). Dementia is a syndrome of decline in one or more cognitive domains (including memory, speech, and language production or comprehension, object naming or recognition, execution of motor activities, abstraction, planning of complex tasks, and judgment). Declines must interfere with daily life and commonly cause difficulty initially with complex tasks, such as driving or managing finances. Later difficulties include more basic activities, such as bathing, dressing, toileting, and eating. Causes of dementia less common than AD include vascular dementia (VD), frontotemporal dementia (FTD), dementia with Lewy bodies (DLB), and Parkinson's disease dementia (PDD). A significant proportion of dementia cases are a mixture of these etiologies.

The number of individuals diagnosed with AD and related dementias in the United States stood at 5.4 million as of 2014, a number expected to rise to about 14 million by 2050 (Thies and Bleiler, 2014). With demographics predicting this rapid rise in the number of older adults with memory loss over the next 20–40 years, interest is growing in the use of healthy lifestyle strategies to protect brain health. As reviewed in this chapter, older adults with conditions ranging from subjective memory impairment to dementia are known to benefit cognitively from healthy lifestyle strategies, including dietary modification and various types of physical exercise.

Nature versus Nurture

A small number of early-onset (< age 65) familial cases of AD (less than 5%) have been linked to specific gene changes involving increased production of pathological forms of beta-amyloid protein, including mutations of Presenilin-1, Presenilin-2, and the Amyloid Precursor Protein (Hsiung and Sadovnick, 2007). Though neither necessary nor sufficient to cause AD, the major known genetic risk factor for AD is the Apolipoprotein E-4 (APOE-4) allele;

APO-E 4 may also increase risk for vascular dementia (Slooter et al., 2004; Li et al., 2008).

Despite these known genetic associations with AD, the landmark McArthur Study of Successful Aging found that, for most people, genetics accounts for only about a third of what contributes to successful aging, defined as both cognitive and physical health (Kahn, 1998). Thus, an entire range of environmental non-genetic factors, including lifestyle choices and changes in habits with aging, combine and interact with an individual's genetics to determine how well that individual will age.

Previous estimates indicate that up to half of AD cases are attributable to known modifiable dementia risk factors (low educational achievement, smoking, physical inactivity, depression, hypertension, diabetes, and obesity) and that a 10%–25% reduction of these risks could potentially prevent 300,000–500,000 cases in the United States and 1–3 million cases worldwide (Barnes and Yaffe, 2011). To support efforts of such modifiable risk factor reduction, there is a growing interest in establishing to what extent lifestyle factors impact AD pathology in pre-dementia states (Williams et al., 2010; Merrill and Small, 2011).

Lifestyle and Brain Aging

A National Institutes of Health review by the Agency for Healthcare Research and Quality, carried out through its Evidence-Based Practice Centers, determined which lifestyle factors showed consistent associations with AD or cognitive decline across multiple observational studies and the available randomized controlled trials at the time (Williams et al., 2010). Factors associated with increased risk of AD and cognitive decline were diabetes, APOE-4, smoking, and depression. Factors consistently associated with a decreased risk of AD and cognitive decline were cognitive engagement and physical activity.

The modification of risk for reported associations in the above-mentioned review was typically small to moderate, and the currently available data were felt to be limited and generally of low strength. The overall conclusion of the review was that further research was necessary before definitive recommendations could be made regarding behavioral and lifestyle modifications/interventions. Here we review data on the major known risk factors for dementia and common lifestyle approaches that diminish the impact of these factors on memory loss with aging.

MEASURING THE IMPACT OF LIFESTYLE ON COGNITIVE AND BIOLOGICAL AGING

Vascular Health

Dementia risk studies implicate conditions related to vascular health and disease, such as hypertension, hyperlipidemia, diabetes, and obesity (Anstey et al., 2008; Beydoun et al., 2008; Lu et al., 2009; McGuinness et al., 2006). Vascular disease adds to memory loss and the development of dementia with aging in a majority of clinical cases (Gorelick et al., 2011; Schneider et al., 2007). Autopsy studies show that cerebral infarctions contribute in an additive fashion to the cognitive impairment caused by markers of AD pathology, such as Aβ plaques and tau neurofibrillary tangles (Schneider et al., 2004). Other prospective clinicopathologic evidence from the Honolulu-Asia Aging Study suggests that elevated cerebrovascular risk, as measured by increased midlife systolic blood pressure, is directly related to later observed brain atrophy, plaques, and tangles at autopsy (Petrovitch et al., 2000).

In living subjects, the impact of vascular health on memory and other aspects of cognition are assessed by several methods. Proxy markers of vascular risk, such as diabetes, smoking status, systolic blood pressure, and midlife total cholesterol level demonstrate a modest relationship to cognition and/or elevated risk of developing dementia (Anstey et al., 2007; Anstey et al., 2008; Kivipelto et al., 2002; Luchsinger, 2010; Williams et al., 2010; Yasar et al., 2011). The Framingham Stroke Risk Profile (FSRP) is a validated index of overall cerebrovascular disease (CVD) that includes several risk factors (e.g., age, systolic blood pressure, diabetes, smoking status) as predictors of 10-year stroke risk (D'Agostino et al., 1994; Wolf et al., 1991).

FSRP correlates with cognitive performance (Elias et al., 2004; Llewellyn et al., 2008) and predicts future cognitive decline (Brady et al., 2001; Unverzagt et al., 2011). Within the Framingham Offspring Study, an inverse association between rising increments in 10-year risk of stroke and lower performance across diverse domains of cognitive performance level was observed for over 2000 subjects in tests of visual-spatial memory, attention, organization, scanning, and abstract reasoning (Elias et al., 2004). FSRP was also used in the Framingham Offspring Study to demonstrate an association between stroke risk factors, smaller total

brain volume, and poorer cognitive function among stroke- and dementia-free subjects (Seshadri et al., 2004). In non-Framingham populations, Brady et al. (2001) found a more circumscribed impact of stroke risk on verbal fluency within a smaller sample; however, study of a larger non-Framingham population found FSRP relating to lowered performance across multiple cognitive domains (Llewellyn et al., 2008).

Structural magnetic resonance imaging (MRI) studies measuring white matter hyperintensities and lacunar strokes have likewise found associations between vascular disease burden and cognitive function (Reed et al., 2004; van der Flier et al., 2005). Midlife vascular risk exposure appears to accelerate structural brain aging and cognitive decline (Debette et al., 2011). Functional MRI has shown that blood pressure and body mass index (BMI), but not total cholesterol, correlate with level of brain activity in older adults (Braskie et al., 2008).

Positron emission tomography (PET) ligands allow in vivo measurement of AD pathology in the brain. The amyloid-β (Aβ) PET ligand Pittsburg compound B (PIB) (Klunk et al., 2004) has been shown at times to correlate with aspects of memory function (Forsberg et al., 2008; Kantarci et al., 2012; Pike et al., 2007; Pike et al., 2011) and predict cognitive decline (Resnick et al., 2010), while other studies show elevated PIB signals in cognitively normal older adults (Aizenstein et al., 2008). Nonetheless, episodic memory deficits have been shown to relate to PIB-PET measured Aβ deposition via a hippocampal-atrophy mediated mechanism (Mormino et al., 2009), and a recent study examining regional PIB-PET binding found that temporal Aβ deposition provided independent contributions to episodic memory deficits in a mixed sample of non-demented older adults, which included subjects with both normal cognition and MCI (Chetelat et al., 2011).

Two additional recent studies examined the relationship between the degree of vascular disease and PIB-PET binding levels. One study in cognitively normal older adults used MRI to define the presence or absence of CVD by measuring white matter hyperintensity burden and/or presence of infarctions. The investigators found that CVD correlated with lower scores on tests of executive function but not episodic memory performance, PIB-PET binding did not relate to cognitive performance, and there was no interaction between CVD and PIB-PET binding (Marchant et al., 2011). A second study combining PIB-PET with Framingham

Coronary Risk Profile (FCRP), a proxy for vascular risk similar to FSRP (focused on cardiac rather than brain risk), found that, when several coronary risk factors were examined together, higher coronary risk was associated with higher cerebral Aβ-levels (Reed et al., 2011). By contrast, when individual components of FCRP were compared against global PIB-PET binding (e.g., hypertension, hyperlipidemia, diabetes), no significant relationships were found.

The PET ligand 2-(1-(6-[(2-[F-18]fluoroethyl)(methyl)amino]-2-naphthyl)ethylidene)malononitrile (FDDNP) provides a measure of both Aβ plaques and tau neurofibrillary tangle binding levels (Shoghi-Jadid et al., 2002). FDDNP-PET binding has previously been shown to correlate with cognitive function in older adults (Braskie et al., 2010; Ercoli et al., 2009) and to predict cognitive decline (Small et al., 2012). In a recently reported sample of healthy non-demented subjects ($n = 75$), FSRP score and FDDNP-PET binding levels each predicted cognitive performance across five tested cognitive domains (i.e., memory, executive function, visuospatial function, language, and attention/processing speed) (Merrill et al., 2013). In a sub-region analysis of this sample, the prior observed associations in frontal and parietal regions (Braskie et al., 2010) were confirmed, and significant association was observed between lateral temporal lobe FDDNP-PET binding levels and performance on executive function and language tasks (Merrill et al., 2013). While findings using FDDNP-PET largely concur with studies of PIB-PET, the observed differences may result from FDDNP-PET binding to both Aβ plaques and tau tangles. These findings in non-demented volunteers suggest that the effects of elevated vascular risk and occult AD pathology become apparent early on in vascular and neurodegenerative disease progression, even before the manifestation of vascular damage or the diagnosis of dementia.

In summary, current findings relating vascular disease to cognition with aging reinforce the importance of managing stroke risk factors to prevent cognitive decline in individuals even before the development of clinically significant dementia. Age is a consistently a significant non-modifiable contributing vascular risk factor, but control of systolic blood pressure through diet, exercise, and the use of antihypertensive medications when indicated associate with preservation of brain health and cognitive function. These findings reinforce the importance of managing stroke risk factors in preventing cognitive decline in individuals even before the development of clinically significant dementia.

Overweight and Obesity

In middle-aged and older adults, increased weight has been associated with greater risk of cognitive decline and conversion to dementia (Elias et al., 2005; Fitzpatrick et al., 2009; Wolf et al., 2007; Xu et al. 2011). For example, being overweight or obese at midlife independently increases risk for dementia, Alzheimer's disease, and vascular dementia (Xu et al., 2011), and a higher BMI at mid-life has been associated with greater cognitive decline after 5 years (Cournot et al., 2006).

Prior work from the neuroimaging arm of the Cardiovascular Health Study indicates that being overweight or obese is an independent predictor of brain atrophy in AD and MCI patients (Ho et al., 2010). Similar results have been found for cognitively normal older adult subjects in the Alzheimer's Disease Neuroimaging Initiative, who demonstrate selective patterns of gray and white matter atrophy that include memory relevant areas (e.g., frontal and temporal lobes) (Raji et al., 2010). A recent MRI study using an arterial spin labeling approach found that increased BMI was selectively related to a decrease in cerebral blood flow in frontal but not parietal or global gray matter of older adults (Zimmerman et al., 2014).

Data relating BMI to AD neuropathology in non-demented older adults are limited. A small neuropathology report that focused on obese, cognitively intact, older adults demonstrated significantly increased brain deposition of amyloid-β plaques and tau-neurofibrillary tangles at autopsy (Mrak, 2009). By contrast, in vivo positron emission tomography (PET) using the amyloid PET-ligand Pittsburgh Compound B (PiB) found an *inverse* relationship between BMI and total brain PiB-PET binding in both demented and non-demented subjects, with higher BMI associated with lower PiB-PET signal (Toledo et al., 2012; Vidoni et al., 2011).

It should be noted that body mass index (BMI), a measure of human body shape based on an individual's weight and height (kg/m^2), has been widely used to measure how much an individual's body weight departs from what is normal for a particular height. BMI is used in many contexts as a readily measurable and simple method to assess body composition and adiposity (Taylor et al., 1998). Though not all experts agree, the most widely adopted upper limit of normal for BMI is 25 (U.S. Department of Agriculture and U.S. Department of Health and Human Services, 2010). BMI has been widely used to define overweight and obesity for investigations of cognitive function in middle-aged and older adults, particularly in the epidemiologic literature. Despite its widespread use, BMI has limitations—for some individuals, their BMI is high, yet they are at a healthy weight if their lean body mass is greater than average. Others may have a BMI in the normal range, but they may have greater than average body fat from central obesity. Aging is also known to result in a gradual decrease in lean body mass; thus, the definition of normal BMI may be higher than 25 in older populations. As such, future work may benefit from relating additional objective physiologic measures, such as waist circumference and those derived from tests of maximal aerobic capacity, accelerometer data, or structured longitudinal dietary assessment.

In summary, successful lifestyle-based efforts to treat overweight and obese individuals in order to normalize body composition could result in a lowered risk of cognitive decline and conversion to dementia, improved brain structure, and lower levels of AD neuropathology in pre-dementia states.

Smoking

Smoking cessation is an important source of behavior change to prevent morbidity and premature mortality in the United States, with smoking-related diseases causing over 400,000 deaths each year (National Institutes of Health, 2010). For the brain, meta-analysis of 10 prospective cohort studies on the potential link between smoking and dementia found an increased risk of dementia with continued smoking (summary RR 1.79; 95% CI: 1.43 to 2.23), while quitting smoking appeared to lessen risk toward the level of risk seen in those who had never smoked (Anstey et al., 2007). While there is insufficient evidence to conclude how much smoking over what time period is necessary to increase risk of dementia, it appears that smoking increases risk for the development of AD and cognitive decline (Williams et al., 2010). The physical and psychological aspects of nicotine addiction need to be addressed during smoking cessation efforts, with greater success found through a combination of nicotine replacement, smoking cessation medications (bupropion or varenicline), and cognitive behavioral therapy.

Alcohol Use

The "French paradox" of regular red wine consumption leading to lower rates of heart disease, despite a high intake of dietary cholesterol and saturated fats, may hold true for the risk of age-related disorders related to brain health. Light to moderate non-risk levels of alcohol consumption (defined as 1–2 drinks per night for men, and 1 drink or less per night for women) have in fact been associated with a decreased risk of developing dementia (Anstey et al., 2009; Orgogozo et al., 1997). It is unclear whether this reflects selection effects in cohort studies commencing in late life, a protective effect of alcohol consumption throughout adulthood, or a specific benefit of alcohol in late life. It would be premature to recommend that all older adults drink wine regularly to prevent dementia. Of course, nutritional deficits associated with severe alcoholism lead to dementia, and acute alcohol intoxication can lead to increased confusion and disinhibition, especially in persons already experiencing memory loss.

Head Trauma and Concussions

Risk for developing Alzheimer's disease later in life doubles with loss of consciousness for an hour or more (Mayeux, 1998). Less severe head trauma, such as repeated concussive and/or sub-concussive injury, may likewise relate to cognitive function over time. A study comparing amateur soccer players to runners and swimmers (who were less likely to have had concussive head injuries) in their mid-twenties found that over 30% of soccer players had memory impairments, compared to less than 10% of the runners and swimmers (Matser et al., 1999). Results of studies examining head injury and risk of dementia have been mixed; however, a meta-analysis of 15 case control studies found an excess history of head injury in those with Alzheimer's disease (Fleminger et al., 2003). Thus, avoiding head trauma appears to be a prudent strategy to maintain brain health throughout life. Brain health can be protected through regular use of seat belts while driving, wearing helmets during contact sports, and minimizing fall risks by "fall proofing" the home (e.g., eliminating throw rugs, minimizing clutter, and optimizing lighting).

Environmental Exposures

Data on environmental exposures and risk for AD and cognitive decline remain limited. One available systematic review of case-control and cohort studies on the association between AD and occupational exposures found increased and statistically significant associations with pesticide exposure (Santibanez et al., 2007). For the remaining exposures studied, the evidence of association was less consistent (for solvents and electromagnetic fields) or absent (for lead and aluminum).

Occupation

Intellectually demanding jobs, including those involving coordination of tasks and management of groups are associated with decreased risk of dementia, whereas simpler occupations are implicated with increased risk (Helmer et al., 2001; Jorm et al., 1998; Stern et al., 1994). Similar to the benefits observed with increased educational level, occupational attainment may reduce the risk of AD by enhancing an individual's cognitive reserve, which delays the onset of clinical signs of disease. Occupation is related to education, which begins to blur the line between a modifiable risk factor versus an active choice or intervention to promote and preserve brain health. We review such strategies in the following sections.

INTERVENTIONAL LIFESTYLE STRATEGIES TO SLOW COGNITIVE AND BIOLOGICAL AGING

Education and Cognitive Training

Risk for developing AD and related dementias has been found to decrease with higher levels of education (Caamano-Isorna et al., 2006). One theory of this effect is increased "cognitive reserve," delaying the clinical deficits of dementia (Ngandu et al., 2007). Animal studies show that environmental enrichment (modeling an increased level of education and/or cognitive training) results in hippocampal neurogenesis, synaptogenesis, and enhanced neuronal plasticity via increased neurotrophin levels including brain derived neurotrophic factor (BDNF) (van Praag et al., 2000). Interestingly, these same neurotrophins are released during cognitive training (Vinogradov et al., 2009), and are related to increased memory performance in older adults who exercise regularly (Erickson et al., 2012); neurotrophin up-regulation is implicated in reversing the neurodegenerative effects of

amyloid plaques in Alzheimer's disease (Burbach et al., 2004).

Twin studies have similarly found that higher midlife engagement in cognitively stimulating activities decreases dementia risk (Carlson et al., 2008; Crowe et al., 2003). Further, individuals who spend time doing complex mental tasks during midlife decrease their dementia risk by as much as 48% (Karp et al., 2009). Prospective studies of late-life cognitive stimulation demonstrate slowing of cognitive decline (Wilson et al., 2003) and overall decreased risk of developing cognitive impairment (Verghese et al., 2006) or dementia (Wilson et al., 2007). Interestingly, when compared to persons who spend time on more intellectually challenging tasks, the relatively undemanding task of watching television increases risk of cognitive decline (J. Y. Wang et al., 2006).

Observational and initial randomized controlled trials (RCTs) of cognitive training in normal aging have found a protective effect of such training on risk of cognitive decline (Acevedo and Loewenstein, 2007; Williams et al., 2010). One landmark study, the Advanced Cognitive Training for Independent and Vital Elderly (ACTIVE) study, demonstrated sustained improvements in the cognitive areas trained (speed of processing, verbal memory, and reasoning compared to a no-contact control condition) at 2 years following the intervention (Ball et al., 2002). While the initial study failed to find transfer of skills to everyday function, a 5-year follow-up of the same group showed that problem-solving training resulted in less functional decline (Willis et al., 2006). More recent work is exploring the possibility of training older adults individually using computer-based training.

Strategy-based memory techniques to improve memory performance, as opposed to repetitive cognitive training, have also previously been used successfully in non-demented older adults as part of healthy lifestyle programs to improve memory performance in interventions lasting from 2 to 6 weeks (Ercoli et al., 2011; Miller et al., 2012; Small et al., 2006). One example of a strategy-based technique includes teaching individuals to stop multitasking while learning new things—that is, to pay full, undivided attention with all senses. This approach can bolster the likelihood of retaining new information.

Taken together, cognitive and memory training interventions in older adults show promise but, similar to the study of physical activity (as discussed later in this chapter), the exact form(s), frequency,

Diet and Nutrition

Increasing attention has been given to dietary modification as an approach to improve and preserve brain function with aging. For example, greater adherence to a Mediterranean diet has been shown to reduce cognitive decline in several large cohort studies (Feart et al., 2009; Tangney et al., 2011). Combining Mediterranean diet with higher rates of physical activity has been shown to further decrease the rate of cognitive decline and conversion of patients from MCI to AD (Scarmeas et al., 2009).

Mediterranean diets typically include high amounts of fruits and vegetables, fish or shellfish twice weekly, olive oil or canola oil, nuts such as walnuts or pecans, moderate amounts of red wine, and plentiful herbs and spices as seasonings. Such diets limit the amounts of added salt and animal fats found in red meats and butter—foods typically associated with increased risk for vascular disease.

Specific components of the Mediterranean diet that add to reduced risk for AD potentially include the antioxidant actions of high intake of monounsaturated fatty acids, olive oil, red wine, and fish (Panza et al., 2006). High antioxidant-capacity foods potentially protecting brain health include blueberries, strawberries, and green vegetables like broccoli and spinach (Joseph, 2002). Currently available observational and clinical trial data support a role of omega-3 fatty acids in slowing cognitive decline in older adults without dementia (Fotuhi et al., 2009). Large clinical trials of extended duration with various dosages and formulations of supplements are needed to provide definitive answers regarding the potential of omega-3 fatty acids for the prevention or treatment of AD and related dementias.

Weekly consumption of baked or broiled fish has recently been shown to correlate with higher gray matter volumes in AD-relevant brain areas, such as the medial temporal and prefrontal lobes (Raji et al., 2014). Conversely, overweight status and obesity are known consequences of a high-fat diet in which differences in amyloid processing, particularly in APOE4 positive individuals, may mediate neurodegeneration over time (Grimm et al., 2012). Diets rich in carbohydrates with high glycemic indices (pretzels, French fries, etc.) can increase the risk for diabetes, and can lead to stroke disease and vascular

dementia (Brand-Miller et al., 1999), while dietary changes can reverse such effects. For example, the combination of weight loss, eating a healthy diet, and exercising regularly has been demonstrated to reduce the risk of developing type-2 diabetes by more than 50% (Eriksson et al., 2001).

Given the association of midlife obesity with increased risk of dementia (Fitzpatrick et al., 2009), a healthy brain diet should emphasize moderate caloric intake with total daily amounts ranging from 2000 to 2500 kcal/day, depending on total body mass and gender. Taken one step further, caloric restriction of roughly 30% has been shown repeatedly across species to increase longevity substantially, apparently through a reduction in both inflammation and oxidative stress (Holloszy and Fontana, 2007). Even without frank caloric restriction, dietary choices can be informed by the above-mentioned evidence and used to mitigate the impact of aging on brain health and function.

Physical Activity and Exercise

There is a growing literature in older adults detailing the benefits of aerobic exercise on cognitive function (Barnes et al., 2003; Erickson et al., 2012; Goodwin et al., 2008; Hillman et al., 2008; Petzinger et al., 2013) and mood (Mead et al., 2009; Sjosten and Kivela, 2006). For example, regular physical exercise was found to lower risk for memory decline in older adults by 46% (Etgen et al., 2010). In general, cohort studies support the conclusion that aerobic physical activities, particularly at high levels, are associated with lower risk of developing AD (Williams et al., 2010). A meta-analysis of randomized controlled trials comparing aerobic physical activity programs with control interventions found that aerobic exercise is protective against loss of cognitive function in healthy older adults (Angevaren et al., 2008). In particular, the meta-analysis demonstrated significant effects of physical activity on motor function, cognitive speed, and auditory and visual attention. In one such study, adults with subjective memory impairment but no dementia showed a modest improvement in cognition at 18-month follow-up after a 6-month program of increased physical activity (Lautenschlager et al., 2008).

In seminal work, neuropsychological examination of healthy adults aged 60–75 found that involvement in an aerobic exercise program (compared to a stretching and toning control group) improved performance on mental tasks involved in frontal lobe function (monitoring, scheduling, planning, inhibition, and memory) (Kramer et al., 1999). Subsequent work has confirmed that exercise improves executive control, visuospatial learning, and memory (Colcombe and Kramer, 2003; Hillman et al., 2008).

Studies examining physical activity level with imaging metrics show that exercise predicts gray matter volume associated with aging (Erickson et al., 2010) and that increased exercise can reverse volume loss and improve memory and other cognitive functions (Erickson et al., 2011; Hillman et al., 2008). A positive association between greater physical activity levels and lower PiB-PET binding has been demonstrated in older adults with normal cognition (Liang et al., 2010). Further, exercise appears to moderate the effect of APOE-4 genotype, with higher PiB binding observed in more sedentary APOE-4 carriers compared with non-carriers (Head et al., 2012). More recently, higher levels of physical activity and lower inflammatory markers such as tumor necrosis factor alpha were shown to correlate with greater brain volumes in normal aging (Braskie et al., 2014).

When laboratory animals exercise regularly, they develop new neurons in the hippocampus, which then form functional connections with other brain cells (Gage, 2002). Physical exercise–induced increases in BDNF support cell survival, dendritic branching, and synaptic plasticity (Bekinschtein et al., 2011), including improved memory performance in older adults who begin exercising regularly (Erickson et al., 2012). Physical exercise may also increase cerebral blood flow, which in turn promotes nerve cell growth and expression of BDNF, further enhancing brain plasticity. BDNF and related neurotrophin up-regulation are implicated in reversing the neurodegenerative effects of amyloid plaques in Alzheimer's disease (Burbach et al., 2004). Animal models further reveal that aerobic exercise acutely increases levels of BDNF levels within 15 minutes of sustained aerobic activity, and BDNF remains elevated during exercise, followed by rapid decline after stopping (i.e., over minutes to hours) (Berchtold et al., 2010; Rasmussen et al., 2009). This BDNF rise is thought to lead to enhancement of memory and mood circuit neuroplasticity, and ultimately, improvement in well-being.

In conclusion, exercise intervention studies with significantly improved cognitive outcomes in older adults typically incorporate sustained aerobic exercise at a minimum duration of 30 minutes, using individualized aerobic targets set at least 50%–80% of the heart rate reserve, providing the feasibility of this low-cost, non-invasive intervention to attenuate cognitive impairment and reduce dementia risk.

Maintaining Social Connections

Forming and maintaining social connections may lower dementia risk. The Kungsholmen Project, a long-term population study in Sweden, demonstrated over 6 years that continuing frequent (daily to weekly) engagement in mental, social, or productive activities during late life was related to a decreased incidence of dementia (H. X. Wang et al., 2002). In contrast, poor or limited social networks increased risk of dementia by 60% (95% CI: 1.2–2.1) in this same Swedish population (Fratiglioni et al., 2000). A study sample of community-dwelling elderly adults in New Haven, Connecticut, found that global social disengagement was a risk factor for developing cognitive impairment (Bassuk et al., 1999). The MacArthur study of successful aging found that staying in close contact with people and remaining involved in meaningful activities predicted successful aging (Kahn, 1998). Level of social engagement has also been related to depression, which may itself be an independent risk factor for dementia (Glass et al., 2006; Ownby et al., 2006).

Stress Reduction

Research has shown that memory function and brain health decline over time with chronic stress. Animal studies of prolonged stress hormone exposure show deleterious effects on the hippocampus, a brain region involved in learning and memory, leading to decreased brain plasticity (Sapolsky, 1999). Human studies demonstrate that exposure to cortisol impairs memory (Newcomer et al., 1999). In contrast, a study of New York City Traffic Enforcement Agents showed that increased levels of workplace support decrease stress levels, as measured by changes in blood pressure, especially during stressful periods (Karlin et al., 2003). Taken together, these findings suggest that minimizing stress may have a beneficial impact on brain health.

Sleep Hygiene and Related CAIM Approaches

Consistent high-quality sleep is critical for peak cognitive function at any age. Aging is known to impact sleep in a number of predictable normative ways, including but not limited to lighter sleep (i.e., increased wakefulness after sleep onset), decreased deep slow-wave stage-3 sleep, decreased and more fragmented REM sleep, and decreased total sleep time (averaging 5–7 hours) (Gooneratne and Vitiello, 2014). Going to bed earlier and waking up earlier (advanced sleep phase) is another common occurrence in older adults, which, when associated with daytime fatigue and impairments, is categorized as a circadian rhythm sleep disorder.

Evaluation of disrupted sleep in older adults needs to include ruling out medical etiologies such as obstructive sleep apnea, restless leg syndrome, periodic limb movement disorder, excessive nocturia, musculoskeletal pain, chronic obstructive pulmonary disease, and medication-induced (i.e., iatrogenic) insomnia. Psychiatric causes of sleep disturbance can include depression, generalized anxiety, grief, and dementing illnesses. Sleep–wake disorders not mentioned thus far include insomnia disorder, hypersomnolence, narcolepsy, and parasomnias such as REM sleep behavior disorder. The evaluation of sleep disorders is often best accomplished by referral to a specialty sleep center.

Complementary and integrative medicine (CAIM) approaches to improving sleep are varied, and the most appropriate choice often depends on the identified etiologies of the sleep disruption. The best evidence is for cognitive behavioral therapy, including sleep hygiene approaches. Getting up out of bed when unable to fall asleep, avoiding bright light exposure (e.g., television or computer) or heavy exercise just before bedtime, having a regular sleep and wake time, and using the bedroom only for sleep are among the various sleep hygiene approaches used with success to improve sleep. Proper sleep hygiene is an important aspect of a healthy brain lifestyle. Additional CAIM approaches to sleep improvement are discussed in Chapter 26 of this volume, and include melatonin, valerian root, magnesium, yoga, tai chi, and cognitive behavioral therapy.

Combining Lifestyle Strategies

An increasing number of studies have examined the impact of combining lifestyle strategies. For example, some studies of physical exercise and cognitive training show a potentially synergistic impact on cognitive functioning (Barnes et al.,

2013; Fabre et al., 2002; Oswald et al., 1996; Shah et al., 2014; Theill et al., 2013). To examine the synergistic effects of a temporally combined intervention, one recent study examined the acute effects of simultaneous treadmill running while performing a verbal working memory task in older adults (compared to patients who did sedentary memory training) (Theill et al., 2013). The study found that the simultaneous training group had significant improvements in paired-associative memory performance compared to the sedentary training group. Engaging in several healthy lifestyle habits may have an additive effect on forestalling symptom onset by several years. A recent study surveyed more than 18,000 Americans and found that the greater the number of healthy lifestyle strategies people practiced, the lower their risk for experiencing memory symptoms (Small et al., 2013).

SUMMARY

Lifestyle medicine encourages addressing age-related changes to memory and cognition via lifestyle-based approaches. Preventive strategies related to healthy lifestyle in aging offer the potential for a major public health impact, with the ability to successfully interrupt progressive age-related memory loss by using widely available and inexpensive behavior-based lifestyle strategies representing an important factor in improving long-term outcomes and reducing the cost of dementia (Thies et al., 2014). Future work should integrate the existent data into an overall clinical and lifestyle-based strategy to reduce risk for and to potentially delay the onset of Alzheimer's disease and related dementia symptoms.

DISCLOSURE STATEMENT

David Merrill has no disclosures or conflicts of interest to report. His salary is funded by his department (Psychiatry) and an institutional KL2 research award (CTSI-NIH funded research center grant).

REFERENCES

Acevedo, A. & Loewenstein, D. A. (2007). Nonpharmacological cognitive interventions in aging and dementia. *J Geriatr Psychiatry Neurol*, 20(4), 239–249.

Aizenstein, H. J., Nebes, R. D., Saxton, J. A., Price, J. C., Mathis, C. A., Tsopelas, N. D., Ziolko, S. K., James, J. A., Snitz, B. E., Houck, P. R., Bi, W., Cohen, A. D., Lopresti, B. J., DeKosky, S. T., Halligan, E. M., & Klunk, W. E. (2008). Frequent amyloid deposition without significant cognitive impairment among the elderly. *Arch Neurol, 65*(11), 1509–1517.

Angevaren, M., Aufdemkampe, G., Verhaar, H. J., Aleman A., & Vanhees, L. (2008). Physical activity and enhanced fitness to improve cognitive function in older people without known cognitive impairment. *Cochrane Database Syst Rev, 3,* CD005381.

Anstey, K. J., Lipnicki, D. M., & Low, L. F. (2008). Cholesterol as a risk factor for dementia and cognitive decline: a systematic review of prospective studies with meta-analysis. *Am J Geriatr Psychiatry, 16*(5), 343–354.

Anstey, K. J., Mack, H. A., & Cherbuin, N. (2009). Alcohol consumption as a risk factor for dementia and cognitive decline: meta-analysis of prospective studies. *Am J Geriatr Psychiatry, 17*(7), 542–555.

Anstey, K. J., von Sanden, C., Salim, A., & O'Kearney, R. (2007). Smoking as a risk factor for dementia and cognitive decline: a meta-analysis of prospective studies. *Am J Epidemiol, 166*(4), 367–378.

Ball, K., Berch, D. B., Helmers, K. F., Jobe, J. B., Leveck, M. D., Marsiske, M., Morris, J. N., Rebok, G. W., Smith, D. M., Tennstedt, S. L., Unverzagt, F. W., & Willis, S. L. (2002). Effects of cognitive training interventions with older adults: a randomized controlled trial. *JAMA, 288*(18), 2271–2281.

Barnes, D. E., Santos-Modesitt, W., Poelke, G., Kramer, A. F., Castro, C., Middleton, L. E., & Yaffe, K. (2013). The Mental Activity and eXercise (MAX) trial: a randomized controlled trial to enhance cognitive function in older adults. *JAMA Intern Med, 173*(9), 797–804.

Barnes, D. E., & Yaffe, K. (2011). The projected effect of risk factor reduction on Alzheimer's disease prevalence. *Lancet Neurol, 10*(9), 819–828.

Barnes, D. E., Yaffe, K., Satariano, W. A., & Tager, I. B. (2003). A longitudinal study of cardiorespiratory fitness and cognitive function in healthy older adults. *J Am Geriatr Soc, 51*(4), 459–465.

Bassett, S. S., & Folstein, M. F. (1993). Memory complaint, memory performance, and psychiatric diagnosis: a community study. *J Geriatr Psychiatry Neurol, 6*(2), 105–111.

Bassuk, S. S., Glass, T. A., & Berkman, L. F. (1999). Social disengagement and incident cognitive decline in community-dwelling elderly persons. *Ann Intern Med, 131*(3), 165–173.

Bekinschtein, P., Oomen, C. A., Saksida, L. M., & Bussey, T. J. (2011). Effects of environmental enrichment and voluntary exercise on neurogenesis, learning and memory, and pattern separation: BDNF as a critical variable? *Semin Cell Dev Biol, 22*(5), 536–542.

Berchtold, N. C., Castello, N., & Cotman, C. W. (2010). Exercise and time-dependent benefits to learning and memory. *Neuroscience, 167*(3), 588–597.

Beydoun, M. A., Beydoun, H. A., & Wang, Y. (2008). Obesity and central obesity as risk factors for incident dementia and its subtypes: a systematic review and meta-analysis. *Obes Rev, 9*(3), 204–218.

Brady, C. B., Spiro, A., 3rd, McGlinchey-Berroth, R., Milberg, W., & Gaziano, J. M. (2001). Stroke risk predicts verbal fluency decline in healthy older men: evidence from the normative aging study. *J Gerontology B, 56*(6), P340–346.

Brand-Miller, J., Volwever, T.M.S., Colaguiri, S., & Foster-Powell, K. (1999). *The glucose revolution.* New York: Marlow.

Braskie, M. N., Boyle, C. P., Rajagopalan, P., Gutman, B. A., Toga, A. W., Raji, C. A., Tracy, R. P., Kuller, L. H., Becker, J. T., Lopez, O. L., & Thompson, P. M. (2014). Physical activity, inflammation, and volume of the aging brain. *Neuroscience, 273,* 199–209.

Braskie, M. N., Klunder, A. D., Hayashi, K. M., Protas, H., Kepe, V., Miller, K. J., Huang, S. C., Barrio, J. R., Ercoli, L. M., Siddarth, P., Satyamurthy, N., Liu, J., Toga, A. W., Bookheimer, S. Y., Small, G. W., & Thompson, P. M. (2010). Plaque and tangle imaging and cognition in normal aging and Alzheimer's disease. *Neurobiology Aging, 31*(10), 1669–1678.

Braskie, M. N., Small, G. W., & Bookheimer, S. Y. (2010). Vascular health risks and fMRI activation during a memory task in older adults. *Neurobiol Aging, 31,* 1532–1542.

Burbach, G. J., Hellweg, R., Haas, C. A., Del Turco, D., Deicke, U., Abramowski, D., Jucker, M., Staufenbiel, M., & Deller, T. (2004). Induction of brain-derived neurotrophic factor in plaque-associated glial cells of aged APP23 transgenic mice. *J Neurosci, 24*(10), 2421–2430.

Caamano-Isorna, F., Corral, M., Montes-Martinez, A., & Takkouche, B. (2006). Education and dementia: a meta-analytic study. *Neuroepidemiology, 26*(4), 226–232.

Carlson, M. C., Helms, M. J., Steffens, D. C., Burke, J. R., Potter, G. G., & Plassman, B. L. (2008). Midlife activity predicts risk of dementia in older male twin pairs. *Alzheimers Dement, 4*(5), 324–331.

Chetelat, G., Villemagne, V. L., Pike, K. E., Ellis, K. A., Bourgeat, P., Jones, G., O'Keefe, G. J., Salvado, O., Szoeke, C., Martins, R. N., Ames, D., Masters, C. L., & Rowe, C. C. (2011). Independent contribution of temporal beta-amyloid deposition to memory decline in the pre-dementia phase of Alzheimer's disease. *Brain, 134*(Pt 3), 798–807.

Christensen, H. (2001). What cognitive changes can be expected with normal ageing? *Aust N Z J Psychiatry, 35*(6), 768–775.

Colcombe, S., & Kramer, A. F. (2003). Fitness effects on the cognitive function of older adults: a meta-analytic study. *Psychol Sci, 14*(2), 125–130.

Cournot, M., Marquie, J. C., Ansiau, D., Martinaud, C., Fonds, H., Ferrieres, J., & Ruidavets, J. B. (2006). Relation between body mass index and cognitive function in healthy middle-aged men and women. *Neurology, 67*(7), 1208–1214.

Crowe, M., Andel, R., Pedersen, N. L., Johansson, B., & Gatz, M. (2003). Does participation in leisure activities lead to reduced risk of Alzheimer's disease? A prospective study of Swedish twins. *J Gerontol B Psychol Sci Soc Sci, 58*(5), P249–255.

D'Agostino, R. B., Wolf, P. A., Belanger, A. J., & Kannel, W. B. (1994). Stroke risk profile: adjustment for antihypertensive medication. The Framingham Study. *Stroke, 25*(1), 40–43.

Debette, S., Seshadri, S., Beiser, A., Au, R., Himali, J. J., Palumbo, C., Wolf, P. A., & DeCarli, C. (2011). Midlife vascular risk factor exposure accelerates structural brain aging and cognitive decline. *Neurology, 77*(5), 461–468.

Elias, M. F., Elias, P. K., Sullivan, L. M., Wolf, P. A., & D'Agostino, R. B. (2005). Obesity, diabetes and cognitive deficit: The Framingham Heart Study. *Neurobiology Aging, 26*(Suppl 1), 11–16.

Elias, M. F., Sullivan, L. M., D'Agostino, R. B., Elias, P.K., Beiser, A., Au, R., Seshadri, S., DeCarli, C., & Wolf, P. A. (2004). Framingham stroke risk profile and lowered cognitive performance. *Stroke, 35*(2), 404–409.

Ercoli, L. M., Cernin, P. A., & Small, G. W. (2011). Peer-led memory training programs to support brain fitness. In P. E. Hartman-Stein and A. LaRue (Eds.), *Enhancing cognitive fitness in older adults* (pp. 213–230). New York: Springer.

Ercoli, L. M., Siddarth, P., Kepe, V., Miller, K. J., Huang, S. C., Cole, G. M., Lavretsky, H., Bookheimer, S. Y., Kim, J., Phelps, M. E., Barrio, J. R., & Small, G. W. (2009). Differential FDDNP PET patterns in nondemented middle-aged and older adults. *Am J Geriatr Psychiatry, 17*(5), 397–406.

Erickson, K. I., Miller, D. L., & Roecklein, K. A. (2012). The aging hippocampus: interactions between exercise, depression, and BDNF. *Neuroscientist, 18*(1), 82–97.

Erickson, K. I., Raji, C. A., Lopez, O. L., Becker, J. T., Rosano, C., Newman, A. B., Gach, H. M., Thompson, P. M., Ho, A. J., & Kuller, L. H. (2010). Physical activity predicts gray matter volume in late adulthood: the Cardiovascular Health Study. *Neurology, 75*(16), 1415–1422.

Erickson, K. I., Voss, M. W., Prakash, R. S., Basak, C., Szabo, A., Chaddock, L., Kim, J. S., Heo, S., Alves, H., White, S. M., Wojcicki, T. R., Mailey, E., Vieira, V. J., Martin, S. A., Pence, B. D., Woods, J. A., McAuley E., & Kramer, A. F. (2011). Exercise training increases size of hippocampus and improves memory. *Proc Natl Acad Sci USA, 108*(7), 3017–3022.

Eriksson, J., Lindstrom, J., & Tuomilehto, J. (2001). Potential for the prevention of type 2 diabetes. *Br Med Bull, 60*, 183–199.

Etgen, T., Sander, D., Huntgeburth, U., Poppert, H., Forstl, H., & Bickel, H. (2010). Physical activity and incident cognitive impairment in elderly persons: the INVADE study. *Arch Internal Med, 170*(2), 186–193.

Fabre, C., Chamari, K., Mucci, P., Massé-Biron, J., & Préfaut, C. (2002). Improvement of cognitive function by mental and/or individualized aerobic training in healthy elderly subjects. *Int J Sports Med, 23*(6), 415–421.

Feart, C., Samieri, C., Rondeau, V., Amieva, H., Portet, F., Dartigues, J. F., Scarmeas, N., & Barberger-Gateau, P. (2009). Adherence to a Mediterranean diet, cognitive decline, and risk of dementia. *JAMA, 302*(6), 638–648.

Fitzpatrick, A. L., Kuller, L. H., Lopez, O. L., Diehr, P., O'Meara, E. S., Longstreth, W. T., Jr., & Luchsinger, J. A. (2009). Midlife and late-life obesity and the risk of dementia: cardiovascular health study. *Arch Neurol, 66*(3), 336–342.

Fleminger, S., Oliver, D. L., Lovestone, S., Rabe-Hesketh, S., & Giora, A. (2003). Head injury as a risk factor for Alzheimer's disease: the evidence 10 years on; a partial replication. *J Neurol Neurosurg Psychiatry, 74*(7), 857–862.

Forsberg, A., Engler, H., Almkvist, O., Blomquist, G., Hagman, G., Wall, A., Ringheim, A., Langstrom, B., & Nordberg, A. (2008). PET imaging of amyloid deposition in patients with mild cognitive impairment. *Neurobiology Aging, 29*(10), 1456–1465.

Fotuhi, M., Mohassel, P., & Yaffe, K. (2009). Fish consumption, long-chain omega-3 fatty acids and risk of cognitive decline or Alzheimer disease: a complex association. *Nat Clin Pract Neurol, 5*(3), 140–152.

Fratiglioni, L., Wang, H. X., Ericsson, K., Maytan, M., & Winblad, B. (2000). Influence of social network on occurrence of dementia: a community-based longitudinal study. *Lancet, 355*(9212), 1315–1319.

Gage, F. H. (2002). Neurogenesis in the adult brain. *J Neurosci, 22*(3), 612–613.

Glass, T. A., De Leon, C. F., Bassuk, S. S., & Berkman, L. F. (2006). Social engagement and depressive symptoms in late life: longitudinal findings. *J Aging Health, 18*(4), 604–628.

Goodwin, V. A., Richards, S. H., Taylor, R. S., Taylor, A. H., & Campbell, J. L. (2008). The effectiveness of exercise interventions for people with Parkinson's disease: a systematic review and meta-analysis. *Mov Disord, 23*(5), 631–640.

Gooneratne, N. S., & Vitiello, M. V. (2014). Sleep in older adults: normative changes, sleep disorders, and treatment options. *Clin Geriatr Med, 30*(3), 591–627.

Gorelick, P. B., Scuteri, A., Black, S. E., Decarli, C., Greenberg, S. M., Iadecola, C., Launer, L. J., Laurent, S., Lopez, O. L., Nyenhuis, D., Petersen, R. C., Schneider, J. A., Tzourio, C., Arnett, D. K., Bennett, D. A., Chui, H. C., Higashida, R. T., Lindquist, R., Nilsson, P. M., Roman, G. C., Sellke, F. W., & Seshadri, S. (2011). Vascular contributions to cognitive impairment and dementia: a statement for healthcare professionals from the american heart association/american stroke association. *Stroke, 42*(9), 2672–2713.

Grimm, M. O., Rothhaar, T. L., Grosgen, S., Burg, V. K., Hundsdorfer, B., Haupenthal, V. J., Friess, P., Kins, S., Grimm, H. S., & Hartmann, T. (2012). Trans fatty acids enhance amyloidogenic processing of the Alzheimer amyloid precursor protein (APP). *J Nutrit Biochem, 23*(10), 1214–1223.

Hanninen, T., Hallikainen, M., Tuomainen, S., Vanhanen, M., & Soininen, H. (2002). Prevalence of mild cognitive impairment: a population-based study in elderly subjects." *Acta Neurol Scand, 106*(3), 148–154.

Head, D., Bugg, J. M., Goate, A. M., Fagan, A. M, Mintun, M. A., Benzinger, T., Holtzman, D. M, & Morris, J. C. (2012). Exercise engagement as a moderator of the effects of APOE genotype on amyloid deposition. *Arch Neurology, 69*(5), 636–643.

Helmer, C., Letenneur, L., Rouch, I., Richard-Harston, S., Barberger-Gateau, P., Fabrigoule, C., Orgogozo, J. M., & Dartigues, J. F. (2001). Occupation during life and risk of dementia in French elderly community residents. *J Neurol Neurosurg Psychiatry, 71*(3), 303–309.

Hillman, C. H., Erickson, K. I., & Kramer, A. F. (2008). Be smart, exercise your heart: exercise effects on brain and cognition. *Nat Rev Neurosci, 9*(1), 58–65.

Ho, A. J., Raji, C. A., Becker, J. T., Lopez, O. L., Kuller, L. H., Hua, X., Lee, S., Hibar, D., Dinov, I. D., Stein, J. L., Jack, C. R., Jr., Weiner, M. W., Toga, A. W., & Thompson, P. M. (2010). Obesity is linked with lower brain volume in 700 AD and MCI patients. *Neurobiol Aging, 31*(8), 1326–1339.

Holloszy, J. O., & Fontana, L. (2007). Caloric restriction in humans. *Exp Gerontol, 42*(8), 709–712.

Hsiung, G. Y., & Sadovnick, A. D. (2007). Genetics and dementia: risk factors, diagnosis, and management. *Alzheimers Dement, 3*(4), 418–427.

Jorm, A. F., Rodgers, B., Henderson, A. S., Korten, A. E., Jacomb, P. A., Christensen, H., & Mackinnon, A. (1998). Occupation type as a predictor of cognitive decline and dementia in old age. *Age Ageing, 27*(4), 477–483.

Joseph, J. A. (2002). *The color code: a revolutionary eating plan for optimal health.* New York: Hyperion.

Kahn, R. L. (1998). *Successful aging.* New York: Pantheon.

Kantarci, K., Lowe, V., Przybelski, S. A., Weigand, S. D., Senjem, M. L., Ivnik, R. J., Preboske, G. M., Roberts, R., Geda, Y. E., Boeve, B. F., Knopman, D. S., Petersen R. C., & Jack, C. R., Jr. (2012). APOE modifies the association between Abeta load and cognition in cognitively normal older adults. *Neurology, 78*(4), 232–240.

Karlin, W. A., Brondolo E., & Schwartz, J. (2003). Workplace social support and ambulatory cardiovascular activity in New York City traffic agents. *Psychosom Med, 65*(2), 167–176.

Kivipelto, M., Helkala, E. L., Laakso, M. P., Hanninen, T., Hallikainen, M., Alhainen, K., Iivonen, S., Mannermaa, A., Tuomilehto, J., Nissinen A., & Soininen, H. (2002). Apolipoprotein E epsilon4 allele, elevated midlife total cholesterol level, and high midlife systolic blood pressure are independent risk factors for late-life Alzheimer disease. *Ann Intern Med, 137*(3), 149–155.

Klunk, W. E., Engler, H., Nordberg, A., Wang, Y., Blomqvist, G., D. P. Holt, D. P., M. Bergstrom, M., I. Savitcheva, I., G. F. Huang, G. F., Estrada, S., Ausen, B., Debnath, M. L., Barletta, J., Price, J. C., Sandell, J., Lopresti, B. J., Wall, A., Koivisto, P., Antoni, G., Mathis, C. A., & Langstrom, B. (2004). Imaging brain amyloid in Alzheimer's disease with Pittsburgh Compound-B. *Ann Neurol, 55*(3), 306–319.

Kramer, A. F., Hahn, S., Cohen, N. J., Banich, M. T., McAuley, E., Harrison, C. R., Chason, J., Vakil, E. Bardell, L., Boileau, R. A., & Colcombe, A. (1999). Ageing, fitness and neurocognitive function. *Nature, 400*(6743), 418–419.

Larrabee, G. J., & Crook, T. H., 3rd (1994). Estimated prevalence of age-associated memory impairment derived from standardized tests of memory function. *Int Psychogeriatr, 6*(1), 95–104.

Lautenschlager, N. T., Cox, K. L., Flicker, L., Foster, J. K., van Bockxmeer, F. M., Xiao, J., Greenop, K. R., & Almeida, O. P. (2008). Effect of physical activity on cognitive function in older adults at risk for Alzheimer disease: a randomized trial. *JAMA, 300*(9), 1027–1037.

Li, H., S. Wetten, S., L. Li, ., P. L. St Jean, P. L., R. Upmanyu, R., L. Surh, L., D. Hosford, D., M. R. Barnes, M. R., J. D. Briley, J. D., M. Borrie, M., N. Coletta, N., . . . Roses, A. D. (2008). Candidate single-nucleotide polymorphisms from a genomewide association study of Alzheimer disease. *Arch Neurol, 65*(1), 45–53.

Liang, K. Y., Mintun, M. A., Fagan, A. M., Goate, A. M., Bugg, J. M., Holtzman, D. M., Morris, J. C., & Head, D. (2010). Exercise and Alzheimer's disease biomarkers in cognitively normal older adults. *Ann Neurol, 68*(3), 311–318.

Llewellyn, D. J., Lang, I. A., Xie, J., Huppert, F. A., Melzer D., & Langa, K. M. (2008). Framingham Stroke Risk Profile and poor cognitive function: a population-based study. *BMC Neurology, 8,* 12.

Lopez, O. L., Jagust, W. J., DeKosky, S. T., Becker, J. T., Fitzpatrick, A., Dulberg, C., Breitner, J., Lyketsos, C., Jones, B., Kawas, C., Carlson, M., & Kuller L. H. (2003). Prevalence and classification of mild cognitive impairment in the Cardiovascular Health Study Cognition Study: part 1. *Arch Neurol, 60*(10), 1385–1389.

Lu, F. P., Lin, K. P., & Kuo, H. K. (2009). Diabetes and the risk of multi-system aging phenotypes: a systematic review and meta-analysis. *PLoS One, 4*(1), e4144.

Luchsinger, J. A. (2010). Diabetes, related conditions, and dementia. *J Neurol Sci, 299*(1–2), 35–38.

Marchant, N. L., Reed, B. R., Decarli, C. S., Madison, C. M., Weiner, M. W., Chui, H. C., & Jagust, W. J. (2011). Cerebrovascular disease, beta-amyloid, and cognition in aging. *Neurobiol Aging. 33*(5), 1006 e25–36

Matser, E. J., Kessels, A. G., Lezak, M. D., Jordan, B. D., & Troost, J. (1999). Neuropsychological impairment in amateur soccer players. *JAMA, 282*(10), 971–973.

Mayeux, R. (1998). Gene-environment interaction in late-onset Alzheimer disease: the role of apolipoprotein-epsilon4. *Alzheimer Dis Assoc Disord, 12*(Suppl 3), S10–15.

McGuinness, B., Todd, S., Passmore, P., & Bullock, R. (2006). The effects of blood pressure lowering on development of cognitive impairment and dementia in patients without apparent prior cerebrovascular disease. *Cochrane Database Syst Rev, 2,* CD004034.

Mead, G. E., Morley, W., Campbell, P., Greig, C. A., McMurdo, M., & Lawlor, D. A. (2009). Exercise for depression. *Cochrane Database Syst Rev, 3,* CD004366.

Merrill, D. A., Siddarth, P., Kepe, V., Raja, P. V., Saito, N., Ercoli, L. M., Miller, K. J., Lavretsky, H., Bookheimer, S. Y., Barrio, J. R., & Small, G. W. (2013). Vascular risk and FDDNP-PET influence cognitive performance. *J Alzheimers Disease, 35*(1), 147–157.

Merrill, D. A., & Small, G. W. (2011). Prevention in psychiatry: effects of healthy lifestyle on cognition. *Psych Clin N Am, 34*(1), 249–261.

Miller, K. J., Siddarth, P., Gaines, Parrish, J. M., Ercoli, L. M., Marx, K., Ronch, J., Pilgram, B., Burke, K., Barczak, N., Babcock, B., & Small, G. W. (2012). The memory fitness program: cognitive effects of a healthy aging intervention. *Am J Geriatr Psychiatry, 20*(6), 514–523.

Mitchell, A. J., & Shiri-Feshki, M. (2009). Rate of progression of mild cognitive impairment to dementia: meta-analysis of 41 robust inception cohort studies. *Acta Psychiat Scand, 119*(4), 252–265.

Mormino, E. C., Kluth, J. T., Madison, C. M., Rabinovici, G. D., Baker, S. L., Miller, B. L., Koeppe, R. A., Mathis, C. A., Weiner, M. W., & Jagust, W. J. (2009). Episodic memory loss is related to hippocampal-mediated beta-amyloid deposition in elderly subjects. *Brain, 132*(Pt 5), 1310–1323.

Mrak, R. E. (2009). Alzheimer-type neuropathological changes in morbidly obese elderly individuals. *Clin Neuropathol, 28*(1), 40–45.

National Institutes of Health, N. C. I. (2010). *Smoking facts and tips for quitting.* http://www.cancer.gov/about-cancer/causes-prevention/risk/tobacco/cessation-fact-sheet

Newcomer, J. W., Selke, G., Melson, A. K., Hershey, T., Craft, S., Richards, K., & Alderson, A. L. (1999). Decreased memory performance in healthy humans induced by stress-level cortisol treatment. *Arch Gen Psychiatry, 56*(6), 527–533.

Ngandu, T., von Strauss, E., Helkala, E. L., Winblad, B., Nissinen, A., Tuomilehto, J., Soininen, H., & Kivipelto, M. (2007). Education and dementia: what lies behind the association? *Neurology, 69*(14), 1442–1450.

Orgogozo, J. M., Dartigues, J. F., Lafont, S., Letenneur, L., Commenges, D., Salamon, R., Renaud, S., & Breteler, M. B. (1997). Wine consumption and dementia in the elderly: a prospective community study in the Bordeaux area. *Rev Neurol (Paris), 153*(3), 185–192.

Oswald, W. D., Rupprecht, R., Gunzelmann, T., & Tritt, K. (1996). The SIMA-project: effects of 1 year cognitive and psychomotor training on cognitive abilities of the elderly. *Behav Brain Res, 78*(1), 67–72.

Ownby, R. L., Crocco, E., Acevedo, A., John, V., & Loewenstein, D. (2006). Depression and risk for Alzheimer disease: systematic review, meta-analysis, and metaregression analysis. *Arch Gen Psychiatry, 63*(5), 530–538.

Panza, F., D'Introno, A., Colacicco, A. M., Capurso, C., Pichichero, G., Capurso, S. A., Capurso, A., & Solfrizzi, V. (2006). Lipid metabolism in cognitive decline and dementia. *Brain Res Rev, 51*(2), 275–292.

Petersen, R. C., Smith, G. E., Waring, S. C., Ivnik, R. J., Tangalos, E. G., & Kokmen, E. (1999). Mild cognitive impairment: clinical characterization and outcome. *Arch Neurol, 56*(3), 303–308.

Petrovitch, H., White, L. R., Izmirilian, G., Ross, G. W., Havlik, R. J., Markesbery, W., Nelson, J., Davis, D. G., Hardman, J., Foley, D. J., & Launer, L. J. (2000). Midlife blood pressure and neuritic plaques, neurofibrillary tangles, and brain weight at death: the HAAS. Honolulu-Asia Aging Study. *Neurobiol Aging, 21*(1), 57–62.

Petzinger, G. M., Fisher, B. E., McEwen, S., Beeler, J. A., Walsh, J. P., & Jakowec, M. W. (2013). Exercise-enhanced neuroplasticity targeting motor and cognitive circuitry in Parkinson's disease. *Lancet Neurol, 12*(7), 716–726.

Pike, K. E., Ellis, K. A., Villemagne, V. L., Good, N., Chetelat, G., Ames, D., Szoeke, C., Laws, S. M., Verdile, G., Martins, R. N., Masters, C. L., & Rowe, C. C. (2011). Cognition and beta-amyloid in preclinical Alzheimer's disease: data from the AIBL study. *Neuropsychologia, 49*(9), 2384–2390.

Pike, K. E., Savage, G., Villemagne, V. L., Ng, S., Moss, S. A., Maruff, P., Mathis, C. A., Klunk, W. E., Masters, C. L., & Rowe, C. C. (2007). Beta-amyloid imaging and memory in non-demented individuals: evidence for preclinical Alzheimer's disease. *Brain, 130*(Pt 11), 2837–2844.

Raji, C. A., Erickson, K. I., Lopez, O. L., Kuller, L. H., Gach, H. M., Thompson, P. M., Riverol, M., & Becker, J. T. (2014). Regular fish consumption and age-related brain gray matter loss. *Am J Prev Med, 47*(4), 444–451.

Raji, C. A., Ho, A. J., Parikshak, N. N., Becker, J. T., Lopez, O. L., Kuller, L. H., Hua, X., Leow, A. D., Toga, A. W., & Thompson, P. M. (2010). Brain structure and obesity. *Human Brain Mapp, 31*(3), 353–364.

Rasmussen, P., Brassard, P., Adser, H., Pedersen, M. V., Leick, L., Hart, E., Secher, N. H., Pedersen, B. H., & Pilegaard, H. (2009). Evidence for a release of brain-derived neurotrophic factor from the brain during exercise. *Exp Physiol, 94*(10), 1062–1069.

Reed, B. R., Eberling, J. L., Mungas, D., Weiner, M., Kramer, J. H., & Jagust, W. J. (2004). Effects of white matter lesions and lacunes on cortical function. *Arch Neurology, 61*(10), 1545–1550.

Reed, B. R., Marchant, N. L., Jagust, W. J., Decarli, C. C., Mack, W., & Chui, H. C. (2011). Coronary risk correlates with cerebral amyloid deposition. *Neurobiol Aging.* 2012, 33(5), 1006 e25–36

Resnick, S. M., Sojkova, J., Zhou, Y., An, Y., Ye, W., Holt, D. P., Dannals, R. F., Mathis, C. A., Klunk, W. E., Ferrucci, L., Kraut, M. A., & Wong, D. F. (2010). Longitudinal cognitive decline is associated with fibrillar amyloid-beta measured by [11C]PiB. *Neurology, 74*(10), 807–815.

Santibanez, M., Bolumar, F., & Garcia, A. M. (2007). Occupational risk factors in Alzheimer's disease: a review assessing the quality of published epidemiological studies. *Occup Environ Med, 64*(11), 723–732.

Sapolsky, R. M. (1999). Glucocorticoids, stress, and their adverse neurological effects: relevance to aging. *Exp Gerontol, 34*(6), 721–732.

Scarmeas, N., Luchsinger, J. A., Schupf, N., Brickman, A. M., Cosentino, A., Tang, M. X., & Stern, Y. (2009). Physical activity, diet, and risk of Alzheimer disease. *JAMA, 302*(6), 627–637.

Schneider, J. A., Arvanitakis, Z., Bang, W., & Bennett, D. A. (2007). Mixed brain pathologies account for most dementia cases in community-dwelling older persons. *Neurology, 69*(24), 2197–2204.

Schneider, J. A., Wilson, R. S., Bienias, J. L., Evans, D. A., & Bennett, D. A. (2004). Cerebral infarctions and the likelihood of dementia from Alzheimer disease pathology. *Neurology, 62*(7), 1148–1155.

Seshadri, S., Wolf, P. A., Beiser, A., Elias, M. F., Au, R., Kase, C. S., D'Agostino, R. B., & DeCarli, C. (2004). Stroke risk profile, brain volume, and cognitive function: the Framingham Offspring Study. *Neurology, 63*(9), 1591–1599.

Shah, T., Verdile, G., Sohrabi, H., Campbell, A., Putland, E., Cheetham, C., Dhaliwal, S., Weinborn, M., Maruff, P., Darby, D., & Martins,

R. N. (2014). A combination of physical activity and computerized brain training improves verbal memory and increases cerebral glucose metabolism in the elderly. *Transl Psychiatry*, 4, e487.

Shoghi-Jadid, K., Small, G. W., Agdeppa, E. D.,Kepe, V., Ercoli, L. M., Siddarth, P., Read, S., Satyamurthy, N., Petric, A., Huang, S. C., & Barrio, J. R. (2002). Localization of neurofibrillary tangles and beta-amyloid plaques in the brains of living patients with Alzheimer disease. *Am J Geriatr Psychiatry*, 10(1), 24–35.

Sjosten, N., & Kivela, S. L. (2006). The effects of physical exercise on depressive symptoms among the aged: a systematic review. *Int J Geriatr Psychiatry*, 21(5), 410–418.

Slooter, A. J., Cruts, M., Hofman, A., Koudstaal, P. J., van der Kuip, D., de Ridder, M. A., Witteman, J. C., Breteler, M. M., Van Broeckhoven, C., & van Duijn, C. M. (2004). The impact of APOE on myocardial infarction, stroke, and dementia: the Rotterdam Study. *Neurology*, 62(7), 1196–1198.

Small, G. W., Rabins, P. V., Barry, P. P., Buckholtz, N. S., DeKosky, S. T., Ferris, S. H., Finkel, S. I., Gwyther, L. P., Khachaturian, Z. S., Lebowitz, B. D., McRae, T. D., Morris, J. C., Oakley, F., Schneider, L. S., Streim, J. E., Sunderland, T., Teri, L. A., & Tune, L. E. (1997). Diagnosis and treatment of Alzheimer disease and related disorders. Consensus statement of the American Association for Geriatric Psychiatry, the Alzheimer's Association, and the American Geriatrics Society. *JAMA*, 278(16), 1363–1371.

Small, G. W., Siddarth, P., Kepe, V., Ercoli, L. M., Burggren, A. C., Bookheimer, S. Y., Miller, K. J., Kim, J., Lavretsky, H., Huang, S. C., & Barrio, J. R. (2012). Prediction of cognitive decline by positron emission tomography of brain amyloid and tau. *Arch Neurol*, 69(2), 215–222.

Small, G. W., Silverman, D. H., Siddarth, P., Ercoli, L. M., Miller, K. J., Lavretsky, H., Wright, B. C., Bookheimer, S. Y., Barrio, J. R., & Phelps, M. E. (2006). Effects of a 14-day healthy longevity lifestyle program on cognition and brain function. *Am J Geriatr Psychiatry*, 14(6): 538–545.

Stern, Y., Gurland, B., Tatemichi, T. K., Tang, M. X., Wilder, D., & Mayeux, R. (1994). Influence of education and occupation on the incidence of Alzheimer's disease. *JAMA*, 271(13), 1004–1010.

Tangney, C. C., Kwasny, M. J., Li, H., Wilson, R. S., Evans, D. A., & Morris, M. C. (2011). Adherence to a Mediterranean-type dietary pattern and cognitive decline in a community population. *Am J Clin Nutrit*, 93(3), 601–607.

Theill, N., Schumacher, V., Adelsberger, R., Martin, M., & Jäncke, L. (2013). Effects of simultaneously performed cognitive and physical training in older adults. *BMC Neurosci*, 14, 103.

Thies, W., & Bleiler, L. (2014). 2014 Alzheimer's disease facts and figures. *Alzheimers Dement*, 10(2), e47–92.

Toledo, J. B., Toledo, E., Weiner, M. W., Jack, C. R., Jr., Jagust, W., Lee, V. M., Shaw, L. M., & Trojanowski, J. Q. (2012). Cardiovascular risk factors, cortisol, and amyloid-beta deposition in Alzheimer's Disease Neuroimaging Initiative. *Alzheimers Dement*, 8(6): 483–489.

U.S. Department of Agriculture and U.S. Department of Health and Human Services (2010). Dietary Guidelines for Americans. 7th Edition. U.S. Government Printing Office. Washington, D.C.

Unverzagt, F. W., McClure, L. A., Wadley, V. G., Jenny, N. S., Go, R. C., Cushman, M., Kissela, B. M., Kelley, B. J., Kennedy, R., Moy, C. S., Howard, V., & Howard, G. (2011). Vascular risk factors and cognitive impairment in a stroke-free cohort. *Neurology*, 77(19), 1729–1736.

van der Flier, W. M., van Straaten, E. C., Barkhof, F., Verdelho, A., Madureira, S., Pantoni, L., Inzitari, D., Erkinjuntti, T., Crisby, M., Waldemar, G., Schmidt, R., Fazekas, F., & Scheltens, P. (2005). Small vessel disease and general cognitive function in nondisabled elderly: the LADIS study. *Stroke*, 36(10), 2116–2120.

van Praag, H., Kempermann, G., & Gage, F. H. (2000). Neural consequences of environmental enrichment. *Nat Rev Neurosci*, 1(3), 191–198.

Verghese, J., LeValley, A., Derby, C., Kuslansky, G., Katz, M., Hall, C., Buschke, H., & Lipton, R. B. (2006). Leisure activities and the risk of amnestic mild cognitive impairment in the elderly. *Neurology*, 66(6), 821–827.

Vidoni, E. D., Townley, R. A., Honea, R. A., & Burns, J. M. (2011). Alzheimer disease biomarkers are associated with body mass index. *Neurology*, 77(21), 1913–1920.

Vinogradov, S., Fisher, M., Holland, C., Shelly, W., Wolkowitz, O., &Mellon, S. H. (2009). Is serum brain-derived neurotrophic factor a biomarker for cognitive enhancement in schizophrenia? *Biol Psychiatry*, 66(6), 549–553.

Wang, H. X., Karp, A., Winblad B., & Fratiglioni, L. (2002). Late-life engagement in social and leisure activities is associated with a decreased risk of dementia: a longitudinal study from the Kungsholmen project. *Am J Epidemiol*, 155(12), 1081–1087.

Wang, J. Y., Zhou, D. H., Li, J., Zhang, M., Deng, J., Tang, M., Gao, C., Lian, Y., & Chen, M.

(2006). Leisure activity and risk of cognitive impairment: the Chongqing aging study. *Neurology*, 66(6), 911–913.

Williams, J. W., Plassman, B.L., Burke, J., Holsinger, T., & Benjamin, S. (2010). *Preventing Alzheimer's disease and cognitive decline.* Evidence Report/Technology Assessment No. 193. (Prepared by the Duke Evidence-based Practice Center under Contract No. HHSA 290-2007-10066-I.) AHRQ Publication No. 10-E005. Rockville, MD: Agency for Healthcare Research and Quality.

Willis, S. L., Tennstedt, S. L., Marsiske, M., Ball, K., Elias, J., Koepke, K. M., Morris, J. N., Rebok, G. W., Unverzagt, F. W., Stoddard, A. M., & Wright, E. (2006). Long-term effects of cognitive training on everyday functional outcomes in older adults. *JAMA*, 296(23), 2805–2814.

Wilson, R. S., Bennett, D. A., Bienias, J. L., Mendes de Leon, C. F., Morris, M. C., & Evans, D. A. (2003). Cognitive activity and cognitive decline in a biracial community population. *Neurology*, 61(6), 812–816.

Wilson, R. S., Scherr, P. A., Schneider, J. A., Tang, Y., & Bennett, D. A. (2007). Relation of cognitive activity to risk of developing Alzheimer disease. *Neurology*, 69(20), 1911–1920.

Wolf, P. A., Beiser, A., Elias, M. F., Au, R., Vasan, R. S., & Seshadri, S. (2007). Relation of obesity to cognitive function: importance of central obesity and synergistic influence of concomitant hypertension. The Framingham Heart Study. *Curr Alzheimer Res*, 4(2), 111–116.

Wolf, P. A., D'Agostino, R. B., Belanger, A. J., & Kannel, W. B. (1991). Probability of stroke: a risk profile from the Framingham Study. *Stroke*, 22(3), 312–318.

Xu, W. L., Atti, A. R., Gatz, M., Pedersen, N. L., Johansson, B., & Fratiglioni, L. (2011). Midlife overweight and obesity increase late-life dementia risk: a population-based twin study. *Neurology*, 76(18), 1568–1574.

Yasar, S., Ko, J. Y., Nothelle, S., Mielke, M. M., & Carlson, M. C. (2011). Evaluation of the effect of systolic blood pressure and pulse pressure on cognitive function: the Women's Health and Aging Study II. *PloS One*, 6(12), e27976.

Zimmerman, B., Sutton, B. P., Low, K. A., Fletcher, M. A., Tan, C. H., Schneider-Garces, N., Li, Y., Ouyang, C., Maclin, E. L., Gratton, G., & Fabiani, M. (2014). Cardiorespiratory fitness mediates the effects of aging on cerebral blood flow. *Front Aging Neurosci*, 6, 59.

SECTION B

MENTAL AND PHYSICAL DISORDERS OF AGING AND INTEGRATIVE THERAPIES

25

COMPLEMENTARY AND ALTERNATIVE THERAPIES FOR MOOD AND ANXIETY DISORDERS IN LATE LIFE

Arun V. Ravindran and Tricia L. da Silva

INTRODUCTION

Depression and anxiety are the most common mental illnesses diagnosed in late life (Kastenschmidt & Kennedy, 2011). The 12-month prevalence of late-life depression has been estimated at 4% to 20%, while that of anxiety conditions ranges from 3% to 17% (Gallo & Lebowitz, 1999; Hybels & Blazer, 2003). While pharmacotherapy is a standard first treatment, patient management can be complicated by comorbid medical conditions and the physiological changes associated with aging (Kastenschmidt & Kennedy, 2011). Up to 50% of these patients also fail to respond to initial treatment, and some medication side effects, such as cognitive and motor impairment, can be serious risks for this population (Kastenschmidt & Kennedy, 2011). Side effects and high prescription costs can also affect compliance (Sajatovic et al., 2011; Zivin et al., 2009).

In seeking other sources of symptom relief, older adults frequently turn to complementary and alternative medicine (CAM) therapies, often in addition to conventional medications, and usually without medical supervision (Astin et al., 2000; Grzywacz et al., 2006). While there is variation in how CAMs are categorized, a common method is to separate them broadly as physical therapies (e.g., exercise, light therapy), nutraceuticals (i.e., dietary/nutritional supplements) and herbal remedies (i.e., plants and plant extracts) (see Figure 25.1). They are often also grouped by key foci, such as conventional physical activities (e.g., aerobic exercise, stretching), mind-body therapies (e.g., tai chi, yoga), whole-system therapies (Ayurveda, traditional Chinese medicine), and so on. However, for the purpose of this review, the use of such a classification may pose some difficulty due to the uneven numbers of publications across topics and the use of English-language publications alone. Therefore, the former, narrower categorization will be used in this chapter. Regardless of how they are grouped, CAMs are often perceived as equivalent in efficacy to medications, but also as more natural, affordable, accessible, and tolerable (Ravindran et al., 2009). Their increasing popularity

Physical Therapies

Acupuncture
Exercise*
Light therapy*
Massage
Qi gong
Relaxation
Sleep deprivation*
Tai chi
Yoga*

Herbal Remedies

Borage
Kava kava
Lavender
Passionflower
Roseroot
St. John's wort*
Saffron

Asian herbs and herbal compounds

Nutraceuticals (Dietary or nutritional supplements)

Acetyl-L-carnitine
Amino acids
B vitamins
Calcium
DHEA*
Folate
Inositol
Magnesium
N-acetylcysteine
Omega-3 fatty acids*
SAM-e*
Tryptophan*
Vitamine D
Zinc

FIGURE 25.1 CAMs that have been researched for benefit in mood and anxiety disorders (not all reviewed in this chapter).

* Reviewed in this book chapter

highlights a need to evaluate their benefits and risks (see Figure 25.1 for a list of various CAMs that have been researched for benefit in mood and anxiety disorders and Box 25.1 for a list on online databases on CAMs).

This book chapter will review the evidence for CAMs as monotherapy or augmentation or combination treatment for depression and anxiety in older adults. Only those CAMs that have a reasonable body of published research and data in older adult populations, thus warranting clinical consideration of their use, will be evaluated. *Integrative medicine* describes the interface of CAMs with conventional medicine. In this chapter, integrative medicine will be addressed by including a critical review of published literature on the use of CAM therapies in combination with evidence-based interventions from Western medicine. In this context, *monotherapy* refers to the use of an agent as sole treatment; *augmentation* describes the addition of an agent to existing treatment; *combination* describes the concurrent use of two or more agents with individual antidepressant or anxiolytic effects; and *add-on* describes either strategy (Lam et al., 2009).

METHODS

A search of the psychiatric literature, using PubMed, was conducted for all articles relating to the use of physical therapies, nutraceuticals, and herbal remedies as treatment for mood and anxiety disorders and published in English up to August 2014. The

Box 25.1 Online Databases on CAM therapies

More information on CAM dosing, side effects, and drug-CAM interactions, related to the CAMs reviewed in this chapter or others of interest to readers, can be found in the following online sources.

AMED—the Allied and Complementary Medicine Database

http://www.ebscohost.com/academic/AMED-The-Allied-and-Complementary-Medicine-Database

Natural Medicines (formerly Natural Standard and Natural Medicines Comprehensive Database)

http://naturalmedicines.therapeuticresearch.com

disorders covered include major depressive disorder (MDD), dysthymia, psychotic depression, treatment resistant depression (TRD), chronic depression, bipolar disorder, seasonal affective disorder, generalized anxiety disorder (GAD), panic disorder (PD), obsessive-compulsive disorder (OCD), social anxiety disorder (SAD) and post-traumatic stress disorder (PTSD). Study results were evaluated using the standard criteria for considering the strength of evidence for efficacy and tolerability. They are discussed in the following sections and are summarized in Table 25.1.

RESULTS AND DISCUSSION

Physical Therapies

EXERCISE

Exercise can be aerobic (exertive) or non-aerobic. Its effect on neurogenesis (particularly increased expression of brain-derived neurotrophic factor, B-endorphins and serotonin) (Lucassen et al., 2010) and reduced inflammation and oxidative stress (Eyre & Baune, 2012) is thought to mediate its antidepressant action. Its anxiolytic benefits may derive from its increase of endocannabinoid and atrial natriuretic peptide (ANP) levels (Dietrich & McDaniel, 2004; Ströhle et al., 2006) and its modulation of hypothalamic-pituitary adrenocortical (HPA) axis activity and cortisol production (Lucassen et al., 2010).

Most data for exercise as an alternative therapy come from studies of depression. In the general population, the evidence for exercise as monotherapy for unipolar depression has been mixed, with meta-analyses and systematic reviews reporting no difference from treatment as usual, no treatment, or placebo (Lawlor & Hopker, 2001; Mead et al., 2008), but also superiority of exercise to no treatment or placebo and equivalence to medication or psychotherapy (Cooney et al., 2013; Larun et al., 2006; Pinquart et al., 2007). There are also mixed data for exercise as augmentation to medication in unipolar depression and sparse data in bipolar disorder (Barbour et al., 2007; Ravindran & da Silva, 2013). Data for exercise in anxiety disorders is also limited, with mixed results as monotherapy or augmentation in PD and GAD, and preliminary evidence for benefit as augmentation in OCD (Ravindran & da Silva, 2013; Ströhle, 2009).

In late-life depression, a systematic review found exercise monotherapy effective in improving unipolar depression compared to wait-list, usual care, social contact, or health education. In addition, this review also noted the limitations of existing research and the need for a systematic comparison of different forms of exercise, and varying durations and intensities of activity, as well as for more long-term follow-up data (Blake et al., 2009). In more recent studies of unipolar depression, a randomized controlled trial (RCT) found balance/strength training as monotherapy no different from social visits (Kerse et al., 2010), but an open trial noted that video-game–directed exercise monotherapy (i.e., Wii Sports tennis, baseball, golf, etc.) alleviated subsyndromal depression (Rosenberg et al., 2010). An RCT of aerobic walking/jogging as monotherapy or augmentation found exercise and medication comparably effective, though also no different from exercise add-on (Blumenthal et al., 1999), while another monotherapy/augmentation RCT found an aerobic-resistance exercise regime no different from usual care (Pfaff et al., 2014). Other RCTs found augmentation with tai chi chih superior to medication alone (Lavretsky et al., 2011) and adjunctive aerobic training superior to health education augmentation (Deslandes et al., 2010). No studies were found for anxiety disorders in older adults.

In summary, exercise has some evidence of benefit as monotherapy for late-life unipolar depression, and specific guidelines for the prescription of exercise can be found in an excellent review by Rethorst and Trivedi (2013). However, variability in exercise forms and regimens affects interpretation. Exercise was well tolerated, but possible side effects include musculoskeletal injury from overexertion, cardiovascular events in vulnerable patients, impact on lithium levels in bipolar patients, and temporary rise in anxiety in those with high anxiety sensitivity (see Ravindran et al., 2009; Ravindran & da Silva, 2013).

YOGA

Yoga's many forms place varying emphasis on the key components of postures, breathing exercises, and meditation, but controlled breathing is thought to be the therapeutic element (da Silva et al., 2009). It is thought to impact positively on emotion regulation and stress responsivity via normalization of the activity of the autonomic, neuroendocrine, monoaminergic, and limbic systems, as well as

Table 25.1. Evidence for CAMs for Late-Life Depression—Unipolar Depression

STUDY	TYPE	n	DURATION	AGENT	COMPARATOR	EFFICACY RESULTS*
			EXERCISE			
Blake et al. (2009)	Systematic review	Total = 11 (≥ 80% of each study sample was ≥ 60 years)	Varying	Exercise	Wait-list, usual care, social contact, health education, tai chi	Exercise monotherapy > control groups*
Blumenthal et al. (1999)	RCT	n = 156 (50–77 years)	16 weeks	Exercise (aerobic walking/jogging)	Sertraline alone Sertraline + exercise	No group differences
Deslandes et al. (2010)	RCT	n = 20 (60+ years)	1 year	Exercise (aerobic training) + medication	Medication alone	Exercise + medication > medication*
Kerse et al. (2010)	RCT	n = 193 (75+ years)	6 months	Exercise (balance/strength training)	Social visits	No group differences
Lavretsky et al. (2011)	RCT	n = 112 (60+ years)	10 weeks	Exercise (tai chi chih) + escitalopram	Health education + escitalopram	Exercise + escitalopram > health education + escitalopram*
Pfaff et al. (2014)	RCT	n = 200 (50+ years) (54% on psychotropics)	12 weeks	Exercise (aerobic + resistance)	Usual care Usual care + exercise	No group differences
Rosenberg et al. (2010)	Open trial	n = 19 (63–94 years)	12 weeks	Exercise (exergames—video game-directed tennis, bowling, baseball, golf, and boxing)	None	Exercise monotherapy effective for subsyndromal depression*

YOGA

Shahidi et al. (2011)	RCT	$n = 60$ (60-80 years)	10 sessions	Laughter yoga	Exercise (aerobic) Usual care	Yoga monotherapy = exercise monotherapy*; both > usual care
Chen et al. (2009)	RCT	$n = 139$ (60+ years)	6 months	Silver yoga	Wait-list	Yoga monotherapy > wait-list for subsyndromal depression*
Chen et al. (2010)	RCT	$n = 69$ (65+ years)	6 months	Silver yoga	Wait-list	Yoga monotherapy > wait-list control for subsyndromal depression*

LIGHT THERAPY

Loving et al. (2005)	RCT	$n = 81$ (60–79 years) (50% on psychotropics)	4 weeks	Bright LT	Dim red light placebo	No group differences
Royer et al. (2012)	RCT	$n = 28$ (75+ years)	4 weeks	Bright LT	Dim red light placebo	No group differences for subsyndromal depression, but LT monotherapy > dim red light for state anxiety*
Tsai et al. (2004)	RCT	$n = 60$ (65+ years)	5 days	Bright LT	No treatment	LT monotherapy > no treatment*

(continued)

Table 25.1. Continued

STUDY	TYPE	n	DURATION	AGENT	COMPARATOR	EFFICACY RESULTS*
			SLEEP DEPRIVATION			
Bump et al. (1997)	Open trial	n = 13 (60+ years)	1 night of TSD + 12 weeks of medication	TSD + paroxetine	None	TSD + paroxetine effective*
Hernandez et al. (2000)	Open trial	n = 15 (60+ years)	1 night of TSD + 12 weeks of medication	TSD + paroxetine	None	TSD + paroxetine effective*
Reynolds et al. (2005)	RCT	n = 80 (60+ years)	1 night of TSD + 2 weeks of medication	TSD + paroxetine	TSD + placebo Paroxetine alone	No group differences
			OMEGA-3 FATTY ACIDS			
Rondanelli et al. (2010)	RCT	n = 46 (66–95 years)	8 weeks	Omega-3 fatty acids	Placebo	Omega-3 fatty acids monotherapy > placebo*
Tajalizadekhoob et al. (2011)	RCT	n = 66 (65+ years)	6 months	Omega-3 fatty acids	Placebo	Omega-3 fatty acids monotherapy > placebo*
			TRYPTOPHAN			
Cooper & Datta (1980)	RCT	n = 20 (60+ years)	6 weeks	L-tryptophan	Placebo	No group differences
Badrasawi et al. (2013)	RCT, cross-over	n = 30 (60+ years) unmedicated	7 weeks	Talbinah cereal (tryptophan-rich) + usual diet	Usual diet	Tryptophan-rich food + usual diet > usual diet*

*Results statistically significant at $p < 0.05$
LT = Light therapy; TSD = Total sleep deprivation

the HPA axis (Brown & Gerbarg, 2005; Streeter et al., 2012).

Systematic reviews and meta-analyses of the general literature have noted that yoga shows reasonable evidence for benefit as monotherapy or augmentation to medication in mild to moderate unipolar depression and preliminary evidence for benefit in GAD and PD (Cabral et al., 2011; Cramer et al., 2013; da Silva et al., 2009; Ravindran & da Silva, 2013).

Data with older adults are very limited and are restricted to depression only. One RCT found laughter yoga (which focuses on yogic breathing) as monotherapy comparable to exercise in improving unipolar depression and both were superior to usual care (Shahidi et al., 2011), while two RCTs found "Silver yoga" (comprising postures, stretching, relaxation, and meditation) as monotherapy superior to wait-list control in reducing subsyndromal depression (Chen et al., 2009; Chen et al., 2010). No data for anxiety disorders in older patients were found.

The data for yoga for late-life unipolar depression are very preliminary, suggesting use as an adjunct strategy only. Heterogeneity in yoga forms and the possible impact of group dynamics also limit the results (Ravindran et al., 2009). Though generally tolerable, rare side effects have included mild physical discomfort due to poor fitness, meditation-induced mania or psychosis in susceptible patients, as well as single cases of artery occlusion or lotus neuropathy, likely resulting from excessive or incorrect yoga practice (see Pilkington et al., 2005).

LIGHT THERAPY

Light therapy (LT) involves daily exposure to artificial bright light via a fluorescent light box or light-emitting diodes (Ravindran et al., 2009; Tuunainen et al., 2004). It is thought to affect the suprachiasmatic nucleus and melatonin production (both involved in circadian rhythm regulation), as well as monoaminergic modulation, thus influencing mood (Pail et al., 2011).

Reviews and meta-analyses of general adult data have reported LT monotherapy superior to placebo for seasonal/unipolar depression, but augmentation studies in seasonal/unipolar and bipolar depression have had mixed results (Even et al., 2008; Golden et al., 2005; Thompson, 2002; Tuunainen et al., 2004). There are no published studies of LT for anxiety disorders.

In older adult samples, available studies are very few. One RCT found bright LT monotherapy superior to no treatment for unipolar depression (Tsai et al., 2004). Two other RCTs found no difference between bright LT monotherapy and dim red light placebo for subsyndromal depression (Royer et al., 2012), or between LT monotherapy/augmentation and dim red light placebo for major or minor depression (Loving et al., 2005). There are no studies involving clinical anxiety conditions in late life, but one RCT noted that bright LT was superior to dim red light placebo in improving state anxiety (Royer et al., 2012).

The evidence for LT for depression or anxiety in late life is too inconsistent to draw conclusions. Data from general adult studies indicate a risk of relapse after LT cessation or manic switch in vulnerable individuals, and mild difficulties with sleep, vision, nausea, and agitation, as well as rare increased suicidality under inadequate treatment conditions, and also LT–medication interactions and psychotropic-linked increase in photosensitivity (see Ravindran et al., 2009; Ravindran and da Silva, 2013).

SLEEP DEPRIVATION

Sleep deprivation (SD) requires patients to remain awake for extended periods, with partial SD allowing 3–4 hours of sleep per night and total SD lasting up to 40 hours (Benedetti & Colombo, 2011). Its impact on mood may be via multimodal effects on HPA axis activity, thyroid hormone levels, and metabolic and monoaminergic functioning (Benedetti & Colombo, 2011; Giedke & Schwarzler, 2002; Parekh et al., 1998; Vgontzas et al., 1999).

Systematic reviews have reported SD augmentation to be beneficial for both unipolar and bipolar depression in adult samples (Dallaspezia & Benedetti, 2011; Giedke & Schwarzler, 2002; Morgan & Jorm, 2008; Ravindran & da Silva, 2013). Data on its benefit as monotherapy for unipolar depression, though positive, is far more preliminary (Ravindran et al., 2009). There are no published data for SD for anxiety disorders.

With older adults with unipolar depression, two open trials found total sleep deprivation (TSD) combined with medication effective (Bump et al., 1997; Hernandez et al., 2000). However, an RCT found no differences between medication alone or in combination with TSD (Reynolds et al., 2005).

No data for anxiety disorders in this population were found.

SD may have some promise as augmentation for unipolar depression in older adults, but more data are needed. Further, the obstacles to applying SD in clinical settings, such as quick relapse after recovery sleep, development of tolerance, and difficulty with sustaining more than brief treatment (Ravindran et al., 2009), would limit its use to third-line adjunct only. Reported side effects include headache and fatigue, and more rarely, gastrointestinal (GI) symptoms, increased depression, and (hypo)mania in vulnerable patients (Giedke & Schwarzler, 2002).

Herbal Remedies

ST. JOHN'S WORT

St. John's wort (*Hypericum perforatum*) is a flowering plant with demonstrated benefits for both depressive and anxiety symptoms. Its key components, hyperforin and hypericin, are thought to act by influencing the activity of the monoaminergic system and HPA axis (Lakhan & Vieira, 2010; Sarris & Kavanagh, 2009).

Several systematic reviews and meta-analyses have found St. John's wort effective as monotherapy for mild to moderate unipolar depression in adult patients, versus both medication and placebo (e.g., Kasper & Dienel, 2002; Linde et al., 2008). While it has shown no benefits as monotherapy for SAD and has mixed data in OCD, there are preliminary positive results in GAD (Ravindran & da Silva, 2013). There are no studies specifically with older adult samples.

Despite the lack of data for St. John's wort in older patients, its significant body of research in unipolar depression supports its use as a third-line strategy in older adults, with caution. There is risk of photosensitivity and drug interactions that may reduce the efficacy of immunoregulatory compounds, anticoagulants, and anti-infective agents (Golan et al., 2007). Serotonin syndrome due to combination with antidepressants, and risk of mania/hypomania induction, have also been reported (Natural Medicines, 2015c).

Nutraceuticals

OMEGA-3 FATTY ACIDS

Polyunsaturated omega-3 fatty acids are involved in multiple biological systems. Highly purified estyl esters of eicosapentanoic acid (EPA) or docosahexaenoic acid (DHA), or a combination, are used in dietary supplements. Their neuropsychiatric benefits are thought to derive from their modulation of neuronal communication and impact on monoaminergic neural systems (Ross et al., 2007).

Meta-analyses of combined unipolar and bipolar depression studies have had mixed results for omega-3 fatty acids as monotherapy or augmentation (e.g., Bloch & Hannestad, 2012; Kraguljac et al., 2009), though more recent meta-analyses in bipolar depression alone have been more positive (Montgomery & Richardson, 2008; Sarris et al., 2012). In anxiety disorders, omega-3s showed no benefits in single augmentation studies in OCD and PTSD (see Ravindran & da Silva, 2013).

In older adults, two RCTs found omega-3 fatty acids as monotherapy superior to placebo for improving unipolar depression (Rondanelli et al., 2010; Tajalizadekhoob et al., 2011). No data for late life anxiety disorders were found.

There is reasonable evidence to support the use of omega-3 fatty acids for unipolar depression in older adults, but due to lack of systematic clinical use, they may be better placed as an augmentation strategy. They are generally well tolerated and have shown cardioprotective properties and mild side effects like nausea and a fishy aftertaste, but patients on anticoagulants or antiplatelet medications may be at risk of increased bleeding (Freeman et al., 2010). Risk of hypomania has also been reported, though not in bipolar patients, thus far (e.g., Montgomery & Richardson, 2008; Sarris et al., 2012).

S-ADENOSYLMETHIONINE

S-adenosylmethionine (SAMe) is a naturally occurring body molecule and a derivative of the amino acid methionine, which is thought to benefit mood by boosting monoaminergic neurotransmission (Alpert et al., 2008). In Europe, where SAMe has been evaluated in a large number of trials, synthetic SAMe is a formally recognized prescription drug that is commonly used to treat depression and medical conditions like arthritis. However, due to limited research and clinical use in North America, it is marketed only as an over-the-counter dietary supplement.

Several systematic reviews of unipolar depression studies in the general population have found SAMe as effective as medication and superior to placebo as monotherapy (e.g., Papakostas et al,

2003; Williams et al, 2005) and it has also shown preliminary benefits as augmentation to medication (Ravindran & da Silva, 2013). It has no published data for anxiety disorders, and no studies specifically with older adult samples.

Although SAMe lacks particular evidence with older adult patients, there is sufficient evidence from general adult trials to support its use as a treatment for unipolar depression in this population, albeit as a third-line augmentation strategy due to lack of wider clinical experience. While usually quite tolerable, side effects can include restlessness and GI symptoms, as well as rare manic induction in vulnerable patients and serotonin syndrome when combined with antidepressants (Natural Medicines, 2015b).

DEHYDROEPIANDROSTERONE

Dehydroepiandrosterone (DHEA), an adrenosteroid precursor of the sex hormones estrogen and testosterone, is a popular dietary supplement. Its benefits for mood are thought to result from its modulation of monoaminergic and glutaminergic neurotransmission, as well as its neuroprotective and antioxidant benefits (Maninger et al., 2009). Though available over the counter in the United States and the United Kingdom, it is available only by prescription in Canada, Australia, and other parts of Europe, where it is considered an anabolic steroid and therefore a controlled substance. The exact reason for such difference in regulatory perception remains unclear.

Data on DHEA are limited, but the very few trials reported in reviews did find DHEA superior to placebo as monotherapy or augmentation for unipolar depression in adult patients (Ravindran et al., 2009; Ravindran & da Silva, 2013). It has no published data for anxiety disorders, and no studies specifically with older adult populations.

There is only preliminary evidence for DHEA in unipolar depression, and it is insufficient to recommend its use in older patients. Though it showed good tolerability in available studies, potential side effects include acne, hirsutism, worsening of prostatis, increased risk of breast cancer and mania, decreased blood clotting, and liver damage (Natural Medicines, 2015a).

TRYPTOPHAN

The dietary amino acid tryptophan is a precursor of 5-hydroxy tryptophan (5-HTP) and serotonin (5-HT), and is available as a supplement as both 5-HTP and L-tryptophan. It is thought to act by enhancing serotonergic neurotransmission (Shaw et al., 2002). Though concerns over side effects led to a ban on its sale in the United States for a period and, until recently, its regulation as a controlled drug in Canada and Europe, it is now available as an over-the-counter dietary supplement in North America and Europe.

Reviews and meta-analyses indicate that tryptophan has mixed evidence for use as monotherapy or augmentation for unipolar depression in adult patients (Ravindran & da Silva, 2013; Ravindran et al., 2009; Shaw et al., 2002; Turner et al., 2006). In anxiety disorders, a single and early RCT reported tryptophan inferior to medication and no different from placebo for PD (Kahn et al., 1987).

In older patients, one early RCT in unipolar depression found L-tryptophan monotherapy no different from placebo (Cooper and Datta, 1980), but a more recent cross-over RCT found tryptophan-rich food superior to usual diet for improving depression in unmedicated patients (Badrasawi et al., 2013). There are no published studies of tryptophan for anxiety disorders in older adults.

The largely mixed evidence prevents recommendation of tryptophan as a treatment for late life unipolar depression. Of note, though it is a serotonin precursor, serotonin syndrome has rarely occurred, and a sole outbreak of eosinophilia-myalgia syndrome in the late 1980s was linked to a single manufacturer and a contaminated batch of tryptophan (Turner et al., 2006). Mild side effects reported include sedation, dry mouth, and GI symptoms (Shaw et al., 2002; Turner et al., 2006).

CONCLUSIONS AND FUTURE DIRECTIONS

Although research on the utility and safety of CAM therapies for mood and anxiety disorders has been increasing, the overall literature is still limited, and studies focusing on older adults are sparse. Data on depressive disorders are also far greater than on anxiety conditions, perhaps due to perceptions of need and illness-related disability. Of interest, however, is that some good foundational work has been done to elucidate the mechanisms of actions of the CAMs reviewed in this chapter, which, based on the research thus far, appear to resemble that of standard antidepressants, that is, impact on neuroplasticity, neurogenesis, and monoaminergic, glutaminergic, and HPA axis activity. These CAMs were also well tolerated.

The complementary, alternative, and integrative medicine with current potential for future use includes exercise, yoga, LT, omega-3 fatty acids, St. John's wort, and SAMe. Most available data with older patient samples were for depressive disorders, with relatively little in anxiety conditions. In unipolar depression, there is reasonable evidence for exercise as monotherapy, mixed evidence for exercise and SD as augmentation, and preliminary evidence for yoga, LT, and omega-3 fatty acids as monotherapy. There is very preliminary data for LT for state anxiety. Despite lack of specific evidence with St. John's wort and SAMe in older patients, the preponderance of positive data from adult patient samples supports their consideration in the treatment of unipolar depression. There is insufficient evidence to support the use of DHEA or tryptophan. Due to the lack of long-term efficacy and safety data (particularly relating to drug–CAM interactions), limited clinical experience, and methodological weaknesses of available studies, these CAMs are often recommended only as third-line augmentation strategies for depression in older adults, following trials of combination and/or augmentation with evidence-based pharmacotherapies and/or psychotherapies. But clinical utility and patient preference also need be taken into account, particularly for older patients who may be prone to adverse effects with psychoactive medications. Thus, clinicians may consider the use of certain CAM therapies at an earlier stage in the treatment algorithm, if there are no medical or medication contraindications, and safety is well established. With the same caveats, they may also opt to use certain CAM therapies in an integrated fashion with conventional interventions early in the treatment phase to treat specific symptoms. More in-depth research on the physiological mechanisms of action of CAMs would also be highly useful to clarify their potential role alongside conventional medicine in treatment plans. Patient interest and promising results with some CAMs also encourage their further exploration in larger RCTs as treatment options for late-life mood and anxiety disorders.

DISCLOSURE STATEMENT

The authors have no conflicts of interest to report. This manuscript was prepared independently without any funding support.

REFERENCES

Alpert, J. E., Papakostas, G. I., & Mischoulon, D. (2008). One-carbon metabolism and the treatment of depression: roles of S-adenosyl-l-methionine and folate. In: D. Mischoulon & J. Rosenbaum (Eds.), *Natural medications for psychiatric disorders: considering the alternatives* (2nd ed., pp. 68–83). Philadelphia: Lippincott Williams and Wilkins.

Astin, J. A., Pelletier, K. R., Marie, A., & Haskell, W. L. (2000). Complementary and alternative medicine use among elderly persons: one-year analysis of a Blue Shield Medicare supplement. *J Gerontol A, 55*, M4–9.

Badrasawi, M.M., Shahar, S., Abd Manaf, Z., & Haron, H. (2013). Effect of Talbinah food consumption on depressive symptoms among elderly individuals in long term care facilities, randomized clinical trial. *Clin Interv Aging, 8*, 279–285.

Barbour, K. A., Edenfield, T. M., & Blumenthal, J. A. (2007). Exercise as a treatment for depression and other psychiatric disorders: a review. *J Cardiopulm Rehabil Prev, 27*, 359–367.

Benedetti, F., & Colombo, C. (2011). Sleep deprivation in mood disorders. *Neuropsychobiology, 64*, 141–151.

Blake, H., Mo, P., Malik, S., & Thomas, S. (2009). How effective are physical activity interventions for alleviating depressive symptoms in older people? A systematic review. *Clinical Rehabil, 23*, 873–887.

Bloch, M. H., & Hannestad, J. (2012). Omega-3 fatty acids for the treatment of depression: systematic review and meta-analysis. *Mol Psychiatry, 17*, 1272–1282.

Blumenthal, J. A., Babyak, M. A., Moore, K. A., Craighead, W. E., Herman, S., Khatri, P., . . . Krishnan, K. R. (1999). Effects of exercise training on older patients with major depression. *Arch Intern Med, 159*, 2349–2356.

Brown, R. P., & Gerbarg, P. L. (2005). Sudarshan Kriya Yoga breathing in the treatment of stress, anxiety and depression: Part I—Neurophysiologic model. *J Alt Compl Med, 11*, 189–201.

Bump, G. M., Reynolds, C. F. 3rd, Smith, G., Pollock, B. G., Dew, M. A., Mazumdar, S., . . . Kupfer, D. J. (1997). Accelerating response in geriatric depression: a pilot study combining sleep deprivation and paroxetine. *Depress Anxiety, 6*, 113–118.

Cabral, P., Meyer, H. B., & Ames, D. (2011). Effectiveness of yoga therapy as a complementary treatment for major depressive disorders: a meta-analysis. *Primary Care Compan CNS Disord, 13*, doi: 10.4088/PCC.10r01068

Chen, K. M., Chen, M. H., Chao, H. C., Hung, H. M., Lin, H. S., & Li, C. H. (2009). Sleep quality, depression state, and health status of older adults after silver yoga exercises: cluster randomized trial. *Int J Nurs Studies, 46*, 154–163.

Chen, K. M., Chen, M. H., Lin, M. H., Fan, J. T., Lin, H. S., & Li, C. H. (2010). Effects of yoga on sleep quality and depression in elders in assisted living facilities. *J Nurs Research, 18*, 53–61.

Cooney, G. M., Dwan, K., Greig, C. A., Lawlor, D. A., Rimer, J., Waugh, F. R., . . . Mead, G. E. (2013). Exercise for depression. *Cochrane Database Syst Rev, 12*(9), CD004366.

Cooper, A.J., & Datta, S.R. (1980). A placebo controlled evaluation of L-tryptophan in depression in the elderly. *Can J Psychiatry, 25*, 386-390.

Cramer, H., Lauche, R., Langhorst, J., & Dobos, G. (2013). Yoga for depression: a systematic review and meta-analysis. *Depression Anxiety, 30*, 1068–1083.

Dallaspezia, S., & Benedetti, F. (2011). Chronobiological therapy for mood disorders. *Expert Rev Neurother, 11*, 961–970.

da Silva, T. L., Ravindran, L. N., & Ravindran, A.V. (2009). Yoga in the treatment of mood and anxiety disorders. *Asian J Psychiatry, 2*, 6–16.

Deslandes, A. C., Moraes, H., Alves, H., Pompeu, F. A., Silveira, H., Mouta, R., . . . Coutinho, E. S. (2010). Effect of aerobic training on EEG alpha asymmetry and depressive symptoms in the elderly: a 1-year follow-up study. *Braz J Med Biol Res, 43*, 585–592.

Dietrich, A., & McDaniel, W. F. (2004). Endocannabinoids and exercise. *Br J Sports Med, 38*, 536–541.

Even, C., Schröder, C. M., Friedman, S., & Rouillon, F. (2008). Efficacy of light therapy in nonseasonal depression: a systematic review. *J Affect Disord, 108*, 11–23.

Eyre, H., & Baune, B. T. (2012). Neuroimmunological effects of physical exercise in depression. *Brain Behav Immun, 26*, 251–266.

Freeman, M. P., Fava, M., Lake, J., Trivedi, M. H., Wisner, K. L., & Mischoulon, D. (2010). Complementary and alternative medicine in major depressive disorder: the American Psychiatric Association Task Force report. *J Clin Psychiatry, 71*, 669–681.

Gallo, J. J., & Lebowitz, B. D. (1999). The epidemiology of common late-life mental disorders in the community: themes for the new century. *Psychiatric Serv, 50*, 1158–1166.

Giedke, H., & Schwarzler, F. (2002). Therapeutic use of sleep deprivation in depression. *Sleep Med Rev, 6*, 361–377.

Golan, D.E., Tashjian, A.H., Armstrong, E.J., Armstrong, A.W. (2007). *Principles of pharmacology: the pathophysiologic basis of drug therapy.* New York, Lippincott, Williams and Wilkins. pp. 49–62.

Golden, R. N., Gaynes, B. N., Ekstrom, R. D., Hamer, R. M., Jacobsen, F. M., Suppes, T., . . . Nemeroff, C. B. (2005). The efficacy of light therapy in the treatment of mood disorders: a review and meta-analysis of the evidence. *Am J Psychiatry, 162*, 656–662.

Grzywacz, J. G., Suerken, C. K., Quandt, S. A., Bell, R. A., Lang, W., & Arcury, T. A. (2006). Older adults' use of complementary and alternative medicine for mental health: findings from the 2002 National Health Interview Survey. *J Alt Compl Med, 12*, 467–473.

Hernandez, C. R., Smith, G. S., Houck, P. R., Pollock, B. G., Mulsant, B., Dew, M. A., & Reynolds, C. F., 3rd (2000). The clinical response to total sleep deprivation and recovery sleep in geriatric depression: potential indicators of antidepressant treatment outcome. *Psychiatry Res, 97*, 41–49.

Hybels, C. F., & Blazer, D. G. (2003). Epidemiology of late-life mental disorders. *Clin Geriatr Med, 19*, 663–696.

Kahn, R. S., Westenberg, H. G., Verhoeven, W. M., Gispen-de Wied, C. C., & Kamerbeek, W. D. (1987). Effect of a serotonin precursor and uptake inhibitor in anxiety disorders; a double-blind comparison of 5-hydroxytryptophan, clomipramine and placebo. *Int Clin Psychopharmacol, 2*, 33–45.

Kasper, S., & Dienel, A. (2002). Cluster analysis of symptoms during antidepressant treatment with hypericum extract in mildly to moderately depressed out-patients. A meta-analysis of data from three randomized, placebo-controlled trials. *Psychopharmacology (Berl.), 164*, 301–308.

Kastenschmidt, E.K., & Kennedy, G.J. (2011). Depression and anxiety in late life: diagnostic insights and therapeutic options. *Mt Sinai J Med, 78*, 527–545.

Kerse, N., Hayman, K. J., Moyes, S. A., Peri, K., Robinson, E., Dowell, A., . . . Arroll, B. (2010). Home-based activity program for older people with depressive symptoms: DeLLITE—a randomized controlled trial. *Ann Family Med, 8*, 214–223.

Kraguljac, N. V., Montori, V. M., Pavuluri, M., Chai, H. S., Wilson, B. S., & Unal, S. S. (2009). Efficacy of omega-3 fatty acids in mood disorders: a systematic review and metaanalysis. *Psychopharmacol Bull, 42*, 39–54.

Lakhan, S.E., & Vieira, K.F. (2010). Nutritional and herbal supplements for anxiety and anxiety-related disorders: systematic review. *Nutr J*, 9, 42.

Lam, R.W., Kennedy, S.H., Grigoriadis, S., McIntyre, R.S., Milev, R., Ramasubbu, R., Parikh, S.V., Patten, S.B., & Ravindran, A.V.; Canadian Network for Mood and Anxiety Treatments (CANMAT) (2009). Canadian Network for Mood and Anxiety Treatments (CANMAT) clinical guidelines for the management of major depressive disorder in adults. III. Pharmacotherapy. *J Affect Disord*, 117 Suppl 1, S26–43.

Larun, L., Nordheim, L. V., Ekeland, E., Hagen, K. B., & Heian, F. (2006). Exercise in prevention and treatment of anxiety and depression among children and young people. *Cochrane Database Syst Rev*, 3, CD004691.

Lavretsky, H., Alstein, L. L., Olmstead, R. E., Ercoli, L. M., Riparetti-Brown, M., Cyr, N. S., & Irwin, M. R. (2011). Complementary use of tai chi chih augments escitalopram treatment of geriatric depression: a randomized controlled trial. *Am J Geriatr Psychiatry*, 19, 839–850.

Lawlor, D. A., & Hopker, S. W. (2001). The effectiveness of exercise as an intervention in the management of depression: systematic review and meta-regression analysis of randomised controlled trials. *Br Med J*, 322, 763–767.

Linde, K., Berner, M. M., & Kriston, L. (2008). St John's wort for major depression. *Cochrane Database Syst Rev*, 4, CD000448.

Loving, R.T., Kripke, D.F., Elliott, J.A., Knickerbocker, N.C., & Grandner, M.A.. (2005). Bright light treatment of depression for older adults [ISRCTN55452501]. *BMC Psychiatry*, 5, 41.

Lucassen, P. J., Meerlo, P., Naylor, A. S., van Dam, A. M., Dayer, A. G., Fuchs, E., . . . Czeh, B. (2010). Regulation of adult neurogenesis by stress, sleep disruption, exercise and inflammation: implications for depression and antidepressant action. *Eur Neuropsychopharmacol*, 20, 1–17.

Maninger, N., Wolkowitz, O. M., Reus, V. I., Epel, E. S., & Mellon, S. H. (2009). Neurobiological and neuropsychiatric effects of dehydroepiandrosterone (DHEA) and DHEA sulfate (DHEAS). *Front Neuroendocrinol*, 30, 65–91.

Mead, G. E., Morley, W., Campbell, P., Greig, C. A., McMurdo, M., & Lawlor, D. A. (2008). Exercise for depression. *Cochrane Database Syst Rev*, 4, CD004366.

Montgomery, P., & Richardson, A. J. (2008). Omega-3 fatty acids for bipolar disorder. *Cochrane Database Syst Rev*, 2, CD005169.

Morgan, A. J., & Jorm, A. J. (2008). Self-help interventions for depressive disorderse and depressive symptoms: a systematic review. *Ann Gen Psychiatry*, 7, 13.

Natural Medicines, 2015a. DHEA professional monograph. Retrieved from https://naturalmedicines.therapeuticresearch.com/default.aspx.

Natural Medicines, 2015b. SAMe professional monograph. Retrieved from https://naturalmedicines.therapeuticresearch.com/default.aspx.

Natural Medicines, 2015c. St. John's wort professional monograph. Retrieved from https://naturalmedicines.therapeuticresearch.com/default.aspx.

Pail, G., Huf, W., Pjrek, E., Winkler, D., Willeit, M., Praschak-Rieder, N., & Kasper, S. (2011). Bright-light therapy in the treatment of mood disorders. *Neuropsychobiology*, 64, 152–162.

Papakostas, G. I., Alpert, J. E., & Fava, M. (2003). S-adenosyl-methionine in depression: a comprehensive review of the literature. *Curr Psychiatry Rep*, 5, 460–466.

Parekh, P. I., Ketter, T. A., Altshuler, L., Frye, M. A., Callahan, A., Marangell, L., & Post, R. M. (1998). Relationship between thyroid hormone and antidepressant responses to total sleep deprivation in mood disorder patients. *Biol Psychiatry*, 43, 392–394.

Pfaff, J. J., Alfonso, H., Newton, R. U., Sim, M., Flicker, L., & Almeida, O. P. (2014). ACTIVEDEP: a randomised, controlled trial of a home-based exercise intervention to alleviate depression in middle-aged and older adults. *Br J Sports Med*, 48, 226–232.

Pilkington, K., Kirkwood, G., Rampes, H., & Richardson, J. (2005). Yoga for depression: the research evidence. *J Affect Disord*, 89, 13–24.

Pinquart, M., Duberstein, P. R., & Lyness, J. M. (2007). Effects of psychotherapy and other behavioral interventions on clinically depressed older adults: a meta-analysis. *Aging Mental Health*, 11, 645–657.

Ravindran, A. V., & da Silva, T. L. (2013). Complementary and alternative therapies as add-on to pharmacotherapy for mood and anxiety disorders: a systematic review. *J Affect Disord*, 150, 707–719.

Ravindran, A. V., Lam, R. W., Filteau, M. J., Lespérance, F., Kennedy, S. H., Parikh, & S. V., Patten, S. B., Canadian Network for Mood and Anxiety Treatments (CANMAT) (2009). Canadian Network for Mood and Anxiety Treatments (CANMAT) clinical guidelines for the management of major depressive disorder in adults. V. Complementary and alternative medicine treatments. *J Affect Disord, 117*(Suppl 1), S54–S64.

Rethorst, C. D., & Trivedi, M. H. (2013). Evidence-based recommendations for the prescription of exercise for major depressive disorder. *J Psychiatric Res, 19*, 204–212.

Reynolds, C. F., Smith, G. S., Dew, M. A., Mulsant, B. H., Miller, M. D., Schlernitzauer, M., . . . Pollock, B. G. (2005). Accelerating symptom-reduction in late-life depression: a double-blind, randomized, placebo-controlled trial of sleep deprivation. *Am J Geriatr Psychiatry, 13*, 353–358.

Rondanelli, M., Giacosa, A., Opizzi, A., Pelucchi, C., La Vecchia, C., Montorfano, G., . . . Rizzo, A. M. (2010). Effect of omega-3 fatty acids supplementation on depressive symptoms and on health-related quality of life in the treatment of elderly women with depression: a double-blind, placebo-controlled, randomized clinical trial. *J Am College Nutrition, 29*, 55–64.

Rosenberg, D., Depp, C. A., Vahia, I. V., Reichstadt, J., Palmer, B. W., Kerr, J., . . . Jeste, D. V. (2010). Exergames for subsyndromal depression in older adults: a pilot study of a novel intervention. *Am J Geriatr Psychiatry, 18*, 221–226.

Ross, B. M., Seguin, J., & Sieswerda, L. E. (2007). Omega-3 fatty acids as treatments for mental illness: which disorder and which fatty acid? *Lipids Health Disease, 6*, 21.

Royer, M., Ballentine, N. H., Eslinger, P. J., Houser, K., Mistrick, R., Behr, R., & Rakos, K. (2012). Light therapy for seniors in long term care. *J Am Med Directors Assoc, 13*, 100–102.

Sarris, J., & Kavanagh, D.J. (2009). Kava and St. John's Wort: current evidence for use in mood and anxiety disorders. *J Altern Complement Med, 15*, 827–836.

Sarris, J., Mischoulon, D., & Schweitzer, I. (2012). Omega-3 for bipolar disorder: meta-analyses of use in mania and bipolar depression. *J Clin Psychiatry, 73*, 81–86.

Sajatovic, M., Levin, J., Fuentes-Casiano, E., Cassidy, K. A., Tatsuoka, C., & Jenkins, J. H. (2011). Illness experience and reasons for nonadherence among individuals with bipolar disorder who are poorly adherent with medication. *Comp Psychiatry, 52*, 280–287.

Shahidi, M., Mojtahed, A., Modabbernia, A., Mojtahed, M., Shafiabady, A., Delavar, A., & Honari, H. (2011). Laughter yoga versus group exercise program in elderly depressed women: a randomized controlled trial. *Int J Geriatr Psychiatry, 26*, 322–327.

Shaw, K., Turner, J., & Del Mar, C. (2002). Are tryptophan and 5-hydroxytryptophan effective treatments for depression? A meta-analysis. *Aust NZ J Psychiatry, 36*, 488–491.

Streeter, C. C., Gerbarg, P. L., Saper, R. B., Ciraulo, D. A., & Brown, R. P. (2012). Effects of yoga on the autonomic nervous system, gamm-aminobutyric-acid, and allostasis in epilepsy, depression, and post-traumatic stress disorder. *Med Hypotheses, 78*, 571–579.

Ströhle, A. (2009). Physical activity, exercise, depression and anxiety disorders. *J Neural Trans, 116*, 777–784.

Ströhle, A., Feller, C., Strasburger, C. J., Heinz, A., & Dimeo, F. (2006). Anxiety modulation by the heart? Aerobic exercise and atrial natriuretic peptide. *Psychoneuroendocrinology, 31*, 1127–1130.

Tajalizadekhoob, Y., Sharifi, F., Fakhrzadeh, H., Mirarefin, M., Ghaderpanahi, M., Badamchizade, Z., & Azimipour, S. (2011). The effect of low-dose omega 3 fatty acids on the treatment of mild to moderate depression in the elderly: a double-blind, randomized, placebo-controlled study. *Eur Arch Psychiatry Clinical Neurosci, 261*, 539–549.

Thompson, C. (2002). Light therapy in the treatment of seasonal and non-seasonal affective disorders: a meta-analysis of randomised controlled trials. In: T. Partonen & A. Magnusson (Eds.), *Seasonal affective disorder. Practice and research*, pp. 149–158. Oxford: Oxford University Press.

Tsai, Y. F., Wong, T. K., Juang, Y. Y., & Tsai, H. H. (2004). The effects of light therapy on depressed elders. *Int J Geriatr Psychiatry, 19*, 545–548.

Turner, E. H., Loftis, J. M., & Blackwell, A. D. (2006). Serotonin a la carte: Supplementation with the serotonin precursor 5-hydroxytryptophan. *Pharmacol Ther, 109*, 325–338.

Tuunainen, A., Kripke, D. F., & Endo, T. (2004). Light therapy for non-seasonal depression. *Cochrane Database Syst Rev, 2*, CD004050.

Vgontzas, A. N., Mastorakos, G., Bixler, E. O., Kales, A., Gold, P. W., & Chrousos, G. P. (1999). Sleep deprivation effects on the activity of the hypothalamic-pituitary-adrenal and growth axes: potential clinical implications. *Clin Endocrinol (Oxford), 51*, 205–215.

Williams, A. L., Girard, C., Jui D., Sabina, A., & Katz, D. L. (2005). S-adenosylmethionine (SAMe) as treatment for depression: a systematic review. *Clin Invest Med, 28*, 132–139.

Zivin, K., Madden, J. M., Graves, A. J., Zhang, F., & Soumerai, S. B. (2009). Cost-related medication nonadherence among beneficiaries with depression following Medicare Part D. *Am J Geriatr Psychiatry, 17*, 1068–1076.

26

COMPLEMENTARY, ALTERNATIVE, AND INTEGRATIVE MEDICINE INTERVENTIONS FOR SLEEP DISORDERS IN OLDER ADULTS

Taya Varteresian and Helen Lavretsky

INTRODUCTION

Insomnia and Sleep Disorders

Sleep disorders include a diverse variety of conditions, many of which do increase with age (Krystal et al., 2012). The *DSM-5* describes a variety of sleep–wake disorders, including insomnia disorder, which is defined by a subjective difficulty with sleep along with functional impairment. However, other noteworthy sleep–wake disorders defined by the *DSM-5* include hypersomnolence disorder, narcolepsy, breathing-related sleep disorder, circadian rhythm sleep–wake disorder, and parasomnias such as nightmare disorder and REM sleep behavior disorder. A commonly occurring circadian rhythm disorder for older adults is advanced sleep phase type, which is defined as having an earlier sleep time than desired by at least 2 hours (APA, 2013). When evaluating a geriatric patient with insomnia, it is important to acknowledge the growing number of medical conditions that

older adults can experience that can adversely affect sleep. Sleep apnea, restless leg syndrome and periodic limb movement disorder, musculoskeletal pain, chronic obstructive pulmonary disease (COPD), nocturia, and menopause are important medical conditions that impact sleep in the elderly and should be acknowledged prior to treating insomnia (Krystal et al., 2012). Additionally, various neuropsychiatric disorders such as bereavement, major depressive disorder, and Alzheimer's disease (AD) are essential to notice in evaluating an older patient with insomnia, as these conditions can affect treatment approach and dosing of medications. The commonly used phrase *sundowning* refers to an increase in confusion and behavioral problems toward evening, when sensory cues are reduced. It should be noted that sundowning can often create insomnia in the patient as well as the caregiver. In order to fully evaluate an older individual with insomnia, sometimes a cognitive assessment is pertinent; in other instances a polysomnography is helpful, especially in the case of diagnosis of obstructive sleep apnea or periodic limb movement disorder. However, having a patient record a sleep diary for 2 weeks is highly recommended (Gooneratne & Vitiello, 2014). When attempting to diagnose a primary insomnia in any population, and particularly in older adults, it is always necessary to rule out a variety of medical and psychiatric disorders.

As individuals age, multiple changes occur normally that affect sleep. When evaluating insomnia in a geriatric patient, it is important to acknowledge that aging involves a decrease in total sleep time compared to younger adults up until about 60 years old, at which time it generally stabilizes at 5–7 hours (Gooneratne & Vitiello, 2014). Other noteworthy changes to sleep with normal aging include increase in wakefulness after sleep onset and a decrease in the deeper sleep called slow wave or stage 3 sleep (Gooneratne & Vitiello, 2014). Sleep latency, however, does not tend to change with aging (Gooneratne & Vitiello, 2014). In order to avoid overmedicating older patients, it is important to consider non-pharmacological interventions that could restore normal sleep physiology, which lends itself nicely to the use of CAIM interventions.

CAIM Interventions for Sleep Disorders

According to the National Health Interview Survey of 2007, 45% of adults suffering from insomnia used complementary and alternative medicine (Bertisch et al., 2012). Another study from the National Center for Complementary and Alternative Medicine and the American Association of Retired Persons examined older adults and found that 54% of the older population was utilizing complementary, alternative, and integrative medicine (CAIM) (Gooneratne, 2008). Therefore when an older adult enters a clinical setting, it is highly likely that he or she might be using a CAIM intervention. This is especially important for clinicians who prescribe medications to notice because most biologically based products are not regulated with the same stringency as traditional medications, which are administered by the US Food and Drug Administration (FDA). The Dietary Supplemental and Education Act of 1994 regulates most natural products and supplements. CAIM provides numerous interventions for health that our older population is utilizing to treat and prevent various disease states. CAIM includes various interventions from natural supplements and herbal remedies to mind–body and manipulative practices. The population over the age of 65 years is rapidly growing and changing. Many older adults are looking toward alternative agents to treat various health conditions due to either lack of efficacy of traditional approaches, intolerability of side effects, or personal preference. Interestingly, back in 1997, older adults comprised 12% of the US population but received 35%–40% of sedatives and hypnotics (King et al., 1997). Safe and effective alternatives to sedative and hypnotics would help our growing elderly population treat an unfortunately common occurrence of aging. This chapter will review the evidence supporting various common CAIM interventions for insomnia in the elderly. Due to limitations in quantity of studies evaluating older adults exclusively, sometimes studies involving mixed-age populations will be discussed.

This chapter provides an overview of the literature on integrative interventions for treating insomnia in older adults (see Table 26.1). The studies were found by performing searches on the PubMed search engine with keywords of "complementary and alternative medicine," and "geriatric," along with more specific key words (e.g., "melatonin," "valerian root," "magnesium," "yoga," "music therapy," and "sleep disorders"). Due to the scarcity of studies utilizing older adults, sometimes studies were included in which the participants did not have insomnia. Special consideration for CAIM interventions that had more studies or stronger research designs were included in this review.

MELATONIN

Melatonin is a hormone that is secreted in the pineal gland and is related to regulating circadian rhythms and therefore can play a role in insomnia. It is plausible that melatonin supplementation would improve insomnia in older adults due to normal age-related decreases in melatonin levels (Gooneratne 2008). Additional risk factors can lead to melatonin deficiency in older adults, including medications, such as benzodiazepines, beta-blockers, and NSAIDS; various medical conditions, such as chronic pain, cerebral vascular accident, and myocardial infarction, can further reduce melatonin levels (Gooneratne, 2008). Additionally, AD has shown decreased amplitude of melatonin secretions, as well as abnormal variations in melatonin, which has been

Table 26.1 Effects from Studies on Various CAIM Interventions for Insomnia

INTERVENTION	REFERENCE	SAMPLE SIZE, CHARACERIZATION	STUDY DESIGN	TREATMENT DURATION	TREATMENT INTERVENTION	RESULTS, EFFECT SIZE	ADVERSE EFFECTS
Melatonin							
		Neurocognitive disorder/Dementia					
	Wade et al. (2014)	$n = 80$ Outpatients AD With & without insomnia	Randomized double blind parallel group	24 weeks	Prolonged release melatonin 2 mg	PSQI improved $(1.62 \pm 2.74)^*$ ADAS-cog improved in those with insomnia $(-3.5 \text{ vs. } +3)^*$	Diarrhea (10.3% vs. placebo 5.5%)
	Singer et al. (2003)	$n = 157$ AD Insomnia Outpatients & long-term care institutions	RCT	2 months	2.5 mg slow released vs. 10 mg vs. placebo	No significant improvement on insomnia	More adverse effects in placebo group compared to treatment groups Elevated daytime melatonin levels
	Dowling et al. (2007)	$n = 50$ AD Long-term care institution	RCT	10 weeks	1 hour morning light exposure (≥ 2500 lux) + 5 mg melatonin vs. placebo vs. light therapy alone	No improvement on insomnia only light therapy + melatonin Reduced daytime sleep (estimate, standard error) $-116.09(24.17)$, $t = -4.80^{**}$ Improved daytime activity scores 30,133.17(9,215.39), $t = 3.27^{**}$	None mentioned

(continued)

Table 26.1. Continued

INTERVENTION	REFERENCE	SAMPLE SIZE, CHARACTERIZATION	STUDY DESIGN	TREATMENT DURATION	TREATMENT INTERVENTION	RESULTS, EFFECT SIZE	ADVERSE EFFECTS
	Riemersma-van der Lek et al. (2008)	*n* = 89 Dementia Group home	RCT	15 months	Whole day bright light (1000 lux) vs. dim light (300 lux) + melatonin 2.5 mg	Melatonin decreased sleep latency by 8.2 minutes (95% CI: 1.08–15.38) Melatonin increased sleep duration 27 minutes (95% CI: 9–46) Melatonin + light decreased CMAI 3.9 points (95% CI: 0.88–6.92) Melatonin + light increased sleep efficiency 3.5% (95% CI: 0.8–6.1) Melatonin + light improved nocturnal restlessness by 1 minute per hour each year (95% CI: 0.26–1.78) When light combined with melatonin, reversed result of decreased mood	Melatonin was associated with worsening scores on Philadelphia Geriatric Centre Affect Rating scale + affect & negative affect increased withdrawn behavior, drowsiness, and irritability
	Serfaty et al. (2002)	*n* = 44 Dementia + sleep disturbance *Non-demented*	RCT cross-over	7 weeks	Slow release melatonin 6 mg vs. placebo	No significant effects of melatonin on total sleep, number of awakenings, or sleep efficiency	None

| Garrido et al. (2013) | $n = 30$
Healthy outpatients (young, middle-aged, elderly)
Most without insomnia | Randomized blind placebo-controlled cross-over | 5 days | Jerte Valley cherry product BID | Sleep efficiency (%) improved compared to pretreatment (71.21 ± 3.27 vs. 79.03 ± 3.40)
Sleep time minutes improved compared to pretreatment (356.79 ± 15.23 vs. 403.17 ± 14.54)
Awakenings decreased compared to pretreatment (12.25 ± 1.75 vs. 10.90 ± 0.36)
Sleep latency improved compared to pretreatment (42.46 ± 5.89 vs. 31.84 ± 2.54)
Assumed sleep (minutes) improved compared to pretreatment (306.39 ± 6.90 vs. 330.90 ± 12.38)
Immobility improved compared to pretreatment (267.50 ± 7.37 vs. 302.27 ± 16.07) | None listed |

(continued)

Table 26.1. Continued

INTERVENTION	REFERENCE	SAMPLE SIZE, CHARACERIZATION	STUDY DESIGN	TREATMENT DURATION	TREATMENT INTERVENTION	RESULTS, EFFECT SIZE	ADVERSE EFFECTS
	Buscemi et al. (2005)	14 RCTs General adult n = 279	Meta-analysis	< 1 week– 5 weeks	< 1 mg–5 mg	Reduced sleep latency (–11.7 minutes; 95% CI: – 18.2, –5.2) Improved sleep latency with those having delayed sleep phase disorder (–38.8 minutes; 95% CI: –50.3, –27.3) No effect on sleep efficiency	Headaches Dizziness Nausea Drowsiness
	Verbeek et al. (2014)	15 RCT n = 718 General adult population, night shift work, with or without insomnia	Meta-analysis		Night after shift work melatonin 1 mg–10 mg	Improved daytime sleep following nightshift (mean difference 24 minutes, 95% CI: 9.8–38.9)	Rare

MAGNESIUM

Study		Design			Results	Adverse effects
Abbasi et al. (2012)	$n = 46$ Older adults	RCT	8 weeks	500 mg magnesium vs. placebo x	No differences between placebo and magnesium group Improvement in pre- and post-treatment group (% change/baseline, 95% CI) ISI −14.4(−31.6, 2.8) Sleep time 12(5.2, 18.9) Sleep onset latency −14 (−30.8, 2.7) Early morning awakening −3(−5.1, −0.8) Sleep efficiency 9.6 (2.5, 16.7) Serum renin 36.7 (18.2, 55.2) Serum melatonin 35 (10.5, 59.5) Serum cortisol −8.2 (−19.6, 3.1)	None reported

AROMATHERAPY

Study		Design			Results	Adverse effects
	Dementia/ Neurocognitive disorder					
O'Connor et al. (2013)	$n = 64$ Nursing home Dementia with agitation	Randomized placebo controlled single-blind cross-over trial	1 mL 30% lavender oil vs. placebo	30–60 minutes	No significant effects on agitation	None listed

(*continued*)

Table 26.1. Continued

INTERVENTION	REFERENCE	SAMPLE SIZE, CHARACERIZATION	STUDY DESIGN	TREATMENT DURATION	TREATMENT INTERVENTION	RESULTS, EFFECT SIZE	ADVERSE EFFECTS
	Ballard et al. (2002)	$n = 72$ Long-term care residents Severe dementia	Double-blind placebo controlled trial	Melissa essential oil vs. placebo	4 Weeks	CMAI improved 35 % vs. 11% placebo (Mann-Whitney U test $Z = 4.1$)*** *Quality of life improved, less socially withdrawn $Z = 2.6$)** More time spent in constructive activities $Z = 3.5$)***	None
	Burns et al. (2011)	$n = 114$ AD with agitation Long-term care facility	Double-blind parallel group placebo randomized trial	Placebo medication + aromatherapy vs. donepezil + placebo aroma-therapy, vs. placebo aroma-therapy + placebo medication *aromatherapy = Melissa	12 weeks	No significant effect of aromatherapy on agitation Large placebo effect	

VALERIAN ROOT

Fernandez-San-Martin et al. (2010)	18 RCTs $n = 1317$ Mixed-age adults with and without insomnia	Meta-analysis	Valerian root 60 mg–600 mg	9 days–56 days	Subjective improvement in insomnia RR 1.37 (95% CI: 1.05–1.78) No significant differences in quantitative measures of sleep	Diarrhea (18% vs. 8%) Other GI effects nausea, heartburn CNS effects headache, nervousness, drowsiness
Maroon et al. (2013)	$n = 91$ General adult population Primary insomnia	Parallel group, double-blind, randomized controlled trial, no placebo group	NSF-3 (valerian root, passiflora, Humulus lupululs) vs. zolpidem	2 weeks	No difference between NSF-3 and zolpidem for total sleep time, sleep latency, # night time awakenings on EPSS Concluded that NSF-3 is as effective as zolpidem	similar frequency of s/e to zolpidem, drowsiness, headache, epigastric pain
Stevinson & Ernst (2000)	9 trials	Meta-analysis	Valerian 400 mg–900 mg	1–28 days	Inconsistencies among trials cause inconclusive results	Dizziness Headache Nausea Tiredness vomiting Hangover

(continued)

Table 26.1. Continued

INTERVENTION	REFERENCE	SAMPLE SIZE, CHARACERIZATION	STUDY DESIGN	TREATMENT DURATION	TREATMENT INTERVENTION	RESULTS, EFFECT SIZE	ADVERSE EFFECTS
	Diaper & Hindmarch (2004)	$n = 16$ Older adults (50–64 years old) Insomnia	Placebo controlled three-way cross-over trial	Valerian 300 mg vs. 600 mg vs. placebo	1 night	No significant differences between valerian dosages and placebo, not effective as acute treatment for insomnia	Drowsiness Headache irritability Mental dullness tiredness Increased sweating Confusion Lightheadedness
	Taavoni et al. (2011)	$n = 100$ Postmenopausal women	RCT	530 mg BID vs placebo	4 weeks	Improved quality of sleep Pittsburgh Sleep Quality Index Pretreatment score 9.8(3.6) vs. posttreatment score 6.02(2.6)*** PSQI mean scores 1.7 ± 1.3 placebo vs. 3.8 ± 1.7 valerian group***	None reported
	Donath et al. (2000)	$n = 16$ General adult population Primary insomnia	RCT	Valerian root 600 mg QHS	14 days	Increased slow wave sleep in valerian group Reduced slow sleep latency (21.3 minutes vs. 13.5 minutes)* Increased slow wave sleep % increased (9.8% vs 8.1%)*	Migraine headache GI complaints

Bent et al. (2006)	16 trials $n = 1093$	Meta-analysis	Valerian root 300 mg–600 mg	1 day–30 days	*Subjective sleep improved when asked on dichotomous variable RR 1.8, 95% CI, 1.2–2.9	Diarrhea
			YOGA			
Halpern et al. (2014)	$n = 67$ Older adults Insomnia	RCT	Yoga postures and meditation 2x/week + daily home practice of meditative yoga	12 weeks	(Pretreatment mean ± standard deviation vs. post-intervention mean ± standard deviation) Improvements for high-compliance group PSQI global score (10.26 ± 3.14 vs. 7.96 ± 3.22) *** PSQI subscales sleep quality, latency, duration, and efficiency improved High-compliance group increased slow wave sleep (minutes) M = 106.67 ± 30.75 vs. M = 120.56 ± 33.45)*	None

(continued)

Table 26.1. Continued

INTERVENTION	REFERENCE	SAMPLE SIZE, CHARACERIZATION	STUDY DESIGN	TREATMENT DURATION	TREATMENT INTERVENTION	RESULTS, EFFECT SIZE	ADVERSE EFFECTS
	Khalsa S. (2004)	$n = 20$ Mixed age Chronic insomnia	Cohort study	1 hour self-study yoga daily vs. pretreatment without yoga sleep wake diaries	8 weeks	Total wake time improved $F(4, 76) = 6.02**$ Sleep efficiency improved $(F(4, 76) = 8.86**$ Sleep onset latency $F(4, 76) = 4.42**$ Wake time after sleep $F(4, 76) = 6.42***$	None reported
	Taibi & Vitiello (2011)	$n = 14$ Older women with osteoarthritis and insomnia	Cohort study	75 minute weekly class + 20 minutes home practice	8 weeks	ISI improved (pretreatment 15 ± 5.7 vs. post-treatment 11.4 ± 4.4; $t = 2.56)*$ Sleep onset latency improved (pretreatment 30.1 ± 21.1 minutes vs. post-treatment 14.3 ± 9.3, $t = 2.65)*$ Sleep efficiency improved pretreatment $75.2 \pm 12.9\%$ vs. post-treatment 84.1 ± 8.9, $t = -3.47)**$	Shoulder soreness Muscle cramps Lumbar soreness Numbness in hands Dizziness
	Manjunath & Telles (2005)	$n = 120$ Residents of long-term care facility Older adults	Randomized	Yoga group vs. Ayurveda vs. wait-list control	1 week	Yoga showed improvement Decreased time to fall asleep (10 minutes)* Increase in total hours slept (60 minutes)*	None reported

MUSIC THERAPY

	Neurocognitive disorder/dementia			
Livingston et al. (2014)	3 RCT Dementia with agitation	Meta-analysis	Music protocol provided by trained therapists	Up to 6 weeks	Improvement in agitation SES = 0.5–0.9
Chang et al. (2010)	$n = 41$ Dementia Agitation during meal times Long-term care facility	Quasi-experimental	1 hour music during meal time	1 week	Improvement in CMAI physically aggressive ($\beta = 0.39$)*, verbally aggressive behavior ($\beta = 0.49$)*
	Non-dementia population				
De Niet et al. (2009)	5 RCTs General adult population $n = 208$	Meta-analysis	20–45 minute sessions	2 days–3 weeks	SMD = −0.74; 95% CI: −0.96, −0.46) on PSQI or RCSQ

(continued)

Table 26.1. Continued

INTERVENTION	REFERENCE	SAMPLE SIZE, CHARACERIZATION	STUDY DESIGN	TREATMENT DURATION	TREATMENT INTERVENTION	RESULTS, EFFECT SIZE	ADVERSE EFFECTS
	Chang et al. (2012)	$n = 50$ General adult population with chronic insomnia	RCT	45 minutes soothing music nocturnal time	4 days	PGS prolonged REM sleep (SES = 0.10) and shortened stage 2 sleep (SES = 0.17)	

PSQI = Pittsburgh Sleep Quality Index
SMD = Standardized Mean Difference
RCSQ = Richard-Campbell Sleep Questionnaire
PSG = Polysomnography
ESS = Epworth Sleepiness Scale
SES = standardized effect size
ADAS-Cog = Alzheimer's Disease Assessment Scale-cognitive
SL = sleep latency
ISI = Insomnia Severity Index
CMAI = Cohen Mansfield Agitation Inventory
$^{*}p < 0.05$, $^{**}p < 0.01$, $^{***}p < 0.001$

associated with insomnia (Mishima et al., 1999). Despite a theoretical basis of melatonin in insomnia for the older adult with and without dementia, the data supporting its use are not as strong as one would have expected.

Studies of Cognitively Impaired Older Adults

Most of the literature examining the impact of melatonin on insomnia for older adults involves those individuals suffering from cognitive disorders. In their Cochrane review, McCleery, Cohen, and Sharpley (2014) reviewed two randomized controlled trials (RCTs) using melatonin in approximately 200 individuals suffering from AD and did not find convincing evidence for support of its use. However, when other studies combined melatonin with bright light therapy (BLT), an improvement in insomnia was seen (Dowling et al., 2008; Riemersma-van der Lek et al., 2008). In the studies, bright light was administered in the morning, > 2500 lux for 1 hour (Dowling et al., 2008) to 1000 lux for 8 hours (Riemersma-van-der Lek et al., 2008). It has been suggested that melatonin used in combination with bright light exposure is important in regulating circadian rhythms (Lewy et al., 1992). Given that the Cochrane database did not find convincing evidence for any traditional or alternative treatment for insomnia in AD, it is worthwhile to look at specific aspects of sleep that may be affected by melatonin use. Studies support melatonin for the benefit of improving sleep latency in older adults with cognitive impairment. A small (n = 12) randomized double-blind controlled study of older adults taking 2 mg of controlled-release melatonin for 3 weeks was performed and measured sleep by wrist actinography (Garfinkel et al., 1995). The results showed a significant advantage of melatonin on sleep efficiency as well as reduced sleep latency. However, total sleep time was not affected. In an RCT with a larger sample (n = 157) using two dosages of melatonin (10 mg vs. 2.5 mg), there was no benefit for insomnia; however, there was a benefit for subjective measures of sleep by caregivers (Singer et al., 2003). Dosages in the studies of melatonin for insomnia in AD ranged from 2.5 mg to 10 mg; however, studies showing a benefit tended to use dosages of 2.5 mg–5 mg of extended-release melatonin. There is evidence to support the use of melatonin when combined with BLT for insomnia in AD, especially with an impact on sleep latency.

Beyond objective and subjective measurements of sleep, there appears to be a possible impact on cognition with melatonin. In a more recent RCT (n = 80) with individuals with AD, there was a benefit on sleep as well as cognition (Wade et al., 2014). The benefit on cognitive impairment was seen on both Mini Mental Status Examination (MMSE) scores and Instrumental Activities of Daily Living (IADLS); however, these results should be interpreted carefully, as there was a decline in these measures in the placebo group and the improvement was very small on cognitive scores (ADAS-cog scores improved 3.5 points and placebo scores worsened by 3 points on a 70-point scale). Although most of the subjects did not suffer in insomnia, a subset analysis on those individuals with AD and insomnia showed benefit in sleep efficiency, as measured by the subjective measurement of global Pittsburgh Sleep Quality Index (PSQI) score (Wade et al., 2014). Given that few treatments for insomnia and AD exist, some supportive evidence exists for treating certain aspects of insomnia in older adults suffering from cognitive disorders.

Studies in Cognitively Intact Adults

Compared to studies examining cognitively impaired individuals with dementia, there are fewer studies including cognitively intact older adults. However, there are several meta-analyses examining the general adult population that may be used to extrapolate effects to the older adult population. A meta-analysis of 14 RCTs of adults being treated with melatonin, dosages of 1 mg–5 mg, showed the strongest effects on improvement in sleep latency among other sleep quality variables (Buscemi et al., 2005). Furthermore, when a subset analysis was performed on individuals suffering from delayed-sleep phase syndrome, compared to other types of insomnia, there was a more robust improvement in sleep latency (38.8 minutes compared to 7.2 minutes) (Buscemi et al., 2005). Another meta-analysis examining 15 RCTs including about 700 cognitively intact individuals supports melatonin in subjects suffering from shift work in that it improves sleep length (Liira et al., 2014). A short study comparing younger adults and older adults showed that Jerte Valley cherry, which consists of high amounts of melatonin, was effective in improving sleep quality (Garrido et al., 2013). Therefore, studies seem to support treating insomnia in the form of sleep onset latency, delayed or advanced sleep phase disorder, or shift work disorder in the general adult population in dosages similar to what has been utilized in cognitively impaired populations (1 mg–5 mg).

Side Effects, Drug Interactions

There are minimal known side effects from melatonin; however, some effects are noteworthy, and the effects of long-term administration is not clearly known. In terms of drug–drug interactions, it is important to recognize that melatonin can interrupt the effect of calcium channel blockers on blood pressure, and in general melatonin can reduce blood pressure in small amounts.

Melatonin has been associated with increased occurrence of urinary tract infections (17.6% compared to 2.5% placebo) and diarrhea and upper respiratory tract infections (Wade et al., 2014), as well as headaches, dizziness, nausea, and drowsiness (Busccemi et al., 2005). A study examining melatonin administration in individuals with dementia showed worsening scores on depression scale, but when bright light was co-administered there were no adverse mood effects (Riemersma-van der Lek et al., 2008). Additionally, when utilized with light, caution must be exerted, as melatonin has caused increased photoreceptor sensitivity in animals (Zhadanova & Friedman, , 2008). It should be noted that in the studies mentioned previously demonstrating the benefit of BLT combined with melatonin, BLT was administered during the day prior to taking melatonin. Melatonin has been found to decrease body temperature in larger dosages, which can be problematic for older adults whose thermoregulation is often quiet fragile (Zhdanova & Friedman, 2008).

Conclusions

In summary, the strongest evidence supports the use of melatonin 2 mg–5 mg for older adults with and without cognitive disorders when used in combination with bright light, who suffer from advanced phase sleep disorders, sleep latency difficulties, or shift work disorder, or AD. Side effects should be routinely monitored, as well as use for the shortest amount of time necessary. Melatonin use provides a non-addictive approach to improving sleep in older adults.

VALERIAN ROOT

Valerian root is an herbal remedy that has been used for hundreds of years as an aid for sleep and had been associated with effects on the GABAergic system, making it a feasible alternative to benzodiazepines for insomnia (Shi et al., 2014).

Studies in Cognitively Intact Older Adults and General Adult Populations

Most studies in the general adult population support using valerian root for insomnia. In a meta-analysis consisting of 18 RCTs, valerian root showed an improvement in participants of general age populations in subjective measurements of sleep but not objective measurements of sleep when using a range of valerian root from 90 mg to 900 mg over varied periods of time (9 days–56 days) (Fernandez-San-Martin et al., 2010). Furthermore, in a small study ($n = 16$) of mixed-age adults (average age 49 years), valerian root showed an improvement in slow wave sleep (Donath et al., 2000). Additionally, long-term use of valerian root produces a small but significant improvement in sleep latency reduction (21.3 minutes vs. 13.5 minutes) as well as an increase in percentage of slow wave sleep (9.8% vs. 8.1%) (Baek et al., 2014; Stevinson & Ernst, 2000). Although acute impact on insomnia has been seen in some studies, it appears that there is a trend for valerian root to be effective for insomnia when administered for longer periods of time, such as 2 weeks, as opposed to acute administration (Baek et al., 2014; Stevinson & Ernst, 2000). Some researchers have supported using valerian root as an alternative to benzodiazepines (Mischoulon, 2008), which is especially helpful when treating older adults, as the concern for cognitive impairment and falls is increased with aging.

There is evidence to support valerian root as being equally effective for insomnia compared to standard insomnia medications. A study compared a mixed-herb combination (consisting of valerian root and other herbs) to zolpidem. The study, conducted in India, utilized a commonly marked insomnia agent called NF3 (valerian root, passiflora, and humulus lupulus [hops]) to zolpidem in a mixed-age population with average age in the late forties (Maroo et al., 2013). Both zolpidem and NF3 showed improvements on subjective measurements of total sleep, sleep latency, and number of awakenings; however, they failed to show a statistical significance on the Epiworth Sleepiness scale (ESS). Interestingly, there were no differences between the zolpidem and the NF3 group; unfortunately, there was no control group, and the elements of NF3 were not examined in isolation. Taken together, there does seem to be a small improvement from using valerian root in the general age population, mostly on subjective markers of insomnia.

Similar to other alternative interventions, fewer data exist for older adults and valerian root. The few studies including older adults show mixed results for the impact of valerian root and insomnia. However, an RCT consisting of 16 older individuals (aged 50years to 64 years) showed no improvement using two dosages of valerian root (300 mg and 600 mg) (Diaper & Hindmarch, 2004) . Another study pertinent to older women involved 100 postmenopausal women aged 50–60 years old who were experiencing insomnia. Valerian root administered at 530 mg twice per day for 4 weeks showed a significant improvement in subjective measurements of sleep, as well as the Pittsburgh sleep quality index scores (Taavoni et al., 2011). Therefore the database examining the effect of valerian root in older adults is small, but if studies including general adults are included, there does appear to be a long-term effect on the use of valerian root for insomnia.

Side Effects and Drug–Drug Interactions

Valerian root appears to be fairly well tolerated; however, there are some side effects that are worth noting. First, valerian is described as having an unpleasant odor (Kuhn & Winston) and for the purposes of research has led to unmasking the blinding effect as placebos. There have been exacerbations of pre-existing migraine headache and gastrointestinal effects (Donath et al., 2000), diarrhea (Fernandez-San Martin et al., 2010), and daytime sedation (Baek et al., 2014).

Conclusions

In conclusion, valerian root appears to be effective at subjective markers of insomnia when given in durations spanning several weeks and appears to be a well-tolerated alternative to benzodiazepines.

Studies for valerian root have included dosages ranging from 60 mg to 1800 mg; however, recommended dosages are 450 mg–600 mg (Mischoulon, 2008).

MAGNESIUM

Magnesium is an essential element that is recommended by the FDA to be consumed in quantities of 420 mg daily for men and 320 mg daily for women. These recommendations do not decrease for the aging process. However, it has been shown that magnesium levels decline with aging, primarily through reduction in consumption of foods with magnesium, but there is also a decline due to the aging process. Magnesium-rich foods include nuts, seeds, beans, whole grains, and dark green leafy vegetables (Abbasi et al., 2012). It is speculated that magnesium plays a role in sleep through being an NMDA antagonist and a GABA agonist. Therefore, due to biologic effects of aging and changes in nutrition throughout life, older adults are more vulnerable to magnesium deficiencies and therefore may be vulnerable to sleep disorders.

Use in Cognitively Intact Older Adults

There are several studies that have examined the impact of magnesium supplementation on insomnia in older adults. An RCT was performed in Iran consisting of 46 adults aged 60–75 years who had a history of low magnesium levels and insomnia. Sleep was assessed by the insomnia severity index (ISI). Magnesium supplementation consisted of 500 mg per day over an 8-week time period. Magnesium supplementation showed statistically significant improvement in subjective measures of increased sleep time and decreased sleep onset latency; however, there were no changes in early morning awakenings or total sleep time. Magnesium supplementation showed elevations in serum serum renin levels, and melatonin as well as decreases in cortisol levels . Renin was assessed due to its relationship with non-rapid eye movement (NREM) sleep, and when renin levels are low, sleep tends to be lighter. Another RCT examining the effect of a lower dosage of magnesium (225 mg) in combination with melatonin 5 mg and zinc 11.25 mg showed beneficial effects on primary insomnia in older adults living in an Italian nursing home. Improvement was seen on the PSQI (Rondanelli et al., 2011). Therefore, there are data to support the use of supplemental magnesium (250 mg–500 mg) in the treatment of insomnia in older adults.

Side Effects, Drug–Drug Interactions

As always, it is important to evaluate the side-effect profile of any agent recommended to an older adult who is also likely to be taking other medications. Oral magnesium supplementation has been fairly well tolerated in the studies looking at older individuals. Although oral magnesium has long been a cause of diarrhea, none of the studies examined showed significant diarrhea. In the study using the combination of magnesium, zinc, and melatonin, there were several cases of headache (Rondanelli et al., 2011).

Conclusions

Magnesium supplementation is a reasonably safe and well-tolerated intervention for insomnia in dosages ranging from 250 mg to 500 mg.

CHAMOMILE

The petals of chamomile flowers have been used to make teas and aromatherapy for relaxation for many years and have been thought to regulate GABA receptors and monoamine neurotransmission (Baek et al., 2014).

Studies in Cognitively Intact Adults and Older Adults

Only one small (n = 34) RCT evaluating the impact of 240 mg twice daily of chamomile on insomnia in a mixed-age population (18–65 years old) has been performed and did not reveal any significant effects in sleep (Zick et al., 2011). Although given that other studies do exist supporting chamomile in anxiety disorders, it is possible that subsequent studies should be performed to better evaluate the impact of this herbal remedy, which is frequently used in teas and aromatherapy already. However, currently there is no convincing evidence that chamomile improves insomnia.

Side Effects, Drug–Drug Interactions

Additionally, there are some CYP-450 isoenzyme interactions with chamomile that have been found in vitro, which should add further caution. Chamomile has been found to have potent inhibition of CYP1A2 and moderate inhibition of CYP3A4 (Baek et al., 2014), which are common enzymes in numerous psychiatric and medical medications that the elderly take on a routine basis.

Conclusions

Chamomile does not have much support for its use in insomnia and could potentially impact the metabolism of other drugs via P450 metabolism and therefore should be discouraged until more convincing evidence is uncovered.

HOPS

Hops, or *Humulus lupulus*, has been thought to enhance GABA and melatonin transmission and therefore plays a role in treating insomnia (Baek et al., 2014). In general, studies evaluating hops tend to include other elements such as valerian root and melatonin (Maroo et al., 2013).

Studies in Cognitively Intact Adults and Older Adults

There is only one RCT that evaluated the impact of hops in isolation in a mixed-age population (25–65 years old) of about 100 individuals, which failed to show any benefit from hops on sleep (Cornu et al., 2010). It should be noted that the placebo group, which received olive oil, also improved during this study, which impacted the results. There is no evidence regarding side effects or drug–drug interactions for hops. Therefore cautious utilization of this agent is suggested, as more studies are definitely needed.

YOGA

Yoga is a series of physical postures and meditation that has been used for thousands of years for the purpose of health. Due to its ability to reduce physiologic arousal, it is logical that yoga could have a role in reducing insomnia (Khalsa, 2004). Previous work has demonstrated that yogic meditation can reverse a series of genetic activation typically associated with stress and inflammation (Black et al., 2012).

Studies in Cognitively Intact Older Adults

There have been benefits of yoga on chronic insomnia (Khalsa, 2004) as well as insomnia associated with osteoarthritis (Taibi & Vitiello, 2011). Two studies are available showing the benefit of yoga on insomnia in older populations. Halpern et al. (2014) demonstrated the successful intervention of yoga in older adults who suffered from insomnia. Yoga consisted of two weekly in-person classes of static yoga postures and relaxation, as well as CD-guided yoga for home use, in total consisting of 25 minutes of yoga performed daily. In addition to improvement in subjective markers of sleep, polysomnography showed a significant increase in slow wave sleep and decrease in REM sleep. Another study examined older adults living in a nursing facility in India and showed significant improvements in sleep latency (10 minutes), sleep duration (1 hour), and subjective improvements in sleep quality (Manjunath & Telles, 2005). Therefore, yoga provides a viable approach to assist in insomnia that does not rely on medications.

Side Effects

Even though studies do adapt yoga to older adults, there were still some adverse effects. In one study of 14 women with pre-existing osteoarthritis, more common side effects included shoulder soreness, muscle cramps, lumbar soreness, numbness in hands, and dizziness (Tabi & Vitiello, 2011). However, given the diversity of yoga practices, it is important to recognize that if one form of yoga is intolerable, other forms may still be possible and helpful. For example, Black et al. (2013) performed Kirtan Kriya meditation, which consisted of meditation chanting as well as yoga mudras that involved finger movements and did not reveal any significant side effects with this type of yoga.

Conclusions

As with many of the manipulative or body-based practices available, it is very difficult to have blinded groups, as having a sham yoga class is relatively impossible, leaving the better studies having to utilize wait-list controls or comparison to aerobic activity or other forms of non-meditative physical activity. Among the studies available, yoga does

appear to offer significant benefits for insomnia in older adults.

TAI CHI

Tai chi is an ancient Chinese exercise program that consists of relatively low-intensity physical exercises combined with meditation (Gooneratne 2008). Studies have shown tai chi to be practical in application to older populations, and it has recently been compared to cognitive behavioral therapy (CBT) in the treatment of insomnia (Irwin et al., 2014). In this RCT, tai chi did show improvements in sleep quality but did not improve insomnia remission, as was seen by CBT (Irwin et al., 2014). There were no observed side effects to tai chi, although physical injury is a plausible consequence. As with other forms of CAIM for insomnia, often the alternative treatment does not out-perform standard of care but rather makes some improvements and can be implemented in those individuals who have either failed traditional approaches or who would like to try an alternative approach.

AROMATHERAPY

Aromatherapy involves the use of plant extracts that exude an odor, which can be absorbed through inhalation or through contact with the skin (Ballard et al., 2002). In general, aromatherapy is thought to be relatively safe; unfortunately, the data evaluating aromatherapy have not provided consistent or significant benefit in treating agitation with neurocognitive disorders. Livingston et al. (2014) reviewed two RCTs evaluating the impact of aromatherapy and agitation with cognitive impairment in patients living in institutions and concluded that there was insufficient evidence to support its use. Because aromatherapy contains multiple types of scents, another RCT evaluated the impact of lavender (*Lavandula angustifolia*) in nursing home patients and also failed to demonstrate efficacy in treating agitation (O'Conner et al., 2013). It is possible that possibly the type of neurocognitive disorder may impact the response to aromatherapy. For example, AD shows early signs of anosmia and therefore these patients might not benefit from aromatherapy as much as those with other forms of neurocognitive disorders might. Based on the evidence available, aromatherapy does not appear to significantly improve agitation in individuals living in institutions with neurocognitive disorders. However, given its safety profile and lack of effective, safe alternatives in treating sundowning syndrome with cognitive impairment, further studies should be encouraged.

MUSIC THERAPY

Music therapy has shown significant benefit to insomnia in the general adult population, as well as for agitation with neurocognitive disorders in the older population. A meta-analysis of three RCTs of institutionalized patients showed significant and immediate impact of music therapy on agitation (Livingston et al., 2014). In another study of agitation with dementia, the impact of music therapy showed a benefit but demonstrated a delayed effect of 1 week (Chang et al., 2010). Another study looking at adults suffering from insomnia in Taiwan showed an impact of music therapy around bedtime in subjective measure of sleep, including a rating on rested feeling, as well as objective measures on polysomnography in terms of increased REM sleep and reduced stage 2 sleep (Chang et al., 2012). Music therapy can be relatively easy to implement for long-term care facilities as well as the home environment and is relatively safe compared to orally ingested products.

SUMMARY

Many of the data on CAIM therapies for insomnia in older adults come from small studies, uncontrolled designs, or short duration, or from mixed-age populations. However, despite the data lacking strong evidence, clinicians should not dismiss their patients when they inquire about or express a desire to use CAIM, as this can be isolating and demeaning for patients. Instead, a clinician should maintain a level of proficiency in the commonly used remedies and therapies, trying to provide a balanced informed view of the existing evidence with some of the unknown effects of the CAIM interventions, along with the potential indications and adverse effects, thus helping patients eliminate extraneous agents that may have worsening effects. The modern cohorts of aging adults and Baby Boomers are well informed about existing therapies via the Internet. The consumers of CAIM frequently strongly believe in the positive effects of the interventions, regardless of their providers' views, beliefs, and recommendations. An informed healthcare provider can help these individuals make safe and informed choices and cut down on unnecessary costs of the CAIM therapies without denying them autonomy and the empowerment of making their own healthcare decisions. This model of cooperative decision-making encourages cooperation, better patient–provider alliance, and adherence to treatment, and promotes preventive care models.

REFERENCES

Abbasi, B., Kimiagar, M., Sadeghniiat, K., Shirazi, M., Hedayati, M., &Rashidkhani, B. (2012). The effect of magnesium supplementation on primary insomnia in elderly: a double-blind placebo-controlled clinical trial. *J Res Med Sci*, 12(12), 1161–1169.

American Psychiatric Association (APA). (2013). *Diagnostic and statistical manual of mental disorders* (5th ed., *DSM-5*). Washington, DC: American Psychiatric Association.

Baek, J., Nierenberg, A., & Kinrys, G. (2014). Clinical applications of herbal medicines for anxiety and insomnia; targeting patients with bipolar disorder. *Aust NZ J Psychiatry*, 48(8), 705–715.

Ballard, C. G., O'Brien, J. T., Reichelt, K., & Perry, E. K. (2002). Aromatherapy as a safe and effective treatment for the management of agitation in severe dementia: the results of a double-blind placebo-controlled trial with Melissa. *J Clin Psychiatry*, 63(7), 553–558.

Bent, S., Padula, A., Moore, D., Patterson, M., & Mehling, W. (2006). Valerian for sleep: a systematic review and meta-analysis. *Am J Med*, 119, 1005–1012.

Bertisch, S. M., Wells, R. E., Smith, M. T., & McCarthy, E. P. (2012). Use of relaxation techniques and complementary and alternative medicine by American adults with insomnia symptoms: results from a national survey. *J Clin Sleep Med*, 8(6), 681–691.

Black, D. S., Cole, S., Irwin, M. R., Breen, E., St Cyr, N. M., Nazarian, N., Khalsa DS. & Lavretsky, H. (2013). Yogic meditation reverses NF-kB and IRF-related transcriptome dynamics in leukocytes of family dementia caregivers in a randomized controlled trial. *Psychoneuroendocrinology*, 38(3), 348–355.

Burns, A., Perry, E., Holmes, C., Francis, P., Morris, J., Howes, M. J., et al. (2011). A double-blind placebo controlled randomized trial of Melissa officinalis oil and donepezil for the treatment of agitation in

Alzheimer's disease. *Dementia Geriatr Cogn Disord*, 31(2), 158–164.

Buscemi, N., Vandermeer, B., Hooton, N., Pandya R, Tjosvold L, Hartling L et al. (2005). The efficacy and safety of exogenous melatonin for primary sleep disorders a meta-analysis. *J Gen Intern Med*, 20, 1151–1158.

Chang, E. T., Lai, H. L., Chen, P. W., Hsieh, Y. M., & Lee, L. H. (2012). The effect of music on the sleep quality of adults with chronic insomnia using evidence from polysomnographic and self-reported analysis: a randomized control trial. *Int J Nurs Studies*, 49, 921–930.

Chang, F. U., Huang, H. C., Lin, K. C., & Lin, L. C. (2010). The effect of a music programme during lunchtime on the problem behaviour of the older residents with dementia at an institution in Taiwan. *J Clin Nursing*, 19, 939–948.

Cornu, C., Remontet, L., Noel-Baron, F., Nicolas, A., Feugier-Favier, N., Roy, P., et al. (2010). A dietary supplement to improve the quality of sleep: a randomized placebo controlled trial. *BMC Compl Alt Med*, 10, 1–9.

de Niet, G., Tiemens, B., Lendemeijer B. & Hutschemaekers G.(2009). Music-assisted relaxation to improve sleep quality: meta-analysis. *J Advan Nurs;* 65(7): 1356-64.

Diaper, A., & Hindmarch, I. (2004). A double-blind, placebo-controlled investigation of the effects of two doses of a valerian preparation on the sleep, cognitive and psychomotor function of sleep-disturbed older adults. *Phytotherapy*, 18, 831–836.

Donath, F., Quispe, S., Diefenbach, K., Maurer, A., Fietze, I., & Roots, I. (2000). Critical evaluation of the effect of valerian extract on sleep structure and sleep quality. *Pharmacopsychiatry*, 33, 47–53.

Dowling, G. A., Burr, R. L., Van Someren, E., Hubbard, E., Luxenber, J. S., et al. (2008). Melatonin and bright-light treatment for rest-activity disruption in institutionalized patients with Alzheimer's disease. *JAGS*, 56, 239–246.

Fernandez-San-Martin, M., Masa-Font, R., Palacios-Soler, L., Sancho-Gomez, P., Calbo-Caldentey, C., & Flores-Mateo, G. (2010). Effectiveness of valerian on insomnia: a metanaylsis of randomized placebo-controlled trials. *Sleep Med*, 11, 505–511.

Garfinkel, D., Laudon, M., Nof D. & Zisapel, N. (1995). Improvement of sleep quality in elderly people by controlled-released melatonin. Lancet; 346(8974): 541-4.

Garrido, M., Gonzales-Gomez, D., Lozano, M., Barriga, C., Paredes, S. D., & Rodriguez, A. B. (2013). A Jerte Valley cherry product provides beneficial effects on sleep quality influence on aging. *J Nutr Health Aging*, 17(6), 553–560.

Gooneratne, N. (2008). Complementary and alternative medicine for sleep disturbances in older adults. *Clin Geriatr Med*, 24(1), 121–138.

Gooneratne, N., & Vitiello, M. (2014). Sleep in older adults normative changes, sleep disorders, and treatment options. *Clin Geriatr Med*, 30, 591–627.

Halpern, J., Cohen, M., Kennedy, G., Reece, J., Cahan, C., & Baharav, A. (2014). Yoga for improving sleep quality and quality of life for older adults. *Altern Ther*, 20(3), 37–46.

Irwin, M. R., Olmstead, R., Carrillo, C., Sadeghi, N., Breen, E. C., Witarama, T., et al. (2014). Cognitive behavioral therapy vs Tai Chi for late life insomnia and inflammatory risk: a randomized controlled comparative efficacy trial. *Sleep*, 37(9), 1543–52.

Liira, J., Verbeek, JH, Costa, G., Driscoll, TR., Sallinen M., Isotalo LK., et al. 2014. *Cochrane Database Systemic review. 8.*

Livingston, G., Kelly, L., Lewis-Holmes, E., Baio, G., Morris, S., Patel, N., et al. (2014). Non-pharmacological interventions for agitation in dementia: systematic review of randomized controlled trials. *Br J Psychiatry*, 205, 436–442.

Khalsa, S. B. (2004). Treatment of chronic insomnia with yoga: a preliminary study with sleep-wake diaries. *Appl Psychophysiol Biofeed*, 29(4), 269–278.

King, A., Oman, R., Brassington, G., Bliwise, D., & Haskell, W. (1997). Moderate-intensity exercise and self-rated quality of sleep in older adults. *JAMA*, 277(1), 32–37.

Krystal, A. D., Edinger, J. D., & Wohlgemuth, W. K. (2012). Sleep and circadian rhythm disorders. In D. G. Blazer & D. C. Steffens (Eds.), *Essentials of geriatric psychiatry* (2nd ed., pp. 209–221).Washington, DC: American Psychiatric Publishing.

Lewy, A., Ahmed, S., Jackson, J., & Sack, R. (1992). Melatonin shifts human circadian rhythms according to a phase response curve. *Chronobiol Int*, 9(5), 380–392.

Manjunath, N. K., & Telles, S. (2005). Influence of yoga and Ayurveda on self-rated sleep in a geriatric population. *Indian J Med Res*, 121(5), 683–690.

Maroo, N., Hazra, A., & Das, T. Efficacy and safety of a polyherbal sedative-hypnotic formulation NSF-3 in primary insomnia in comparison to zolpidem: a randomized controlled trial. 2013. *Indian J Pharmacol*, 45(1), 34–39.

McCleery, J., Cohen, D. A., & Sharpley, A. (2014). Pharmacotherapies for sleep disturbances in Alzheimer's disease. *Cochrane database;*3.

Mischoulon, D. (2008). Herbal remedies for anxiety and insomnia: kava and valerian. In D. Mischoulon & J. F. Rosenbaum (Eds.), *Natural medications for psychiatric disorders* (2nd ed., pp. 119–139). Philadelphia: Lippincott, Williams & Wilkins.

Mishima, K., Tozawa, T., Satoh, K., Matsumoto, Y., Hishikawa, Y., & Okawa, M. (1999). Melatonin secretion rhythm disorders in patients with senile dementia of Alzheimer's type with disturbed sleep-waking. *Soc Biol Psychiatry, 45,* 417–421.

O'Connor, D., Eppingstall, B., Taffe, J., & van der Ploeg, E. (2013). A randomized, controlled cross-over trial of dermally-applied lavender (lavanduala angustifolia) oil as a treatment of agitated behaviour in dementia. *BMC Compl Alt Med, 13,* 315.

Riemersma-van der Lek, R., Swaab, D. F., Twisk, J., Hol, E. M., Hoogendijk, W., & Van Someren, E. J. W. (2008). Effect of bright light and melatonin on cognitive and noncognitive function in elderly residents of group care facilities. *JAMA, 299*(22), 2642–2655.

Rondanelli, M., Opizzi, A., Monteferrario, F., Antoniello, N., Manni, R., & Klersy, C. (2011). The effect of melatonin, magnesium, and zinc on primary insomnia in long-term care facility residents in Italy: a double-blind placebo-controlled clinical trial. *JAGS, 59,* 82–90.

Shi, Y., Dong, J. W., Zhao, J. H., Tang, L. N., & Zhang, J. J. (2014). Herbal insomnia medications that target GABAergic systems: a review of the psychopharmacological evidence. *Curr Neuropharmacol, 12,* 289–302.

Singer, C., Tractenberg, R. E., Kaye, J., Schafer, K., Gamst, A., Grudman, M., et al. (2003). A multicenter, placebo-controlled trial of melatonin for sleep disturbance in Alzheimer's disease. *Sleep, 26*(7), 893–901.

Serfaty, M., Kennell-Webb, S., Warner, J., Blizard, R., & Raven, P. (2002). Double blind randomized placebo controlled trial of low dose melatonin for sleep disorders in dementia. *Int J Geriatr Psychiatry, 17,* 1120–1127.

Stevinson, C., & Ernst, E. (2000). Valerian for insomnia: a systematic review of randomized clinical trials. *Sleep Med, 1,* 91–99.

Taavoni, S., Ekbatani, N., Kashaniyan, M., & Haghani, H. (2011). Effect of valerian on sleep quality in postmenopausal women: a randomized placebo-controlled clinical trial. *Menopause, 18*(9), 951–955.

Taibi, D., & Vitiello, M. (2011). A pilot study of gentle yoga for sleep disturbance in women with osteoarthritis. *Sleep Med, 12*(5), 512–517.

Wade, A. G., Farmer, M., Harari, G., Fund, N., Laudon, M., & Nir, T. (2014). Add-on prolonged release melatonin for cognitive function and sleep in mild to moderate Alzheimer's disease: a 6 month, randomized, placebo-controlled, multicenter trial. *Clin Intervent Aging, 9,* 947–961.

Zhadanova, I. V., & Friedman, L. (2008). Therapeutic potential of melatonin in sleep and circadian disorders. In D. Mischoulon & J. F. Rosenbaum (Eds.), *Natural medications for psychiatric disorders* (2nd ed., pp. 140–160). . Philadelphia: Lippincott Williams & Wilkins.

Zick, S., Wright, B., Sen, A., & Arnedt, T. (2011). Preliminary examination of the efficacy and safety of a standardized chamomile extract for chronic primary insomnia: a randomized placebo-controlled pilot study. *BMC Compl Alt Med, 11,* 1–8.

27

ACUPUNCTURE TREATMENT FOR PAIN AND RELATED PROBLEMS IN THE ELDERLY

Shu-Ming Wang and Brenda Golianu

OVERVIEW

Globally, the population is aging rapidly. As of 2008, the number of people aged 65 years and older was estimated at 506 million. By 2040 this number will likely increase to 1.3 billion (1). In 2008, the US Census Bureau asserted that there were 38.9 million people aged 65 and older, making up 12.8% of the total population. Of this population, 5.7 million are 85 years and older, and this number is growing (1). As the United States evolves into a nation with an older population, greater attention should focus on healthcare problems in the elderly.

Epidemiological data also suggest that there is an increasing prevalence of chronic pain and frailty with advancing age (2). The prevalence of pain in older people living in the community ranged from 25% to 76%, while that of those living in residential care ranged from 83% to 93% (3). Common chronic pain among the elderly includes arthritis/joint pain, peripheral neuropathy, fibromyalgia, central pain

syndromes, repetitive strain injury, lingering pain from ligament tear or fracture, cancer pain, and somatic pain related to psychological issues.

While it is important to include both physiological and medical conditions, the psychological well-being of the elderly should not be ignored in managing pain. Inappropriate management of pain in the elderly can lead to serious health consequences, such as depression, anxiety, decreased mobility, social isolation, poor sleep, and related health risks.

BARRIERS IN TREATING PAIN IN OLDER ADULTS

Several barriers influence the effective treatment of pain in the elderly. Elderly patients often do not present with typical signs and symptoms of pain; thus it is difficult to make a timely and accurate diagnosis. In addition, functional decline of organ function and coexisting chronic conditions may not only lead to the development and maintenance of pain but also interfere with treatment.

Pain medications may interact with other medications that patients are already receiving for other chronic medical conditions (4). Some medications, such as benzodiazepines or opioids for example, may have much longer half-life due to declining hepatic function in the elderly, while organ function may itself be adversely affected by the administration of pain medications such as non-steroidal anti-inflammatory agents, which adversely affect kidney function. Pain medications may have a disproportionate effect on the mental functioning of elderly patients, especially if cognitive decline is already present. Patients may refuse to take pain medications due to fears of adverse effects, fear of impairment, difficulty in communication, decline in mental status, or simply because they believe that pain is a natural consequence of old age.

Although elderly patients may have frequent office visits for their chronic medical conditions, many healthcare providers focus only on the pathophysiolological conditions, and do not inquire about related pain. Some practitioners may believe that pain is a "normal" part of aging; others may have concerns about possible physical dependence or psychological addiction to pain medications, or have lack of experience in pain assessment and treatment. All of these factors may limit practitioners' engagement in the pain management process (5). Consequently, pain in the elderly is largely undertreated.

To overcome these barriers, the National Institutes of Health has created a Pain Consortium to help study all aspects of pain prevention and treatment. This interdisciplinary Consortium is composed of 18 different Institutes and Centers that help coordinate planning for key research opportunities in every aspect of pain, including pain assessment (6).

PAIN ASSESSMENT IN THE ELDERLY

Pain, especially chronic long-lasting pain, is prevalent across many different diseases and conditions. When caring for elderly patients, one should carefully assess physical symtpoms of pain but also explore the mental impact of pain, and patients' attitude, beliefs, level of knowledge, and previous experiences with pain and pain management. For older adults with cognitive dysfunction or dementia, and those who are not able to communicate, extra attention should be paid to any changes in functioning and behavior.

Similar to routine pain assessment of any age, it is recommended that tools assessing various psychological and physical conditions be included (7). Body drawing or verbal report provides useful information. Instruments such as the McGill Pain Questionnaire (8,9) contain a variety of verbal descriptors that help to distinguish between musculoskeletal and nerve-related pain. Typically, patients describe deep tissue pain as dull, aching, and cramping, while nerve-related pain tends to be more sporadic, shooting, or burning (10,11). For patients with severe cognitive impairment, specialized tools have been created and validated to assess pain. These include the Pain Assessment Checklist for Seniors with Limited Ability to Communicate, the Pain Assessment in Advanced Dementia, and the Doloplus-2 scale (12).

MULTIDISCIPLINARY PAIN MANAGEMENT FOR THE ELDERLY

In synthesizing a realistic pain management plan for elderly patients with pain, several important questions should be included (see Box 27.1; modified from Carr DR, Jacox AK, Chapman CR, et al. AHCPR Pub No 92-0032; Public Health Service) (6).

SPECIAL CONSIDERATION IN ASSESSING AND MANAGING PAIN IN THE ELDERLY

Due to multiple comorbidities, decreased organ function, and potential drug interactions, special considerations are needed in assessing and managing pain in the elderly.

The selection of an assessment tool should be based on the patient's cognitive level and functional states to meet the unique characteristics and needs of that patient. For example, healthcare providers can use a simple tool such as happy/sad faces and have the family use the same tool at home to record the patient's pain, thus facilitating the tracking of pain over time.

There is a high incidence of visual, hearing, and motor impairment among elderly patients

Box 27.1 Assessing the Impact of Pain on the Elderly Individual

a. Does the patient have any significant previous and/or ongoing instances of pain?
b. How does pain affect the patient?
c. What are the patient's underlying mental and physical conditions, as well as comorbidities?
d. What are the aggravating and alleviating factors that affect the level of pain?
e. How does the patient describe or communicate the experience of pain?
f. What are previously used methods for pain control that the patient has found either helpful or unhelpful?
g. What is the patient's attitude toward the experience of pain and the use of opioids, anxiolytics, or other medications or any history of substance abuse?
h. What is the patient's typical coping response for stress or pain, including the presence or absence of psychiatric disorders such as depression, anxiety, or psychosis?
i. What are the family expectations and beliefs concerning pain, stress, and the overall effects?
j. What does the patient know about pain?
k. What are the patient's expectations and preferences of treatment for pain and receiving information about pain management?
l. What are the goals of pain management for the patient and family?
m. What are the steps needed to focus on enhancing the elderly pain patient's daily functions, maintaining a positive affect or mood, and improving sleep?

that can interfere with self-report and requires a quiet and distraction-free environment for full expression. In addition, ample amount of time must be allowed to explore the pain symptoms fully and perform an thorough assessment. When an elderly patient cannot communicate verbally, alternative methods should be utilized, such as paying attention to the patient's behavioral cues and facial expression. For example, an elderly patient with cognitive impairment may become quiet but not complain about pain when he or she is experiencing pain.

Family members may be more familiar with the member's specific pain presentation and can be particularly helpful in the pain assessment. A multidisciplinary approach should be considered to achieve adequate pain control, and the quality of pain management should be monitored closely (13). This approach includes an assessment of physical functioning, not only from a rehabilitation perspective (i.e., physical and occupational therapy), but also psychological and psychiatric assessment when indicated. Depression, anxiety, and sleep disorders frequently accompany pain and should be assessed routinely and treated appropriately (14).

INTEGRATIVE THERAPIES FOR PAIN DISORDERS

Non-pharmacological integrative therapies, such as acupuncture, guided imagery, chiropractic treatment, yoga, hypnosis, biofeedback, aromatherapy, relaxation, herbal remedies, massage, and others, have increasingly been utilized alongside pharmacologic therapies in the management of chronic pain. Additionally, for the management of pain related to arthritis, an individualized approach consisting of daily physical activity in a manner that does not promote further injury, dietary interventions, weight loss where appropriate, adequate footwear, and assistive devices can be of significant benefit (15).

Here, we will focus on the use of acupuncture because there is ample scientific and clinical evidence in supporting acupuncture analgesia for chronic pain in older adults. In addition, acupuncture has been found to have high safety profile when performed by trained acupuncturists (16,17). Furthermore, there are some clinical data to support acupuncture used in other chronic medical conditions that may contribute to elderly patients' pain and psychological conditions related to pain.

WHAT IS ACUPUNCTURE?

Acupuncture is an ancient Chinese medical practice, first described more than 2000 years ago. This intervention consists of applying physical stimuli to specific points on the body to prevent and treat various conditions. Over the years, various stimulation techniques have been incorporated into acupuncture. Including direct pressure, needling, moxibustion, vacuum, injection, laser, electrical stimulation, laser, and ultrasound. All of these stimulating techniques are commonly used in clinical acupuncture practice for various conditions (18). The term *acupuncture* will be used to refer any of these techniques in the rest of this chapter.

Thus far, the exact mechanism of acupuncture has remained elusive however, several theories have been proposed:

1. *Endorphin theory*: Acupuncture point stimulation triggers the release of endogenous opioids into the central nervous system. Low-frequency electrical stimulation (2Hz) applied via acupuncture points triggers the release of endorphins, while high-frequency stimulation (100 Hz) triggers dynorphin release (19,20).

2. *Modulation of the adrenergic system*: In this theory, acupuncture point stimulation activates the autonomic nervous system through cutaneous-visceral reflexes and through actions on the hypothalamic-pituitary axis and thereby helps to restore homeostasis in the body and facilitate the healing process. There is some evidence that acupuncture does have significant effects on the autonomic nervous system (21,22).

3. *Spinal mechanisms*: These include gate control, long-term depression, propriospinal inhibition, and the balance between long-term depression and long-term potentiation (23).

4. *Supraspinal mechanisms*: These include the descending pain inhibitory system, diffuse noxious inhibitory control, and the modulation of default mode network connectivity (23–25).

5. *Morphogenetic theory*: Acupuncture points are singular points in a surface bioelectric field. This bioelectric field exerts an effect on growth control and morphogenesis of the growing organism. Organizing centers have high electric conductance, and acupuncture points are felt to coincide with these organizing centers. This theory, while attractive from a theoretical viewpoint, is difficult to test from an experimental approach (26).

6. *Mechanical signaling through connective tissue, anti-inflammatory effects*: Acupuncture activates fibroblasts in connective tissue, leading to local and systemic effects (25,27).

The schematic illustration (Figure 27.1) summarizes some of the neurophysiologic mechanisms of acupuncture analgesia. Thus far, there is ample evidence, derived from both animals and human experiments, that acupuncture stimulation triggers a series of neurohormone release (30,31) activation of c-fos gene expression in the central nervous system (32), and normalizes neuroplasticity (e.g., 5 weeks of acupuncture treatment can normalize the somatotopic representation of digits 2 and 3 in patients with carpal tunnel syndrome) (33). Interestingly, anticipation and belief of a patient might also affect the level of acupuncture therapeutic outcome, though the effect of expectancy is different from that of acupuncture analgesia (34,35). Acupuncture also has been used in prevention and treatment for more than 40 various medical conditions clinically (36).

ACUPUNCTURE USE FOR CHRONIC PAIN

Based on the data published in the literature, acupuncture was found to be an effective treatment for musculoskeletal pain (neck, shoulder, and back pain), headache, and osteoarthritis. In fact, in the headache category, acupuncture has achieved the strongest evidence-based medical practice recommendation. A systematic review with 31 randomized controlled trials found that acupuncture was effective in treating chronic headaches. The combined response rate in the acupuncture group was significantly higher compared with sham acupuncture, both at the early follow-up period (risk ratio [RR]: 1.19; 95% confidence interval [CI]: 1.08 to 1.30) and late follow-up period (RR: 1.22; 95% CI: 1.04 to 1.43). Its effect was superior to medications for headache intensity (weighted mean difference: -8.54 mm; 95% CI: -15.52 to 1.57), frequency

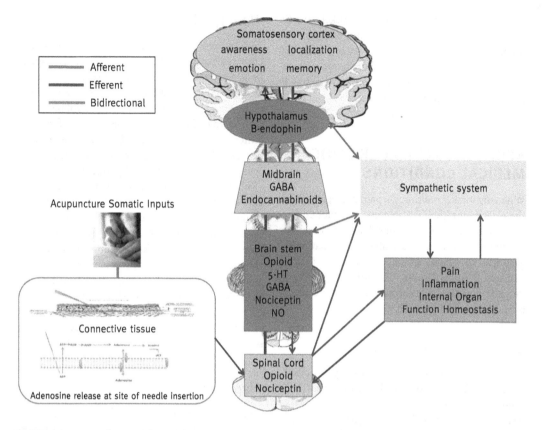

FIGURE 27.1   Schematic drawing representing the potential mechanisms of acupuncture analgesia

(standard mean difference: −0.70; 95% CI: −1.38 to −0.02), physical function (weighted 4.16; 95% CI: −1.38 to −0.02), and responses (RR: 1.49; 95% CI: 1.02 to 2.17) (37).

Subsequently, Vickers and colleagues (38) performed a meta-analysis on data derived from 29 eligible randomized control trails with a total of 17,922 patients. This meta-analysis showed that acupuncture was superior to sham control condition, that is, effect sizes were 0.23 (95% CI: 0.13 to 0.33) for neck and back pain; 0.16 (95% CI: 0.07 to 0.25) for osteoarthritis, and 0.15 (95% CI: 0.07 to 0.24) for chronic headache. Similarly, when comparing acupuncture with no acupuncture control, the effect sizes were 0.55 (95% CI: 0.51 to 0.58) for neck and back pain, 0.57 (95% CI: 0.50 to 0.64) for osteoarthritis, and 0.42 (95% CI: 0.37 to 0.46) for chronic headache.

Acupuncture has been shown to improve health-related quality of life in many chronic pain conditions. Wondering and colleagues conducted a cost-effectiveness analysis of a randomized

controlled trial consisting of 401 patients with chronic headache. They found that total costs during the study period were on average higher for the acupuncture group than control group due to the costs of acupuncture treatment, but cost per quality-adjusted life-year dropped substantially (39).

Witt and colleagues (40,41) performed a study of the effectiveness of acupuncture in the management of various chronic pain conditions such as osteoarthritis pain and chronic neck pain. They found that acupuncture improves health-related quality of life at a small additional cost and is relatively cost-effective compared with a number of other interventions (42).

Pragmatic trials consistently demonstrate that acupuncture complimentary to routine care improves quality of life and is cost-effective in treating osteoarthritis (40), neck pain (41), and chronic low back pain (43). Acupuncture is an effective non-pharmacological or complementary treatment for headache, osteoarthritis, and musculoskeletal pain. In addition, acupuncture does not interact with other drugs that elderly patients may be taking and has no lingering side effects. Furthermore, techniques such as acupressure can easily be taught to patients, family members or caregivers, allowing additional therapeutic benefits.

ACUPUNCTURE FOR CHRONIC MEDICAL CONDITIONS

When organizing multimodal pain management for the elderly, one should also consider other comorbid chronic medical conditions that may worsen the symptoms of pain, such as diabetic neuropathy and gastroparesis, which are common in long-standing diabetes in older adults. The following sections describe chronic medical conditions for which acupuncture may be beneficial.

Gastrointestinal Disorders

Acupuncture has been used to treat gastrointestinal dysmotility, related to diabetes mellitus (DM); abnormal myoelectrical disturbances with either high (tachygastric) or low (bradygastric) slow frequencies are commonly observed in DM patients. Chang and colleagues (43) applied acupuncture at the Zu San Li point (ST36) to 15 type II DM patients who suffered from dyspeptic symptoms for more than 3 months. The study showed that acupuncture at the Zusanli point could increase the percentage of normal electrogastrography frequency and decrease the percentage of tachygastric/bradygastric frequency in diabetic patients. In addition, there was an increased level of serum human pancreatic polypeptide during acupuncture treatment. The researchers suggest that acupuncture may enhance the regularity of gastric myoelectrical activity in diabetic patients.

A systematic review was performed to assess the evidence for the effectiveness of acupuncture treatment in gastrointestinal diseases (44). This review included 18 relevant trials meeting the inclusion criteria, and all the trials demonstrated significantly improved quality of life in patients with a history of gastrointestinal diseases. Similarly, acupuncture effectively improved disease activity scores when used as a treatment for both Crohn's disease and in colitis trials (45–48).

Neuropathy

Acupuncture has been used as an adjuvant or complementary treatment for chronic neuropathy in DM patients. Abuaish and colleagues (49) evaluated the efficacy and long-term effectiveness in 46 diabetic individuals with chronic painful peripheral neuropathy. Over 18–52 weeks, 67% of patients either reduced or stopped taking medications because of significant improvement of their clinical symptoms of pain. Studies by Tesfaye and Ahmed (50) also showed short-term relief in various acute and chronic pain syndromes (51). Hamza performed a randomized, controlled, cross-over study on a group of patients suffering from neuropathy pain (52). After 3 weeks of acupuncture, patients showed a significant improvement in both visual analogue pain and sleep score. Patients must discuss their use of acupuncture or other nonpharmacological therapies with their physician, and reduce or discontinue medications only under direct physician supervision.

Hypertension

Hypertension is one of the risk factors for serious cardiovascular events or stroke. Unfortunately, many elderly patients have hypertension that is poorly controlled by medical management. In addition, anti-hypertension medications have many side effects, such as fatigue, dizziness, weakness, headache, cold hands and feet, sleep disturbance, and joint pain. Acupuncture also has been used as an adjunctive treatment for hypertension. Cevik and Iseri (53) have performed acupuncture on a group of 34 hypertension patients whose blood pressures were well controlled by more than one medication. Acupuncture was performed at Tai Xi (KI3), Tai Chong (LI 3), Yin Ling Quan (SP 9), He Gu (LI 4, HT7), Zu San Li (ST36), San-Yin Jiao (SP6), Fu Liu (KI 7), and Tai Yuan (LU 9) acupuncture points once every 2 days for a month for a total of 15 sessions. All these patients had significant normalization of blood pressure. As a result, the researchers concluded that acupuncture facilitates a significant reduction of blood pressure and decreases the usual complaints associated with medications. Currently there is a large multicenter randomized control trial ongoing in the People's Republic of China to determine the efficacy of acupuncture as a treatment for patients with mild hypertension (54). As above, utilizing acupuncture as an adjuvant in the management of hypertension must be done only following discussion with and oversight of one's physician.

ACUPUNCTURE FOR COGNITIVE AND PSYCHOLOGICAL SYMPTOMS AND ILLNESSES

Many elderly patients have suffered from declining mental acuity, insomnia, sleep disturbance, depression, and anxiety as a result of underlying medical conditions. A recently released Center for Mental Health Services (CMHS) Fact Sheet devotes the entire issue to information on self-help, diet and nutrition, expression therapies, acupuncture, yoga, and relaxation and stress reduction techniques that can be used as complementary approaches to mental health care. Kessler and his colleagues (55) report that in a representative sample of 2055 respondents, 66.7% of those seen by a conventional provider for severe depression and 65.9% of those seen by a conventional provider for anxiety attacks used complementary and alternative therapies.

A recent document by the National Survey of Alternative Health Care Practice and Their Perceived Effect on Functional Recovery indicated that a growing number of people use complementary and alternative practices for psychiatric disorders. Anecdotal data suggest that these alternative practices may supplement traditional mental health and rehabilitation services. Existing literature suggests that acupuncture may ameliorate some symptoms commonly associated with vascular dementia, depression and anxiety.

Vascular Dementia

Yu and colleagues (56) performed a clinical trial including a total of 60 patients, randomized to acupuncture or control group. Patients in the acupuncture groups received acupuncture at Dang Zhong (CV17), Zhong Wan (CV12), Qi Hai (CV6), ST36, and Xue Hai (SP10). The researchers discovered that Mini-Mental Status Examination (MMSE), Hasegawa's Dementia Scale (HDS-R), and activities of daily living (ADL) scores were significantly improved in the acupuncture group as compared to those of the control group. Guo and colleagues (57) performed a meta-analysis to determine the effect of acupuncture on dementia and found that acupuncture demonstrated efficacy for delaying cognitive decline. In a study comparing the cerebral effects of acupuncture for vascular dementia (VaD), acupuncture increased glucose metabolism as measured by positron emission tomography (PET) scan in the temporal lobe of the unaffected hemisphere and in the lentiform nucleus of the affected sphere (58). Additional needling in VaD-specific points rendered higher metabolism bilaterally in the frontal lobes and the thalamus and in the temporal lobe and the lentiform nucleus of the of the unaffected hemisphere (59). Acupuncture applied to Waiguan (TE5) has a balancing effect on regional brain metabolism using positron emission tomography (PET) that may related to the recovery of post-stroke patients (60). These preliminary indicators that acupuncture may have some clinical effectiveness in the treatment of dementia must be confirmed and further studied in randomized controlled trials prior to incorporation into standard treatment protocols, however may be considered as an adjuvant to minimize doses of pharmacological agents or in refractory cases/

Depression

Mukaino and colleagues (61) performed a systematic review of the randomized controlled trials and suggested that the therapeutic effect of acupuncture is similar to conventional antidepressants in depressive disorders. While the data on the use of acupuncture for mood disorders is significant, it must be underscored that depression and anxiety must be closely assessed and monitoried by a treating primary care physician or psychiatrist and appropriate management must be considered even as this adjuvant therapy is being implemented.

Impaired Cognition

A number of controlled and uncontrolled clinical studies demonstrated that acupuncture therapy may be able to improve the cognitive function of patients with mild cognitive impairment and various forms of dementia (62–64). The reduced severity of cognitive symptoms correlated with the fMRI changes in brain regions associated with learning and memory processes (65,66). Although the exact mechanism remains unclear, many animal studies have indicated that the effect of acupuncture might be associated with the inhibition of cytokine-mediated neuronal cell apoptosis, inflammatory reaction, and oxidative cellular injury, among others (67–69).

ACUPUNCTURE FOR PHYSICAL FATIGUE

Fatigue is a significant geriatric syndrome, which has only recently been defined in the elderly population, and it can affect work performance, family life, and social relationships negatively (70). Yiu and colleagues (71) conducted a single-blinded, randomized controlled trial of acupuncture for chronic fatigue syndrome. A total of 99 participants who met the inclusion criteria were randomized into acupuncture or control group. Acupuncture stimulations were applied to Zu San Li (ST36), San Yin Jiao (SP6), and Bai Hui (GV 20) in sequence. The treatment continued for 4 weeks, with twice a week acupuncture sessions. The research team found that acupuncture significantly improved physical and mental fatigue, as well as health-related quality of life. Recently, Ng and Yiu (72) reported the acupuncture group demonstrated moderate effect sizes in physical and mental fatigue and in the physical component of health-related qualify of life. A pragmatic randomized controlled trial was conducted to assess the effectiveness of acupuncture for cancer-related fatigue. The research team found that acupuncture is an effective intervention for managing the symptom of cancer-related fatigue and improving patients' quality of life (73).

ACUPUNCTURE FOR INSOMNIA

Insomnia and sleep disorder in the elderly are often mistakenly considered a normal part of aging. More than 50% of the elderly have insomnia or sleep disturbances that do not receive treatment. Sleep disturbance in the elderly is associated with decreased memory, impaired concentration, and impaired functional performance (74). Insomnia also contributes to an increased risk of accidents, falls, and chronic fatigue (74). Sok and colleagues (75) evaluated the effects of acupuncture therapy on insomnia, suggesting that acupuncture may be an effective intervention for the relief of insomnia. Additional research is necessary to determine the effectiveness of acupuncture. More work is also needed to promote the long-term therapeutic effects of acupuncture and to compare it with other therapies for insomnia. A recent systematic review of randomized controlled trails by Cao and colleagues (76) indicated a beneficial effect of acupuncture compared with no treatment (MD -3.28; 95% CI: -6.10 to -0.46; $p = 0.02$; 4 trials) and real acupressure compared with sham acupressure (MD -2.94; 95% CI: -5.77 to -0.11; $p = 0.04$; 2 trials) on total scores of Pittsburgh Sleep Quality Index. Acupuncture was superior to medications regarding the number of patients with total sleep duration increased for > 3 hours (RR 1.53; 95% CI: 1.24 to 1.88; $p < 0.0001$). However, there was no difference between acupuncture and medications in average sleep duration (MD -0.06; 95% CI: -0.30 to 0.18; $p = 0.63$). Acupuncture plus medications showed better effect than medications alone on total sleep duration (MD 1.09; 95% CI: 0.56 to 1.61; $p < 0.0001$). Similarly, acupuncture plus herbs was significantly better than herbs alone on increase of sleep rates (RR 1.67; 95% CI: 1.12 to 2.50; $p = 0.01$). There were no serious adverse effects related to acupuncture treatment in the included trials. Currently a multicenter randomized controlled trial is ongoing in China to determine the effects of acupuncture treatment on depression related insomnia (77).

SUMMARY

In summary, acupuncture is commonly used for the management of pain and comorbid medical and mental disorders in older adults. Thus far, there is strong scientific and clinical evidence supporting the use of this intervention for pain. Acupuncture can be used for associated mild depression and anxiety, insomnia, fatigue, and cognitive symtpoms in conjunction with or as an adjuvant to regular treatments. Other advantages of using acupuncture as a treatment in elderly patients with pain and chronic medical conditions are several. First, acupuncture is usually well tolerated, with minimal reported adverse effects (e.g., fear of needles, minor bleeding at the site). In addition, the non-invasive stimulating techniques such as acupressure (direct finger pressure, or press beads) can easily be taught to caregivers or patients for self-administration at regular frequencies. Acupuncture may play an essential role in caring for the elderly with chronic pain conditions and many other medical and psychological conditions such as fatigue, depression, and cognitive impairment. Health care practitioners should consider acupuncture as part of multimodal integrative pain management for older adults.

DISCLOSURE STATEMENT

Brenda Golianu has no financial interest to disclose. She has received funding from NIH. Dr. Shu-Ming Wang does not have anything to disclose.

REFERENCES

1. Kaye AD, Baluch A, Scott JT. Pain management in the elderly population: a review. *Ochsner J.* 2010;10(3):179–187.
2. Rastogi R, Meek BD. Management of chronic pain in elderly, frail patients: finding a suitable, personalized method of control. *Clinical Intervent Aging.* 2013;8:37–46.
3. Abdula A, Adams N, Bone M et al. Guidance on the management of pain in older people. *Age Ageing.* 2013;42:i1–i57.
4. Jacox A, Carr DB, Payne R, et al. *Management of cancer pain.* Clinical Practice Guideline No. 9. AHCPR Publication No. 84-0592, 1994.
5. Tracy B, Morrison RS. Pain management in older adults. *Clin Ther.* 2013;35(11):1659–1668.
6. Carr DR, Jacox AK, Chapman CR, et al. *Acute pain management: operative or medical procedures and trauma.* No 1. Rockville, MD: US Department of Health and Human Services; 1992. AHCPR Pub No 92-0032; Public Health Service.
7. Gordon DB, Dahl J, Miaskowski C, et al. American pain society recommendations for improving the quality of acute and cancer pain management. *Arch Intern Med.* 2005;165:1574–1580.
8. Melzack R. The McGill Pain Questionnaire: major properties and scoring methods. *Pain.* 1975;1:277–299.
9. Melzack R. The short-form McGill Pain Questionnaire. *Pain.* 1987;30:191–197.
10. Bouhassira D, Attal N, Alchaar H, et al. Comparison of pain syndromes associated with nervous or somatic lesions and development of a new neuropathic pain diagnostic questionnaire (DN4). *Pain.* 2005;114(1–2):29–36.
11. Wilkie DJ, Huang H, Reilly N, Cain K. Nociceptive and neuropathic pain in patients with lung cancer: a comparison of pain quality descriptors. *J Pain Symptom Manage.* 2001;22(5):899–910.
12. Herr K, Coyne PJ, McCaffery M, et al. Pain assessment in the patient unable to self-report: position statement with clinical practice recommendations. *Pain Manag Nurs.* 2011;12:230–250.
13. Makris UE, Abrams RC, Gurland B, et al. Management of persistent pain in the older patient: a clinical review. *JAMA.* 2014;312(8):825–835.
14. Sanders JB, Comijs HC, Bremmer MA, et al. A 13-year prospective cohort study on the effect of aging and frailty on the depression-pain relationship in older adults. *Int J Geriatr Psych.* 2015;7:751–7.
15. Fernandes L, Hagen KB, Bijlsma JWJ, et al. EULAR recommendations for non-pharmacological core management of hip and knee osteoarthritis. *Ann Rheum Dis.* 2013;72:1125–1135.
16. Yamashita H, Tsukayama H, White AR, Tanno Y, Sugishita C, Ernst E. Systematic review of adverse events following acupuncture: the Japanese literature. *Complement Ther Med.* 2001;9:98–104.
17. Lao L, Hamilton GR, Fu J, Berman BM. Is acupuncture safe? A systematic review of case reports. *Altern Ther Health Med.* 2003;9:72–83.
18. White A. A cumulative review of the range and incidence of significant adverse events associated with acupuncture. *Acupunct Med.* 2004;22:122–133.
19. Han JS. Acupuncture and endorphins. *Neurosci Lett.* 2004;361(1–3):258–261.
20. Han JS. Acupuncture: neuropeptide release produced by electrical stimulation of different frequencies. *Trends Neurosci.* 2003;26:17–22.
21. Longhurst J. Acupuncture's cardiovascular actions: a mechanistic perspective. *Med Acup.* 2013;25(2):101–113.
22. Longhurst JC, Tjen-A-Looi S. Acupuncture regulation of blood pressure: two decades of research. *Int Rev Neurobiol.* 2013;111:259–271.
23. Carlsson C. Acupuncture mechanisms for clinically relevant long-term effects. *Acupunct Med.* 2002;20(2–3):82–99.
24. Zhao L, Liu JX, Zhang F et al. Effects of long-term acupuncture treatment on resting-state brain activity in migraine patients: a randomized controlled trial on active and inactive acupoints. *PLOS One.* 2014 Jun 10;9(6):e99538.
25. Leung L. Neurophysiological basis of acupuncture induced analgesia: an updated review. *J Acup Meridian Studies.* 2012;5(6):261–270.
26. Shang C. Singular point, organizing center and acupuncture point. *Am J Chin Med.* 1989;17:119–127.
27. Langevin HM, Churchill DL, Cipolla MJ. Mechanical signaling through connective tissue: a mechanism for the therapeutic effect of acupuncture. *FASEB J.* 2001;15:2275–2282.
28. Wang SM, Harris RE, Lin YC, Gan TJ. Acupuncture in 21st century anesthesia: Is there a needle in the haystack? *A&A.* 2013;116(6):1356–1359.
29. Lee JH, Beitz AJ. The distribution of brain-stem and spinal cord nuclei associated with different

frequencies of electroacupuncture analgesia. *Pain*. 1993;52:11–28.

30. Han JS. Acupuncture: neuropeptide release produced by electrical stimulation of different frequencies. *Neuroscience*. 2003;26:17–22.

31. Han JS, Sun SL. Differential release of enkephalin and dynorphin by low and high frequency electroacupuncture in the central nervous system. *Acupunct Sci Int J*. 1990;1:19–27.

32. Guo HF, Tian JH, Wang X, Fang Y, Hou Y, Han J. Brain substrates activated by electroacupuncture of different frequencies. I. Comparative study on the expression of oncogene c-fos genes coding for three opioid peptides. *Brain Res Mol Brain Res*. 1996;43:157–166.

33. Napadow V, Kettner N, Liu J, Li M, Kwong KK, Hui KKS, Audette J. somatosensory cortical plasticity in carpal tunnel syndrome treated by acupuncture. *Hum Brain Mapp*. 2007;28:159–171.

34. Pariente J, White P, Frackowiak RSJ, Lewith G. Expectancy and belief modulate the neuronal substrates of pain treated by acupuncture. *Neuroimage*. 2005;25:1161–1167.

35. Kong J, Kaptchuk TJ, Polich G, Kirsch I, Vangel M, Zyloney C, Rosen B, Gollub RL. An fMRI study on the interaction and dissociation between expectation of pain relief and acupuncture treatment. *Neuroimage*. 2009;47:1066–1076.

36. World Health Organization. *Acupuncture: review and analysis of reports on controlled clinical trial*. WHO Library Cataloguing-in-Publication Data. Geneva: World Health Organization, 2003.

37. Sun Y, Gan TJ. Acupuncture for the management of chronic headache: a systematic review. *Anesth Analg*. 2008;107:2038–2047.

38. Vickers AJ, Cronin AM, Maschino AC, Lewith G, Macpherson H, Foster NE, Sherman KJ, Witt CM, Linde K. Acupuncture for chronic pain: individual patient data meta-analysis. *Arch Intern Med*. 2012;172:1444–1453.

39. Wonderling D, Vicker AJ, Grieve R, McCaryney R. Cost effectiveness analysis of a randomized trial of acupuncture for chronic headache in primary care. *BMJ*. 2004;328:747.

40. Reinhold T, Witt CM, Jena S, Brinkhaus B, Willich SN. Quality of life and cost-effectiveness of acupuncture in patients with osteoarthritis pain. *Eur J Health Ecom*. 2008;9:209–219.

41. Willich SN, Reinhold T, Selim D, Jena S, Brinkhaus B, Witt CM. Cost-effectiveness of acupuncture treatment in patients with chronic neck pain. *Pain*. 2006;125:107–113.

42. Witt CM, Jena S, Selim D, Brinkhaus B, Reinhold T, Wruck K, Liecker B, Linde K, Wegscheider

K, Willich SN. Pragmatic randomized trial evaluating the clinical and economic effectiveness of acupuncture for chronic low back pain. *Am J Epidemiol*. 2006;164:487–496.

43. Chang C-S, Ko C-W, Wu C-Y, Chen G-H. Effect of electrical stimulation on acupuncture points in diabetic patients with gastric dysrhythmia: a pilot study. *Digestion*. 2001;64(3):184–190.

44. Schneider A, Streitberger K, Joos S. Acupuncture treatment in gastrointestinal diseases: systematic review. *World J*. 2007;13(25):3417–3424.

45. Joos S, Brinkhaus B, Maluche C, Maupai N, Kohnen R, Kraehmer N, Hahn EG, Schuppan D. Acupuncture and moxibustion in the treatment of active Crohn's disease: a randomized controlled study. *Digestion*. 2004; 69: 131–139.

46. Joos S, Wildau N, Kohnen R, Szecsenyi J, Schuppan D, Willich SN, Hahn EG, Brinkhaus B. Acupuncture and moxibustion in the treatment of ulcerative colitis: a randomized controlled study. *Scand J Gastroenterol*. 2006; 41: 1056–1063

47. Yang C, Yan H. Observation of the efficacy of acupuncture and moxibustion in 62 cases of chronic colitis. *J Tradit Chin Med*. 1999; 19: 111–114

48. Yue Z, Zhenhui Y. Ulcerative colitis treated by acupuncture at Jiaji points (EX-B2) and tapping with plum-blossom needle at Sanjiaoshu (BL22) and Dachangshu (BL 25): a report of 43 cases. *J Tradit Chin Med*. 2005; 25: 83–84

49. Abuaisha BB, Costanzi JB, Boulton AJM. Acupuncture for the treatment of chronic painful peripheral diabetic neuropathy: a long-term study. *Diabetes Res Clin Pract*. 1998;39:115–121.

50. Tesfaye S, Watt J, Benbow SJ, Pang KA, Miles J, MacFariane IA. Electrical spinal cord stimulation for painful diabetic peripheral neuropathy. *Lancet*. 1996;348:1696–1701.

51. Ahmed HE, Craing WF, White PF. Percutaneous electrical nerve stimulation (PENS): a complementary therapy for the management of pain secondary to bone metastasis. *Clin J Pain*. 1998:14:320–323.

52. Hamza MA, White PF, Craig WF, Ghoname ES, Ahmed HE, Proctor TJ, et al. Percutaneous electrical nerve stimulation: a novel analgesic therapy for diabetic neuropathic pain. *Diabetes Care*. 2000; 23: 365–370.

53. Cervik C, Iseri SO. The effect of acupuncture on high blood pressure of patients using antihypertensive drugs. *Acupunct Electrother Res*. 2013; 38: (1–2): 1–15.

54. Li J, Zheng H, Zhao L, Li Y, Chang X, Wang R, Shi J, Huang Y, Li X, Chen J, Li D, Liang F. Acupuncture for patients with mild hypertension: study protocol of an open-label

multicenter randomized controlled trail. *Trail.* 2013; 14: 380

55. Kessler RC, Soukup J, Davis RB, Foster DF, Wilkey SA, Van Rompay MI, Eisenberg, DM. The use of complementary and alternative therapies to treat anxiety and depression in the United States. *Am J Psychiatry.* 2001;158(2):289–294.

56. Yu J, Zhang X, Liu C, Meng Y, Han J. Effect of acupuncture treatment on vascular dementia. *Neurol Res 2006.* 2006;28(1):97–103.

57. Cuo XX, Jin HS, Huo L, Zheng J, Zhou XM. Meta-analysis on acupuncture for treatment of dementia. *Chinese Acupunct Moxibust.* 2008;28:140–144.

58. Zhang L, Wang J, Yao K, Zhang J. The treatment of vascular dementia in acupuncture based on syndromes differentiation in Acupuncture - Clinical Practice, Particular Techniques, and Special Issues. Edited by Marcelo Saad. Published by InTech. September 06, 2011, p. 62 under CC BY-NC-SA 3.0 license.

59. Huang Y, LI DJ, Tang AW, Li QS, Xia DB, Xie YN, Gong W, Chen J. Effect of scalp acupuncture on glucose metabolism in brain of patients with depression. *Zhongguo Zhong Xi Yi Jie He Za Zhi.* 2005 Feb;25(2):119–122.

60. Huan Y, Tang C, Wang S, Lu Y, Shen W, Yang J, C, hen J, Lin R, Cui S, Xiao H, Qu S, Lai X, Shan B. Acupuncture regulates the glucose metabolism in cerebral functional regions in chronic stage ischemic stroke patients: a PET-CT cerebral functional image study. *BMC Neurosci.* 2012;13:75. http://www. biomedcemtral.com/1471-2202/13/75.

61. Mukaino Y, Park J, White A, Ernst E. The effectiveness of acupuncture for depression - a systematic review of randomized controlled trials. Acupunct Med 2005;23(2):70–6.

62. Chou P, Chu H, Lin JG. Effects of electroacupuncture treatment on impaired cognition and quality of life in Taiwanese stroke patients. *J Altern Complement Med.* 2009;15(10):1067–1073.

63. Wang Z, Nie B, Li D, Zhao Z, Han Y, Song H, Xu J, Shan B, Lu J, Li K. Effect of acupuncture in mild cognitive impairment and Alzheimer disease: a functional MRI study. *PLoS One.* 2012;7(8):e42730.

64. Zhang H, Zhao L, Yang S, Chen Z, Li Y, Peng X, Yang Y, Zhu M. Clinical observation on effect of scalp electroacupuncture for mild cognitive impairment. *J Tradit Chin Med.* 2013;33(1):46–50.

65. Feng Y, Bai L, Ren Y, Chen S, Wang H, Zhang W, Tian J. FMRI connectivity analysis of acupuncture effects on the whole brain network

in mild cognitive impairment patients. *Magn Reson Imaging.* 2012;30(5):672–682.

66. Wang Z, Nie B, Li D, Zhao Z, Han Y, Song H, Xu J, Shan B, Lu J, Li K. Effect of acupuncture in mild cognitive impairment and Alzheimer disease: a functional MRI study. *PLoS One.* 2012;7(8):e42730.

67. Feng S, Wang Q, Wang H, Peng Y, Wang L, Lu Y, Shi T, Xiong L. Electroacupuncture pretreatment ameliorates hypergravity-induced impairment of learning and memory and apoptosis of hippocampal neurons in rats. *Neurosci Lett.* 2010;478(3):150–155.

68. Feng X, Yang S, Liu J, Huang J, Peng J, Lin J, Tao J, Chen L. Electroacupuncture ameliorates cognitive impairment through inhibition of NF-κB-mediated neuronal cell apoptosis in cerebral ischemia-reperfusion injured rats. *Mol Med Rep.* 2013;7(5):1516–1522.

69. Liu CZ, Li ZG, Wang DJ, Shi GX, Liu LY, Li QQ, Li C. Effect of acupuncture on hippocampal Ref-1 expression in cerebral multi-infarction rats. *Neurol Sci.* 2013;34(3):305–312.

70. Rosenthal TC, Majeroni BA, Pretorius R. et al. Fatigue: an overview. *Am Fam Physician.* 2008;78:1173–1179.

71. Yiu YM, Ng SM, Tsui YL, Chan YL. A clinical trial of acupuncture for treating chronic fatigue syndrome in Hong Kong. *Zhong Xi Yi Jie Xue Bao.* 2007;5(6):630–633.

72. Ng SM, Yiu YM. Acupuncture for chronic fatigue syndrome: a randomized, sham-controlled trial with single-blinded design. *Altern Ther Health Med.* 2013;19940;21–26.

73. Molassiotis A, Brady J, Finnegan-John J, Mackereth P, Ryder DW, Fllshle J, Ream E, Richardson A. Acupuncture for cancer-related fatigue in patients with breast cancer: a pragmatic randomized controlled trial. *J Clin Onco.* 2012;30(36):4470–4476.

74. Kamel NS, Gammack Jk. Insomnia in the elderly: cause, approach, and treatment. *AMJ.* 2006;119:463–469.

75. Sok SR, Erien J, Kim KB. Effects of acupuncture therapy on insomnia. *J Adv Nurs.* 2003;44(4): 375–384.

76. Cao H, Pari X, Li H, Liu J. Acupuncture for treatment of insomnia: a systematic review of randomized controlled trails. *J Altern Complement Med.* 2009;15(11):1171–1182.

77. Chen YF, Liu JH, Xu NG, Liang ZH, Xu ZH, Xu SJ, Fu WB. Effects of acupuncture treatment on depression insomnia: a study protocol of a multicenter randomized controlled trial. *Trials.* 2013 Jan 3;14:2. doi: 10.1186/1745-6215-14-2.

28

COMPLEMENTARY AND INTEGRATIVE INTERVENTIONS FOR ARTHRITIS AND BACK PAIN

Karen J. Sherman and Michelle L. Dossett

INTRODUCTION

Chronic pain is common in older adults, affecting up to 50% of community-dwelling seniors and up to 80% of seniors living in residential housing (1). Arthritis, especially osteoarthritis, and back pain are the most common pain conditions in older adults. Complementary and integrative medicine (CIM) is often used for symptom relief in these conditions. In this chapter, we will briefly describe the epidemiology of these pain conditions in older adults and review the evidence for the efficacy and safety of CIM in patients with osteoarthritis and back pain, focusing whenever possible on studies of older adults.

ARTHRITIS

Osteoarthritis is one of the most common musculoskeletal diseases and is characterized by progressive loss of articular cartilage in synovial joints, joint space narrowing, hypertrophy of surrounding bones, and thickening of the joint capsule (2). The resulting changes frequently result in pain, impaired mobility and activities of daily living, and reduced quality of life (2). The most commonly affected joints are the knees, hips, and hands. Risk factors include older age, obesity, female gender, history of heavy work or joint trauma, and genetics. The World Health Organization estimates that worldwide 10% of men and 18% of women over the age of 60 have symptomatic osteoarthritis, and that 80% of those with osteoarthritis have limitations in movement and 25% cannot perform everyday activities (3). In adults 75 years and older the prevalence of knee and hip osteoarthritis is 40% and 10%, respectively (3). The overall prevalence of osteoarthritis is expected to increase given the rise in obesity and the aging population.

Management approaches aim to reduce pain and to improve function, as no substantial disease-modifying interventions have been described. For severe pain, joint replacement surgery is usually recommended. Recently, a number of professional societies have updated their recommendations on the non-surgical management of osteoarthritis (4). They endorse weight loss, exercise, education, and self-management, as well as analgesics (e.g., acetaminophen and non-steroidal anti-inflammatory drugs [NSAIDs]) and assistive devices (e.g., canes) when necessary (4). Recommendations for the use of CIM therapies vary, though generally they are not recommended, or no specific recommendation is made. Notably, the effect sizes of available interventions (both conventional and complementary) are generally low to moderate (0.2–0.4) (4). Use of NSAIDs is limited by the risk of GI bleeding and is generally discouraged in the elderly. Recently, the European Society for Clinical and Economic Aspects of Osteoporosis and Osteoarthritis (ESCEO) published a stepwise algorithm (5) for the management of knee osteoarthritis, which includes a number of CIM therapies: acupuncture, manual therapy, tai chi, and prescription glucosamine sulfate and chondroitin sulfate.

Acupuncture

Acupuncture is one of the most studied interventions for osteoarthritis as well as other types of chronic pain. Manheimer and colleagues (6) published a review of trials of acupuncture for peripheral joint osteoarthritis that included 16 trials and 3498 participants. The mean age of the trial participants was in the early to mid-sixties for most trials. They found that for sham-controlled trials, acupuncture showed statistically significant, but clinically irrelevant, short-term benefits. Of note, however, the largest and best controlled trial included in this analysis was also the one most likely to have a partially active sham acupuncture arm, and the primary pain measurement occurred 7 weeks after treatment, thus potentially underestimating the effect of real acupuncture (6,7). Acupuncture provided both statistically and clinically relevant improvements in pain compared to wait-list controls and some other active treatments. The benefits of acupuncture were similar to that of exercise programs but appeared to have no benefit as an adjuvant to exercise. A subgroup analysis suggested that trials with an insufficient number of treatment sessions yielded fewer benefits than studies with an adequate number of treatment sessions (6).

Vickers and colleagues (8) obtained individual patient data to conduct a meta-analysis of acupuncture compared to sham acupuncture and to no treatment control (29 studies, n = 17,922) for chronic pain conditions. They chose only large, high-quality studies for their analysis. For studies of osteoarthritis, they found an effect size of 0.57 (95% CI: 0.50 to 0.64) for acupuncture compared to no treatment control (6 studies, n = 1968) and 0.26 (95% CI: 0.17 to 0.34) for acupuncture compared to sham acupuncture (5 studies, n = 1487). They found similar effect sizes for studies of acupuncture for other chronic pain conditions.

Corbett and colleagues (7) used a network meta-analysis approach to compare the efficacy of acupuncture to a variety of other conservative physical treatments that have not been directly compared in head-to-head trials. They did this by comparing relative improvements in short-term pain relief in the active arms to changes in usual care and placebo groups. In their primary analysis of 114 trials (9709 patients), eight treatments had a mean effect suggesting improved pain relief over usual care: interferential therapy, acupuncture, transcutaneous electrical nerve stimulation (TENS), pulsed electrical stimulation (PES), balneotherapy, aerobic exercise, sham acupuncture, and muscle-strengthening exercise. Using acupuncture as the comparator, acupuncture was significantly better at reducing pain than sham acupuncture, muscle-strengthening exercise, weight loss, pulsed electromagnetic fields (PEMF), placebo, insoles, neuromuscular electrical stimulation (NMES), and no intervention.

The authors also conducted a pre-specified sensitivity analysis of better quality studies that included 35 trials (11 of acupuncture and 9 of muscle-strengthening exercise) and 3499 patients. Compared to standard of care, the interventions that resulted in statistically significant better pain relief were acupuncture, balneotherapy, sham acupuncture, and muscle-strengthening exercise. In addition, acupuncture resulted in significantly better pain relief than sham acupuncture, muscle-strengthening exercise, weight loss, aerobic exercise, and no intervention. For studies compared to placebo-controls, inferential therapy (one study) also showed a strong effect. Of note, the studies included in this analysis were quite heterogeneous. Most were low-quality studies, and even some of the better quality studies were pragmatic studies where blinding was not possible.

Overall, these studies suggest that compared to sham acupuncture, verum acupuncture likely significantly improves osteoarthritis pain, in the short to medium term, although the overall effect size may be small. In addition, sham acupuncture significantly improves pain in many trials, and whether this is entirely placebo effect or a partially active intervention is unclear, as the types of sham controls used vary widely. Of note, few of the most common treatments for osteoarthritis, including NSAIDS, meet the cutoff for clinically meaningful effect sizes (6), and the effect size for acupuncture versus sham acupuncture is similar to that of NSAIDS versus placebo (SMD 0.32; 95% CI: 0.24 to 0.3 (7). Moreover, while the overall effectiveness of acupuncture may be limited, it is one of the more effective treatment options for short-term relief of osteoarthritis-related pain and has an excellent safety profile. The treatment frequency in these trials varied from one to three times a week and from 3 to 26 weeks. The optimal treatment frequency for pain relief has not been determined, nor has the average duration of treatment effect.

Two pragmatic studies (one from Germany and one from the UK) (9) examined the cost-effectiveness of acupuncture treatment for osteoarthritis and found that the cost per quality-adjusted life year (QUALY) (in 2013 US dollars) ranged from $6000 to $24,900, indicating good value.

Mind–Body Exercise

Three different meta-analyses have examined the effects of tai chi on pain in osteoarthritis (3,10,11). Two of these meta-analyses also examined physical function and stiffness (10,11). The trials included in these analyses are only partially overlapping and include wait-list as well as attention control groups. Two of these analyses included studies on hip (in addition to knee) osteoarthritis (3,11). All three analyses demonstrated short-term improvements in pain with tai chi relative to control groups, and improvements in physical function and stiffness were found as well (10,11). The authors encouraged the incorporation of tai chi into standard rehabilitation programs (11), yet cautioned that results may be limited by potential biases. There are insufficient data on the long-term benefits of tai chi practice for osteoarthritis. Nonetheless, this slow, meditative mind–body movement-based practice seems uniquely suited for the elderly and those whose health poses physical limitations.

Though exercise programs are commonly recommended for patients with osteoarthritis, there are relatively few published randomized controlled trials, and their structure and content are very heterogeneous. Escalante and colleagues concluded that overall, exercise programs based on tai chi had better results than mixed exercise programs, but without clear differences. There are little data at this time to support the use of yoga for relief of osteoarthritis pain; however, a few studies have been conducted (12).

Manual Therapies

One small systematic review (2) has examined the effects of manual therapy on hip (1 trial) or knee (3 trials) osteoarthritis. Recently, three additional studies assessing the effect of manual therapies on knee osteoarthritis (13), hip osteoarthritis (14), or either joint (15) have been published. Together, these studies have included a range of different manual techniques (physiotherapy, massage, chiropractic) and have suggested that these techniques may be more effective than usual care and possibly cost-effective as well (16). A dose finding study of massage therapy for knee osteoarthritis demonstrated maximum pain relief at 8 weeks with 60 minutes of treatment once weekly compared to usual care (13). However, this improvement was not sustained at 24 weeks.

Dietary Supplements and Herbs

DIETARY SUPPLEMENTS

The most studied supplements for osteoarthritis are glucosamine and chondroitin. Glucosamine is an amino sugar and an important component of glucosaminoglycans, a component of cartilage (17). As a dietary supplement, it is available as both glucosamine hydrochloride and glucosamine sulfate. Data suggest that the sulfate form is more effective; however, there are likely differences in bioavailability across glucosamine sulfate preparations (17,18). Chondroitin is a type of glycosaminoglycan found in articular cartilage, and the bioavailability of chondroitin sulfate also varies across manufacturers. Both glucosamine sulfate and chondroitin sulfate are available by prescription in Europe. The proposed mechanism of action of these compounds includes decreasing inflammation, increasing synthesis of cartilage precursors, and altering chondrocyte activity (17).

Numerous randomized controlled trials and meta-analyses have been conducted using these compounds, either alone or in combination with both positive and negative results. Trial heterogeneity (e.g., supplement formulation, dose, length of intervention, population, outcomes) and the poor quality of early studies in this field have been major limitations to understanding the true effect of these compounds (17). Overall, their safety profile is similar to that of placebo (17).

Many of the RCTs of glucosamine have been performed using a product by Rottapharm/Madaus, which appears to be more active than other products that have been tested and is purported to be in a more bioavailable form. In 12 trials of this product for osteoarthritis-related pain, the effect size was −1.05 (95% CI: −1.43 to −0.68) compared to an effect size of −0.11 (95% CI: −0.46 to 0.24) in 13 trials of other products (18). When the authors restricted their analysis only to studies with low risk of bias, the effect sizes were −0.27 (95% CI: −0.43 to −0.12, 3 trials) and 0.02 (95% CI: −0.08 to 0.12, 5 trials). The standard dose was 1500 mg of glucosamine sulfate once daily. There does not appear to be any benefit for hip-related osteoarthritis pain (17).

A meta-analysis of 20 trials (3846 patients, median age 61) examined chondroitin sulfate for treating osteoarthritis-related pain (19). Doses ranged from 800 to 2000 mg per day. The effect size was −0.75 (95% CI: −0.99 to −0.50). However, there was a high degree of trial heterogeneity that was largely explained by three study characteristics: concealment of allocation, intention-to-treat analysis, and sample size. Studies that reported analgesic co-interventions also showed smaller benefits of chondroitin. When the authors restricted their analysis to three large, higher quality trials that included 40% of the patients, the effect size was −0.03 (95% CI: −0.13 to 0.07). Notably, while more recent trials were generally of higher quality, they also tended to enroll patients with less severe disease (19).

In addition to assessing pain outcomes, some of the longer term trials have examined structural effects by assessing changes in joint space narrowing. A meta-analysis (20) assessing this outcome concluded that glucosamine sulfate had no effect on joint space narrowing over the first year of treatment, but had a small to moderate protective effect after 3 years of daily dosing (SMD 0.432; 95% CI: 0.235 to 0.628, p < 0.001). Similar results were observed for chondroitin sulfate, which had a small but significant protective effect after 2 years (SMD 0.261; 95% CI: 0.131 to 0.392, p < 0.001) (20). Thus, both of these compounds may delay radiologic progression of osteoarthritis after daily administration for 2–3 years.

A few studies have examined the use of other sulfur-containing compounds such as S-adenosylmethionine (SAMe) and methylsulfonylmethane (MSM) for the treatment of osteoarthritis-related pain. While initial studies appear promising, there are insufficient data to recommend the routine use of these products (21).

HERBAL SUPPLEMENTS

A growing number of herbal preparations are being investigated for osteoarthritis treatment, many with promising results in initial studies. Recently two Cochrane reviews have examined the body of evidence for oral and topical herbal therapies for osteoarthritis (22,23).

Cameron and Chrubasik (22) examined 49 studies of oral preparations of 33 different plants, used individually or in combination, for the treatment of osteoarthritis. There were no serious adverse events for any of the herbal products tested, and some appeared to have safety profiles that were better than NSAIDs. Many of these studies had a high risk of bias, and there were only a sufficient number and quality of studies to form definitive conclusions about two agents. They concluded that there is high-quality evidence that Boswellia serrata slightly improves pain and function in individuals with osteoarthritis. Individuals taking 100 mg of enriched Boswellia serrata extract rated their pain 17 points lower (on a 100-point scale) than individuals taking placebo at 90 days. The number needed to treat for an additional beneficial outcome (NNTB) was 2. Quality of life and joint changes were not examined.

They also concluded that there was moderate evidence that the avocado-soybean unsaponifiables (ASU) product Piascledine probably improves pain and function slightly but does not decrease joint space narrowing (22). People taking Piascledine rated their joint pain 8 points lower at 3 to 12 months compared to those taking a placebo. NNTB was 8. While there was no increased incidence of adverse events compared to placebo in the studies examined, a pharmacovigilance analysis has noted 117 post-marketing reports of adverse events with this product.

In their analysis of studies of topical herbal preparations, Cameron and Chrubasik (23) examined seven studies of seven different interventions including 785 participants in total. From a single study each, they concluded that topical arnica extract gel probably improves pain and function as well as topical 5% ibuprofen, that comfrey extract gel probably improves pain more than placebo, and that topical capsicum extract gel will likely not improve pain or function better than placebo. Side-effect profiles were similar for arnica and comfrey compared to placebo but were significantly higher for capsicum extract. As these authors used a strict definition of herbal preparation, they did not include studies of pharmaceutical preparations of topical capsaicin. In a separate review (24), they concluded from five studies of capsaicin ($n = 456$) that there was moderate evidence that 4 times daily use of topical capsaicin (0.025% w/v) cream over 3–4 weeks significantly reduces osteoarthritis pain (mean difference from placebo –7.65 on a 100-point VAS scale, 95% CI: –12.69 to –2.61).

Summary

Osteoarthritis is a major source of pain and disability in elders, and its prevalence is expected to increase in the next decade. The majority of studies in this field are focused on treatments for knee osteoarthritis (see Table 28.1 for a summary). The mean age of participants in most studies is in the early to mid-sixties; however, tai chi studies tended to enroll older adults with a mean age closer to 70. The effect sizes for both conventional and complementary non-surgical management approaches are low to moderate. Within complementary approaches, acupuncture, tai chi, massage, glucosamine sulfate, and condroitin sulfate (both pharmaceutical grade), *Boswellia serrata* extract, and possibly topical arnica and comfrey extract may play a role in pain reduction. It is important to note that placebo effects can be large in many trials of CIM for osteoarthritis, may be long lasting, and that this effect represents real relief of symptoms (4). Importantly, the safety profile of these approaches is generally better than

that of NSAIDs, an important consideration in the elderly population. Preliminary data suggest that acupuncture treatment may be cost-effective. Further studies assessing the cost-effectiveness of other approaches are necessary. At present, none of these complementary approaches are covered by Medicare (social insurance program for the elderly in the US), thus keeping these treatments out of reach for most senior citizens in the United States.

BACK PAIN

Back pain, typically affecting the lower back, is common among adults, with up to 80% of individuals reporting it at some point in their lives. A national survey found that about 30% of community-dwelling adults over the age of 65 reported back pain in the prior 3 months (25), with 6%–12% of all adults reporting disabling back pain (26). In adults of all ages, about 85% of back pain cannot be given a pathophysiological diagnosis, but in older adults, specific causes, including disc degeneration, disc herniation, soft tissue disorders (e.g., myofascial pain, sacroiliac joint dysfunction), spinal stenosis, and vertebral fractures, are more common (27).

Among older adults with chronic low back pain, Rundell et al. (28) found that both pain and back-related dysfunction were more severe as age increased. Only about 40% of patients reported a clinically important improvement in their back pain at 3 or 12 months, and about 35% had clinically significant improvement in their back-related dysfunction at these time points. Roughly 25% reported that their back pain had resolved by 12 months.

Risk factors for new onset back pain include previous back pain, depression, and poor self-rated health (29). Being female, presence of concomitant leg pain, worse baseline levels of pain and dysfunction, longer duration of symptoms, presence of pain in other sites, and a diagnosis of lumbar spinal stenosis are associated with persistent pain and disability (28).

Typical care for back pain is designed to reduce pain and improve functional status and should address other symptoms associated with pain, including psychological distress, impaired sleep, reduced appetite, and inappropriate increases in healthcare utilization. Rates of lumbar spinal fusion have skyrocketed more than increases in the prevalence of low back pain, even though they are not indicated for the

Table 28.1.   Summary of Data on CIM Therapies for Osteoarthritis (OA)–Related Pain

THERAPY	EFFECT SIZE (95% CI)	CAUTIONS AND CONTRAINDICATIONS	DOSING/NOTES
Acupuncture	0.42 (0.15 to 0.70) (reference 7) 0.16 (0.07 to 0.25) compared to sham (6)	Caution in individuals at high risk for bleeding and those prone to vasovagal episodes.	Studies included knee and hip OA with treatments ranging 1–3 times per week and 3–26 weeks; 6 treatments or less may be suboptimal.
Tai chi	0.45 (0.70 to 0.20) (11)	Individuals with severe pain in weight-bearing joints may have difficulty.	Studies included knee and hip OA with treatments ranging 1–3 times per week and 8–24 weeks.
Yoga	Insufficient data	May require modification or be contraindicated in individuals with cardiovascular disease or osteoporosis.	Insufficient data
Manual therapy	Between 0.48 (0.08 to 0.87) and 0.94 (0.44 to 1.44) (2)	Caution in individuals with cancer. Avoid if local open wound or infection.	60 minutes once a week for 8 weeks for massage for knee OA (13); 25 minutes twice a week for 5-6 weeks for combined manual therapy for hip OA (2,14).
Glucosamine sulphate	Between 1.05 (1.43 to 0.68 and 0.27 (95% CI: 0.43 to 0.12) (18)	Avoid in individuals with shellfish allergy.	1500 mg/day. May reduce joint space narrowing when taken over years. Non-pharmaceutical grade products may not be active. Benefit only demonstrated for knee OA.
Chondroitin sulfate	Between 0.75 (0.99 to 0.50) and 0.03 (0.13 to −0.07) (19)	Avoid in individuals with shellfish allergy and with prostate cancer (theoretical increased risk of spread).	800–2000 mg/day. May reduce joint space narrowing when taken over years. Unclear if reduces pain. Non-pharmaceutical grade products may not be active. Studied in hip and knee OA.
SAMe, MSM*	Insufficient data	Avoid use of SAMe in individuals with bipolar disorder due to risk of hypomania.	Insufficient data

Boswellia serrata	16.57 (24.67 to 8.47) (22) Improvement on VAS pain scale at 90 days	Caution, inhibits some CYP enzymes.	100 mg daily. NNT = 2. Only studied in knee OA.
Avocado-soybean unsaponifiables (ASU) product Piascledine	8.47 (15.90 to 1.04) (22) Improvement on VAS pain scale	Adverse events in post-marketing studies.	300 mg daily. NNT = 8. Hip or knee OA.
Arnica	3.80 (10.10 to 2.50) (23) Improvement on VAS pain scale compared to topical ibuprofen	Side-effect profile similar to topical ibuprofen gel.	Tincture applied topically 3 times daily. Single study ($n = 204$) of an herbal extract for hand OA.
Comfrey	41.50 (48.39 to 34.61) (23) Improvement on VAS pain scale compared to placebo	No	2 g applied topically 3 times daily. Single study ($n = 200$) of an herbal extract for knee OA.
Capsicum	1.00 (6.76 to −4.76) (23) Improvement in VAS pain scale compared to placebo	Causes skin irritation and burning.	2 inches of gel applied topically 3 times daily. Single study ($n = 100$) of an herbal extract for knee OA.
Capsaicin	7.65 (12.69 to 2.61) (24) Mean difference in VAS pain scores compared to placebo	Causes skin irritation and burning.	0.025% ointment (4 studies, 1 study 0.075%) applied topically 4 times daily. 5 studies of a pharmaceutical preparation for multiple joint sites.

*SAMe = S-adenosylmethionine, MSM = methylsulfonylmethane.

majority of older adults with chronic low back pain (26). Non-surgical management of low back pain includes medications plus a number of evidence-based non-pharmacological therapies, including exercise and physical therapy (1,30). Some medications typically used for back pain, such as non-steroidal anti-inflammatory drugs (NSAIDs) and opioids, are potentially problematic in older adults. However, the 2007 guidelines released by the American Pain Society/American College of Physicians recommended eight evidence-based non-pharmacological therapies for back pain. Four of these therapies were CIM therapies (i.e., acupuncture, massage therapy, spinal manipulation, and yoga). Effect sizes are typically moderate, with no clear evidence of superiority of one therapy over another.

A large number of alternative treatments, primarily non-pharmacological, are being used by individuals with back pain. Herein we review those that are most popular and contain the largest evidence base (i.e., acupuncture, massage therapy, spinal manipulation as well as chiropractic and osteopathic care, and yoga), as well as some promising therapies with emerging evidence (Alexander Technique, herbal medicine, meditation and tai chi).

Acupuncture

Reviews of acupuncture papers have been compiled for acute low back pain, sciatica, spinal stenosis, and non-specific chronic low back pain, as well as back pain in general. Overall, while these studies include needle acupuncture, they vary in the specific location and number of acupoints needled, the use of adjunctive treatments such as heat, the number of treatments per week, and the number of weeks of treatment. This variation, coupled with differences in the comparators used and the schedule of outcome assessments, which typically include pain intensity or pain bothersomeness as well as back-related dysfunction, makes summary of the results challenging.

In 2013, Lee and colleagues (31) reviewed 11 trials with 1139 participants who had acute low back pain. Eight of the trials were from China, one from Japan, and two from Europe. The dose varied from one treatment to up to 12 over a period of 4 to 6 weeks. While there were substantial methodological limitations, there were statistically

significant benefits of acupuncture for pain (mean difference = −9.38; 95% CI: −17.00 to −1.76) but not function compared to sham acupuncture, and modest but significant benefits compared to NSAIDS (RR 1.11; 95% CI: 1.06 to 1.16). In a network meta-analysis of patients with sciatica, Lewis (32) found that acupuncture and four other treatments (among 21 treatments from 90 trials and quasi-trials that were included in the analysis) were statistically superior to usual care or an inactive control. In a systematic review that included six trials from China (and 582 patients), Kim et al. (33) found positive results for "treatment success" for acupuncture for adults with lumbar spinal stenosis on pain, symptoms, and function, but given the poor quality and heterogeneity of the trials were unwilling to draw firm conclusions.

Lam et al. (34) included 32 studies in their systematic review of chronic non-specific low back pain, which found acupuncture effective for pain reduction compared to no treatment, medications, or sham acupuncture, but noted methodological weaknesses in many studies. Improvement in back-related dysfunction was evident among acupuncture patients compared with no treatment and medications (34). Compared to patients receiving usual care alone, those who were randomized to acupuncture plus usual care reported less pain and improved back-related dysfunction (34). Finally, Lam (34) found that patients receiving electro-acupuncture had less pain and improved back-related dysfunction. In an individual patient–level meta-analysis of high-quality randomized trials of chronic non-specific low back pain, Vickers et al. (2012) (8) found that acupuncture was superior to both sham acupuncture (effect size = 0.20; 95% CI: 0.09 to 0.31; 5 trials, $n = 1068$) and a no-acupuncture control (effect size = 0.46; 95% CI: 0.4 to 0.51; 5 trials, $n = 3864$). The vast majority of patients in most trials were under 65 years of age, though the trials that included older adults were also positive. Overall, acupuncture trials have been associated with a favorable safety profile.

The cost-effectiveness of acupuncture treatment for low back pain has been studied in two pragmatic studies (one from Germany and one from the UK) (9). The cost per QUALY (in 2013 US dollars) ranged from $7370 to $13,800, indicating good value by US standards.

Chiropractic, Osteopathy, and Spinal Manipulation

In a review of spinal manipulation for chronic low back pain that included 26 randomized controlled trials (6070 patients), Rubinstein et al. (35) found high-quality evidence that spinal manipulation had statistically significant, but clinically irrelevant, benefits on pain relief (mean difference = −4.16; 95% CI: −6.97 to −1.36) and on back-related dysfunction (standardized mean difference = −0.22; 95% CI: −0.36 to −0.07) compared to other interventions. When added to another intervention, spinal manipulation showed statistically significant improvement in pain and back-related disability in the short term. Very low-quality evidence found spinal manipulation not superior to sham manipulation or inert interventions for short-term pain relief or back-related dysfunction. No serious adverse events were associated with spinal manipulation.

In a review of spinal manipulation for acute low back pain that included 20 trials (2674 patients) (36), spinal manipulation was not superior to inert therapies or other recommended therapies. They noted that the number of trials for each specific comparison was small, however.

One trial reviewed by Rubinstein (35) focused on adults at least 55 years old and found that the typical technique of spinal manipulation used by chiropractors (HVLA, high velocity, low amplitude) had similar effects to a more gentle technique (LVLA, low velocity, low amplitude); both were moderately sized at the end of treatment. Three other trials of spinal manipulation in older adults are ongoing, but lack results.

Chiropractors can use a variety of manipulative and non-manipulative techniques that would be suitable for older adults who have special needs, such as frailty, severe osteoporosis and other bone diseases, or use of anticoagulant therapy. There has been considerable concern about the possibility that spinal manipulation is dangerous for older adults. Using Medicare administrative data on office visits, Whedon and colleagues (37) found that beneficiaries with neuromusculoskeletal complaints who made a chiropractic visit for their complaint were 76% less likely to have an injury to their head, neck, or body (trunk) in the following week compared to those who made a primary care visit for the same complaint.

In a systematic review of cost-effectiveness for guideline-endorsed back pain treatments, Lin (38) found that spinal manipulation was cost-effective for subacute and chronic low back pain. The cost-effectiveness of spinal manipulation for acute low back pain is presently unclear.

Massage Therapy

Kumar (39) identified nine systematic reviews of various types of massage for low back pain. Among those, Furlan (40) found two poor-quality trials (n = 158 patients) focused on massage for acute or sub-acute low back pain that found short-term benefits compared to inactive controls. For chronic low back pain (overall more than 1000 patients across the various studies), Kumar concluded that massage therapy may be effective in improving short-term pain and function compared to sham or placebo interventions, but is not consistently better than other active interventions. In a large trial of 401 patients, Cherkin (41) found that both relaxation and focused structural massage were superior to usual care in improving both pain and back-related function, with functional benefits persisting to one year, especially for relaxation massage. Older adults were not prominently featured in any of these trials, which had few adverse events, none of which was serious. A clinical trial of 140 Thai adults at least 60 years of age with chronic back pain randomized to receive 5 weeks of twice weekly 30-minute treatments of either Swedish massage with aromatic ginger oil or traditional Thai massage found that both groups improved their pain intensity and back-related dysfunction by the end of the treatment series (42). However, those randomized to Swedish massage had more significant reductions in pain and dysfunction, which persisted for 9 additional weeks.

Mind–Body Therapies

MEDITATION

Cramer et al. (43) identified three trials of mindfulness-based stress reduction (MBSR; total of 117 patients) for chronic low back pain. Compared to no treatment, MBSR was associated with clinically important short-term improvements in pain intensity, pain acceptance, and back-related dysfunction in patients with failed back surgery. Two trials of older adults with chronic back pain found that MBSR did not improve pain or back-related dysfunction compared to either health education or wait-list control. However, one of those trials found improved pain acceptance with MBSR. Two large trials of MBSR for individuals with chronic back pain are currently ongoing (44,45) and should offer more definitive conclusions about the value of MBSR for patients with chronic back pain. One trial (44) is recruiting 300 adults 65 years and older and randomizing them to a mindfulness intervention or an education control, while the other (45) has completed recruitment of 341 participants with chronic low back pain up to age 70 years who were randomized to MBSR, cognitive behavioral therapy, or usual care.

YOGA

Cramer and colleagues (46) conducted a systematic review and meta-analysis on the effectiveness of yoga for low back pain. They included 10 trials with 967 patients who had chronic low back pain, all under the age of 65. They reported strong evidence of yoga's short- and long-term benefits on pain reduction (standard mean difference = −0.48; 95% CI: −0.65 to −0.31; and SMD= -0.33; 95% CI: −0.59 to −0.07, respectively). For back-specific function, they found strong evidence for short-term improvement (SMD = −0.59; 95% CI: −0.87 to −0.30) and moderate evidence for long-term improvement (SMD = −0.35; 95% CI: −0.55 to −0.15). They found no effects on health-related quality of life, nor did they report serious adverse effects. One large trial included an economic analysis suggesting that yoga is cost-effective because it is well below the US thresholds of $50,000 to 100,000 per QUALY.

Since the publication of the Cramer review, several other trials have been published. In a study of 80 patients with chronic low back pain randomized to a comprehensive week-long residential retreat focused on either yoga or physical exercise, Tekur et al. (47) found those randomized to comprehensive yoga had significantly greater improvements in pain, anxiety, depression, and spinal mobility. In a trial of 95 patients with chronic low back pain, Saper (48) found equivalent benefits for yoga classes given once or twice weekly for 12 weeks. None of these trials has included adults over the age of 65 years.

TAI CHI

Compared to a wait-list control, Hall et al. (49) found that community volunteers with persistent back pain (up to age 70) had improvement in back pain intensity, bothersomeness, and back-related dysfunction after a 10-week course of tai chi (n = 160). Longer term follow-up was not available.

ALEXANDER TECHNIQUE

Little et al. (50) published a study that included 579 patients under age 66 randomized to either 6 or 24 lessons in the Alexander Technique, massage, or usual care, with half of the patients in each intervention receiving an exercise prescription as well. Patients randomized to both doses of Alexander Technique or to exercise (or Alexander Technique plus exercise) showed clinically important improvement at both 3 months and 1 year. The strongest effects were found in the group receiving 24 Alexander Technique lessons, regardless of exercise prescription. No adverse events were reported for the Alexander Technique.

Dietary Supplements and Herbs

DIETARY SUPPLEMENTS

Stuber et al. (51) conducted a systematic review to examine the evidence for the use of glucosamine, chondroitin sulfate, and methylsulfonylmethane (MSM) for patients with spinal degenerative joint disease and degenerative disc disease. One high-quality study with 34 patients (23 of whom had spinal degenerative joint disease) found no difference between the group receiving a combination of glucosamine, chondroitin, and manganese ascorbate and placebo. The second study, which included 80 patients with knee or low back pain, randomized patients to a combination of glucosamine, procine skin collagen, compos mucopolysaccharide, and vitamin C or a non-supplemented control group found decreases in pain intensity and increases in lumbar bone mineral density. They concluded that this contradictory evidence was insufficient to support the use of these supplements for spine degenerative joint disease.

HERBAL SUPPLEMENTS

Oltean et al. (52) recently updated a Cochrane review of herbal supplements for low back pain. They included 14 randomized controlled trials (with 2050 adults with acute or chronic low back pain) for six different herbs. Eleven of these studies had a low risk of bias, but even they had serious methodological flaws (e.g., lack of control for co-interventions, unknown allocation concealment). All studies were 6 weeks or less, thus providing only short-term data. Very few adverse events were reported, largely transient gastrointestinal complaints and irritations of the skin.

Devil's claw (*Harpagophytum procumbens*) was studied in three trials (*n* = 403 participants) as an oral herbal medication for chronic low back pain. Two trials with 315 patients found that doses standardized to 50 mg or 100 mg harpagoside were superior to placebo for pain relief and the need for rescue medication. A third trial of devil's claw with 88 patients found it equivalent to 12.5 mg of rofecoxib.

Three trials of willow bark (*Salix alba*) included 489 patients. Among those, two found that daily doses standardized to 120 mg or 240 mg of salicin were superior to placebo for pain relief and the need for rescue medication. A third trial that included 228 patients found that willow bark was equivalent to 12.5 mg of rofecoxib. One severe allergic reaction was seen, but other adverse events were relatively mild.

Five trials tested cayenne (*Capsicum frutescens*) in several forms, including plaster or creams (three trials with 755 participants who had chronic low back pain and one trial with 40 participants who had acute low back pain) and a gel form (one trial with 161 participants having either acute back pain or acute flare-ups of chronic back pain where the control group was a homeopathic gel). The four placebo-controlled trials found cayenne superior to placebo for pain relief with only minor adverse effects. The gel trial found pain relief from the cayenne gel preparations similar to the homeopathic gel preparation.

Three additional trials of lavender essential oil, Brazilian arnica, and topical comfrey (one for each herbal preparation) had high risk of bias, and their results are not described further.

Summary

Back pain, especially chronic pain, is the most common musculoskeletal complaint in older adults.

In addition to pain intensity and bothersomeness, older adults with back pain may suffer from impaired physical function and back-related disability, as well as difficulties with sleep, mood, appetite, social interactions, and reduced quality of life. While there have been a substantial number of studies of CIM therapies for chronic low back pain and a good number of studies of CIM therapies for acute low back pain, most studies have typically focused on adults under the age of 65 (see Table 28.2). The effect sizes for both conventional and CIM non-pharmacological therapies are comparable, typically of moderate size and all with favorable safety profiles. Currently, the most extensive and compelling evidence of benefits exists for acupuncture, spinal manipulation, massage, and yoga in the short term. However, yoga classes as typically offered in community settings and yoga studios would need extensive modification for many seniors, especially those with a variety of health conditions besides back pain. Most yoga instructors would not be qualified to do this, although there are some instructors who have extensive experience working with older adults and others who have a healthcare background. While limited evidence exists for benefits from herbal and dietary supplements, the short-term effect sizes appear comparable to those for medications, with likely better safety profiles than for NSAIDs or opioids. Economic analyses of acupuncture, spinal manipulation, and yoga suggest that they are cost-effective. At present, only spinal manipulation is a Medicare benefit, thus making most of these treatments inaccessible for most older adults in the United States.

SUGGESTIONS FOR FUTURE RESEARCH

Further research on CIM therapies for both osteoarthritis and back pain are warranted. For both conditions, studies in older adults are needed that focus on evaluating (1) additional CIM therapies, (2) the appropriate dose for all CIM therapies, (3) the full range of outcomes that CIM therapies might impact, (4) safety and adverse events associated with CIM therapies, and (5) the effects of CIM therapies over the longer term. Additional information on cost-effectiveness and cost savings, if any, would be useful. For osteoarthritis, further studies targeting older adults with hip osteoarthritis and hand osteoarthritis would be desirable. For back pain, further

Table 28.2.   Summary of Data on CIM Therapies for Low Back-Related Pain (LBP)*

THERAPY	EFFECT SIZE (95% CI)	CAUTIONS AND CONTRAINDICATIONS	DOSING/NOTES
Acupuncture	0.20 (0.09 to 0.31) compared to sham (8); 0.46 (0.4 to 0.51) compared to no treatments (8)	Caution in individuals at high risk for bleeding and those prone to vasovagal episodes.	Typically 10 to 12 treatments (1 or 2x/week); range was 1 to 20 treatments.
Chiropractic, osteopathy, and spinal manipulation	−0.22 (−0.36 to −0.07) for chronic LBP (35)	Caution in individuals with severe osteoporosis; chiropractor may modify treatment	Multiple doses/week more effective at the beginning of treatment for both chronic and acute back pain.
Massage therapy	Number needed to treat = 4.1 (41)	Caution in individuals with cancer. Avoid if local open wound or infection.	8 to 10 treatments may be needed. Inclusion of self-care most effective treatment.
Meditation	Inadequate data	May want to omit yoga exercises for older adults.	Typically use mindfulness-based stress reduction with 8 classes.
Yoga	−0.59 (−0.87 to −0.30) (46)	May require modification or be contraindicated in individuals with cardiovascular disease or osteoporosis.	Typically once or twice weekly classes for 8 to 12 weeks, sometimes supplemented with home practice.
Devil's claw	Inadequate data	High doses may cause mild stomach problems, long-term safety unknown; may lower blood sugar.	50 mg or 100 mg harpagoside
Willow bark	Inadequate data	Do not use if allergic or sensitive to salicylates (e.g., aspirin).	120 mg or 240 mg of salicin
Capsicum	Number needed to treat of 5 for plaster (52)	Cream may occasionally cause itching or burning on the skin.	

*Only CIM therapies with at least 3 studies are included here.

studies targeting older adults with specific causes of back pain, including disc disease and spinal stenosis, would be valuable. Studies that focus on special populations of older adults, such as frail elderly, individuals who are depressed, or those who have mild cognitive impairment, are needed. A focus on pragmatic trials with a broad range of the elderly is appropriate in all these settings. With the large increase in the proportion of adults over the age of 65 in the Western world, the need for additional research on these topics is even more compelling.

DISCLOSURE STATEMENT

Karen J. Sherman, PhD, MPH: Research grants: from the National Center for Complementary and Integrative Health and the Patient Centered Outcomes Research Institute. Consultant: on several NIH grants.

Michelle L. Dossett, MD, PhD, MPH, has no relevant financial conflicts of interest related to this chapter. She has served as a consultant for TJL Enterprises and has received grant funding from the National Center for Complementary and Integrative Health.

REFERENCES

1. Weiner DK. Office management of chronic pain in the elderly. *Am J Med*. 2007 Apr;120(4):306–315.
2. French HP, Brennan A, White B, Cusack T. Manual therapy for osteoarthritis of the hip or knee: a systematic review. *Man Ther*. 2011 Apr;16(2):109–117.
3. Escalante Y, Saavedra JM, Garcia-Hermoso A, Silva AJ, Barbosa TM. Physical exercise and reduction of pain in adults with lower limb osteoarthritis: a systematic review. *J Back Musculoskel Rehabil*. 2010;23(4):175–186.
4. Block JA. Osteoarthritis: OA guidelines: improving care or merely codifying practice? *Nature Rev Rheumatol*. 2014 Jun;10(6):324–326.
5. Bruyère O, Cooper C, Pelletier JP, et. al., An algorithm recommendation for the management of knee osteoarthritis in Europe and internationally: a report from a task force of the European Society for Clinical and Economic Aspects of Osteoporosis and Osteoarthritis (ESCEO). *Semin Arthritis Rheum*. 2014 Dec;44(3):253–263.
6. Manheimer E, Cheng K, Linde K, et al. Acupuncture for peripheral joint osteoarthritis. *Cochrane Database Syst Rev*. 2010(1):CD001977.
7. Corbett MS, Rice SJ, Madurasinghe V, et al. Acupuncture and other physical treatments for the relief of pain due to osteoarthritis of the knee: network meta-analysis. *Osteoarthr Cartilage*. 2013 Sep;21(9):1290–1298.
8. Vickers AJ, Cronin AM, Maschino AC, et al. Acupuncture for chronic pain: individual patient data meta-analysis. *Arch Intern Med*. 2012 Oct 22;172(19):1444–1453.
9. Kim SY, Lee H, Chae Y, Park HJ, Lee H. A systematic review of cost-effectiveness analyses alongside randomised controlled trials of acupuncture. *Acupunct Med*. 2012 Dec;30(4):273–285.
10. Lauche R, Langhorst J, Dobos G, Cramer H. A systematic review and meta-analysis of Tai Chi for osteoarthritis of the knee. *Complement Ther Med*. 2013 Aug;21(4):396–406.
11. Yan JH, Gu WJ, Sun J, Zhang WX, Li BW, Pan L. Efficacy of Tai Chi on pain, stiffness and function in patients with osteoarthritis: a meta-analysis. *PLoS One*. 2013;8(4):e61672.
12. Cramer H, Lauche R, Langhorst J, Dobos G. Yoga for rheumatic diseases: a systematic review. *Rheumatology (Oxford)*. 2013 Nov;52(11):2025–2030.
13. Perlman AI, Ali A, Njike VY, et al. Massage therapy for osteoarthritis of the knee: a randomized dose-finding trial. *PLoS One*. 2012;7(2):e30248.
14. Poulsen E, Hartvigsen J, Christensen HW, Roos EM, Vach W, Overgaard S. Patient education with or without manual therapy compared to a control group in patients with osteoarthritis of the hip: a proof-of-principle three-arm parallel group randomized clinical trial. *Osteoarthr Cartilage*. 2013 Oct;21(10):1494–1503.
15. Abbott JH, Robertson MC, Chapple C, et al. Manual therapy, exercise therapy, or both, in addition to usual care, for osteoarthritis of the hip or knee: a randomized controlled trial. 1: clinical effectiveness. *Osteoarthr Cartilage*. 2013 Apr;21(4):525–534.
16. Pinto D, Robertson MC, Abbott JH, Hansen P, Campbell AJ, Team MOAT. Manual therapy, exercise therapy, or both, in addition to usual care, for osteoarthritis of the hip or knee. 2: economic evaluation alongside a randomized controlled trial. *Osteoarthr Cartilage*. 2013 Oct;21(10):1504–1513.

17. Ragle RL, Sawitzke AD. Nutraceuticals in the management of osteoarthritis: a critical review. *Drugs Aging*. 2012 Sep;29(9):717–731.

18. Eriksen P, Bartels EM, Altman RD, Bliddal H, Juhl C, Christensen R. Risk of bias and brand explain the observed inconsistency in trials on glucosamine for symptomatic relief of osteoarthritis: a meta-analysis of placebo-controlled trials. *Arthritis Care Res (Hoboken)*. 2014 Dec;66(12):1844–1855.

19. Reichenbach S, Sterchi R, Scherer M, et al. Meta-analysis: chondroitin for osteoarthritis of the knee or hip. *Ann Intern Med*. 2007 Apr 17;146(8):580–590.

20. Lee YH, Woo JH, Choi SJ, Ji JD, Song GG. Effect of glucosamine or chondroitin sulfate on the osteoarthritis progression: a meta-analysis. *Rheumatol Int*. 2010 Jan;30(3):357–363.

21. Vangsness CT, Jr., Spiker W, Erickson J. A review of evidence-based medicine for glucosamine and chondroitin sulfate use in knee osteoarthritis. *Arthroscopy*. 2009 Jan;25(1):86–94.

22. Cameron M, Chrubasik S. Oral herbal therapies for treating osteoarthritis. *Cochrane Database Syst Rev*. 2014;5:CD002947.

23. Cameron M, Chrubasik S. Topical herbal therapies for treating osteoarthritis. *Cochrane Database Syst Rev*. 2013;5:CD010538.

24. Cameron M, Gagnier JJ, Little CV, Parsons TJ, Blumle A, Chrubasik S. Evidence of effectiveness of herbal medicinal products in the treatment of arthritis. Part I: Osteoarthritis. *Phytotherapy research: PTR*. 2009 Nov;23(11):1497–1515.

25. Strine TW, Hootman JM. US national prevalence and correlates of low back and neck pain among adults. *Arthritis Rheum*. 2007 May 15;57(4):656–665.

26. Freburger JK, Holmes GM, Agans RP, et al. The rising prevalence of chronic low back pain. *Arch Intern Med*. 2009 Feb 9;169(3):251–258.

27. Weiner DK, Sakamoto S, Perera S, Breuer P. Chronic low back pain in older adults: prevalence, reliability, and validity of physical examination findings. *J Am Geriatr Soc*. 2006 Jan;54(1):11–20.

28. Rundell S, Sherman KJ, Heagerty PJ, Mock CN, Jarvik JG. The clinical course of pain and function in older adults with a new primary care visit for low back pain. *J Am Geriatr Soc*. 2015 Mar;63(3):524–530.

29. Docking RE, Fleming J, Brayne C, et al. Epidemiology of back pain in older adults: prevalence and risk factors for back pain onset. *Rheumatology (Oxford)*. 2011 Sep;50(9):1645–1653.

30. Chou R, Huffman LH. Nonpharmacologic therapies for acute and chronic low back pain: a review of the evidence for an American Pain Society/American College of Physicians clinical practice guideline. *Ann Intern Med*. 2007 Oct 2;147(7):492–504.

31. Lee JH, Choi TY, Lee MS, Lee H, Shin BC, Lee H. Acupuncture for acute low back pain: a systematic review. *Clin J Pain*. 2013 Feb;29(2):172–185.

32. Lewis RA, Williams NH, Sutton AJ, et al. Comparative clinical effectiveness of management strategies for sciatica: systematic review and network meta-analyses. *Spine J*. 2015 June 1; 15(6):1461–1477.

33. Kim KH, Kim TH, Lee BR, et al. Acupuncture for lumbar spinal stenosis: a systematic review and meta-analysis. *Complement Ther Med*. 2013 Oct;21(5):535–556.

34. Lam M, Galvin R, Curry P. Effectiveness of acupuncture for nonspecific chronic low back pain: a systematic review and meta-analysis. *Spine (Phila Pa 1976)*. 2013 Nov 15;38(24):2124–2138.

35. Rubinstein SM, van Middelkoop M, Assendelft WJ, de Boer MR, van Tulder MW. Spinal manipulative therapy for chronic low-back pain. *Cochrane Database Syst Rev*. 2011(2):CD008112.

36. Rubinstein SM, Terwee CB, Assendelft WJ, de Boer MR, van Tulder MW. Spinal manipulative therapy for acute low-back pain. *Cochrane Database Syst Rev*. 2012;9:CD008880.

37. Whedon JM, Mackenzie TA, Phillips RB, Lurie JD. Risk of traumatic injury associated with chiropractic spinal manipulation in Medicare Part B beneficiaries aged 66–99. *Spine (Phila Pa 1976)*. 2015 Feb 15;40(4):264–270.

38. Lin CW, Haas M, Maher CG, Machado LA, van Tulder MW. Cost-effectiveness of guideline-endorsed treatments for low back pain: a systematic review. *Eur Spine J*. 2011 Jul;20(7):1024–1038.

39. Kumar S, Beaton K, Hughes T. The effectiveness of massage therapy for the treatment of nonspecific low back pain: a systematic review of systematic reviews. *Int J Gen Med*. 2013;6:733–741.

40. Furlan AD, Yazdi F, Tsertsvadze A, et al. A systematic review and meta-analysis of efficacy, cost-effectiveness, and safety of selected complementary and alternative medicine for neck and low-back pain. *Evid Based Complement Alternat Med*. 2012;2012:953139.

41. Cherkin DC, Sherman KJ, Kahn J, et al. A comparison of the effects of 2 types of massage

and usual care on chronic low back pain: a randomized, controlled trial. *Ann Intern Med.* 2011 Jul 5;155(1):1–9.

42. Sritoomma N, Moyle W, Cooke M, O'Dwyer S. The effectiveness of Swedish massage with aromatic ginger oil in treating chronic low back pain in older adults: a randomized controlled trial. *Complement Ther Med.* 2014 Feb;22(1):26–33.

43. Cramer H, Haller H, Lauche R, Dobos G. Mindfulness-based stress reduction for low back pain. A systematic review. *BMC Complement Altern Med.* 2012;12:162.

44. Morone NE, Greco CM, Rollman BL, et al. The design and methods of the aging successfully with pain study. *Contemp Clin Trials.* 2012 Mar;33(2):417–425.

45. Cherkin DC, Sherman KJ, Balderson BH, et al. Comparison of complementary and alternative medicine with conventional mind-body therapies for chronic back pain: protocol for the Mind-body Approaches to Pain (MAP) randomized controlled trial. *Trials.* 2014;15:211.

46. Cramer H, Lauche R, Haller H, Dobos G. A systematic review and meta-analysis of yoga for low back pain. *Clin J Pain.* 2013 May;29(5):450–460.

47. Tekur P, Nagarathna R, Chametcha S, Hankey A, Nagendra HR. A comprehensive yoga programs improves pain, anxiety and depression in chronic low back pain patients more than exercise: an RCT. *Complement Ther Med.* 2012 Jun;20(3):107–118.

48. Saper RB, Boah AR, Keosaian J, Cerrada C, Weinberg J, Sherman KJ. Comparing once- versus twice-weekly yoga classes for chronic low back pain in predominantly low income minorities: a randomized dosing trial. *Evid Based Complement Alternat Med.* 2013;2013:658030.

49. Hall AM, Maher CG, Lam P, Ferreira M, Latimer J. Tai chi exercise for treatment of pain and disability in people with persistent low back pain: a randomized controlled trial. *Arthritis Care Res (Hoboken).* 2011 Nov;63(11):1576–1583.

50. Little P, Lewith G, Webley F, et al. Randomised controlled trial of Alexander technique lessons, exercise, and massage (ATEAM) for chronic and recurrent back pain. *BMJ.* 2008;337:a884.

51. Stuber K, Sajko S, Kristmanson K. Efficacy of glucosamine, chondroitin, and methylsulfonylmethane for spinal degenerative joint disease and degenerative disc disease: a systematic review. *J Can Chiropr Assoc.* 2011 Mar;55(1):47–55.

52. Oltean H, Robbins C, van Tulder MW, Berman BM, Bombardier C, Gagnier JJ. Herbal medicine for low-back pain. *Cochrane Database Syst Rev.* 2014;12:CD004504.

29

COMPLEMENTARY, ALTERNATIVE, AND INTEGRATIVE MEDICINE IN THE TREATMENT AND MANAGEMENT OF DEMENTIA

Bruce J. Diamond, Susan K. Johnson, Katelyn Van Clef,
Stephanie Magou, and Briana Stanfield

INTRODUCTION

Dementia-related disorders have profound medical, psychological, social, and economic consequences for the healthcare system and for caregivers. The United States alone will be faced with the burden of 14 million individuals by the year 2050 with Alzheimer's disease. In that time, there will be 135.5 million people worldwide with dementia-related disorders in developed and developing nations. Why explore complementary, alternative, and integrative medicine (CAIM) approaches to treating and managing dementia? The answer lies in the fact that pharmacological interventions for the treatment of dementia-associated psychosis have shown limited efficacy, and many of these pharmacotherapies exhibit adverse effects. Depression is associated with decreased quality of life, reduced independence, faster rates of cognitive decline, higher mortality, and greater burdens on caregivers and society (Starkstein, Mizrahi & Power, 2008). However, there is no clear indication that antidepressants are effective in patients with depression *and* dementia (Bains, Birks, & Dening, 2002).

Moreover, pharmaceutical approaches for treating dementia using US Food and Drug Administration (FDA)–approved drugs have primarily provided only short-term efficacy. The impetus has, therefore, intensified for exploring alternative, complementary, and integrative approaches for managing and treating dementia, including pharmacotherapies and non-pharmacotherapies, which are generally better tolerated.

DEMENTIA IN CONTEXT

Alzheimer's disease (AD) accounts for the majority of dementia cases, followed by vascular dementia (VaD) (33% of dementias). In AD, histologic evidence generally shows amyloid angiopathy, gliosis, granulovacuolar degeneration, neuritic plaques, neuronal cell loss, and neurofibrillary tangles. Neurofibrillary tangles concentrate in hippocampal pyramidal cells, amygdala, and neocortex and can be observed in the locus coeruleus and raphe nucleus of the brain stem. Neuritic plaques predominate in the hippocampus and cerebral cortex, but may also be observed in the amygdala, thalamus, and corpus striatum (Zhang et al., 2013). Damage to the locus coeruleus is implicated in AD-related depression, and the plaque buildup and apoptosis associated with AD may be mediated by free radical activity associated with the aging process. This may explain why substances exhibiting antioxidant activity demonstrate beneficial effects (Diamond et al., 2003). While the pathogenesis of neuronal injury in AD is unclear, evidence suggests that Na+-K+-ATPase plays an important role and may exert neuroprotective modulating effects against AD (Zhang et al., 2013).

Vascular-based dementias are the second most frequent form of dementia, and multi-infarct dementia (MID) is the most common form (Diamond et al., 2003). Cerebral vascular insufficiency is a diagnostic category used in Germany, and it is characterized by 12 primary symptoms, including absent-mindedness, poor concentration and memory, confusion, lack of energy, fatigue, decreased physical performance, depressive mood, anxiety, vertigo, tinnitus, and headache (Diamond et al., 2000).

Dementia also includes Lewy body types of dementia (LBD), Parkinson's disease dementia (PDD), and frontotemporal dementias. Common symptoms of dementia include anterograde memory and attentional impairments and the behavioral and psychological symptoms of dementia (BPSD) (e.g., psychosis, agitation, anxiety, sleep disorders, and depression), which, if not effectively treated, can lead to institutionalization (Bains et al., 2002). Up to 70% of individuals with dementia exhibit disturbed sleep patterns, bedtime agitation, and night–day reversal leading to wandering, accidents, and disruptive behaviors (Diamond et al., 2003).

Diagnosis of Dementia

In the *DSM-5* (American Psychiatric Association, 2013), dementia is subsumed under neurocognitive disorders (NCDs), which are classified based on the putative etiological and pathological mechanisms underlying cognitive decline from previous levels of performance in one or more domains (e.g., complex attention, executive function, learning and memory, language, perceptual-motor or social cognition).

NCDs also include AD, vascular disease, traumatic brain injury, substance/medication induced states, HIV infection, Pick's, Creutzfeldt-Jacob, and Prion disease, and BPSD do not occur exclusively in the course of a delirium (American Psychiatric Association, 2013).

Underlying Mechanisms and Implications for Treatment

The mechanisms underlying dementia are not well characterized with the exception of hereditary AD and the vascular risk factors for VaD. While the multiple pathologies associated with the wide spectrum of dementias present treatment challenges, they also provide opportunities because there are potentially multiple therapeutic targets. These include, but are not limited to, β-amyloidosis and abnormal tau (AD), angiogenic and ischemic lesions (VaD), α-synucleinopathy (LBD), neurotransmitter abnormalities (glutamatergic and serotonergic), and cholinergic mechanisms. Inadequate cerebral blood supply, hypoxia-induced cellular membrane damage, oxygen free radical production during the re-oxygenation-reperfusion phase following ischemia, inflammatory mechanisms, apoptosis, and attenuated neuroplasticity (synaptic and dendritic proteins, trophic factors, and neurogenesis) are implicated in the aetiology of dementia as well (Perry & Howes, 2011).

Based on the premise that oxidative stress and the accumulation of free radicals contribute to neurodegeneration in AD, substances with antioxidant properties may slow the rate of dementia progression (Diamond et al., 2003) via the reduction of free radicals and products of oxidative metabolism. Overall, while individual response is variable, interventions that enhance cholinergic function by inhibiting acetylcholinesterase (AChE) activity show consistent and strong effects, with some evidence for positive effects on disease progression (Munoz-Torrero, 2008; Perry & Howes, 2011).

It is within this context that we explore alternative, complementary, and integrative (ACI) substances, techniques, and interventions, their underlying mechanisms of action, and their safety in the management and treatment of the cognitive, psychiatric, and behavioral symptoms associated with dementia.

INTERVENTIONS: PHARMACOLOGICAL AND NON-PHARMACOLOGICAL

Based on reviews and meta-analyses of controlled clinical studies, select well-tolerated herbals show promise in treating and managing dementia (Man et al., 2008; Perry & Howes, 2011). In addition, many AChE inhibitory alkaloids have been discovered in plant sources and their synthetic derivatives, such as vinpocetine (*Vinca*-derived alkaloids) and galantamine (originally from the snowdrop *Galanthus woronowii*) that also occurs in species of *Narcissus* and *Leucojum aestivum* (summer snowflakes) will be examined.

However, the therapeutic options for managing and treating the cognitive, behavioral, and psychological symptoms of dementia extend beyond pharmacotherapies that are ingested or include endogenous substances and/or their precursors or derivatives. Management options also encompass a variety of non-pharmacological interventions including body work, light therapy, meditation, music, movement therapy, and animal-assisted therapy, among others.

Taken together, a number of pharmacological and non-pharmacological interventions that have been examined in controlled studies show promise in ameliorating and managing, at least, some of the symptoms of dementia.

Pharmacological Interventions

OVERVIEW OF MECHANISMS

There are a variety of plants that have shown cognitive-enhancing effects and/or alleviate or mitigate behavioral and psychological symptoms in dementia trials. Naturally derived compounds utilizing a variety of mechanisms of action, such as acetylcholinesterase (AChE), protein kinase C (PKC), and glycogen synthase kinase-3 (GSK3) inhibition, neuroregenerative characteristics, and ion channel modulation may play a role in treating AD (Williams, Sorribas, & Howes, 2011).

The use of substances that enhance cholinergic function show treatment potential based on findings that volume loss of the cholinergic basal forebrain region is associated with cognitive decline in the elderly (Muth, Schönmeyer, Matura, Haenschel, Schröder, & Pantel, 2010). In fact, recent work

suggests that substances that enhance cholinergic function via the inhibition of cholinesterase activity have shown the greatest promise in treating dementia, primarily AD (e.g., the cholinesterase inhibitors [ChEIs] donepezil, galantamine, and rivastigmine). By inhibiting acetylcholinesterase (AChE) and butyrylcholinesterase (BChE), which break down acetylcholine (ACh), higher concentrations of ACh accumulate in affected regions. While they have shown efficacy in LBD and some evidence supports their use in VaD, evidence supporting their use to slow disease progression is equivocal (Howes & Perry, 2011).

Several plants and their extracts have shown promise in ameliorating cognitive impairments in dementia patients, for example, saffron (*Crocus sativus*), ginseng (*Panax species*), sage (*Salvia species*), and lemon balm (*Melissa officinalis*). The alkaloid physostigmine, a ChEI from the calabar bean (*Physostigma venenosum*) has been used as a template for the development of synthetic derivatives (e.g., rivastigmine) based on its acetylcholinesterase-inhibiting properties. ChEI alkaloids that have shown efficacy in improving cognition in AD include huperzine A (from *Huperzia serrata*) and galantamine, originally from the snowdrop (*Galanthus woronowii*). The cannabinoids (e.g., cannabidiol from *Cannabis sativa*) are potential therapeutic agents for BPSD. Resveratrol (plant constituent) and curcumin (from turmeric) (*Curcuma longa*) have been examined for their potential ameliorative effects in delaying dementia progression (Howes & Perry, 2011). Acetyl L-carnitine (ALc) has a chemical structure similar to acetylcholine and acts as a postsynaptic cholinergic agonist by increasing acetylcholine release and choline acetyltransferase activity (the main enzyme in acetylcholine synthesis). It also promotes cell membrane stabilization and stimulates nerve growth factor levels, as well as functioning as a free radical scavenger in mitochondria.

Several controlled trials suggest that ALc slows AD progression, but there is also a 1-year multicenter randomized placebo controlled (RPC) trial with negative findings. However, a post hoc subgroup analysis of one of the trials indicated that participants with AD onset before age 66 had a slowing in the progression of AD, while those with onset after age 66 declined faster than the placebo group. ALc is generally well tolerated but depression, nausea, vomiting, mania, confusion, and aggression in

AD patients have been reported (Sierpina, Sierpina, Loera, & Grumbles, 2005).

ADVERSE EFFECTS AND QUALITY CONTROL

Cholinesterase inhibitors (ChEIs) are associated with gastrointestinal and other adverse effects that can limit their desirability, thus providing an impetus for developing ChEIs with improved pharmacokinetic and tolerability profiles. Given the heterogeneity of phytochemicals derived from plant extracts, quality control over components and concentrations requires standardization procedures in order to ensure safety and efficacy. Continuing research on adverse effects and drug–phytochemical interactions, pharmacokinetics (i.e., blood–brain barrier permeability), and efficacious dosages is essential (Diamond et al., 2003; Howes & Perry, 2011).

LEMON BALM (*MELISSA OFFICINALIS*)

Lemon balm is reported to enhance memory and to exert calming, antidepressant, and anti-anxiety effects. In a double-blind random clinical trial (RCT), it was reported that *M. officinalis* enhanced cognitive function and reduced agitation in AD patients over the course of 4 months (Perry & Howes, 2011).

Putative mechanisms of action include AChE inhibition and antioxidant effects (essential oil and extract). In addition, it exerts effects on nicotinic and muscarinic receptor binding. The 5-HT1A, 5-HT2A, and GABAA binding activity of the essential oil and GABAA-mediated transmission are associated with reduced spontaneous synaptic transmission. Dosages range from 1 to 4g per day (Wong, Smith, & Boon, 1998).

While adverse effects are not generally reported, insufficient data support lemon balm's broad use during pregnancy and lactation. Moreover, it may also potentiate the effects of CNS depressants and interact with thyroid medications.

SAGE (*SALVIA OFFICINALIS L.* AND *S. LAVANDULIFOLIA*)

Sage is reported to exert memory-enhancing effects as well as exhibiting a variety of neurobiological activities. The extracts and/or essential oil monoterpenoids from *S. officinalis* and *S. lavandulifolia* have been shown to exhibit anti-AChE activity, anti-inflammatory (*S. lavandulifolia* oil), antioxidant effects (extracts, terpenoids, and salvianolic acids), and neuroprotective activity (rosmarinic acid from *S. officinalis*) (Howes & Perry, 2011). Indications commonly include treating disorders of memory and circulation. Dosages commonly include 320 mg divided in 3–4 doses of dry extract and 20 drops three times per day of liquid extract (Committee of Herbal Medicinal Products, 2009). While generally safe, caution is advised when taken with substances acting via GABA receptors, such as barbiturates and benzodiazepines (Wong, Smith, & Boon, 1998).

In a double-blind RCT with AD patients, a higher incidence of agitation was reported in the placebo group, suggesting that *S. officinalis* extract may alleviate or reduce BPSD (Howes & Perry, 2011). In another RCT in AD, the results indicated positive cognitive and behavioral effects, although in mild cognitive impairment (MCI; a condition with intermediate symptomatology between the cognitive changes associated with normal aging and the symptoms of dementia) in Parkinson's disease, a pilot RCT involving 25 patients did not demonstrate a significant cognitive advantage over placebo (Perry & Howes, 2011).

GALANTAMINE

Two of the drugs that have been licensed to treat the cognitive symptoms of dementia include cholinesterase inhibitors (ChEIs) that are naturally derived: galantamine and the synthetic derivative rivastigmine. Galantamine is extracted from snowdrop, narcissus, and lily species. It is an AChE inhibitor and a sensitizer of nicotinic receptors, which allosterically modifies nicotinic ACh receptors, potentiating the presynaptic response to ACh. Galantamine has a half-life of 5 to 6 hours and is metabolized by the same CYP-450 enzymes as donepezil (Akhondzadeh & Abbasi, 2006).

Dosage is usually 50 mg/day and it has not been associated with hepatotoxicity in clinical trials. While synthetic AChE inhibitors are known to cause GI upset, particularly nausea and vomiting, as well as more serious effects such as liver toxicity and heart rate irregularities, the toxicity level of galantamine appears lower than many similarly acting substances, while still providing significant benefit.

Although sample size was small and the follow-up time of 4 months short, correlations have been reported between improved cognitive performance in AD subjects receiving galantamine and increased hippocampal glutamate, which was thought to result from potentiation of presynaptic nAChRs, thereby increasing glutamatergic neurotransmission (Kennedy, Haskell, Wesnes & Scholey, 2004).

Meta- and pooled-data analyses of methodologically rigorous studies showed benefit in mild, moderate, and severe AD patients, with some work suggesting that the largest mean treatment effect sizes in cognitive improvement over 6 months were found in advanced moderate AD patients (i.e., patients with MMSE scores ≤ 12). Moreover, maintenance of functional abilities and delay of problematic behavioral symptoms were also significantly higher in the galantamine versus the placebo group. Additional support for this finding appears in work suggesting that galantamine delayed the time until patients required full-time care by 10%, and there is evidence that patients who cannot tolerate or did not respond to other AChE inhibitors benefit from galantamine treatment (Diamond et al., 2003). In RPC trials involving patients with vascular dementia or SDAT combined with vascular dementia, and using dosages of 24 mg two times per day of oral galantamine or placebo for 6 months, the treatment group displayed improvements in activities of daily living as well as behavior, with a significantly greater proportion of the treatment group exhibiting improvements on the ADAS-cog scale at 6 months (Diamond et al., 2003).

MELATONIN

Melatonin, an endogenous hormone that is produced by the pineal gland, is thought to be a prime mediating factor in regulating the sleep–wake cycle. It is a derivative of serotonin and appears to exert serotonergic receptor modulating effects, tuberhypophyseal and tuberoinfundibular dopamine and pituitary hormone releasing effects, as well as displaying antioxidant properties. However, while showing promise, there is evidence of potential serious side effects and drug and disease interactions, including heightened depression in those with depression and in those susceptible to it, thus precluding its routine use. Adverse effects associated with higher doses (suggested dose is 1–3 mg hs) may also include confusion (Diamond et al., 2003).

Day–night reversal and sundowning are often observed in demented patients and are associated with patient institutionalization. Deficiencies in melatonin appear to play a role in sleep disorders in the elderly, which suggests that melatonin may be a useful therapeutic agent. In patients with dementia who were given 3 mg of melatonin orally for 21 days, sleep quality improved overall. In addition, there was a decrease in the number of awakenings and nighttime agitated behaviors following 2–3 days of treatment (Diamond et al., 2003).

A recent study provides additional support for this finding. That is, in order to evaluate the efficacy of low-dose exogenous melatonin in decreasing delirium, an RPC trial involving 145 individuals aged 65 years or over who were admitted to the emergency department of a tertiary care center were administered either 0.5 mg of melatonin or placebo nightly for 14 days or until they were discharged. The primary outcome measure was the occurrence of delirium as assessed by the Confusion Assessment Method criteria. Melatonin was associated with a lower risk of delirium, thus providing support for the idea that disturbance in the metabolism of tryptophan and tryptophan-derived compounds (e.g., melatonin) may play a role in the pathogenesis of delirium (Al-Aama et al., 2011). Further support for this finding is found in a recent RPC trial that examined whether ramelteon, a melatonin agonist, was effective for preventing delirium.

Sixty-seven patients ranging from 65 to 89 years of age were randomly assigned to receive ramelteon (8 mg/d; 33 patients) or placebo (34 patients) every night for 7 days. The authors concluded that ramelteon may provide protection against delirium, which may support the idea of a pathogenic role of melatonin neurotransmission in delirium (Hatta et al., 2014).

In an RPC nutritional intervention trial involving 25 elderly subjects (86 ± 6 years; 20 females, 5 males) with mild cognitive impairment (MCI), who were randomly assigned to supplement their diet with either an oily emulsion of docosahexaenoic acid (DHA)-phospholipids containing melatonin and tryptophan (11 subjects) or a placebo (14 matched subjects) for 12 weeks, there was significant improvement on the Mini-Mental State Examination (MMSE) and a positive trend for semantic verbal fluency in the treatment group (Rondanelli et al., 2012).

In an RPC trial using bright light therapy and melatonin (2.5 mg/day) involving 24 patients of whom 10 had dementia and motor restlessness, in the six demented participants who completed the trial, the use of melatonin was not supported, but there was some support for light therapy (Haffsman, Sival, Lucius, Cats & van Gelder, 2001).

In several studies involving patients with AD who received dosages of melatonin ranging from 9 to 40 mg per day for durations of 22–35 months, sleep quality improved, neuropsychological functioning remained unchanged, and pineal gland function appeared compromised in demented but not depressed and normal subjects. This may suggest that the pineal gland may be functionally compromised in dementia (Diamond et al., 2003).

KAVA

Kava has been used as an anxiolytic and a relaxant in Europe and North America. Current evidence for herbals supports the use of *Piper methysticum* (kava) for generalized anxiety (Sarris & Kavanagh, 2009).

Mechanisms of action may be mediated by kava lactones, which potentiate GABA receptors and kavapyrones, producing an effect similar to that of benzodiazepines. Dosage is usually 70 mg 3 times per day. Adverse effects may include yellowing of the skin, exacerbation of symptoms of Parkinson's disease, hepatitis in rare cases, withdrawal symptoms similar to a benzodiazepine if the substance is terminated abruptly, and interactions with sedatives, hypnotics, and antipsychotics.

Systemic reviews have reported mild gastrointestinal complaints, headaches, dizziness, allergic reactions, dermatological reactions including flushing and itchy rashes, extrapyramidal reactions (oral and lingual dykinesias), disorientation (after taking kava and alprazolam), and potential liver damage. In fact, the FDA issued a safety alert to consumers and healthcare professionals (March 26, 2002), stating that "persons who have liver disease or liver problems or are taking drugs that can affect the liver, should consult a physician before using kava-containing dietary supplements" (US Food and Drug Administration, 2002). Kava-containing products have been associated with liver-related injuries, including hepatitis, cirrhosis, and liver failure in over 25 reports worldwide.

A number of RPC trials have reported that when compared to oxazepam (a benzodiazepine agonist anxiolytic), kava was more efficacious in improving performance on a visual search task. When kava (6 weeks, 120 mg/day) was compared to valerian (600 mg/day) in patients with stress-induced insomnia, both compounds were equally efficacious in relieving stress severity and insomnia with side effects reported by ~42% of the patients (e.g., vivid dreams: valerian; and dizziness: kava). It should also be noted that in an RPC trial using 300 mg of kava daily, there was no effect on optical orientation, concentration, reaction time, vigilance, and motor coordination (Diamond et al., 2003).

ST. JOHN'S WORT

Depression is often underdiagnosed in dementia, yet in Alzheimer's disease, 20%–30% of patients will develop a major depression. In dementia patients, the classic symptoms of depression, such as sadness and crying, may not be present, but instead symptoms such as pessimism, guilt, hopelessness, dwelling on past failures, and anhedonia are evident. St. Johns's wort (SJW) is, in fact, the most commonly used herb for mild depression (Diamond et al., 2003).

While the active component underlying the antidepressant activity of SJW is unknown, the mechanism of action is thought to be inhibition of reuptake of serotonin, norepinephrine, and dopamine, as well as an MAO inhibition-type mechanism. Active ingredients thought to mediate SJW's therapeutic action are the napthodianthrones, hypericin and pseudohypericin. Dosages are 0.3% hypericum, 300 mg three times per day. A recent review concluded that passion flower and valerian exhibited potential as sedatives, and St. John's wort and sadenosylmethionine as antidepressants, with selenium and folate complementing the antidepressants (Werneke, Turner, & Priebe, 2006).

Herbals may provide a safer pharmacological strategy for treating some of the behavioral and psychological symptoms of dementia, as many pharmaceutical antidepressants interact with other medications. Adverse effects of SJW are generally low, with photosensitivity, headache, dry mouth, dizziness, and various gastrointestinal symptoms reported. However, side effects are generally similar to those experienced by placebo groups.

A meta-analysis of 23 randomized trials of SJW found that SJW was superior to placebo and comparable to tricyclic antidepressants, with systematic reviews of RPC trials concluding that SJW is more effective than placebo in the treatment of mild to moderate depression. However, the response rate of SJW ranged from 23% to 55% higher than placebo, but 6% to 18% below tricyclic antidepressants (Gaster & Holroyd, 2000).

Several large-scale RPC multi-site studies, ranging from 6 to 8 weeks in duration, that included 587 patients with mild to moderate depression reported that SJW and imipramine were equally efficacious relative to placebo at reducing Hamilton Depression Rating Scale scores (HAM-D), with SJW exhibiting good tolerability.

However, SJW does not always exert beneficial effects. Several RPC trials involving over 500 patients, treated for 8 weeks, did not find any advantage for SJW over placebo or sertraline in reducing HAM-D scores. It is thought that patient populations in the United States may be more severely depressed and chronically resistant to treatment than the groups recruited in German and European studies (Diamond et al., 2003).

It should be noted that earlier meta-analyses and reviews evaluated studies that had methodological weaknesses, including diagnostically heterogeneous groups, short duration, and non-standardized rating instruments.

PANAX GINSENG

Panax ginseng acts as an anti-anxiety/antidepressant and has been used for treatment of cerebrovascular disease. *Panax ginseng*'s mechanism of action is thought to be via ginsenosides, with effects due to antioxidant activity and nitric oxide production. Adverse effects include swollen tender breasts, lowering of blood glucose, and interactions with antidepressants, sedatives, hypnotics, caffeine, and alcohol. Reviews of well-controlled clinical trials do provide some support for the efficacy of ginseng.

Recent open-label and single-blind trials in AD or MCI show some evidence for improved cognition in AD patients, although the evidence for efficacy in AD is limited. While reviews of several RCTs examining *Panax ginseng* in people with AD conclude significant effect in favor of ginseng, there were serious methodological flaws (Perry & Howes, 2011)

HUPERZINE A

Huperzine A (HupA) is a club moss, a naturally occurring novel Lycopodium alkaloid, also referred to as *Huperzia serrata* or *qian chen ta*, which is extensively used in China for treating Alzheimer's disease (AD), vascular dementia (VaD), and memory

problems. The active ingredient is huperzine alkaloid, which acts as an acetylocholinesterase AChE inhibitor (Diamond et al., 2003). It is a potent, selective, and well-tolerated AChE inhibitor with a longer duration of action and a higher therapeutic index than tacrine and donezpil. Therapeutic properties are thought to be based on its ability to regulate beta-amyloid precursor protein (APP) metabolism, and to protect against oxidative stress, apoptosis, and mitochondrial dysfunction, as well as anti-inflammation (Zhang et al., 2008). While having fewer side effects than tacrine and donezpil, adverse effects can include nausea, vomiting, and depression.

Huperzine A may offer some therapeutic benefits for mitigating mild cognitive impairment. RPC trials comparing huperzine A with placebo in patients to MCI are virtually absent in the literature (Yue et al., 2012). In RPC trials involving 126 participants with AD, MID, and senile memory disorder, extending from 3 days to 8 weeks, using dosages ranging from .03 mg two times per day to 0.4 mg three times per day, most patients showed improvements in memory, cognition, and behavioral functions compared to controls. However, studies generally have small sample size and short interval, and intervention timing is variable.

ESTROGEN

Some clinical trials report that estrogen may improve cognitive function in AD, although the evidence is equivocal. Estrogen modulates cholinergic and serotonergic function, influencing choline acetyltransferase production and 5HT2 binding. It can also increase blood flow and may increase the number of gliacytes as well as suppress the apolipoproteinE (ApoE), which precipitates the amyloid B-protein in senile plaques. Dosages can range from .0625mg/day to 1.25 of conjugated estrogen.

Adverse effects may include increased risk for breast and endometrial cancer, blood clots in the lungs and veins, breast tenderness, and uterine bleeding. Selective estrogen receptor modulators, such as raloxifene, may reduce the potential risk of breast cancer.

A number of case-controlled and RPC studies involving women diagnosed with AD (both with and without depression) and extending for durations of a few weeks to up to 4 months who were administered estrogen replacement therapy (ERT) (e.g., conjugated estrogen of 1.25 - ~.06254 mg/day) (Honjo et al., 2001) including transdermal estrogen (0.05/day dosage of 17B estradiol) in postmenopausal women with AD (Asthana et al., 1999) concluded that estrogen may improve cognitive performance. Improvements were reported on semantic memory (Boston Naming Test), verbal memory, orientation, calculation, and a brief cognitive screening instrument, with plasma levels of estradiol associated with better performance and combination therapy (i.e., tacrine and ERT) more effective than tacrine alone.

However, not all studies have found ERT to be efficacious. RPC trials involving participants with mild to moderate AD administered conjugated estrogen (1.25 mg/day for 16 weeks and 0.625 mg/day) have not reported improvements in cognitive function or in slowing cognitive decline (Diamond et al., 2003).

While some reports suggest that estrogen stimulates ACH metabolism, improves cerebral blood flow, increases the number of gliacytes, and suppresses apolipoprotein E., other reports do not substantiate these findings.

BACOPA MONNIERI

Bacopa monnieri (BM, or bramhi), which is rooted in Ayurvedic medicine (a 3000-year-old Eastern belief system for viewing disease and health that promotes the use of herbal compounds, special diets, and other unique health practices), has been used to treat a variety of neurologic and behavioral impairments. Putative mechanisms of action include antioxidant neuroprotective effects (via redox and enzyme induction), acetylcholinesterase inhibition and/or choline acetyltransferase activation, β-amyloid reduction, neurotransmitter modulation (acetylcholine [ACh], 5-hydroxytryptamine [5-HT], dopamine [DA]) and increased cerebral blood flow. Dosages range from 30 mg/day to 450 mg extract per day (Pase et al., 2012).

While long-term studies of toxicity in humans need to be conducted, human and animal models generally indicate that BM exhibits low toxicity (Aguiar & Borowski, 2013). However, *Bacopa* has caused gastrointestinal tract (GIT) side effects (e.g., increased stool frequency, abdominal cramps, and nausea) (Morgan & Stevens, 2010).

Several RPC trials have supported BM's nootropic usefulness with evidence suggesting that it can attenuate some of the adverse effects of dementia (Aguiar & Borowski, 2013). Systematic reviews of RPC trials in healthy individuals using dosages of 300–450 mg extract per day for durations of 12 weeks indicate that BM improved free recall performance on a majority of tests but with little evidence of enhancement in any other cognitive domain (Pase et al., 2012).

AD has been associated with type 2 diabetes mellitus at both the molecular and biochemical level, with amyloids forming in neurons and amylin forming in pancreatic cells, thus representing a potential link between these disorders. While there is no well-established treatment for either of these disorders, nanoparticles and *Bacopa monnieri* (Rasool et al., 2013) have been used as therapeutic agents.

In a meta-analysis of RPC trials using standardized extracts of *Bacopa monnieri* for ≥ 12 weeks, nine studies consisting of 437 eligible subjects reported improved cognition on the shortened Trails B test and faster choice reaction time (Kongkeaw, Dilokthornsakul, Thanarangsarit, Limpeanchob, & Norman, 2014). A recent review suggests that BM could play a role in improving memory performance in AD, exerting protective effects by increasing expression or activity of Na^+ and K^+-ATPase (Zhang et al., 2013). Some reports suggest that bramhi improved the retention of new information and in decreasing forgetting of newly learned material with no effect on attention, verbal, and visual short-term memory and retrieval of pre-intervention knowledge.

In an RPC trial involving individuals over 55 years of age, 81 healthy individuals were administered an extract of *Bacopa monnieri* (300 mg/day) or an identical placebo for 12 weeks. BM significantly improved verbal learning, memory acquisition, and delayed recall, as measured by the Rey Auditory Verbal Learning Test (AVLT). *Bacopa* versus placebo was associated with gastrointestinal tract (GIT) side effects (increased stool frequency, abdominal cramps, and nausea) (Morgan & Stevens, 2010). A recent review concludes that herbals including BM show potential efficacy in mitigating AD pathology and associated cognitive, behavioral, and psychological symptoms (Howes & Houghton, 2012). However, while *Bacopa monnieri* shows potential, larger trials are needed to support this conclusion.

ACETYL L-CARNITINE

Acetyl L-carnitine (ALC) has been used to improve short- and long-term memory. Dosages have been reported in the range of 1.5–3.0 g/day, and the mechanism of action is thought to be mediated by improvements in neuronal repair and the modification of acetylcholine production. Research reports generally suggest that ALC is well tolerated.

Enhanced alertness among patients with AD has been reported using 2500–3000 mg/day for 3 months, with some reports suggesting that ALC was associated with a slowing of AD progression when administered for a duration of 12 months (Diamond et al., 2003). A meta-analysis of RPC, parallel group comparison studies, where ALC was administered for durations of 3–12 months, showed a greater clinical and psychometric test summary effect versus placebo in mild AD (Montgomery, Thal, & Amrein, 2003).

VINPOCETINE

Vinpocetine, a synthetic ethyl ester of apovincamine, is a vinca alkaloid derived from the leaves of the lesser periwinkle (*Vinca minor*). The mechanisms of action are thought to be through enhanced brain circulation and oxygen utilization, inhibitory effects on phosphodiesterase enzyme (PDE), and inhibition of the aggregation of thrombocytes. It may also inhibit the operation of voltage-dependent neuronal Na+ channels, inhibit slow-inactivating potassium currents, and improve mitochondrial function, oxidative stress, and toxicity in cells treated with β amyloid. Based on vinpocetine's ability to improve streptozotocin-induced memory and learning impairments following 21 days of treatment in an animal model, it has been hypothesized that the mediating mechanism may be reduced oxidative-nitrosative stress, and restoration of glutathione (GSH), acetylcholinesterase, and lactate dehydrogenase levels (Deshmukh, Sharma, Mehan, Sharma & Bedi, 2009).

Vinpocetine exhibits cerebral blood flow enhancing and neuroprotective effects, which suggest a possible role in mitigating the adverse cognitive sequelae (e.g., memory) associated with cerebral ischemia and chronic hypoperfusion. Support for its potential use in dementia is based on the idea that reductions in blood flow and cerebral metabolism caused by cerebrovascular accidents may be mediating factors in the development of certain types of dementia (Patyar, Prakash, Medhi, & Modi, 2011).

The Cochrane Dementia and Cognitive Improvement Group's Specialized Register for human RPC trials, in which treatment with vinpocetine or placebo was administered to patients with Alzheimer's dementia, vascular dementia, or mixed Alzheimer's and other dementias for more than a day, concluded that among three studies comprising 728 individuals and one 16-week double-blind, placebo-controlled study, consisting of 203 people with mild to moderate dementia, there was significant benefit in the treated group. There were also benefits associated with vinpocetine treatment (30mg/day and 60 mg/day) compared with placebo in another trial.

No significant side effects related to vinpocetine have been reported, and it is generally considered to be safe for long-term use (Patyar, Prakash, Medhi, & Modi, 2011), particularly at reported dosages (Szatmári & Whitehouse, 2003). Taken together, given vinpocetine's role in oxidative stress and the fact that reactive oxygen species (ROS) play a prominent role in neuronal damage and apotosis, vinpocetine may provide potential neuroprotective effects (Patyar, Prakash, Medhi, & Modi, 2011). However, clinical trials have had methodological limitations, and the evidence supporting vinpocetine's use in dementia remains inconclusive (Szatmári & Whitehouse, 2003).

GINKGO BILOBA

Ginkgo biloba (EGb 761) has been used for dementia (e.g., Alzheimer's disease, vascular, and mixed disease), with RPC trials generally showing support in alleviating and mitigating symptoms and possibly slowing disease progression, although not all studies support Ginkgo's efficacy.

EGb 761, which is a Ginkgo extract manufactured to pharmaceutical standards by Dr. Wilmar P. Schwabe Company, Gmb, Germany, is used in most RPC trials and standardized to 24% ginkgo-flavone glycosides and 6% terpenoids, in addition to a number of other constituents (Diamond et al., 2000). EGb 761 may be administered intravenously in liquid form or through tablets or capsules in dosages ranging from 120 to 240 mg, although acutely administered dosages of up to 400 mg have been used.

The putative mechanisms mediating ginkgo's ameliorative effects on vascular dementia include reducing ischemia reperfusion injury, enhancing blood flow, and inhibiting platelet formation, while the hypothesized neuroprotective mechanisms in Alzheimer's disease include protection against mitochondrial dysfunction (implicated in AD), amyloidogenesis, and Aβ aggregation, ion homeostasis, modulation of phosphorylation of tau protein and possibly induction of growth factors, in addition to antioxidative, anti-apoptotic, and anti-inflammatory properties (Diamond & Bailey, 2013). Ginkgo's anti-apoptotic actions may be mediated via intracellular signaling pathways involving flavonoid and terpene fractions.

Orally administered extract of dry Ginkgo leaves administered to possible or probable AD patients is absorbed, metabolized, and crosses the blood–brain barrier within 3 hours, based on observed EEG changes. Ginkgo whole extract or its constituents have exhibited half-lives ranging from 2 to 4 hours and activity levels that peak at 1.5 to 3 hours in animal and human models (Diamond et al., 2000).

The evidence is equivocal for a causal association between Ginkgo and bleeding, as well as for changes in blood coagulation parameters. Given that Ginkgo intake may lead to inhibition of platelet aggregation and increased bleeding time, patients should be advised that there is an increased risk of bleeding, particularly when Ginkgo is used with medications exerting synergistic effects. However, Ginkgo has a long history of use, and a large number of studies suggest that it is generally safe, with few verified adverse drug interactions (Diamond & Bailey, 2013).

Clinical indications include dementia-related symptoms associated with AD, normal aging, traumatic brain injury, stroke, multi-infarcts, cerebral atherosclerosis, and cerebral insufficiency. Meta-analyses indicate that the cognitive domains yielding the largest proportion of significant effects compared with placebo are selective attention, executive functions (e.g., planning, working memory, cognitive flexibility, and information-processing speed), fluid intelligence, and short-term and long-term visual and verbal memory (Diamond & Bailey, 2013).

Recent RPC studies with AD, including a study conducted over a 26-week period, reported that EGb 761 produced significant improvements in cognitive function compared to a placebo group, while displaying a safety record comparable to placebo. Recent comprehensive surveys of multiple clinical trials have reported similar results with EGb 761

(Akhondzadeh & Abbasi, 2006). EGb 761 has also improved BPSD in dementia patients compared to placebo; in an RPC trial with 400 patients diagnosed with AD or VaD, using 240 mg/day for 22 weeks, the Ginkgo group was superior to placebo on the Neuropsychiatric Inventory (NPI) and an activities-of-daily-living scale. In an RPC trial with AD patients showing neuropsychiatric features, treatment with either donepezil or EGb 761 and in combination significantly improved cognition and neuropsychiatric symptoms (Perry & Howes, 2011).

Several Cochrane reviews report mixed results, some reporting improvement in cognition and activities of daily living, or no or inconsistent evidence for Ginkgo's clinical benefits. However, psychological data from 29 pooled RPC trials suggest that EGb 761 exerted positive therapeutic effects versus placebo on selective attention and executive function (Kaschel, 2009). Similar positive effects in AD and VaD were also observed in another study, with fewer side effects reported than placebo (Napryeyenko & Borzenko, 2007).

While controlled studies generally support Ginkgo's efficacy and safety in healthy and clinical populations, efficacy has not always been demonstrated with some reports, indicating that Ginkgo was no more effective than either nicergoline or dihydroergotoxine in treating cerebrovascular disease or in treating the symptoms of vascular dementia (Diamond et al., 2000).

Taken together, over the last several decades, reviews and meta-analyses of RPC trials with clear inclusion, exclusion, and diagnostic criteria over durations of 1–6 months, using dosages of 120–240 mg/day of standardized extract suggest that Ginkgo was effective in improving neurologic functions (e.g., cognitive, mood, motor, headache, motivational, EEG activation) across a diverse etiological spectrum (e.g., cerebral insufficiency, Alzheimer's disease, multi-infarct dementia). However, reviews by the Cochrane Collaboration conclude that cholinesterase inhibitors exhibit greater consistency and robust effects on cognition, with some investigators suggesting that cholinesterase inhibitors be used in preference to Ginkgo biloba in patients with mild to moderate AD (Akhondzadeh & Abbasi, 2006).

HERBAL AND DRUG INTERACTIONS

A majority of dementia patients will be prescribed numerous drugs, thereby increasing the probability of herbal–drug interactions and possible adverse events. Because most patients do not report herbal or alternative therapy use to their physicians, the incidence of adverse events from herb–drug interactions is difficult to determine.

Systematic reviews have, however, identified interactions between herbs (e.g., SJW, gingko, kava, valerian, and ginseng) and conventional drugs. For example, SJW reduces the concentrations of cyclosporine, protease inhibitors, and digoxin in blood. Conversely, SJW may enhance the effects of selective serotonin reuptake inhibitors (SSRIs) to the level of a "serotonin syndrome." Cases of tremor, gastrointestinal symptoms, restlessness, myalgia, headache, and confusion have been reported. There may also be an increased risk of bleeding, particularly when Ginkgo is used with medications exerting inhibitory effects on platelet aggregation (Diamond & Bailey, 2013) (see Table 29.1).

Non-Pharmacologic Complementary and Alternative Medical (CAM) Approaches for Managing and Treating Dementia

Non-pharmacological interventions may provide complementary tools and techniques for reducing behavioral and mood disturbances in dementia, improving social interactions and stabilizing or improving cognitive problems.

ANIMAL-ASSISTED INTERVENTIONS

Animal-assisted interventions (AAI), consisting of therapy and activities, have gained in popularity in recent years. Animal contact can provide social interaction, stimulate conversation, and reduce anxiety in persons with dementia. AAI also has the potential to lower disturbing behaviors. In a 2010 review paper, O'Haire summarized results from three studies demonstrating that AAIs could decrease agitation and aggression, and increase socialization and nutritional intake in Alzheimer's disease care units. Possible mechanisms of action include b-endorphin, oxytocin, prolactin, phenylacetic acid, and dopamine increases and a significant decrease in cortisol in humans, accompanied by decreases in blood pressure (Odendaal, 2000).

However, AAIs can introduce liability issues associated with using live animals, such as inducing fear, invoking allergies, and the risk of infections or accidents for nursing home residents. Robotic pets may provide a viable alternative to live animals (Kramer, Friedmann, & Bernstein, 2009). A study conducted in nursing home residents compared one visit a week for 3 weeks with either a human visitor, a live pet and human visitor, or a robotic pet and human visitor. Results indicated that while all three visits stimulated social interactions, the robotic dog stimulated the most, followed by the live dog. This suggests that novel interactions with animals, whether robotic or live, have the potential to stimulate social interactions in those with dementia.

Other studies have demonstrated the effectiveness of various dog-related stimuli on social engagement in those with dementia (Marx, Cohen-Mansfield, Regier, Dakheel-Ali, Srihari, & Thein, 2010). The stimuli consisted of a dog coloring book, a robotic dog, a plush dog, a puppy video, a small dog, a medium dog, and a large dog. Results showed that the puppy video engaged the participants for the longest duration, with the large dogs following behind. However, the real dogs garnered the most positive attitudes, with the large dog receiving the most positive responses out of the three dog types. The robotic dog garnered a positive response as well. Although bringing real dogs to nursing homes may not always be possible, dog-related stimuli such as robotic dogs and videos may be a viable option to provide interaction and stimulation.

Aquariums are an innovative and cost-effective way for animals and nature to be introduced into dementia units. Edwards, Beck, and Lim (2014) reported that after the introduction of aquariums, residents showed improvements in cooperativeness and sleep and decreases in irrational thinking and inappropriate behaviors. Importantly, the staff's satisfaction score significantly improved as well. Animals have provided comfort to humans since earliest recorded history, particularly for people who are socially isolated because of severe cognitive impairment. This type of nonverbal comfort and stimulation may be particularly appropriate and effective.

MUSIC AND MOVEMENT THERAPY

Another approach for providing stimulation and social interaction and improving mood in the nonverbal sphere could be music and movement interventions. Researchers have examined whether music therapy could have beneficial effects on

Table 29.1.   Pharmacologic Interventions

INTERVENTION	INDICATIONS	MECHANISMS	DOSE/ DURATION	ADVERSE EFFECTS	AUTHORS
Lemon balm	Memory, mood	Nicotinic and muscarinic receptor binding	1–4g per/day	Potentiate CNS depressants; unsupported for use during pregnancy	Howes & Perry (2011); Wong, Smith, Boon (1998)
Sage	Memory	Anti-AChE	Dry extract: 320 mg divided in 3–4 doses. Liquid: 20 drops 3x day	Generally safe but caution when used with substances acting via GABA receptors	Howes & Perry (2011); Wong, Smith, Boon (1998)
Galantamine	Cognitive symptoms	AChE inhibitor, nicotinic and ACh receptor modifier	50 mg/day	Nausea, vomiting, liver toxicity, heart irregularities	Akhondzadeh & Abbasi (2006); Kennedy et al. (2004)
Melatonin	Sleep quality, nighttime agitation, delirium	Antioxidant, modulates serotonergic receptors	1–3 mg/day	Depression, confusion	Al-Aama et al. (2011); Diamond et al. (2003); Haffsman, Sival, Lucius, Cats, & van Gelder,(2001); Rondanelli et al. (2012)
Kava	Anxiety, mood, relaxant	Potentiates GABA receptors	70 mg/3x day	Jaundice, exacerbation of: Parkinson's disease, hepatitis, liver disease. Interaction with sedatives, hypnotics, and antipsychotics. Withdrawal effects	Sarris (2009); Diamond et al. (2003)
St John's wort	Depression, behavioral symptoms	Inhibits serotonin, norepinephrine and dopamine reuptake. MAO inhibitor	300 mg/3x day	Photosensitivity, headache, dry mouth, dizziness, GI symptoms	Gaster & Holroyd (2000); Werneke, Turner, & Priebe (2006)
Panax ginseng	Anxiety, depression	Antioxidant activity, nitric oxide production		Swollen/tender breasts, low blood glucose. Interacts with antidepressants, sedatives, hypnotics, caffeine, alcohol	Perry & Howes (2011)

Supplement	Target	Mechanism	Dosage	Side effects	References
Huperzine A	Memory, cognitive and behavioral functioning	AChE inhibitor	0.3–0.4 mg/2x day	Nausea, vomiting, depression	Diamond et al. (2003); Yue et al. (2012); Zhang et al. (2008);
Estrogen	Cognition	Modulates cholinergic and serotonergic function, increases blood flow and gliacytes, suppresses APoE	30–450 mg/day	Increases risk for breast and endometrial cancer, blood clots in the lungs and veins, breast tenderness and uterine bleeding	Asthana et al. (1999); Diamond et al. (2003); Honjo et al. (2001)
Bacopa monnieri	Memory: Recall	Antioxidant effects, acetylcholinesterase inhibition, choline acetyltransferase activation, beta-amyloid reduction, increased cerebral blood flow	30–450 mg/day	GI effects	Aguiar & Borowski (2013); Howes & Houghton (2012); Morgan & Stevens (2010); Pase et al. (2012)
Acetyl L-carnitine	Short-term and long-term memory, alertness	Neuronal repair, modification of acetylcholine production	2500–3000 mg/day	Generally well tolerated	Diamond et al. (2003) Montgomery, Thal. & Amrein (2003)
Vinpocetine	Memory and cognition	Increased cerebral blood flow, inhibitory effects on phosphodiesterase enzyme, inhibition of thrombocyte aggregation	30–60 mg/day	Generally safe for long-term use	Deshmukh, Sharma, Mehan, Sharma, & Bedi (2009); Patyar, Prakash, Medhi, & Modi (2011); Szatmari & Whitehouse (2003)
Gingko biloba	Neurologic function, mood, memory	Reduces ischemia reperfusion injury, increases blood flow, anti-platelet, protection against mitochondrial dysfunction, antioxidant, anti-apoptotic and anti-inflammatory	120–400mg/day	Changes in blood coagulation. Caution when used with medications exerting antiplatelet properties.	Diamond et al. (2000); Diamond & Bailey (2013); Napryyenko & Borzenko (2007); Kaschel (2009)

the psychological problems associated with AD. Music therapy can be administered in two ways, either through a participant listening to music or a participant performing music. The therapeutic effects of music therapy may be mediated by several mechanisms, including modulating effects on attention, cognition (memory processes), and emotion (via limbic and paralimbic brain structures) (Koelsch, 2009).

Svansdottir and Snaedal (2006) examined the performance type of music therapy in a RCT using the BEHAVE-AD scale at baseline and at 6- and 10-week intervals. The control group received no treatment and the music therapy group received three 30-minute music therapy sessions per week for 6 weeks. The results showed a decrease in activity disturbances, aggressiveness, and anxiety, as rated by the BEHAVE-AD scale, in the experimental group and not the control group. These benefits disappeared 4 weeks after stopping music therapy sessions.

Guetin et al. (2009) examined music therapy for decreasing anxiety and depression in AD. The study consisted of an active control group who received weekly reading sessions and the experimental group who received weekly individual listening-type music therapy customized to their musical taste. The sessions lasted 16 weeks. Assessments were obtained at 0-, 4-, 8-, 16-, and 24-week intervals, using the Hamilton Anxiety Scale, Geriatric Depression Scale, and the MMSE. Between week 0 and 16, the anxiety levels of the patients in the music group decreased significantly compared to the control group at 16 weeks and at the 24-week follow-up. While not statistically significant, depression was lower in the experimental versus the control group. Music therapy appears to have beneficial effects on the psychological symptoms associated with dementia and can be administered easily without adverse effects.

The combination of music and social interaction may improve mood, communication, and levels of engagement, which could reduce agitation in dementia. A Taiwanese RCT (Sung, Chang, Lee, & Lee, 2006) randomly assigned participants in the experimental condition to group music and movement intervention twice a week for 4 weeks. The participants listened to familiar music and were encouraged to move around to the rhythm of the songs. The Modified Cohen-Mansfield Agitation Inventory was used to measure agitation. Participants in the experimental group exhibited a decrease in agitation at 2 weeks and a significant

decrease at 4 weeks compared to controls (Sung et al., 2006).

People with dementia often have difficulties communicating emotions, which can exacerbate agitation and aggression. Gotell, Brown, and Ekman (2009) examined improving emotional engagement in Swedish nursing home residents with dementia by having them listen to singing. There were three conditions: no music, background music, and a caregiver singing, with all conditions taking place during morning care sessions. It was reported that communication improved and there was less aggression and more expression of positive emotions between caregivers and participants when they listened to their caregiver singing and to background music. There was also an increase in intimacy between caregivers and patients when participants listened to their caregiver sing (Gotell, Brown, & Ekman, 2009).

Interactive live music performances can increase levels of engagement in dementia patients. A live performance by professional singers for patients with moderate to severe dementia from six different nursing homes in the Netherlands was evaluated by caregivers and family members using observational scales a day after the performance. Results indicated that mental well-being and social engagement both improved significantly in patients with mild dementia, while social engagement improved significantly in those with severe dementia (van der Vleuten, Visser, & Meeuwesen, 2012).

Dance therapy has also been attempted with dementia patients. Putative mechanisms of action may be based on beneficially modulating serotonin and dopamine concentrations (Jeong, Hong, Lee, Park, Kim, & Suh, 2005). In a pilot study conducted in England, the effects of 10 weekly sessions of guided circle dancing were examined in people with moderate to severe dementia (Hamill, Smith, & Rohrict, 2011). The MMSE, Quality of Life Scale (QOL) in AD, and General Health questionnaire were used to measure participants' mood and QOL at baseline and after the dancing sessions. Results demonstrated that the circle dancing group displayed improved mood, concentration, and communication (Hamill et. al., 2011).

Mind–body movement practices have also shown some promise in older community-residing adults. For example, Siddarth, Siddarth, and Lavretsky (2014) found that yoga and tai chi improved mood and sleep problems in older adults. Taken together, mind–body approaches may offer potential benefits for people in the early stages of dementia.

LIGHT THERAPY

Degenerative changes in the suprachiasmic nucleus of the hypothalamus appear to be a biological basis for circadian disturbances in people with dementia. Accordingly, bright light therapy (BLT) was proposed for improving agitation and sleep disturbances in people with dementia, and some early studies appear promising. Light therapy may exert effects via entrainment of the circadian melatonin rhythm. Melatonin, which is a derivative of serotonin, is thought to mediate regulation of the sleep–wake cycle (Diamond et al., 2003).

A Cochrane review in 2004 found only 60% of the studies of sufficient quality and concluded that there was insufficient evidence that BLT affected sleep, behaviors, or mood in dementia (Forbes et al., 2004). Subsequent studies similarly found only limited evidence for effectiveness in depression (Hickman et al., 2007) or reduction in agitation (Burns, Allen, Tomenson, Duignan, & Byrne, 2009).

Nonetheless, Riemersma-van der Lek et al. (2008) found that all-day light, combined with melatonin, reduced agitation. Given these mixed findings, Barrick et al. (2010) used a cluster-unit cross-over design with multiple light dosage regimens while controlling for confounding factors such as staff interaction. They found no ameliorative effect for BLT on agitation and that BLT could increase agitation in mild/moderate dementia patients. It appears that BLT must be combined with melatonin in order to reduce agitation. Furthermore, an updated Cochrane review (Forbes, Blake, Thiessen, Peacock, & Hawranik, 2014) found that only 1/10 of the randomized controlled trials supported any positive results. In most studies, the treatment groups received light therapy ranging from 2500 to 10,000 lux either in the morning or evening for durations of 1–2 hours for 10 days to 2 months. The one positive study found a reduction in the development of activities of daily living (ADL) limitations at three out of five time points. However, the preponderance of evidence does not support BLT as a useful alternative for problem behaviors in people with dementia.

ACUPUNCTURE

Acupuncture researchers have proposed that specific acupoint stimulation could stimulate neural pathways and neurochemical activity, producing benefits in people with AD. Animal models have been promising, demonstrating changes such as enhanced cholinergic neurotransmission, reduced apoptotic and oxidative damage, improved synaptic plasticity, and decreased levels of Aβ proteins in the hippocampus and other relevant brain regions. These biochemical modulations by acupuncture in animal models have also been correlated with cognitive improvement.

In AD patients, several functional brain imaging studies have demonstrated that acupuncture increased activity in the temporal lobe and prefrontal lobes, areas that are related to memory and cognitive function (Zeng, Salvage, & Jenner, 2013). However, much of the literature claiming positive effects of acupuncture in dementia is in traditional Chinese medicine journals. English-language acupuncture studies have primarily explicated the rationale behind acupuncture rather than perform controlled studies of its effects on cognition and problematic behaviors. Along these lines, Wang et al. (2014) used fMRI to compare the effects of acupuncture stimulation in 14 AD and 14 healthy elders, using acupuncture stimulation on the Tai chong and He gu acupoints. They reported that during the resting state, several frontal and temporal regions showed decreased hippocampal connectivity in AD patients relative to control subjects. Following acupuncture, AD patients showed increased connectivity in most of these hippocampus-related regions compared to the first resting state. These results may suggest that acupuncture can enhance hippocampal connectivity in AD patients. Whether these findings will have any practical application in improving cognition or reducing problem behaviors remains to be seen.

Several studies have examined acupuncture for reducing sleep problems. Kwok et al. (2013) employed a cross-over design with twice weekly acupuncture sessions for 6 weeks in a community-dwelling dementia population with sleep disturbances. Sleep parameters were measured by caregivers and wrist actigraphy. The researchers found significant gains in resting time and total sleep time for the treatment time compared to the control period. Rodríguez-Mansilla et al. (2013) performed an RCT of massage versus ear acupuncture on sleep and behavioral disturbances in 120 institutionalized elderly with dementia. Results from caregivers indicated that 97% of massage and 92% of the ear acupuncture group showed improvement in sleep disturbance compared to 0% in the control group.

Although these studies appear promising, acupuncture is a very new treatment in dementia populations. Acupuncture studies such as those cited here need replication and extension, using larger multi-site studies as well as employing sham acupuncture control groups.

AROMATHERAPY

Aromatherapy's route of administration is the nasal-respiratory system and in the form of essential oil applied to the skin. Stimulation of the olfactory bulb and modulation of the limbic system are presumed mechanisms of action (Diamond et al., 2003).

Aromatherapy appears to have a calming effect on behavioral and psychological problems in patients with dementia. A decrease in agitation in Chinese patients with moderate to severe dementia was observed in a cross-over RCT of *lavandula* (lavender) compared to sunflower inhalation by Lin, Chan, Fung-leung, & Lam, (2007). After 3 weeks, agitation decreased in the *lavandula* group patients, as measured by the Cohen-Mansfield Agitation Inventory and Neuropsychiatric Inventory (Lin et al., 2007). In a Japanese RCT, Fujii et al. (2008) examined the effects of lavender aromatherapy on dementia patients. After receiving lavender aromatherapy three times a day for 4 weeks, there were no significant changes in ADLs or MMSE. However, there were significant differences in the Neuropsychiatric Inventory, showing that the experimental group demonstrated decreases in hallucinations, agitation, aggression, and irritability (Fujii et al., 2008).

Results such as those cited in this section spurred a number of trials using aromatherapy in dementia units. Forrester, Maayan, Orrell, Spector, Buchan, and Soares-Weiser (2014) performed a Cochrane review considering all trials using fragrances from plants defined as aromatherapy as an intervention with people with dementia. They uncovered a total of seven studies with 428 participants, but determined that only two studies, Ballard, O'Brien, Reichelt, and Perry (2002) and Burns, Perry, Holmes, Francis, Morris, Howes, et al. (2011), had published usable results. Ballard et al.'s (2002) study applied essential *Melissa* oil (lemon balm) to the skin twice a day for 4 weeks and found a statistically significant treatment effect in favor of the aromatherapy intervention on measures of agitation and behavioral symptoms compared to placebo sunflower oil. Burns et al. (2011) used *Melissa* oil in a double blind, placebo-controlled RT across

three UK centers. They found no difference in agitation, behavioral symptoms, ADLs, or quality of life. Forrester et al. (2014) concluded that the benefits of aromatherapy for people with dementia are equivocal based on the seven trials included in this review.

In a newer study that was not included in this review, Fu, Moyle, and Cooke (2013) attempted to correct the confounds and methodological limitations in prior work. Fu sprayed lavender oil on one group, while a comparison group received lavender oil with hand massage and a control group received water spray. They found no difference in adverse behaviors when aromatherapy was compared to placebo.

Most aromatherapy studies suffer from methodological difficulties such as small sample sizes, unblinded raters, lack of control for antipsychotic use, and a lack of standardized dosage information. Furthermore, olfactory function may be impaired in dementia, limiting the benefits expected from a scent-based intervention. Even with so many statistically non-significant results, there are often individuals within an intervention group who benefit, suggesting that interventions need to be tailored to individual needs and wishes.

MEDITATION

Meditation is an accessible adjunct treatment with potential for attenuating cognitive and mood problems in dementia. There are a number of meditation methods and styles that have been utilized in research studies. Meditation may reduce stress by decreasing rumination, enhancing emotional regulation, and improving general coping mechanisms (Keng, Smoski, & Robins, 2011). Quantifiable changes have been demonstrated in meditators in brain locations that influence attention skills, awareness, and control over emotion states (Keng et al., 2011; Tang, Lu, Fan, Yang, & Posner, 2012).

Recent reviews of the literature suggest that meditation training can offset cognitive decline and may even improve cognition in aging adults (Gard, Holzel, & Lazar, 2014) and may hold promise for treating neurodegenerative diseases (Marciniak et al., 2014; Newberg et al., 2014). These reviews present a rationale for why meditation may be effective in treating dementia, along with demonstrable evidence from cognitive testing to neuroimaging showing superiority in meditators. Nonetheless, only a handful of studies have actually trained dementia patients in meditation.

Newberg et al. (2014) trained 14 participants with memory problems (three had AD) in an 8-week trial using the Kirtan Kriya method that entails a repetitive mantra and finger sequences. The meditation group showed significantly higher cerebral blood flow (CBF) in frontal and parietal lobe regions on single photon emission computed tomography (SPECT) compared to the music-listening controls. There were trends for meditators toward improved scores on working memory and logical memory tasks (verbal information), but the only significant improvement was on verbal fluency. Notably, one AD patient had to be dropped for inability to adequately perform the meditation. Meditation is likely only to be effective in mild cognitive impairment and the early stages of dementia because of the effort and attention skills required to successfully engage in meditation. Ernst et al. (2008) examined a modified version of mindfulness-based stress reduction (MBSR) in German nursing home residents and found improvements in physical health and depressed mood in participants compared to controls, but no differences between groups on the MMSE. These studies suggest that meditation potentially may improve quality of life, reduce anxiety, and strengthen cognitive skills but probably needs to be customized for dementia populations.

ADVERSE EVENTS

No significant adverse events or injuries have been reported in the studies reviewed in the preceding sections on non-pharmacological interventions for dementia, except for the Barrick et al. (2010) study, which found increased agitation with BLT. In evaluating adverse events, defined as any unfavorable and unintended sign, symptom, or disease presenting during or after treatment with acupuncture regardless of causal relationship, events were categorized into syncope, organ or tissue injury, infection, and others (Hempel et al., 2013). Acupuncture generally appears safe across a variety of clinical applications. However, there are reviews reporting some fatalities with causes and mechanisms unclear. While rates for adverse events are generally low and symptoms minor, such symptoms have included vascular and tissue/organ injury, infections and bruising, nausea, temporary pain, and dizziness or faintness in treating pain. The frequency of adverse events is uncertain because of a lack of standardization in reporting adverse events across a global medical community.

The majority of the studies cited find that dropout rates were low and compliance was generally high. However, as Olazarán et al. (2010) note, in most non-pharmacological intervention studies persons with medical illness, sensory impairments, non-native speakers, and those with severe dementia are excluded from the sample. Therefore, it is important to consider that sample selection constraints may reduce the generalizability of positive findings.

Overall, these studies suggest that select non-pharmacologic interventions and therapies show promise in ameliorating many of the cognitive, behavioral, and psychological symptoms associated with dementia (see Table 29.2).

Summary

Taken together, the data derived from epidemiological studies and controlled clinical trials for select herbal and non-pharmacotherapies for the symptomatic relief of cognitive, psychological, and behavioral impairments in dementia are sufficiently promising to warrant prospective intervention studies. The use of CAIM approaches in dementia is still in the embryonic stages of research development. Important considerations in future pharmacological research include the standardization of herbal medicines for the purpose of enhancing safety and comparing findings across studies; and the identification of active constituents, mechanisms, and drug–herbal interactions and the determination of efficacious dosages. A limitation of much of the research using herbals and their derivatives is a lack of data regarding effect sizes, numbers needed to treat/harm, or identification of subgroup responders. However, it should be noted that meta-analyses of RPC trials involving Ginkgo biloba extract showed significant differences in pooled effect size favoring treatment versus placebo, and while differences were modest, it was concluded that the findings were clinically relevant (Diamond et al., 2003). Additionally, meta- and pooled-data analyses of rigorous studies using galantamine identified subgroups of AD patients who showed the largest mean treatment effects in various cognitive domains.

Overall, interventions with elderly normal populations at the earliest stages of disease, using standardized botanicals that ameliorate individual rather than a broad spectrum of symptoms, may also be an effective treatment strategy (Perry & Howes, 2011).

Table 29.2. Non-Pharmacologic Interventions

INTERVENTION	INDICATIONS	MECHANISMS	DOSAGE/DURATION	ADVERSE EFFECTS	AUTHORS
Animal-assisted therapy	Anxiety; facilitate social interaction	Increases in b-endorphin, oxytocin, prolactin, dopamine phenylacetic acid and a decrease in cortisol	One visit in 3 weekly sessions/long-term exposure (aquarium)	Allergies/infections from live animals	Edwards et al. (2014); Kraemer et al. (2009); Odendaal (2000); O'Haire (2010)
Music therapy and social interaction	Anxiety, depression; enhance mental well-being and social engagement; communication	Modulation of attention, memory and emotion (via limbic and paralimbic system)	One interactive performance. Weekly sessions from 4–24 weeks	No adverse effects reported	Guetin et al. (2009); Koelsch (2009); Sung et al. (2006); Van der vleuten et al. (2012)
Movement therapy	Mood, concentration, sleep	Modulation of serotonin and dopamine	4–10 weekly sessions	No adverse effects reported	Hamill et al. (2001); Jeong et al. (2005); Siddartha et al. (2014)
Light therapy with melatonin	Limited support: mood, sleep, agitation, depression	Entrainment of circadian/melatonin rhythm	2500–10,000 lux, am or pm; 1–2 hours for 10 days–2 months.	Increased agitation in subgroups	Barrick et al. (2010); Burns et al. (2009); Diamond et al. (2003); Forbes et al. (2014); Hickman et al. (2007)

Acupuncture	Cognition	Increased activity in temporal and prefrontal lobes. Enhanced hippocampal connectivity.	One session	Organ and tissue injury, infection, and syncope have been reported. Frequency of adverse events are low.	Hempel et al. (2013); Kwok et al. (2013); Rodriguez-Mansilla et al. (2013); Wang et al. (2014); Zeng et al. (2013)
Aromatherapy	Behavioral and psychological problems	Stimulates olfactory bulb, modulates limbic system, influences pyriform cortex, right amygdala, anterior cingulate, and left insular cortex	5–10 drops (inhalation) 4 days–4 weeks	Contact dermatitis	Ballard (2002); Diamond et al. (2003); Lin et al. (2007)
Meditation	Cognition, stress emotional regulation, coping, mood	Higher cerebral blood flow in frontal and parietal lobe	2–8 weekly sessions	No adverse effects reported	Keng et al. (2007); Newberg et al. (2014)

Non-pharmacological CAIM interventions share many of the same methodological weaknesses with herbal therapies. For example, many trials are pilot studies with small numbers of participants comparing baseline to post-test designs, rather than RPC trials. Large-scale studies with active control groups and sensitive standardized outcome measures are needed in order to assess the feasibility, effectiveness, and safety of these interventions.

There are compelling reasons to expand complementary, alternative, and integrative research into dementia populations. Approaches such as physical restraints and highly sedating antipsychotics are problematic methods for managing disruptive behaviors, and new approaches are sorely needed. Many of the FDA-approved drugs for treating dementia and associated symptoms have shown limited efficacy. Moreover, pharmaceutical approaches have primarily provided only short-term efficacy, and some have been accompanied by adverse side effects. While generally better tolerated, possible herbal–drug interactions must be carefully monitored by healthcare providers. In achieving this, patients need to openly communicate their use of such therapies.

We may also see the phenomenon of initially promising findings giving way after more robust, tightly controlled replications at different research sites fail to find significant differences for treated groups. For example, this appears to be the case for BLT, one of the most rigorously researched approaches aimed at improving problematic behaviors. Nonetheless, virtually all of the non-pharmacological interventions are safe, well-tolerated, and relatively inexpensive, and many of the herbal therapies have either a long history of safe use or they can be safely administered under proper medical supervision. Patients and/or caregivers should still include discussion of any CAIM techniques that have been used when developing comprehensive treatment plans with their healthcare providers.

The pathophysiological mechanisms mediating dementia are multifaceted, and the diverse treatment and intervention options provided by CAIM techniques may provide symptomatic relief for various types of dementia, levels of severity, and disease stages. Moreover, it should be emphasized that interventions with results that are not statistically significant can still confer clinical benefits for subsets of dementia patients and make life easier for their caregivers. Even if these interventions provide only mild improvement in the early stage of dementia or subtle changes in later stage patients, they could still provide much-needed quality of life benefits. Clinical trials are, therefore, worth pursuing with the goal of improving quality of life in dementia, which is a worthwhile goal for those directly and indirectly affected by these devastating diseases.

ACKNOWLEDGMENT

The authors wish to acknowledge the editorial support of Victoria Leonardo and Diana Teluk, as well as Dr. Samuel C. Shiflett, where it all began.

REFERENCES

Aguiar, S., & Borowski, T. (2013). Neuropharmacological review of the nootropic herb Bacopa monnieri. *Rejuvenation Res, 16*(4), 313–326.

Akhondzadeh, S., & Hesameddin Abbasi, S. (2006). Herbal medicine in the treatment of Alzheimer's disease. *Am J Alzheimers Dis, 21*(2), 113–118.

Al-Aama, T., Brymer, C., Gutmanis, I., Woolmore-Goodwin, S. M., Esbaugh, J., & Dasgupta, M. (2011). Melatonin decreases delirium in elderly patients: a randomized, placebo-controlled trial. *Int J Geriatr Psychiatry, 26,* 687–694.

American Psychiatric Association. (2013). *Diagnostic and statistical manual of mental disorders* (5th ed.; *DSM-5*). Arlington, VA: American Psychiatric Publishing.

Asthana, S., Craft, S., Baker, L. D., Raskind, M.A., Bimbaum, R. S., Lofgreen, C. P., Veith, R. C., & Plymate, S. R. (1999). Cognitive and neuroendocrine response to transdermal estrogen in postmenopausal women with Alzheimer's disease: results of a placebo-controlled, double-blind, pilot study. *Psychneuroendocrinology, 24*(6), 657–678.

Bains, J., Birks, J. S., & Dening, T. R. (2002). The efficacy of antidepressants in the treatment of depression in dementia. *Cochrane Database Syst Rev, 4,* CD003944.

Ballard, C. G., O'Brien J. T., Reichelt, K., & Perry, E. K. (2002). Aromatherapy as a safe an effective treatment for the management of agitation in severe dementia: the results of a double-blind placebo-controlled trial with Melissa. *J Clin Psychiatry, 63*(7), 553–558.

Barrick, A. L., Sloane, P. D., Williams, C. S., Mitchell, C. M., Connell, B. R., Wood, W., Hickman, S. E., Preisser, J. S., & Zimmerman, S. (2010). Impact of ambient bright light on agitation in dementia. *Int J Geriatr Psychiatry, 25,* 1013–1021, doi: 10.1002/gps.2453.

Burns, A., Allen, H., Tomenson, B., Duignan, D., & Byrne, J. (2009). Bright light therapy for agitation in dementia: a randomized controlled trial. *Int Psychogeriatrics, 21*(04), 711–721.

Burns A., Perry E., Holmes C., Francis P, Morris J., Howes, M. J. R., et al. (2011). A double-blind placebo-controlled randomized trial of Melissa officinalis oil and donepezil for the treatment of agitation in Alzheimer's disease. *Dementia Geriatr Cogn Disord, 31,* 158–164.

Committee of Herbal Medicinal Products (2009). *Community herbal monograph on* Salvia officinalis L., *folium.* London: European Medicines Agency.

Consumer Advisory Center for Food Safety and Applied Nutrition, US Food and Drug Administration. (2002). *Kava-containing dietary supplements may be associated with severe liver injury.* Retrieved from www.cfsan.fda.gov.

Deshmukh, R., Sharma, V., Mehan, S., Sharma, N., & Bedi, K.L. (2009). Amelioration of intracerebroventricular streptozotocin induced cognitive dysfunction and oxidative stress by vinpocetine: a PDE1 inhibitor. *Eur J Pharmacol, 620,* 49–56.

Diamond, B. J., & Bailey, M. R. (2013). Integrative psychiatry and Ginkgo biloba: clinical indications, mechanisms and safety issues. *Integr Psychiatry Psychiatr Clin N Am, 36*(1), 73–83.

Diamond, B. J., Johnson, S. K., Torsney, K., Morodan, J., Davidek, D., Kramer, P., & Prokoff, B. (2003). Complementary and alternative medicines in the treatment of dementia: an evidenced based review. *Drugs Aging, 20*(13), 981–998.

Diamond, B. J., Shiflett, S. C., Feiwel, N., Matheis, R., Noskin, O., Richards, J., & Schoenberger, N. (2000). Ginkgo biloba extract: mechanisms and clinical indications. *Arch Phys Med Rehabil, 81,* 668–678.

Edwards, N. E., Beck A. M., & Lim E. (2014). Influence of aquariums on resident behavior and staff satisfaction in dementia units. *Western J Nurs Res., 36* (10,)1309–22.

Ernst, S., Welke, J., Heintze, C., Gabriel, R., Zöllner, A., Kiehne, S., Schwantes, U., & Esch, T. (2008). Effects of mindfulness-based stress reduction on quality of life in nursing home residents: a feasibility study. *Forsch Komplementärmed, 15,* 74–81. doi: 10.1159/000121479.

Forbes, D., Blake, C. M., Thiessen, E. J., Peacock, S., & Hawranik, P. (2014). Light therapy for improving cognition, activities of daily living, sleep, challenging behaviour, and psychiatric disturbances in dementia. *Cochrane Database Syst Rev, 2,* CD003946. doi: 10.1002/14651858. CD003946.pub4.

Forbes, D., Morgan, D. G., Bangma, J., Peacock, S., Pelletier, N., & Adamson, J. (2004). Light therapy for managing sleep, behavior, and mood disturbances in dementia. *Cochrane Database Syst Rev, 2.* CD003946, doi: 10.1002/14651858

Forrester, L. T., Maayan, N., Orrell, M., Spector, A. E., Buchan, L. D., & Soares-Weiser, K. (2014). Aromatherapy for dementia. *Cochrane Database Syst Rev, 25*(2), CD003150. doi: 10.1002/14651858.CD003150.pub2.

Fu, C. Y., Moyle, W., & Cooke, M. (2013). A randomized controlled trial of the use of aromatherapy and hand massage to reduce disruptive behavior in people with dementia. *BMC Compl Alt Med, 13,* 165–174.

Fujii, M., Hatakeyama, R., Fukuoka, Y., Yamamoto, T., Sasaki, R., Moriya, M., Kanno, M., & Sasaki, H. (2008). Lavender aroma therapy for behavioral and psychological symptoms in dementia patients. *Geriatr Gerontol Int, 8,* 136–138.

Gard, T., Holzel, B. K., & Lazar, S. W. (2014). The potential effects of meditation on age-related cognitive decline: a systematic review. *Ann N Y Acad Sci, 1307*(1), 89–103. doi: 10.1111/nyas.12348.

Gaster, B., & Holroyd, J. (2000). St John's wort for depression: a systematic review. *Arch Intern Med, 160*(2), 152–156.

Gotell, E., Brown, S., & Ekman, S. (2009). The influence of caregiver singing and background music on vocally expressed emotions and moods in dementia care. *Int J Nurs Studies, 46*(4), 422–430.

Guetin, S., Portet, F., Picot, M. C., Pomme, C., Messaoudi, M., Djabelkir, L., Olsen, A. L., Cano, M. M., Lecourt, E., & Touchon, J. (2009). Effect of music therapy on anxiety and depression in patients with Alzheimer's type dementia: randomised, controlled study. *Dement Geriatr Cogn Disord, 28*(1), 36–46.

Haffsman, P. M., Sival, R. C., Lucius, S. A., Cats, Q., & van Gelder, L. (2000). Bright light therapy and melatonin in motor restless behavior in dementia: a placebo-controlled study. *Int J Geriatr Psychiatry, 16*(1), 106–110.

Hamill, M., Smith, L., & Rohrict, F. (2011). "Dancing down memory lane": circle dancing as a psychotherapeutic intervention in dementia: a pilot study. *Dementia.* 11(6), 709–724. doi: 10.1177/1471301211420509.

Hatta, K., Kishi, Y., Wada, K., Takeuchi, T., Odawara, T., Usui, C., Nakamura, H., & DELIRIA-J Group.

(2014). Preventive effects of ramelteon on delirium: a randomized placebo-controlled trial. *JAMA Psychiatry* 71(4), 397–403. doi: 10.1001/jamapsychiatry.2013.3320.

Hempel, S., Taylor, S. L., Solloway, M., Miake-Lye, I. M., Beroes, J. M., Shanman, R., Booth, M. J., Siroka, A. M., & Shekelle, P. G. (2013). *Evidence map of acupuncture*. VA-ESP Project #05-226. URL: http://www.hsrd.research.va.gov/publications/esp/acupuncture.pdf

Hickman, S. E., Barrick, A. L., Williams, C. S., Zimmerman, S., Connell, B. R., Preisser, J. S., & Sloane, P. D. (2007). The effect of ambient bright light therapy on depressive symptoms in persons with dementia. *J Am Geriatr Soc*, 55(11), 1817–1824.

Honjo, H., Kikuchi, N., Hosoda, T., Kariya, K., Kinoshita, Y., Iwasa, K., Ohkubu, T., Tanaka, K., Tamura, T., Urabe, M., & Kawata, M. (2001). Alzheimer's disease and estrogen. *J Steroid Biochem Mol Biology*, 76(1–5), 227–230.

Howes, M-J., & Houghton P. J. (2012). Ethnobotanical treatment strategies against Alzheimer's disease. *Curr Alzheimer Res*, 9(1), 65–85.

Howes, M-J. R., & Perry, E. (2011). The role of phytochemicals in the treatment and prevention of dementia. *Drugs Aging*, 28(6), 439–468.

Jeong, Y. J., Hong, S. C, Lee, M. S, Park, M. C., Kim, Y. K., & Suh, C. M. (2005). Dance movement therapy improves emotional responses and modulates neurohormones in adolescents with mild depression. *Int J Neurosci*, 115(12), 1711–1720.

Kaschel, R. (2009). *Ginkgo biloba*: Specificity of neuropsychological improvement: a selective review in search of differential effects. *Hum Psychopharmaol*, 24, 345–370.

Keng, S.-L., Smoski, M. J., & Robins, C. J. (2011). Effects of mindfulness on psychological health: a review of empirical studies. *Clin Psychol Rev*, 31(6), 1041–1056.

Kennedy, D. O., Haskell, C. F., Wesnes, A. L., & Scholey, A. B. (2004). Improved cognitive performance in human volunteers following administration of guaraná (*Paullinia cupana*) extract: comparison and interaction with *Panax ginseng*. *Pharmacol Biochem Behav*, 79, 401–411.

Koelsch, S. (2009). A neuroscientific perspective on music therapy. *Ann NY Acad Sci*, 1169, 374–384.

Kongkeaw, C., Dilokthornsakul, P., Thanarangsarit, P., Limpeanchob, N., & Norman Scholfield, C. (2014). Meta-analysis of randomized controlled trials on cognitive effects of Bacopa monnieri

extract. *J Ethnopharmacol*, 151(1), 528–535. doi: 10.1016/j.jep.2013.11.008.

Kramer, S. C., Friedmann, E., Bernstein, P. L. (2009). Comparison of the effect of human interaction, animal-assisted therapy, and AIBO-assisted therapy on long-term care residents with dementia. *Anthrozoos*, 22, 1: 43–57. http://dx.doi.org/10.2752/175303708X390464.

Kwok, T., Leung, P. C., Wing, Y. K., Ip, I., Wong, B., Ho, D. W., Wong, W. M., & Ho, F. (2013). The effectiveness of acupuncture on the sleep quality of elderly with dementia: a within subjects trial. *Clin Intervent Aging*, 8, 923–929. doi: 10.2147/CIA.S45611.

Lin, P. W. K., Chan, W., Ng, B. F. L., & Lam, L. C. W. (2007). Efficacy of aromatherapy (Lavandula angustifolia) as an intervention for agitated behaviours in Chinese older person with dementia: a cross-over randomized trial. *Int J Geriatric Psychiatry*, 22, 405–410.

Man, S. C., Sundara, K., Durairajan, W. F. K., Hong Lu, J., Dong Huang, J., Ching Fung, C., Ching, V., Xu, M., & Min, L. (2008). Systematic review on the efficacy and safety of herbal medicines for Alzheimer's disease. *J Alzheimers Dis*, 14, 209–223.

Marciniak, R., Sheardova, K., Cermakova, P., Hudecek, D., Sumec, R., & Hort, J. (2014). Effect of meditation on cognitive functions in context of aging and neurodegenerative diseases. *Front Behav Neurosci*, 8, 1–8. doi: 10.3389/fnbeh.2014.00017

Marx, M. S., Cohen-Mansfield, J., Regier, N. G., li, M., Srihari, A., & Thein, K. (2010). The impact of different dog-related stimuli on engagement of persons with dementia. *Am J Alzheimers Dis*, 25, 37–45.

Montgomery, S. A., Thal, L. J., & Amrein, R. (2003). Meta-analysis of double blind randomized controlled clinical trials of acetyl-L-carnitine versus placebo in the treatment of mild cognitive impairment and mild Alzheimer's disease. *Int Clin Psychopharmacol*, 18(2) 61–71.

Morgan, A., & Stevens, J. (2010). Does Bacopa monnieri improve memory performance in older persons? Results of a randomized, placebo-controlled, double-blind trial. *J Alt Compl Med*, 16(7), 753–759.

Munoz-Torrero, D. (2008). Acetylcholinesterase inhibitors as disease-modifying therapies for Alzheimer's disease. *Curr Med Chem*, 15, 2433–2455.

Muth, K., Schönmeyer, R., Matura, S., Haenschel, C., Schröder, J., & Pantel, J. (2010). Mild cognitive impairment in the elderly is associated with volume loss of the cholinergic basal forebrain region. *Biol Psychiatry*, 67, 588–591.

Odendaal, J. S. J. (2000). Animal-assisted therapy: magic or medicine? *J Psychosomat Res, 49,* 275–280.

Olazarán, J., Reisberg, B., Clare, L., Cruz, I., Peña-Casanova, J., Del Ser, T., & Muñiz, R. (2010). Nonpharmacological therapies in Alzheimer's disease: a systematic review of efficacy. *Dement Geriatr Cognit Disord, 30,* 161–178. doi: 10.1159/000316119.

Napryeyenko, O., & Borzenko, I. (2007) *Ginkgo biloba* special extract in dementia with neuropsychiatric features: a randomised, placebo-controlled, double-blind clinical trial. *Arzneimittelforschung, 57,* 4–11.

Newberg, A. B., Serruya, M., Wintering, N., Moss, A. S., Reibel, D., & Monti, D. A. (2014). Meditation and neurodegenerative diseases. *Ann NY Acad Sci, 1307,* 112–123. doi: 10.1111/nyas.12187.

O'Haire, M. (2010). Companion animals and human health: benefits, challenges and the road ahead. *J Vet Behav, 5,* 226–234. doi: 10.10116/j.jveb.2010.02.002.

Pase, M. P., Kean, J., Sarris, J., Neale, C., Scholey, A. B., & Stough C. (2012). The cognitive-enhancing effects of Bacopa monnieri: a systematic review of randomized, controlled human clinical trials. *J Alt Compl Med, 18*(7), 1–6.

Patyar, S., Prakash, A., Medhi, M., & Modi, B. (2011). Role of vinpocetine in cerebrovascular diseases. *Pharmacol Reports, 63*(3), 618–628.

Perry, E., & Howes, M-J. R. (2011) Medicinal plants and dementia therapy: herbal hopes for brain aging? *CNS Neurosci Therapeut, 17,* 683–669.

Rasool, M., Malik, Q., Sheikh, I. A., Manan, A., Shaheen, S., Qazi, M. H., Chaudhary, A. G., Abuzenadah, A. M., Asif, M., Algahtani, M. H., Igbal, Z., Shaik, M. M., Gan, S. H., Kamal, M. A. (2013). Current view from Alzheimer disease to type 2 diabetes mellitus. *CNS Neurol Disord Drug Targets, 13*(3), 533–542.

Rodríguez-Mansilla, J., González-López-Arza, M. V., Varela-Donoso, E., Montanero-Fernández, J., Jiménez-Palomares, M., Garrido-Ardila, E. M. (2013). Ear therapy and massage therapy in the elderly with dementia: a pilot study. *J Tradit Chinese Med, 33,* 461–467.

Riemersma-van Lek, R. F., Swaab, D. F., Twisk, J., Hol, E. M., Hoogendijk, W. J. G., & van Someren, E. J. W. (2008). Effect of bright light and melatonin on cognitive and noncognitive function in elderly residents of group care facilities: a randomized controlled trial. *JAMA, 299*(22), 2642–2655.

Rondanelli, M., Opizzi, A., Faliva, M., Mozzoni, M., Antoniello, N., Cazzola, R., Savarè, R.,

Cerutti, R., Grossi, E., & Cestaro, B. (2012). Effects of a diet integration with an oily emulsion of DHA-phospholipids containing melatonin and tryptophan in elderly patients suffering from mild cognitive impairment. *Nutr Neurosci, 15*(2), 46–54.

Sarris, J., & Kavanagh, D. J. (2009). Kava and St. John's wort: current evidence for use in mood and anxiety disorders. *J Alt Compl Med, 15*(8), 827–836.

Siddarth, D., Siddarth, P., & Lavretsky, H. (2014). An observational study of the health benefits of yoga or tai chi compared with aerobic exercise in community-dwelling middle-aged and older adults. *Am J Geriatr Psychiatry, 22*(3), 272–273. doi:10.1016/j.jagp.2013.01.065.

Sierpina, V., Sierpina, M., Loera, J. A., & Grumbles, L. (2005). Complementary and integrative approaches to dementia. *Southern Med J, 98*(6), 645.

Starkstein, S. E., Mizrahi, R., & Power, B. D. (2008) Depression in Alzheimer's disease: phenomenology, clinical correlates and treatment. *Int Rev Psychiatry, 20,* 382–388.

Sung, H., Chang, S., Lee, W., & Lee, M. (2006). The effects of group music with movement intervention on agitated behaviors of institutionalized elders with dementia in Taiwan. *Compl Ther Med, 14,* 113–119.

Svansdottir, H. B., & Snaedal, J. (2006). Music therapy in moderate and severe dementia of Alzheimer's type: a case-control study. *Int Psychogeriatric, 18,* 613–621.

Szatmári, S., & Whitehouse, P. (2003). Vinpocetine for cognitive impairment and dementia. *Cochrane Database Syst Rev, 1.* Art. no.: CD003119. doi: 10.1002/14651858.CD003119.

Tang, Y. Y., Lu, Q., Fan, M., Yang, Y., & Posner, M. I. (2012). Mechanisms of white matter changes induced by meditation. *Proc Natl Acad Sci USA, 109*(26), 10570–10574. doi: 10.1073/pnas.1207817109.

van der Vleuten, M., Visser, A., Meeuwesen, L. (2012). The contribution of intimate live music performances to the quality of life for persons with dementia. *Patient Educ Couns, 89,* 484–488.

Wang, Z., Liang, P., Zhao, Z., Han, Y., Song, H., Xu, J., Lu, J., & Li, K. (2014). Acupuncture modulates resting state hippocampal functional connectivity in Alzheimer disease. *PLoS One, 6,* 9(3), e91160. doi: 10.1371/journal.pone.0091160.

Werneke, U., Turner, T., & Priebe, S. (2006). Complementary medicines in psychiatry: Review of effectiveness and safety. *Br J Psychiatry, 188*(2), 109–121.

Williams, P., Sorribas, A., & Howes, M-J. R. (2011). Natural products as a source of Alzheimer's drug leads. *Natural Products Rep, 28*, 48–77.

Wong, A. H. C, Smith, M., Boon, H. S. (1998). Herbal remedies in psychiatric practice. *Arch Gen Psychiatry, 55*(11), 1033–1044.

Yue J., Dong, B. R., Lin, X., Yang, M., Wu, H. M., & Wu, T. (2012). Huperzine A for mild cognitive impairment. *Cochrane Database oSyst Rev, 12*. Art. no.: CD008827. doi: 10.1002/14651858. CD008827.pub2.

Zeng, B. Y., Salvage, S., & Jenner, P. (2013) Effect and mechanism of acupuncture on Alzheimer's disease. *Int Rev Neurobiol, 111*, 181–195. doi: 10.1016/ B978-0-12-411545-3.00009-2.

Zhang, H. Y., Zheng, C. Y., Yan, H., Wang, Z. F., Tang, L. L., Gao, X., & Tang, X. C. (2008). Potential therapeutic targets of huperzine A for Alzheimer's disease and vascular dementia. *Chemico-Biol Interact, 175*(1–3), 396–402.

Zhang, L. N., Sun, Y. J., Pan, S., Li, J. X., Qu, Y. E., Li, Y., Wang, Y. L., & Gao, Z. B. (2013). Na+-K+-ATPase, a potent neuroprotective modulator against Alzheimer disease. *Fundam Clin Pharmacol, 27*(1), 96–103. doi: 10.1111/fcp.12000.

ACRONYMS AND ABBREVIATIONS

AAI = Animal-assisted interventions

$A\beta$ = Amyloid-beta

AChE = Acetylcholinesterase

ACh = Acetylcholine

ACI = Alternative, complementary, and integrative

AD = Alzheimer's disease

ADAS-cog scale = Alzheimer's Disease Assessment Scale

ADL = Activities of Daily Living

ALc = Acetyl L-carnitine

ApoE = ApolipoproteinE\

APP = Beta-Amyloid precursor protein

AVLT = Rey Auditory Verbal Learning Test

BChE = Butyrylcholinesterase

BEHAVE-AD = Behavioral Pathology in Alzheimer's Disease

BLT = Bright Light Therapy

BM = *Bacopa monnieri*

BPSD = Behavioral and psychological symptoms of dementia

CAM = Complementary and alternative medicine

CBF = Cerebral blood flow

CGI =- Clinical Global Impression Scale

ChEIs = Cholinesterase inhibitors

CNS = Central nervous system

CPT-450 = Cytochromes P450

DA = Dopamine

DHA = Docosahexaenoic Acid

DSM-5 - *Diagnostic and Statistical Manual of Mental Disorders* (5th ed.)

EEG = Electroencephalography

EGb 761 = Standardized extract of Ginkgo biloba

ERT = Estrogen replacement therapy

FDA = Food and Drug Administration

fMRI = Functional magnetic resonance imaging

GABA = Gamma-amino butyric acid-A

GI = Gastrointestinal

GSH = Glutathione

GSK3 Inhibitor = Glycogen synthase kinase 3

HAM-D =- Hamilton Rating Scale of Depression

LBD = Lewy body type dementia

MAO Inhibitor = Monoamine oxidase inhibitor

MBSR = Mindfulness-based stress reduction

MCI = Mild cognitive impairment

MID = Multi-infarct dementia

MMSE = Mini-Mental State Examination

nAChRs = Nicotinic acetylcholine receptor

Na+-K+-ATPase = Sodium-potassium adenosine triphosphatase

NCDs = Neurocognitive disorders

NPI = Neuropsychiatric inventory

PDD = Parkinson's disease dementia

PDE = Phosphodiesterase enzyme

PKC inhibitor = Protein kinase C inhibitor

QOL = Quality of life

RCT = Randomized clinical trial

ROS = Reactive oxygen species

RPC = Randomized placebo controlled

SDAT = Senile dementia of Alzheimer's type

SJW = St. John's wort

SPECT = Single photon emission computed tomography

SSRI = Selective serotonin reuptake inhibitor

VaD = Vascular dementia

5-HT = 5-hydroxytryptamine

30

MIND–BODY THERAPIES FOR CANCER SURVIVORS

EFFECTS OF YOGA AND MINDFULNESS MEDITATION ON CANCER-RELATED PHYSICAL AND BEHAVIORAL SYMPTOMS

Chloe C. Boyle and Julienne E. Bower

INTRODUCTION

Cancer is primarily a disease of aging, and the majority of cancer diagnoses occur among individuals over 65 years of age. Fortunately, advances in cancer detection and treatment have resulted in longer survival times for individuals diagnosed with cancer. As a consequence, there are a growing number of cancer survivors in the United States, most of whom are older adults. Indeed, of the current 14.5 million cancer survivors in the United States, approximately 60% are 65 years and older, and nearly a quarter were diagnosed more than 15 years prior (DeSantis et al., 2014).

Older survivors typically demonstrate better psychological adjustment than younger survivors, perhaps because they have had experience confronting other major life stressors and health challenges. However, they are at risk for physical problems and limitations following cancer diagnosis and treatment (Reeve et al., 2009). These include declines in physical functioning as well as cancer-related

fatigue, pain, and sleep disturbance (Bellury et al., 2011). Depression is also prevalent in cancer patients and survivors, including elderly cancer survivors (Mitchell et al., 2011). All of these symptoms have a negative impact on quality of life and may also predict shorter survival (Groenvold et al., 2007).

The management of physical and behavioral symptoms among older survivors is an important challenge for researchers and clinicians (Rowland & Bellizzi, 2014). Medications used to treat pain and sleep problems have unwanted side effects, and pharmacological approaches have shown limited efficacy in treating symptoms like cancer-related fatigue (Bower, 2014). Further, patients may be reluctant to take additional medications to manage the side effects of their cancer treatments (Naeim et al., 2014; Rao & Cohen, 2004). Mind–body therapies are purported to target a wide array of mental and physical ailments, and have shown efficacy in alleviating psychological distress among cancer survivors (e.g., Buffart et al., 2012; Ledesma & Kumano, 2009). Two of the most common mind–body therapies used in cancer populations are yoga and mindfulness meditation. Here, we consider the evidence that these therapies influence cancer-related physical and behavioral symptoms that are common among older cancer survivors, including physical and functional well-being, fatigue, sleep disturbance, pain, and depression. We first present a general overview of these symptoms, then review the results of randomized controlled trials (RCTs) assessing the efficacy of yoga and mindfulness-based interventions on these symptoms. As of yet, there is very little research on whether mind–body approaches are specifically helpful for older cancer survivors. Indeed, older adults remain consistently underrepresented in both research and intervention trials of all types (Rowland & Bellizzi, 2014). Thus, we consider all RCTs conducted with adult cancer survivors, regardless of age at diagnosis, that have examined effects on the symptoms of interest. To identify studies for inclusion, we searched MEDLINE, PsychInfo, and ISI through December 2014. Searches were limited to human studies and the English language. We searched using the following terms: "mindfulness," "meditation," "yoga," "cancer," and "randomized controlled trial." We also screened the reference lists of selected reviews and primary articles for additional publications.

OVERVIEW OF CANCER-RELATED SYMPTOMS

Physical and Functional Well-Being

Physical and functional well-being may include mobility, muscle strength, stamina, the ability to perform activities of daily living, and the extent to which declines in physical health interfere with important life roles (Stein et al., 2008). Prospective studies indicate that older survivors report significantly worse physical functioning than cancer-free controls. These differences are small, but may persist for up to 10 years past diagnosis and beyond (Lazovich et al., 2009; Reeve et al., 2009; Stein et al., 2008). Difficulties with physical function may be amplified by comorbid medical conditions among older cancer survivors, the most common of which are diabetes, chronic obstructive pulmonary disease, and congestive heart failure (Edwards et al., 2014; Rowland & Bellizzi, 2014). As many as 40% of cancer survivors over the age of 65 have at least one comorbidity, and this number increases with age (Edwards et al., 2014).

Functional decline has reciprocal relations with other cancer-related symptoms. Patients who experience fatigue, pain, or depression may decrease their physical activity, placing them at greater risk for functional problems (Bellury et al., 2011). In turn, functional problems may interfere with participation in valued activities or may create dependency on others, leading to isolation, loneliness, and psychological distress (Stein et al., 2008).

Fatigue

Fatigue is one of the most common and distressing side effects of cancer and its treatment, and may endure for months or years after treatment completion (Bower, 2014). Indeed, up to one-third of cancer survivors report persistent post-treatment fatigue. Patient reports suggest that cancer-related fatigue is more severe, more persistent, and more debilitating than "normal" fatigue caused by lack of sleep or overexertion and is not relieved by adequate sleep or rest (Poulson, 2001). Cancer-related fatigue is multidimensional and may have physical, mental, and emotional manifestations, including generalized weakness, diminished concentration or attention, decreased motivation or interest to engage in usual activities, and emotional lability (Bower, 2014).

Younger survivors typically report higher levels of fatigue than older survivors (Champion et al., 2014). However, fatigue is still prevalent in older survivors and is associated with lower levels of physical activity and reduced muscle strength in this population (Winters-Stone et al., 2008). Thus, fatigue may be a risk factor for physical deconditioning and frailty in older patients. Comorbidities may also increase the risk for fatigue in older survivors.

Sleep

Sleep disturbance is common in cancer patients, including difficulty getting to sleep and maintaining sleep during the night (e.g., frequent awakenings, difficulty resuming sleep, waking early). Sleep disturbance may be present before, during, and after treatment (Irwin, 2013). In a recent population-based longitudinal study of 962 patients, over 50% reported insomnia symptoms after diagnosis, which persisted at 18 months post-diagnosis in 36% of survivors (Savard et al., 2011). Of note, 21% of survivors in this study met criteria for clinically significant insomnia, that is, sleep problems that are severe and persistent enough to cause impairments in daytime functioning. Similarly high prevalence estimates have been observed in longer-term survivors, including those over age 60, suggesting that sleep problems may be enduring without treatment (Bardwell & Profant, 2008; Savard et al., 2001).

Like fatigue, rates of insomnia tend to be higher in younger than older survivors (Irwin, 2013), but older survivors may still fare worse than age-matched controls with no cancer history. In one study of older lung cancer survivors an average of 8 years past treatment, 56.5% reported poor sleep quality, compared to 30% in controls (Gooneratne et al., 2007).

Pain

Pain is one of the most feared symptoms for cancer patients and survivors, and more than one-third of post-treatment survivors report moderate to severe pain (van den Beuken-van Everdingen et al., 2007). Longer-term survivors are also at risk, with 5%–10% reporting chronic pain severe enough to interfere with functioning (Glare et al., 2014). Chronic pain may arise from surgery, chemotherapy, or radiation therapy, and treatment combinations (which are frequent in modern cancer treatment) may increase the likelihood of pain (Glare et al., 2014). Up to 40% of postmenopausal breast cancer survivors report arthralgias, or joint pain and stiffness, following hormonal therapies such as aromatase inhibitors; this is particularly problematic given that current guidelines recommend that women take these medications for up to 10 years post-treatment (Glare et al., 2014).

The relationship between age and pain is not clear. Older age is a risk factor for chemotherapy-induced peripheral neuropathy, but in general, studies have found less, more, and equivalent levels of pain among younger and older cancer patients (Glare et al. 2014; van den Beuken-van Everdingen et al., 2007). Nociception does not appear to change with age, but older adults may report less pain, perhaps from an unwillingness to complain, lower expectations for pain control, or an assumption that pain is age related and normative (Rao & Cohen, 2004). Older adults are more vulnerable to increased toxicity from pharmacological approaches to pain treatment (Rao & Cohen, 2004).

Depression

Cancer survivors are at substantially increased risk for depression. While estimates of prevalence vary, approximately 20% of all cancer patients are likely to experience depression or significant depressive symptoms (Irwin, 2013; Mitchell et al., 2011). Rates of depression are highest at diagnosis and treatment and typically decline across the survivorship period (Mitchell et al., 2013). A recent meta-analysis found no relationship between age and depression among cancer survivors (Mitchell et al., 2011).

Despite its prevalence, depression likely remains underrecognized and undertreated, particularly among older cancer survivors (Weinberger et al., 2011). Assessing depression can be particularly difficult in older adults; presentation of symptoms may be subclinical or atypical, characterized by somatic complaints and anhedonia rather than sadness (Naeim et al., 2014). Even when detected, older cancer survivors may be less likely than younger survivors to be referred for psychological treatment by healthcare providers (Weinberger et al., 2011).

Summary

The literature on cancer-related physical and behavioral symptoms indicates that these symptoms are common among older cancer survivors and occur at higher rates than individuals with no cancer history. Importantly, these symptoms may persist for years after successful treatment, creating an enduring burden for otherwise healthy survivors and for those who are managing other health conditions. Thus, targeted interventions may be required to improve symptoms and to prevent declines in physical function. The possibility that yoga and mindfulness-based interventions may be helpful in alleviating cancer-related symptoms is considered in the following sections.

YOGA INTERVENTIONS: EFFECTS ON BEHAVIORAL AND PHYSICAL SYMPTOMS IN CANCER SURVIVORS

Description of Interventions

We focus here on RCTs of yoga conducted with cancer survivors—that is, individuals who have completed primary cancer treatment with surgery, radiation, and/or chemotherapy. We have included studies with a primary focus on yoga that examined effects on physical function and/or behavioral symptoms, and we report on these outcomes in Table 30.1. Of note, because self-report measures

Table 30.1.   Description of Randomized Controlled Yoga Interventions

AUTHOR, YEAR	POPULATION	TIME POST-DIAGNOSIS OR TREATMENT	NUMBER OF PARTICIPANTS (YOGA, CONTROL), % FEMALE	AGE (MEAN)	INTERVENTION TYPE AND DURATION	CONTROL GROUP	CONTROL ASSESSMENTS*	OUTCOMES**	BETWEEN GROUP DIFFERENCE***	EFFECT SIZE FOR BETWEEN GROUP DIFFERENCE (COHEN'S D)
Banasik (2011)	Breast cancer survivors	At least 2 months post-treatment	18 (9Y, 9C), 100% female	Y: 62.4 yrs (SD = 7.3); C: 63.3 yrs (SD = 6.9)	Iyengar yoga, 8 weeks, 2x/week. Intervention described as an "active" practice, with physically demanding poses. Primarily focused on poses, no meditation.	Wait list	Baseline, post-intv	Physical well-being (FACT)	NS	NR
								Functional well-being (FACT)	NS	NR
								Fatigue	Y > C	NR
Bower (2012)	Breast cancer survivors with fatigue	Median = 1.7 yrs post-treatment (range = 0.7–18.3 yrs)	31 (16Y, 15C), 100% female	54.4 yrs (eligible range 40–65 yrs)	Iyengar yoga, 12 weeks, 2x/week. Intervention focused on poses thought to be beneficial for fatigue, including passive inversions, backbends, and restorative poses.	Health education	Baseline, post-intv, 3 mo FU	Fatigue (FSI)	Y > C at post-intv and 3 mo FU	1.5
								Vitality (MFSI-SF)	Y > C at post-intv and 3 mo FU	1.2
								Depression (BDI-II)	Y > C at post-intv only	NR
								Sleep Quality (PSQI)	NS	NR

Author (Year)	Population	Time since diagnosis	N	Age	Intervention	Control	Assessment	Outcome	Results	
Carson (2009)	Breast cancer survivors with hot flashes	Mean = 4.9 yrs post-diagnosis (SD = 2.4)	37 (17Y, 20C), 100% female	54.4 yrs (SD = 7.5)	"Yoga of Awareness" program, 8 weeks, 1x/week. Intervention focused on postures thought to be beneficial for hot flashes, fatigue, and mood disturbance. Described as "gentle stretching poses," done either on mat or in chair. Intervention also included breathing, study, and group discussion.	Wait list	Baseline, post-intv, 3 mo FU	Fatigue (daily diary)	Y > C at post-intv and 3 mo FU	NR
								Vigor (daily diary)	Y > C at post-intv and 3 mo FU	NR
								Joint pain (daily diary)	Y > C at post-intv and 3 mo FU	NR
								Sleep disturbance (daily diary) **note that hot flashes also improved in yoga group vs. controls	Y > C at post-intv only	NR
Culos-Reed (2006)	Mixed cancer survivors, 85% breast	Mean = 55.95 months post-diagnosis	38 (20Y, 18C), 92% female	51.2 yrs (SD = 10.3)	Yoga, 7 weeks, 1x/week. Intervention described as gentle stretching and strengthening exercises, included poses and breathing.	Wait list	Baseline, post-intv	Physical function (EORTC QLQ-C30)	NS	NR
								Pain (EORTC QLQ-C30)	NS	NR
								Fatigue (EORTC QLQ-C30 and POMS)	NS	NR
								Vigor (POMS)	NS	NR
								Depression (POMS)	Y > C (trend)	NR
								Sleep disturbance (EORTC QLQ-C30)	NS	NR

(continued)

Table 30.1. Continued

AUTHOR, POPULATION	TIME POST-DIAGNOSIS OR TREATMENT	NUMBER OF PARTICIPANTS (YOGA, CONTROL), % FEMALE	AGE (MEAN)	INTERVENTION TYPE AND DURATION	CONTROL GROUP	ASSESSMENTS*	OUTCOMES**	BETWEEN GROUP DIFFERENCE***	EFFECT SIZE FOR BETWEEN GROUP DIFFERENCE (COHEN'S D)
Kiecolt-Glaser (2013) Breast cancer survivors	Mean = 10.9 months post-treatment (SD = 7.9)	200 (100Y, 100C), 100% female	51.6 yrs (SD = 9.2); range 27–76 yrs	Hatha-based yoga, 12 weeks, 2x/week Intervention focused on postures thought to improve depression, fatigue, and immune function. Included poses on the floor, standing poses, and restorative poses.	Wait list	Baseline, post-intv, 3 mo FU	Fatigue (MFSI-SF)	NS at post-intv; Y > C at 3 mo FU	0.22 at post-intv; −0.36 at FU
							Depression (CESD)	NS	−0.13 at post-intv; −0.16 at FU
							Vitality (SF-36)	Y > C at post-intv and 3 mo FU	0.31 at post-intv; 0.32 at FU
							Sleep quality (PSQI)	Y > C at post-intv and 3 mo FU	NR
Littman (2011) Breast cancer survivors with BMI > or = 24	Y: Mean = 6 yrs post-diagnosis; C: Mean = 6.5 yrs post-diagnosis (range = 0.5–22.9 yrs)	63 (32Y, 31C), 100% female	Y: 60.6 yrs (SD = 7.1); C: 58.2 yrs (SD = 8.8); eligible range 21–75 yrs	Hatha-based yoga, 6 months, 5x/week Intervention based on viniyoga, a Hatha-based therapeutic style of yoga, developed for overweight/obese cancer survivors. Poses included seated and standing poses; also breathing and meditation.	Wait list	Baseline, post-intv	Physical well-being (FACT)	NS	NR
							Functional well-being (FACT)	NS	NR
							Fatigue (FACIT)	NS	NR

Mustian (2013)	Mixed cancer survivors, 75% breast, with sleep problems	Mean = 16.3 months since first treatment (SD = 0.85)	410 (206Y, 204C), 96% female	54.1 yrs (SE = .51)	Hatha and restorative-based yoga, 4 weeks, 2x/week Intervention included seated, standing, and supine poses, with emphasis on restorative poses. Also included breathing and mindfulness.	Wait list	Baseline, post-intv	Global sleep quality (PSQI)	Y > C	NR

Abbreviations: BDI-II = Beck Depression Inventory II; C= Control group; CESD = Center for Epidemiologic Studies-Depression Scale; EORTC QLQ-30 = European Organization for Research and Treatment of Cancer-Quality of Life; FACIT = Functional Assessment of Chronic Illness Therapy; FACT = Functional Assessment of Cancer Therapy; FSI =Fatigue Symptom Inventory; FU = Follow- up; intv = intervention; MFSI-SF = Multidimensional Fatigue Symptom Inventory- Short Form; mo = month; NR = not reported; NS = non-significant; PSQI = Pittsburgh Sleep Quality Index; POMS = Profile of Mood States; SD = standard deviation; SF-36 = Short-Form Health Survey; Y = Yoga group.

*Follow-up data calculated as time since intervention completion.

**We focus here on physical and behavioral symptoms; many trials also included other outcomes.

***Statistical significance was defined as *p* < .05.

Table 30.2. Description of Randomized Controlled Mindfulness-Based Interventions

AUTHOR, POPULATION YEAR	TIME POST-DIAGNOSIS OR TREATMENT	NUMBER OF PARTICIPANTS (MINDFULNESS, CONTROL), % FEMALE	AGE (MEAN)	INTERVENTION TYPE AND DURATION	CONTROL GROUP	ASSESSMENTS*	OUTCOMES**	BETWEEN GROUP DIFFERENCE***	EFFECT SIZE FOR BETWEEN GROUP DIFFERENCE (COHEN'S D)
Andersen (2013); Würtzen (2013)[†]	Mean = 7.68 months since diagnosis (SD = 5.05)	336 (168M, 168C), 100% female	54.14 yrs (SD = 10.3), eligible range 18–75 yrs	MBSR, 8 weeks, 1x/week, 5-hr silent retreat MBSR includes mindfulness meditation exercises, group discussion. emphasis on mindfulness in daily living and practice, didactic material on relations between stress and health.	Usual care	Baseline, post-intv, 4 and 10 mo FU	Sleep problems (MOS-SS)	M > C at post-intv only	0.24
							Depression (CESD)[†]	M > C at post-intv, 4 and 10 mo FU	NR
							Depression (SCL-90R)[†]	M > C (trend) at post-intv, M > C at 4 and 10 mo FU	NR
Bower (2014)	Mean = 4.1 years since diagnosis (SD = 2.43)	71 (39M, 32C), 100% female	46.83 yrs (SD = 7.27), range 28–60 yrs	Mindful awareness practices (MAPs) program tailored for younger survivors; 6 weeks, 1x/week, no retreat MAPs is a standardized program that cultivates formal and informal mindfulness; also provided education on health and preventing cancer recurrence.	Wait list	Baseline, post-intv, 3 mo FU	Pain (BCPT)	NS	NR
							Fatigue (FSI)	M > C at post-intv only	NR
							Depression (CESD)	M > C (trend) at post-intv only	0.54
							Sleep quality (PSQI)	M > C at post-intv only	NR
Bränström (2010, 2012)	49 participants diagnosed within last 2 years; 22 diagnosed more than 2 years ago.	71 (32M, 39C), 99% female	51.8 yrs (SD = 9.86), range 30–65 yrs	MBSR, 8 weeks, 1x/week, no retreat Intervention followed MBSR curriculum but had no retreat	Wait list	Baseline, post-intv, 3 mo FU	Depression (HADS)	M > C (trend) at post-intv only	0.28

Study	Sample	Time since diagnosis	N	Age	Intervention	Control	Assessment points	Outcome (measure)	Results	Effect size
Foley (2010)	Mixed cancer patients and survivors, 42% breast	M: Mean = 2.2 yrs post-diagnosis (SD = 2.56); C: Mean = 2 yrs post-diagnosis (SD = 4.08)	115 (55M, 60C), 77% female	55.18 yrs (SD = 10.6) range 24–78 yrs	MBCT, 8 weeks, 1x/week, 5-hr silent retreat. MBCT is similar to MBSR but incorporates elements of cognitive therapy; in this trial, didactic material was modified to address challenges often faced in the cancer context.	Wait list	Baseline, post-intv, 3 mo FU	Depression (HAM-D)	M > C at post-intv and 3 mo FU	1.41
Garland (2014)	Mixed cancer survivors, 48% breast, with sleep disturbance	Mean = 3.19 yrs post-diagnosis (SD = 4.03), range = 0.17–30 yrs	111 (64M, 47C), 72% female	58.9 yrs (SD = 11.08), range 35–88 yrs	Mindfulness-based cancer recovery (MBCR), 8 weeks, 1x/week, 6-hr silent retreat. MBCR is a standardized program modeled after MBSR, and adapted for cancer patients and survivors (e.g., highlights challenges often faced by cancer survivors).	Cognitive behavioral therapy for insomnia (C)	Baseline, post-intv, 3 mo FU	Sleep disturbance (ISI)	C > M over the two post-intv assessments	NR
								Sleep quality (PSQI)	C > M over the two post-intv assessments	NR
Henderson (2012)	Breast cancer patients and survivors	Diagnosed within last 2 yrs	163 (53M, 58C, 52NEP), 100% female	49.8 yrs (SD = 8.4), range 20–65 yrs	MBSR, 7 weeks, 1x/week, 7.5-hr silent retreat; plus three monthly sessions following the intervention	Nutrition education program (NEP); Usual Care (C)	Baseline, post-intv, 8 mo and 20 mo FU	Depression (SCL-90R)	M > NEP at post-intv only	NR
								Depression (BDI)	NS	NR
Hoffman (2012)	Breast cancer survivors, seeking psychological services	M: Mean = 17.4 months post-diagnosis (SD = 13) C: Mean = 18.9 months post-diagnosis (SD = 15)	229 (114M, 115C), 100% female	M: 49 yrs (SD = 9.26); C: 50.1 yrs (SD = 9.14), eligible range 18–80 yrs	MBSR, 8 weeks, 1x/week, 6-hr silent retreat. Intervention closely followed MBSR.	Wait list	Baseline, post-intv, 1 mo FU	Functional well-being (FACT-B)	M > C at post-intv and 1 mo FU	NR
								Physical well-being (FACT-B)	M > C at post-intv and 1 mo FU	NR
								Fatigue (POMS)	M > C at post-intv and 1 mo FU	NR
								Vigor (POMS)	M > C at post-intv and 1 mo FU	NR
								Depression (POMS)	M > C at post-intv only	NR

(continued)

Table 30.2.   Continued

AUTHOR, YEAR	POPULATION	TIME POST-DIAGNOSIS OR TREATMENT	NUMBER OF PARTICIPANTS (MINDFULNESS, CONTROL), % FEMALE	AGE (MEAN)	INTERVENTION TYPE AND DURATION	CONTROL GROUP	ASSESSMENTS*	OUTCOMES**	BETWEEN GROUP DIFFERENCE***	EFFECT SIZE FOR BETWEEN GROUP DIFFERENCE (COHEN'S D)
Johns (2015)	Mixed cancer survivors, 85.7% breast, with fatigue	Mean = 51.3 months post-treatment (SD = 39.3)	35 (18M, 17C), 94% female	M: 58.8 yrs (SD = 9.3); C: 55.7 yrs (SD = 9.3)	MBSR - CRF, 7 weeks, 1x/week, no retreat Intervention closely followed MBSR but was adapted to the cancer context and included psychoeducation related to cancer-related fatigue.	Wait list	Baseline, post-intv, 1 mo FU (6 mo FU for mindfulness group only)	Fatigue severity (FSI)	M > C at post-intv and 1 mo FU	−1.55 at post-intv; −1.54 at FU
								Fatigue interference (FSI)	M > C at post-intv and 1 mo FU	−1.43 at post-intv; −1.34 at FU
								Vitality (SF-36)	M > C at post-intv and 1 mo FU	1.29 at post-intv; 1.73 at FU
								Depression (PHQ-8)	M > C at post-intv and 1 mo FU	−1.3 at post-intv; −1.71 at FU
								Sleep disturbance (ISI)	M > C at post-intv and 1 mo FU	−0.74 at post-intv; −1.0 at FU

Study	Population	Time since treatment	N	Age	Intervention	Comparison	Assessment	Outcome (measure)	Result	
Lengacher (2009, 2012)‡	Breast cancer survivors	Mean = 18.8 weeks post-treatment (SD = 17.4)	84 (41M, 43C), 100% female	57.5 yrs (SD = 9.4), 27% > 65 years	MBSR - BC (Breast Cancer), 6 weeks, 1x/week, no retreat. MBSR - BC includes original MBSR material but highlights psychological and physical symptoms common for breast cancer survivors (e.g. fear of recurrence, pain).	Wait list	Baseline, post-intv	Physical functioning (MOS-SF)	M > C	NR
								Physical health–role limitations (MOS-SF)	M > C	NR
								Pain (MOS-SF, MDASI†)	M > C (trend) NS‡	NR
								Energy (MOS-SF)	M > C	NR
								Fatigue (MDASI)‡	M > C	NR
								Depression (CESD)	M > C	NR
								Sleep disturbance (MDASI)‡	NS	NR
Lengacher (2015)	Breast cancer survivors	Between 2 weeks and 2 years post-treatment	79 (38M, 41C), 100% female	57 yrs (SD = 9.7)	MBSR - BC, 6 weeks, 1x/week, no retreat	Wait list	Baseline, post-intv, 6 week FU	Sleep quality (PSQI)	NS	NR
Lerman (2012)	Mixed cancer survivors, 70.6% breast	M: Mean = 3.9 yrs post-diagnosis (SD = 5.1); C: Mean = 3.7 yrs post-diagnosis (SD = 3.5)	77 (53M, 24C), 100% female	M: 57.5 yrs (SD = 10.5); C: 56.4 yrs (SD = 9.8)	MBSR-based cancer recovery and wellness intervention, 8 weeks, 1x/week, 4-hr retreat Intervention included group discussion on body image and sexuality; used mindful breast self-examination and writing.	Wait list	Baseline, post-intv	Functional quality of life (EORTC QLQ-30)	NS	NR

(continued)

Table 30.2. Continued

AUTHOR, YEAR	POPULATION	TIME POST-DIAGNOSIS OR TREATMENT	NUMBER OF PARTICI-PANTS (MIND-FULNESS, CONTROL), % FEMALE	AGE (MEAN)	INTERVENTION TYPE AND DURATION	CONTROL GROUP	ASSESS-MENTS*	OUT-COMES**	BETWEEN GROUP DIFFERENCE***	EFFECT SIZE FOR BETWEEN GROUP DIFF-ERENCE (COHEN'S D)
Nakamura (2013)	Mixed cancer survivors, 54% breast, with sleep disturbance	M: Median = 2.8 yrs post-diagnosis; MB: Median = 3.6 yrs post-diagnosis; SH: Median = 4.17 yrs post-diagnosis	57 (20M, 19MB, 18SH); 75% female	M: 50.8 yrs (SD = 9.1); MB: 55.4 yrs (SD = 9.6); SH: 51.6 yrs (SD = 10.7); eligible range 18–75 yrs	Mindfulness Meditation (MM), 3 weeks, 1x/week, no retreat MM is a shortened version of MBSR, with no yoga, optional homework, and an expressive writing exercise. Group discussion was adapted to address sleep and cancer in relation to mindfulness.	Mind–Body Bridging (MB); Sleep Hygiene Education (SHE)	Baseline, post-intv, 2 mo FU	Sleep disturbance (MOS-SS)	M > SHE (trend) at post-intv; M > SHE at 2 mo FU	0.7
								Depression (CESD)	NS	0.06
Speca (2000)	Mixed cancer patients and survivors, 42% breast	Open to participants at any stage, at any point in treatment; no mean/range given	109 (61M, 48C), 79% female	51 yrs; range 25–75 yrs	MBSR, 7 weeks, 1x/week, no retreat Intervention modeled after MBSR, adapted for cancer patients and survivors.	Wait list	Baseline, post-intv	Vigor (POMS)	M > C	NR
								Fatigue (POMS)	NS	NR
								Depression (POMS)	M > C	NR

| Van der Lee (2012) | Mixed cancer survivors, 58% breast, with fatigue | Mean = 3 yrs post-treatment (SD = 2.3) | 100 (72M, 28C), 86% female | 53.1 yrs (SD = 9.1) | MBCT 8 weeks, 1x/week, 6hr retreat, follow-up session at 2 months post-intv. MBCT is similar to MBSR but includes elements of cognitive therapy, such as learning to identify and detach from negative thoughts; this trial also included didactic material on fatigue. | Wait list | Baseline, post-intv (6 mo FU for MBCT group only) | Fatigue severity (CIS) | M > C at post-intv | 0.74 |
| | | | | | | | | Functional impairment (SIP) | NS | NR |

Abbreviations: BCPT = Breast Cancer Prevention Trial Symptom Checklist; C= Control group; CESD = Center for Epidemiologic Studies-Depression Scale; CIS = Checklist Individual Strength; CRF = Cancer-related fatigue; EORTC QLQ-30 = European Organization for Research and Treatment of Cancer-Quality of Life; FACT-B = Functional Assessment of Cancer Therapy-Breast Symptom Index; FSI =Fatigue Symptom Index; FU = Follow-up; HADS = Hospital Anxiety and Depression Scale; HAM-D = Hamilton Rating Scale for Depression; intv = intervention; ISI = Insomnia Severity Index; M = Mindfulness group; MAPs = Mindful Awareness Practices; MBCT = Mindfulness-Based Cognitive Therapy; MBSR = Mindfulness-Based Stress Reduction; MDASI = M.D. Anderson Symptom Inventory; mo = month; MBB = Mind-Body Bridging; MOS-SF = Medical Outcomes Study Short-Form General Health Survey; MOS- SS = Medical Outcomes Study Sleep Scale; NEP = Nutrition Education Program; NR = not reported; NS = non-significant; PHQ-8 = Patient Health Questionnaire; PSQI = Pittsburgh Sleep Quality Index; POMS = Profile of Mood States; SD = standard deviation; SF-36 = Short-Form Health Survey; SHE = Sleep Hygiene Education; SIP = Sickness Impact Profile.

*Follow-up data calculated as time since intervention completion.

**We focus here on physical and behavioral symptoms; many trials also included other outcomes.

***Statistical significance was defined as p < .05.

† Andersen 2013 and Würtzen 2013 report from the same randomized controlled trial; Würtzen 2013 results are indicated with a dagger symbol.

‡ Lengacher 2009 and Lengacher 2012 report from the same randomized controlled trial; Lengacher 2012 results are indicated with a double dagger symbol.

are the gold standard for the assessment of subjective symptoms, we focused on these outcomes for the purposes of this review.

We identified seven published RCTs that met these criteria. Most of the trials were quite small, and only two had sample sizes larger than 100. All but one used a wait-list control group. In terms of participant characteristics, the samples were primarily composed of breast cancer survivors; five studies included only breast cancer survivors, and two included a heterogeneous sample of cancer survivors that consisted primarily of women with breast cancer. The average age of study participants ranged from 51.2 to 62.9 years old.

The yoga interventions evaluated in these reports ranged from 4 weeks (Mustian et al., 2013) to 6 months (Littman et al., 2012), though most were in the 8–12-week range with classes held two times per week. Interventions were typically based on Hatha yoga and included postures and breathing exercises. Some also included meditation (Littman et al., 2012) or mindfulness (Mustian et al., 2013), and one study included study and group discussion (Carson et al., 2009). One of the notable features of these trials is that many focused on particular problems or symptoms, rather than addressing general quality of life. This focus guided enrollment and intervention content, as the interventions emphasized poses thought to be beneficial for the symptom of interest. For example,

Bower et al. (2012) enrolled breast cancer survivors who reported persistent cancer-related fatigue and tested an Iyengar-based intervention that focused on postures thought to address this symptom (i.e., supported back bends and inversions). Similarly, Carson and colleagues (2009) enrolled breast cancer survivors who were experiencing hot flashes and tested an intervention that targeted this symptom. Many of the practices were gentle or restorative in nature, though others were more physically demanding (e.g., Banasik et al., 2011).

Intervention Effects

When evaluating intervention effects, we focused on differences between the yoga and control groups at post-intervention. Overall, the most consistent positive effects were seen for fatigue and sleep disturbance. Six trials reported effects on fatigue, with four showing beneficial effects on this outcome in the yoga group versus controls. Of note,

three of the four studies that found positive results specifically targeted fatigued survivors and/or included poses that targeted this symptom (Bower et al., 2012; Carson et al., 2009; Kiecolt-Glaser et al., 2014). Further, the study by Bower and colleagues included an active control condition to control for nonspecific aspects of the intervention, providing a more stringent evaluation of intervention efficacy. In the fourth positive study, a small ($n = 19$) trial conducted by Banasik and colleagues (2011) that used a physically demanding, Iyengar-based intervention, fatigue was the only outcome that improved. In contrast, the two trials that did not show beneficial effects on fatigue also found no effects on other outcomes (Culos-Reed et al., 2006; Littman et al., 2012). The study by Littman and colleagues emphasized home practice and recommended that participants attend one facility-based class per week along with four weekly sessions of home practice. Those who attended more facility-based classes, which was standard for the other trials, showed greater reductions in fatigue over the 6-month intervention period.

A similar pattern of results was observed for sleep disturbance. Of the four trials that reported effects on sleep, three showed beneficial effects for yoga versus controls. One of these trials specifically focused on sleep and showed improvements in both self-reported sleep quality and objective sleep measures, as well as decreased use of sleep medications (Mustian et al., 2013).

More mixed results were seen for other outcomes, including depressive symptoms, pain, and physical function. Of the three studies that reported effects on depressive symptoms, only one reported positive results (Bower et al., 2012), which appeared to be time limited. Specifically, Bower and colleagues found that yoga led to a greater decrease in depressive symptoms than health education immediately post-treatment, but this difference disappeared by the 3-month follow-up. Of the two studies that reported effects on pain, only one found positive results (Carson et al., 2009). In this case, the trial that yielded positive effects specifically targeted breast cancer survivors with hot flashes, many of whom also experience joint pain, and found that daily reports of joint pain improved in the yoga group relative to wait-list controls. In contrast, the study that reported negative results assessed general pain and pain-related impairment, and saw no effects (Culos-Reed et al., 2006). In terms of physical function, three trials assessed physical and/or functional well-being using validated quality of life measures (EORTC, FACT). None of these trials found positive effects of yoga on these outcomes. Of note, two of these trials did not find positive effects on any outcome (Culos-Reed et al., 2006; Littman et al., 2012).

Summary of Results

Overall, findings from these trials suggest that yoga is a feasible, acceptable, and safe intervention for cancer survivors. Three of the studies reviewed included information about adverse events (Bower et al., 2012; Kiecolt-Glaser et al., 2014; Mustian et al., 2013); among the 641 individuals included in these trials, only three intervention-related events were reported, which were recurrence of chronic back and/or shoulder problems. It is important to note that most of these trials used highly trained yoga instructors and administered carefully designed, "gentle" intervention protocols, which likely contributed to the lack of adverse events.

In terms of efficacy, the most consistent beneficial effects were seen for fatigue and sleep disturbance. Only a few trials assessed depressive symptoms or pain, and findings were quite mixed. This is interesting because the broader literature on yoga has reported positive effects on depression and pain (Cramer et al., 2013), although these trials focused on patients who were experiencing clinically relevant levels of these symptoms (e.g., individuals with clinically diagnosed musculoskeletal conditions). In contrast, none of the studies with cancer survivors reviewed here specifically recruited patients with elevated pain or depressive symptoms. In general, targeted yoga trials appear to be more effective.

The lack of effects on physical function were notable, particularly since this is an area where older survivors show more pronounced impairments. It is possible that longer interventions may be required to improve physical function (e.g., Oken et al., 2006), or that combined interventions that include strength training in addition to yoga may be more effective. We would encourage investigators to include objective measures of physical function, including performance-based measures (in addition to self-report) in future yoga trials.

MINDFULNESS INTERVENTIONS: EFFECTS ON BEHAVIORAL AND PHYSICAL SYMPTOMS IN CANCER SURVIVORS

Description of Interventions

We identified 14 mindfulness-based RCTs that assessed effects on self-reported behavioral symptoms and/or physical and functional well-being in cancer survivors. Most trials were conducted with breast cancer survivors, and four (Andersen et al., 2013; Foley et al., 2010; Henderson et al., 2012; Speca et al., 2000) included patients as well as post-treatment survivors. Five interventions targeted a specific population or symptom: one for younger breast cancer survivors (Bower et al., 2015), two for survivors with cancer-related fatigue (Johns et al., 2015; Van der Lee et al., 2012), and two for survivors with sleep disturbance (Garland et al., 2014; Nakamura et al., 2013). The average age of participants ranged from 46 to 59 years. All but three trials (Garland et al., 2014; Henderson et al., 2012; Nakamura et al., 2013) used a wait-list control group.

The studies included in this review were modeled after two of the most common standardized mindfulness programs, mindfulness-based stress reduction (MBSR) and mindfulness-based cognitive therapy (MBCT) (Kabat-Zinn, 1990; Teasdale et al., 1995). In general, mindfulness interventions teach individuals to cultivate mindfulness and bring attention to present-moment experiences with openness, curiosity, and non-judgment (Kabat-Zinn, 1990). Most include psychoeducation, group discussion, informal and daily home practice, and meditation exercises (e.g., mindful breathing, sitting/walking meditation, mindful Hatha yoga). In contrast to yoga interventions, gentle yoga in this context is used primarily as a means to foster mindful awareness of the body. The majority of the reviewed trials were modified in some way to address the specific needs of cancer survivors, for example, by providing education about maintaining health and preventing cancer recurrence (Bower et al., 2015) or by discussing body image and sexuality concerns (Lerman et al., 2012). Many of the interventions were also shorter than the standard 8-week

MBSR intervention. A more detailed overview of the studies, including effects on the symptoms of interest, is presented in Table 30.2.

Intervention Effects

Across studies, the most consistent positive effects were seen for fatigue and depression. All of the six studies that assessed fatigue found improvements in fatigue, energy, vigor, or vitality in the mindfulness group versus controls at post-intervention. The sustained and clinically significant effects seen in the trials by Van der Lee and Garssen (2012) and Johns and colleagues (2015) are particularly notable. Both interventions targeted survivors with cancer-related fatigue and provided brief psychoeducation on the relation between cancer and fatigue. While Johns et al. (2015) used a modified MBSR program, Van der Lee et al. (2012) used a modified MBCT program that included elements of cognitive therapy, but omitted gentle yoga. The success of both programs suggests that targeted mindfulness interventions are beneficial in addressing fatigue in this population, despite variations in approach.

Similarly, 9 of the 10 trials that examined effects on depressive symptoms found improvements in this outcome at post-intervention (three marginally so: Bower et al., 2015; Bränström et al., 2010; Wurtzen et al., 2013). The one study that did not see a significant effect for mindfulness meditation was an abbreviated 3-week intervention, and it still noted significant within-group improvement (Nakamura et al., 2013). These positive effects on depression are consistent with the broader literature on mindfulness for cancer patients and other clinical populations (Goyal et al., 2014; Ledesma & Kumano, 2009). However, improvements were not consistently maintained in the months after treatment completion. Only three out of eight studies that included a follow-up assessment saw sustained improvement in depression (Foley et al., 2010; Johns et al., 2015; Würtzen et al., 2013). It may be worthwhile to consider whether modifications such as booster sessions or online programs can facilitate enduring practice and continued improvement in well-being.

The seven studies assessing subjective sleep quality showed more mixed effects. Five of these studies compared mindfulness interventions to a wait-list control group; three reported significantly reduced sleep problems in the mindfulness group

versus controls at post-intervention (Andersen et al., 2013; Bower et al., 2015; Johns et al., 2015), and two found no group differences in subjective sleep problems at post-intervention (Lengacher et al., 2012; Lengacher et al., 2015). The remaining two trials targeted survivors with sleep disturbance, and both found mindfulness to show weaker or delayed effects in comparison to an active comparison group. In the study conducted by Nakamura and colleagues (2013), "Mind–Body Bridging" was more effective than mindfulness meditation at post-intervention, although both were superior to sleep hygiene education at a 2-month follow-up. In a comparative effectiveness trial, Garland and colleagues (2014) randomized participants to a mindfulness-based cancer recovery program (MBCR) or cognitive-behavioral therapy for insomnia (CBT-I). They found that CBT-I improved subjective sleep quality significantly more than the mindfulness program at post-intervention and at a 3-month follow-up. The mindfulness group did demonstrate clinically relevant improvement at the follow-up; however, the CBT-I worked more quickly and had more lasting and robust effects.

The evidence that mindfulness interventions improve physical function and symptoms in cancer survivors is similarly mixed. Four studies assessed self-reported physical and functional well-being, and two saw improvement for the mindfulness group versus controls on these outcomes (Hoffman et al., 2012; Lengacher et al., 2009). In addition, two studies conducted with breast cancer survivors assessed and found improvements in menopausal symptoms (Bower et al., 2015; Hoffman et al., 2012). This is a notable finding, as these symptoms often result from endocrine therapy, and may be associated with non-adherence to treatment (Murphy et al., 2012).

By contrast, mindfulness interventions have not demonstrated positive effects on pain in cancer survivors. Neither of the two trials assessing musculoskeletal pain (Bower et al., 2015) and bodily pain/pain severity (Lengacher et al., 2009; Lengacher et al., 2012) found significant improvement. Both trials did show effects on other symptoms, suggesting that they were generally effective interventions. These results are somewhat surprising, as mindfulness was initially proposed as a way to facilitate self-regulation of stress and chronic pain (Kabat-Zinn, 1990). Further, a recent meta-analysis found moderate evidence for pain improvement in clinical populations following mindfulness meditation (Goyal et al., 2014).

Summary of Results

Overall, results from these trials suggest that mindfulness-based interventions are safe, feasible, and acceptable for older cancer survivors. No adverse effects were found in the few studies that reported on them. In terms of efficacy, mindfulness showed consistently positive effects on fatigue and depressive symptoms, mixed evidence for effects on sleep and physical function, and no effect on pain. Several studies noted an association between the extent of mindfulness practice and positive treatment effects (Hoffman et al., 2012; Lengacher et al., 2009; Lerman et al., 2012; Speca et al., 2000), suggesting that there may be a dose-response relationship. It is important to note that none of these trials specifically targeted older survivors, though individuals up to age 88 were included in the research.

SUMMARY

Our review of the literature on yoga and mindfulness-based therapies for cancer survivors suggests that these approaches are feasible, acceptable, and safe for this population, and may lead to improvements in fatigue, sleep problems, and depression (mindfulness-based interventions only).

It is important to note that this is a developing area of research, and many of the studies included in this review were designed to provide an initial demonstration of intervention feasibility and preliminary efficacy, rather than a definitive evaluation of intervention effects. As such, many were limited by small sample sizes, single-site design, use of wait-list control conditions, and limited (if any) follow-up. The studies are also limited in generalizability, due to the overrepresentation of breast cancer survivors and underrepresentation of minorities. In addition, poor or incomplete reporting of statistical analyses rendered a number of studies difficult to evaluate. Future studies that use multisite designs (e.g., Carlson et al., 2013) with longer-term follow-up (e.g., Andersen et al., 2013) and active control conditions (e.g., Bower et al., 2012) and that include more representative samples of cancer survivors will allow a clearer evaluation of the effectiveness and durability of these interventions. Although we focused here on self-report measures, which are the gold standard for assessing subjective physical and behavioral symptoms, several trials also assessed relevant objective measures (e.g., actigraphy, physical performance measures); inclusion of these measures in future research would enhance our understanding of intervention effects.

In addition to these general recommendations, we believe that interventions may be enhanced by consideration of the specific needs and issues faced by older cancer survivors. In many cases, interventions have already been adapted for individuals with cancer (e.g., mindfulness-based cancer recovery); additional modifications for older survivors may improve the efficacy of these interventions and ensure safety in this potentially vulnerable group. Several mindfulness-based and yoga interventions have already been designed to accommodate older adults (e.g., Morone & Greco, 2014; Park et al., 2014), which could be used to inform programs targeting older cancer survivors. For mindfulness-based interventions, very simple and minor changes are typically made. For example, sitting meditation and mindful yoga may be done in chairs rather than on the floor, and participants with hearing difficulties sit closer to the instructor. Given the physical nature of yoga interventions, more extensive modifications may be required. In general, older adults are at greater risk for musculoskeletal side effects from yoga, and this may be exacerbated in cancer survivors who have undergone treatments that may accelerate biological aging processes. For example, treatment with aromatase inhibitors in women with breast cancer and treatment with androgen deprivation therapy in men with prostate cancer can accelerate bone loss and increase risk of fractures (Naeim et al., 2014). Thus, yoga interventions focusing on older cancer survivors need to be carefully designed to minimize these risks, including safety screening of potential participants, careful selection and sequencing of poses, detailed pose modifications for participants with physical limitations, and use of instructors who have experience with both cancer survivors and older adults, among other considerations (Krucoff et al., 2010). Preliminary work suggests that modified yoga programs are effective for older individuals (e.g. Morone & Greco, 2014; Park et al., 2014), supporting their potential usefulness with older cancer survivors.

Although our review has focused on behavioral and physical outcomes, yoga and mindfulness may also lead to improvements in aspects of psychological functioning relevant for older survivors, including reduced fear of recurrence and enhanced perceptions of peace and meaning in life (Bower et al., 2015; Lengacher et al., 2009). In addition, these approaches may influence cancer-relevant biological outcomes, including inflammatory processes. A growing body of research suggests that mind–body therapies, including yoga, mindfulness, and tai chi/qi gong, may reduce inflammatory activity (Morgan et al., 2014), and work conducted by our group suggests that these effects may extend to cancer survivors. For example, we have shown that yoga (Bower et al., 2014), mindfulness (Bower et al., 2015), and tai chi (Irwin et al., 2014) are associated with reduced inflammatory signaling in randomized controlled trials conducted with breast cancer survivors. There is also evidence that mind–body therapies may have positive effects on other biological processes relevant for older cancer survivors, including anti-viral immunity (Morgan et al., 2014) and biomarkers of bone health (Jahnke et al., 2010).

Cancer survivors are avid consumers of mind–body therapies, and these approaches may offer considerable benefits for this large and growing population. We recommend that researchers and clinicians carefully consider the use of mind–body approaches for older cancer survivors and develop targeted approaches that address the needs of this group in creative and thoughtful ways. For example, investigators may want to consider combining strength training with mind–body approaches to enhance effects on physical outcomes. Along these lines, although not considered in this review, tai chi/qi gong may be an attractive mind–body option for older cancer survivors. In particular, the movements and postures in tai chi/qi gong may be a helpful way to improve balance and incorporate gentle weight-bearing exercise, both of which are increasingly important with greater age (Jahnke et al., 2010). Indeed, preliminary trials have shown beneficial effects of qi gong on mental well-being and fatigue in older survivors (e.g., Campo et al., 2014). Given the growing number of older survivors in the United States, the development and implementation of interventions that improve psychological and physical well-being in this group is of critical importance.

FUNDING

Julienne E. Bower was supported by the Breast Cancer Research Foundation and by NIH/NCI R01 CA160427. Chloe C. Boyle was supported by the NIH/NIMH Predoctoral Fellowship 5T32MH015750-35, "Biobehavioral Aspects of Mental and Physical Health."

DISCLOSURE STATEMENT

The authors declare that they had no conflicts of interest with respect to their authorship or the publication of this article.

REFERENCES

Andersen, S. R., Würtzen, H., Steding-Jensen, M., Christensen, J., Andersen, K. K., Flyger, H., . . . Dalton, S. O. (2013). Effect of mindfulness-based stress reduction on sleep quality: results of a randomized trial among Danish breast cancer patients. *Acta Oncologica, 52*, 336–344.

Banasik, J., Williams, H., Haberman, M., Blank, S. E., & Bendel, R. (2011). Effect of Iyengar yoga practice on fatigue and diurnal salivary cortisol concentration in breast cancer survivors. *J Am Acad Nurse Prac, 23*(3), 135–142.

Bardwell, W., & Profant, J. (2008). The relative importance of specific risk factors for insomnia in women treated for early-stage breast cancer. *Psycho-Oncology, 17*(1), 9–18.

Bellury, L. M., Ellington, L., Beck, S. L., Stein, K., Pett, M., & Clark, J. (2011). Elderly cancer survivorship: an integrative review and conceptual framework. *Eur J Oncol Nurs, 15*(3), 233–242.

Bower, J. E. (2014). Cancer-related fatigue: mechanisms, risk factors, and treatments. *Nature Reviews. Clin Oncol, 11*(10), 597–609. doi: 10.1038/nrclinonc.2014.127.

Bower, J. E., Crosswell, A. D., Stanton, A. L., & Crespi, C. M., Winston, D., Arevalo, J., Ma, J., Cole, S. W., & Ganz, P. A. (2015). Mindfulness meditation for younger breast cancer survivors : a randomized controlled trial. *Cancer, 121*(8), 1231–1240.

Bower, J. E., Garet, D., Sternlieb, B., Ganz, P. A, Irwin, M. R., Olmstead, R., & Greendale, G. (2012). Yoga for persistent fatigue in breast cancer survivors: a randomized controlled trial. *Cancer, 118*(15), 3766–3775. doi: 10.1002/cncr.26702.

Bower, J. E., Greendale, G., Crosswell, A. D., Garet, D., Sternlieb, B., Ganz, P. A, . . . Cole, S. W. (2014). Yoga reduces inflammatory signaling in fatigued breast cancer survivors: a randomized controlled trial. *Psychoneuroendocrinology*. doi: 10.1016/j.psyneuen.2014.01.019.

Bränström, R., Kvillemo, P., Brandberg, Y., & Moskowitz, J. T. (2010). Self-report mindfulness as a mediator of psychological well-being in a stress reduction intervention for cancer patients: a randomized study. *Ann Behav Med, 39*(2), 151–161.

Bränström, R., Kvillemo, P., & Moskowitz, J. T. (2012). A randomized study of the effects of mindfulness training on psychological well-being and symptoms of stress in patients treated for cancer at 6-month follow-up. *Int J Behav Med, 19,* 535–542.

Buffart, L. M., van Uffelen, J. G. Z., Riphagen, I. I., Brug, J., van Mechelen, W., Brown, W. J., & Chinapaw, M. J. M. (2012). Physical and psychosocial benefits of yoga in cancer patients and survivors: a systematic review and meta-analysis of randomized controlled trials. *BMC Cancer, 12*(1), 559. doi: 10.1186/1471-2407-12-559.

Campo, R. A., Agarwal, N., LaStayo, P. C., O'Connor, K., Pappas, L., Boucher, K. M., . . . Kinney, A. Y. (2014). Levels of fatigue and distress in senior prostate cancer survivors enrolled in a 12-week randomized controlled trial of Qigong. *J Cancer Surviv, 8*(1), 60–69. doi: 10.1007/s11764-013-0315-5.

Carson, J. W., Carson, K. M., Porter, L. S., Keefe, F. J., & Seewaldt, V. L. (2009). Yoga of Awareness program for menopausal symptoms in breast cancer survivors: results from a randomized trial. *Support Care Cancer, 17*(10), 1301–1309.

Carlson, L. E., Doll, R., Stephen, J., Faris, P., Tamagawa, R., Drysdale, E., & Speca, M. (2013). Randomized controlled trial of mindfulness-based cancer recovery versus supportive expressive group therapy for distressed survivors of breast cancer (MINDSET). *J Clin Oncol 31*(25), 3119 -3126.

Champion, V. L., Wagner, L. I., Monahan, P. O., Daggy, J., Smith, L., Cohee, A., . . . Sledge, G. W. (2014). Comparison of younger and older breast cancer survivors and age-matched controls on specific and overall quality of life domains. *Cancer, 120*(15), 2237–2246. doi: 10.1002/cncr.28737.

Cramer, H., Lauche, R., Langhorst, J., & Dobos, G. (2013). Yoga for depression: a systematic review and meta-analysis. *Depress Anxiety, 30*(11), 1068–1083. doi: 10.1002/da.22166.

Culos-Reed, S. N., Carlson, L. E., Daroux, L. M., & Hately-Aldous, S. (2006). A pilot study of yoga for breast cancer survivors: physical and psychological benefits. *Psycho-Oncology, 15*(10), 891–897.

DeSantis, C. E., Lin, C. C., Mariotto, A. B., Siegel, R. L., Stein, K. D., Kramer, J. L., . . . Jemal, A. (2014). Cancer treatment and survivorship statistics, 2014. *CA: Cancer Journal for Clinicians, 64,* 252–271. doi: 10.3322/caac.21235.

Edwards, B. K., Noone, A.-M., Mariotto, A. B., Simard, E. P., Boscoe, F. P., Henley, S. J., . . . Ward, E. M. (2014). Annual Report to the Nation on the status of cancer, 1975–2010, featuring prevalence of comorbidity and impact on survival among persons with lung, colorectal, breast, or prostate cancer. *Cancer, 120*(9), 1290–1314. doi: 10.1002/cncr.28509.

Foley, E., Baillie, A., Huxter, M., Price, M., & Sinclair, E. (2010). Mindfulness-based cognitive therapy for individuals whose lives have been affected by cancer: a randomized controlled trial. *J Consult Clin Psychol, 78*(1), 72–79. doi: 10.1037/a0017566.

Garland, S. N., Carlson, L. E., Stephens, A. J., Antle, M. C., Samuels, C., & Campbell, T. S. (2014). Mindfulness-based stress reduction compared with cognitive behavioral therapy for the treatment of insomnia comorbid with cancer: a randomized, partially blinded, noninferiority trial. *J Clin Oncol, 32*(5), 449–457.

Glare, P. A, Davies, P. S., Finlay, E., Gulati, A., Lemanne, D., Moryl, N., . . . Syrjala, K. L. (2014). Pain in cancer survivors. *J Clin Oncol, 32*(16), 1739–1747.

Gooneratne, N., Dean, G., & Rogers, A. (2007). Sleep and quality of life in long-term lung cancer survivors. *Lung Cancer, 58*(3), 403–410.

Goyal, M., Singh, S., Sibinga, E. M. S., Gould, N. F., Rowland-Seymour, A., Sharma, R., . . . Haythornthwaite, J. A. (2014). Meditation programs for psychological stress and well-being. *JAMA Internal Med, 21287,* 1–11. doi: 10.1001/jamainternmed.2013.13018.

Groenvold, M., Petersen, M. A., Idler, E., Bjorner, J. B., Fayers, P. M., & Mouridsen, H. T. (2007). Psychological distress and fatigue predicted recurrence and survival in primary breast cancer patients. *Breast Cancer Res Treat, 105*(2), 209–219. doi: 10.1007/s10549-006-9447.

Henderson, V. P., Clemow, L., Massion, A. O., Hurley, T. G., Druker, S., & Hébert, J. R. (2012). The effects of mindfulness-based stress reduction on psychosocial outcomes and quality of life in early-stage breast cancer patients: a randomized trial. *Breast Cancer Res Treat, 131*(1), 99–109. doi: 10.1007/s10549-011-1738-1.

Hoffman, C. J., Ersser, S. J., Hopkinson, J. B., Nicholls, P. G., Harrington, J. E., & Thomas, P. W. (2012). Effectiveness of mindfulness-based stress reduction in mood, breast- and endocrine-related quality of life, and well-being in stage 0 to III breast cancer: a randomized, controlled trial. *J Clin Oncol, 30*(12), 1335–1342. doi: 10.1200/JCO.2010.34.0331.

Irwin, M. R. (2013). Depression and insomnia in cancer: prevalence, risk factors, and effects on cancer outcomes. *Curr Psychiatry Rep, 15*(404), 1–9. doi: 10.1007/s11920-013-0404-1.

Irwin, M. R., Olmstead, R., Carrillo, C., Sadeghi, N., Breen, E. C., Witarama, T., . . . Nicassio, P. (2014). Cognitive behavioral therapy vs. tai chi for late life insomnia and inflammation: a randomized controlled comparative efficacy trial. *Sleep, 37*(9), 1543–1552.

Jahnke, R., Larkey, L., Rogers, C., Etnier, J., & Lin, F. (2010). A comprehensive review of health benefits of qigong and tai chi. *Am J Health Promot, 24*(6), 1–37. doi: 10.4278/ajhp.081013-LIT-248.A.

Johns, S. A., Brown, L. F., Beck-Coon, K., Monahan, P. O., Tong, Y., & Kroenke, K. (2015). Randomized controlled pilot study of mindfulness-based stress reduction for persistently fatigued cancer survivors. *Psycho-Oncology.* 24,885–893. doi: 10.1002/pon.3648.

Kabat-Zinn, J. (1990). *Full catastrophe living: using the wisdom of your body and mind to face stress, pain, and illness.* New York: Delta.

Kiecolt-Glaser, J. K., Bennett, J. M., Andridge, R., Peng, J., Shapiro, C. L., Malarkey, W. B., . . . Glaser, R. (2014). Yoga's impact on inflammation, mood, and fatigue in breast cancer survivors: a randomized controlled trial. *J Clin Oncol, 32*(10), 1040–1049. doi: 10.1200/JCO.2013.51.8860.

Krucoff, C., Carson, K., Peterson, M., Shipp, K., & Krucoff, M. (2010). Teaching yoga to seniors: essential considerations to enhance safety and reduce risk in a uniquely vulnerable age group. *J Alt Compl Med, 16*(8), 899–905.

Lazovich, D., Robien, K., Cutler, G., Virnig, B., & Sweeney, C. (2009). Quality of life in a prospective cohort of elderly women with and without cancer. *Cancer, 115*(18 Suppl), 4283–4297.

Ledesma, D., & Kumano, H. (2009). Mindfulness-based stress reduction and cancer: a meta-analysis. *Psycho-Oncology, 18*(6), 571–579. doi:10.1002/pon.1400

Lengacher, C. A., Johnson-Mallard, V., Post-White, J., Moscoso, M. S., Jacobsen, P. B., Klein, T. W., . . . Kip, K. E. (2009). Randomized controlled trial of mindfulness-based stress reduction (MBSR) for survivors of breast cancer. *Psycho-Oncology, 18*(12), 1261–1272. doi: 10.1002/pon.1529.

Lengacher, C. A., Reich, R. R., Paterson, C. L., Jim, H. S., Ramesar, S., Alinat, C. B., . . . Kip, K. E. (2015). The effects of mindfulness-based stress reduction on objective and subjective sleep parameters in women with breast cancer: a randomized controlled trial. *Psycho-Oncology, 24*(4), 424–432. doi: 10.1002/pon.3603.

Lengacher, C. A., Reich, R. R., Post-White, J., Moscoso, M., Shelton, M. M., Barta, M., . . . Budhrani, P. (2012). Mindfulness based stress reduction in post-treatment breast cancer patients: an examination of symptoms and symptom clusters. *J Behav Med, 35*, 86–94.

Lerman, R., Jarski, R., Rea, H., Gellish, R., & Vicini, F. (2012). Improving symptoms and quality of life of female cancer survivors: a randomized controlled study. *Ann Surg Oncol, 19*, 373–378.

Littman, A. J., Bertram, L. C., Ceballos, R., Ulrich, C. M., Ramaprasad, J., McGregor, B., & McTiernan, A. (2012). Randomized controlled pilot trial of yoga in overweight and obese breast cancer survivors: effects on quality of life and anthropometric measures. *Support Care Cancer, 20*(2), 267–277.

Mitchell, A. J., Chan, M., Bhatti, H., Halton, M., Grassi, L., Johansen, C., & Meader, N. (2011). Prevalence of depression, anxiety, and adjustment disorder in oncological, haematological, and palliative-care settings: a meta-analysis of 94 interview-based studies. *Lancet Oncology, 12*(2), 160–174. doi: 10.1016/S1470-2045(11)70002-X.

Mitchell, A. J., Ferguson, D. W., Gill, J., Paul, J., & Symonds, P. (2013). Depression and anxiety in long-term cancer survivors compared with spouses and healthy controls: a systematic review and meta-analysis. *Lancet Oncology, 14*(8), 721–732. doi: 10.1016/S1470-2045(13)70244-4.

Morgan, N., Irwin, M. R., Chung, M., & Wang, C. (2014). The effects of mind-body therapies on the immune system: meta-analysis. *PloS One, 9*(7), e100903. doi: 10.1371/journal.pone.0100903.

Morone, N. E., & Greco, C. M. (2014). Adapting mindfulness meditation for the older adult. *Mindfulness, 5*(5), 610–612. doi: 10.1007/s12671-014-0297-z.

Murphy, C. C., Bartholomew, L. K., Carpentier, M. Y., Bluethmann, S. M., & Vernon, S. W. (2012). Adherence to adjuvant hormonal therapy among breast cancer survivors in clinical practice: a systematic review. *Breast Cancer Res Treat, 134*(2), 459–478. doi: 10.1007/s10549-012-2114-5.

Mustian, K. M., Sprod, L. K., Janelsins, M., Peppone, L. J., Palesh, O. G., Chandwani, K., . . . Morrow, G. R. (2013). Multicenter, randomized controlled trial of yoga for sleep quality among cancer survivors. *J Clin Oncol, 31*(26), 3233–3241.

Naeim, A., Aapro, M., Subbarao, R., & Balducci, L. (2014). Supportive care considerations for older adults with cancer. *J Clin Oncol, 32*(24), 2627–2634. doi: 10.1200/JCO.2014.55.3065.

Nakamura, Y., Lipschitz, D. L., Kuhn, R., Kinney, A. Y., & Donaldson, G. W. (2013). Investigating efficacy of two brief mind–body intervention programs for managing sleep disturbance in cancer survivors: a pilot randomized controlled trial. *J Cancer Surviv, 7*, 165–182.

Oken, B., Zajdel, D., & Kishiyama, S. (2006). Randomized, controlled, six-month trial of yoga in healthy seniors: effects on cognition and quality of life. *Altern Ther Health Med, 12*(1), 40–47.

Park, J., Mccaffrey, R., Newman, D., Cheung, C., & Hagen, D. (2014). The effect of sit 'n' fit chair yoga among community-dwelling older adults with osteoarthritis. *Holist Nurs Pract 28*(4), 247–257.

Poulson, M. J. (2001). Not just tired. *J Clin Oncol, 19*(21), 4180–4181.

Rao, A., & Cohen, H. J. (2004). Symptom management in the elderly cancer patient: fatigue, pain, and depression. *J Natl Cancer Inst Monographs*, (32), 150–157.

Reeve, B. B., Potosky, A. L., Smith, A. W., Han, P. K., Hays, R. D., Davis, W. W., . . . Clauser, S. B. (2009). Impact of cancer on health-related quality of life of older Americans. *J Natl Cancer Inst, 101*(12), 860–868. doi:10.1093/jnci/djp123

Rowland, J. H., & Bellizzi, K. M. (2014). Cancer survivorship issues: life after treatment and implications for an aging population. *J Clin Oncol, 32*(24), 2662–2668.

Savard, J., Ivers, H., Villa, J., Caplette-Gingras, A., & Morin, C. M. (2011). Natural course of insomnia comorbid with cancer: an 18-month longitudinal study. *J Clin Oncol, 29*(26), 3580–3586.

Savard, J., Simard, S., Blanchet, J., Ivers, H., & Morin, C. M. (2001). Prevalence, clinical characteristics, and risk factors for insomnia in the context of breast cancer. *Sleep, 24*(5), 583–590.

Speca, M., Carlson, L. E., Goodey, E., & Angen, M. (2000). A randomized, wait-list controlled clinical trial: the effect of a mindfulness meditation-based stress reduction program on mood symptoms of stress in cancer outpatients. *Psychosom Med, 62*(12), 613–622.

Stein, K. D., Syrjala, K. L., & Andrykowski, M. A. (2008). Physical and psychological long-term and late effects of cancer. *Cancer, 112*(11 Suppl), 2577–2592. doi: 10.1002/cncr.23448.

Teasdale, J. D., Segal, Z., & Williams, J. M. G. (1995). How does cognitive therapy prevent depressive relapse and why should attentional control (mindfulness) training help?. *Behav Res Ther, 33*(1), 25–39.

van den Beuken-van Everdingen, M. H. J., de Rijke, J. M., Kessels, A. G., Schouten, H. C., van Kleef, M., & Patijn, J. (2007). Prevalence of pain in patients with cancer: a systematic review of the past 40 years. *Ann Oncol, 18*(9), 1437–1449. doi: 10.1093/annonc/mdm056.

Van der Lee, M. L. & Garssen, B. (2012). Mindfulness-based cognitive therapy reduces chronic cancer-related fatigue: a treatment study. *Psycho-Oncology, 21*(3), 264–272. doi. org/10.1002/pon.1890

Weinberger, M. I., Bruce, M. L., Roth, A. J., Breitbart, W., & Nelson, C. J. (2011). Depression and barriers to mental health care in older cancer patients. *Int J Geriatr Psychiatry, 26*(1), 21–26. doi: 10.1002/gps.2497.

Winters-Stone, K. M., Bennett, J. A., Nail, L., & Schwartz, A. (2008). Strength, physical activity, and age predict fatigue in older breast cancer survivors. *Oncol Nurs Forum, 35*(5), 815–821.

Würtzen, H., Dalton, S. O., Elsass, P., Sumbundu, A. D., Steding-Jensen, M., Karlsen, R. V., . . . Johansen, C. (2013). Mindfulness significantly reduces self-reported levels of anxiety and depression: results of a randomised controlled trial among 336 Danish women treated for stage I-III breast cancer. *Eur J Cancer, 49*(6), 1365–1373. doi: 10.1016/j.ejca.2012.10.030.

SECTION C

INTEGRATIVE MEDICINE AND END-OF-LIFE CARE

31

HOSPICE AND PALLIATIVE SETTINGS

Emily A. Meier, Lori P. Montross Thomas, Natasha Ghani, Jarred V. Gallegos, and Scott A. Irwin

HOSPICE AND palliative care teams specialize in addressing the medical *and* psychosocial needs of patients and families. Hospice and palliative care patients often report pain, weakness/fatigue, feeling as though they are a burden to others, loss of hope, meaning, and dignity, and concerns about the future as some of their most severe concerns (Chochinov, 2002; Chochinov, Wilson, Enns, & Lander, 1998; De Faye, Wilson, Chater, Viola, & Hall, 2006). In fact, the prevalence of psychological distress, specifically depression and anxiety, is present in approximately 30%–60% of palliative care patients (Ewing, Todd, Rogers, Barclay, & McCabe, 2004; Steifel, Die Trill, Berney, Olarte, & Razavi, 2001). Improving end-of-life care for patients has become a priority in the United States, with a focus on providing physical, psychological, social, and spiritual support for patients and families through the use of interdisciplinary teams (Robert Wood Johnson Foundation, 1998). An important element of improving quality of care at the end of life is the inclusion of integrative medicine services. Research demonstrates that integrative medicine services can be integrated into standard hospice and palliative care and that they are beneficial and effective for addressing patient concerns (Lewis, de Vedia, Reuer, Schwan, & Tourin, 2003).

HISTORY OF THE HOSPICE MOVEMENT AND PALLIATIVE CARE

The origin of the term "hospice" derives from the Latin expression *hospis* ("hospitality") and dates back to medieval times when weary or ill travelers sought out shelter to rest when on a long journey (National Hospice and Palliative Care Organization, 2014). The concept of hospice as a place for individuals to be cared for while sick and dying arose in fourth-century Rome under the direction of Fabiola, who was a member of the Roman patrician class and was well known as a caregiver and comforter to those who were sick and dying. In 1842 the term "hospice" was identified as a place to care for chronically ill and dying patients in France, and Jeanne Gamier was credited with establishing a hospice institution. Soon after, in 1879, hospice was started in Ireland by nuns from the Irish Sisters of Charity and quickly expanded to England (Simms, 2007).

The birth of the modern hospice movement is credited to British physician Dame Cicely Saunders. Saunders began her work with the terminally ill in 1948 and created the first modern hospice institution, St. Christopher's Hospice, in London. During her work with thousands of cancer patients, Saunders discovered that patients were not only concerned about physical symptoms, but spoke of loneliness, spiritual pain, fears, and feelings of abandonment. She witnessed the destruction of families through terminal disease that led to financial and psychological burden. Through her experience she discovered that terminal cancer was not simply a disease, but consisted of multiple tragedies that should be seen as a whole, multifaceted condition (Ford, 1998).

In 1963, during a lecture at Yale University for medical, nursing, social work, and chaplaincy students, Saunders discussed her belief and practice of specialized care for the dying. During her lecture she incorporated photographs of terminally ill cancer patients and their families in order to demonstrate the "before and after" effects of specialized symptom control care (NHPCO, 2014). Saunder's inspiring lecture launched a series of events that led to the creation of the hospice movement as we know it today in the United States.

Hospices provide enhanced palliative care for those individuals near the end of life, in which the focus is on comfort. Palliative care has been increasingly applied earlier in progressive, potentially life-limiting illnesses with the same focus on decreasing pain and suffering while improving quality of life for both patients and family members. Palliative care can be provided along with curative treatment and is appropriate for individuals of any age and at any stage of disease. Several studies have established that palliative care is beneficial in three domains: the relief of physical and emotional suffering; improving patient–physician communication and decision-making; and continuity of care (National Palliative Care Research Center, 2012).

Both hospice care and palliative care are approaches for healthcare delivery. The mission of hospice and palliative care is to enhance quality of life while decreasing pain and suffering (NHPCO, 2014). Hospice care and palliative care both utilize an interdisciplinary approach, which encompasses the emotional, physical, psychosocial, and spiritual needs of each individual. Though we have many pharmacological avenues that are effective for managing symptoms, often integrative medicine and other non-pharmacological approaches can be used effectively to manage physical, mental, spiritual, and social aspects of pain and suffering, often with fewer side effects and burdens of treatment.

INTEGRATIVE MEDICINE SERVICES

The utilization of integrative medicine within hospice and palliative care is fitting given the philosophical approach of addressing mind, body, and spirit among all patients. During the last decade, integrative medicine has been incorporated into various aspects of health care (Kozak et al., 2009). Integrative medicine provides care that is patient centered and healing oriented, using therapeutic approaches originating from mostly Eastern, non-traditional medicine (Maizes, Rakel, & Niemiec, 2009). Services often provided by integrative medicine include acupuncture, aromatherapy, biofield therapies, hypnotherapy, massage therapy, or music therapy.

The overall interest in integrative medicine has increased in recent years. According to the 2007 National Health Interview Survey ($n = 23,000$), 38% of US adults reported using integrative medicine in the previous 12 months, with the highest rates among people aged 50–59 (44%). Additionally, AARP and the National Center for Complementary and Alternative Medicine (NCCAM) conducted a national survey report of integrative medicine usage in adults aged 50 and older ($n = 1,013$). Just over half (53%) of people 50 and older reported using integrative medicine therapies at some point in their lives, and nearly as many (47%) reported using it in the past 12 months. The most common reason cited for the use of integrative medicine by individuals over the age of 50 was to prevent illness and to promote general wellness (77%). The second most common reason cited was to reduce pain or treat painful conditions (73%). Other popular uses of integrative medicine therapies in the 50 and older adult population were to treat a specific health condition (59%) or to supplement conventional medicine (53%) (AARP and NCCAM Annual Survey

Report, 2011). The most common integrative medicine modalities utilized among adults over the age of 50 in the United States are presented in Figure 31.1.

Recent systematic reviews indicate the efficacy of various non-pharmacological, integrative approaches for pain management in hospitalized patient populations, including obstetrics, surgical, and postoperative and cancer-related nausea and vomiting (Dusek, Finch, Plotnikoff, & Knutson, 2010). Research studies of non-pharmacological, integrative methods to manage pain have also shown both efficacy and the potential for a reduced risk of side effects (Dusek et al., 2010). Previous studies of inpatient integrative medicine services have demonstrated that integrative medicine therapies can lower patient pain scores on average by 55% (Dusek et al., 2010), and reduce the average inpatient medication costs by 47% (Kliger et al., 2011).

Hospice and palliative care patients also utilize integrative medicine therapies for a multitude of reasons. Some patients may pursue integrative medicine with the hope of curing their illness when traditional medicines and interventions are no longer viable (Lewis et al., 2003). Additionally, integrative medicine therapies may be sought as a way to relieve pain and suffering and improve quality of life (Lewis et al., 2003). More specifically, integrative medicine therapies often encourage relaxation, reduce stress and anxiety, enhance well-being, offset adverse side effects of treatments and medications, and improve sleep (Ernst, 2001). Additionally, hospice and palliative care patients often report feeling cared for during and after the delivery of integrative medicine therapies and report the ability to progress beyond their physical symptoms in order to connect with the emotional, psychosocial, and spiritual facets of their lives (Nelson, 2006). Consequently, when integrative medicine therapies are offered as an adjunct to traditional hospice services, there is the potential to decrease physical and psychological suffering while improving overall quality of life for patients (Demmer, 2004).

In the United States, increasing attention is focused on integrative medicine for hospice and palliative care patients. Demmer (2004) conducted a national survey to gather information on integrative medicine therapies provided by hospices. A total of 300 hospices were randomly selected across the nation, of which 169 responded; 60% of these hospices offered integrative medicine therapies to their

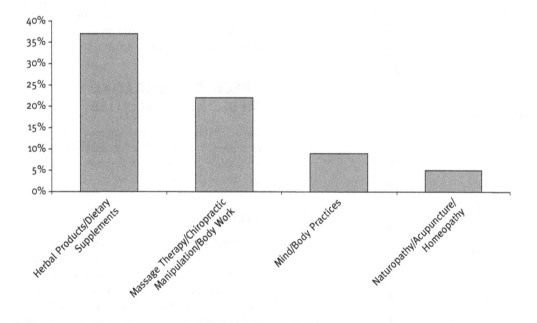

FIGURE 31.1   Type of integrative medicine modalities used in the past 12 months among adults 50 and older ($n = 1013$)

Source: AARP/NCCAM Survey of U.S. Adults 50+ (2010)

*Mind/Body practices consisted of hypnotherapy and meditation

patients. Demmer (2004) discovered that 56% of hospices that offered these therapies were older (had been in operation for 15 or more years) and served a larger number of patients (438 vs. 159). The most common integrative medicine therapies offered in hospice and palliative care organizations in the United States are presented in Table 31.1.

However, the majority (73%) of hospices surveyed that reported offering integrative medicine therapies reported that less than one-quarter of patients actually received these services. On average, these therapies were received by patients for less than 1 month (28%), 1–2 months (33%), and 3 or more months (7%); conversely, many hospices were unsure as to the duration (length of sessions) of these therapies (32%).

Additional studies have been conducted in Illinois, Nevada, Montana, Texas, and Washington State to survey the use of integrative medicine usage

Table 31.1. Most Common Types of Integrative Medicine Services offered at Hospices across the United States (n = 102)

CATEGORY	PERCENTAGE[a]
Massage therapy	83
Music therapy	50
Therapeutic touch	49
Pet therapy	48
Guided imagery	45
Reiki	36
Aromatherapy	30
Harp music	23
Reflexology	20
Art therapy	20
Hypnotherapy	4
Yoga therapy	3
Acupuncture	1
Humor therapy	1

[a]Multiple Responses
Source: Demmer, C. (2004). A survey of complementary therapy services provided by hospices. J Palliat Med, 7(4), 510–516.

among hospice and palliative care patients (Kozack et al., 2009; Oluto, Brown, Lawson, & Barner, 2014; Running, Shreffler-Grant, & Andrews, 2008; Van Hyfte, Kozak, & Lepore, 2013). These studies found that 56%–90% of hospice and palliative care organizations offered integrative medicine therapies to their patients. The most commonly cited reason for utilizing integrative medicine therapies in Nevada and Montana was to reduce emotional and spiritual pain (Running et al., 2008). Table 31.2 provides percentages on the most commonly offered integrative medicine therapies to hospice and palliative care patients among these states. Table 31.3 provides information on the key integrative medicine studies conducted in the United States in hospice and palliative care.

The findings from these studies of integrative medicine usage in Illinois, Nevada, Montana, Texas, and Washington State among hospice and palliative care patients were consistent with the national survey conducted by Demmer (2004) and the National Home and Hospice Care Survey (2007), which was conducted by the Centers for Disease Control and Prevention, and also found that 41% of hospice organizations offered integrative medicine therapies, with the most popular services being massage therapy (71%), supportive group therapy (69%), music therapy (62%), pet therapy (58%), and guided imagery or relaxation (52%) (Bercovitz, Sengupta, Jones & Harris-Kojetin, 2011).

SPECIFIC INTEGRATIVE MEDICINE MODALITIES

The following sections provide an overview of the five most common and well-researched integrative medicine therapies provided to hospice and palliative care patients in the United States.

Acupuncture

Acupuncture consists of placing small needles into target points within the body in order to aid in controlling various physical and psychological symptoms. As a result of increasing interest in acupuncture, research has greatly expanded. Hospice and palliative care patients are becoming increasingly interested in utilizing acupuncture services for symptom management. Faily and Oneschuk (2007) gauged palliative cancer care patients' understanding and interest in acupuncture and found that 54%

Table 31.2.   Most Common Types of Integrative Medicine Services Offered
in Illinois, Nevada, Montana, Texas, and Washington State Hospices

INTEGRATIVE MEDICINE MODALITY	ILLINOIS (n = 28)	NEVADA/ MONTANA (n = 70)	TEXAS(n = 62)	WASHINGTON STATE(n = 36)
Acupuncture	-	-	-	32%
Aromatherapy	-	-	-	45%
Art therapy	29%	-	-	22%
Compassionate touch	-	-	-	42%
Energy healing	25%	-	-	65%
Guided imagery	-	48%	-	45%
Hypnotherapy	-	-	-	16%
Massage therapy	54%	59%	67%	87%
Meditation	-	-	-	29%
Music therapy	61%	48%	61%	74%
Pet therapy	64%	-	45%	32%
Reflexology	-	-	-	19%
Relaxation	-	-	56%	-
Spiritual healing	-	-	51%	-

(n = 27) of patients provided an accurate understanding of acupuncture. However, only 30% of patients had previous experience using acupuncture to treat non-cancer medical issues, and 10% of patients had used acupuncture for cancer-related symptoms. Additionally, 80% of patients would be interested in meeting with an acupuncture provider if available.

The use of acupuncture in hospice and palliative care settings has significant value. Research has demonstrated acupuncture to be beneficial in areas such as pain relief, dyspnea, nausea and vomiting, dry mouth, and other cancer-related symptoms (Standish et al., 2008). Leng (1999) conducted a study of palliative care patients receiving acupuncture in order to identify which conditions were most commonly treated and patients' responses to treatment. The most common reason for utilizing acupuncture was to manage pain, with 62% reporting an excellent or good response to acupuncture (n = 50).

Further, Lim, Wong, and Aung (2011) conducted a study comparing acupuncture to nurse-led supportive care. Patients (n = 20) were randomized into one of the two groups in order to investigate improvement among nine common symptoms: anxiety, depression, drowsiness, lack of well-being, loss of appetite, nausea, pain, shortness of breath, and tiredness. All nine symptoms were found to improve immediately for patients in the acupuncture group. These symptoms continued to improve at a 6-week follow-up, with the exception of pain, nausea, and loss of appetite. In the nurse-led supportive care group, patients immediately improved on six of the nine symptoms (tiredness, nausea, and depression did not show immediate improvement). However, at the 6-week follow-up, all nine symptoms continued to show improvement, suggesting that acupuncture may provide more immediate symptom improvement, whereas nurse-led supportive interventions may be effective in improving symptoms

Table 31.3. Key Integrative Medicine Studies across the United States in Hospice and Palliative Care Organizations

CITATION	n	% HOSPICES THAT OFFER INTEGRATIVE MEDICINE	TOP THREE MODALITIES	LIMITATIONS OF OFFERING INTEGRATIVE MEDICINE THERAPIES
Bercovitz et al. (2011)	Data from 2007 National Home and Hospice Care Survey (NHHCS) conducted by the Center for Disease Control and Prevention's National Center for Health Statistics	41%	Massage therapy (71%) Supportive group therapy (69%) Music therapy (62%)	Did not address
Demmer (2004)	300 surveys mailed to randomly selected hospice organizations in the United States; 169 returned surveys	69%	Massage therapy (83%) Music therapy (50%) Therapeutic touch (49%)	Program constraints related to funding, staffing, knowledge and dissemination of integrative medicine therapies
Kozak et al. (2009)	36 hospice organizations offering inpatient and outpatient care in Washington State surveyed by phone	86%	Massage therapy (87%) Music therapy (74%) Energy healing (65%)	Lack of insurance reimbursement for integrative medicine therapies; relying predominantly on volunteers and small grants to fund program
Olotu et al. (2014)	369 surveys mailed to hospice organizations in Texas; 110 surveys returned	56%	Massage hherapy (67%) Music therapy (61%) Relaxation (56%)	Length of stay by patients; funding; lack of qualified personnel and insufficient knowledge and dissemination of integrative medicine therapies
Running et al. (2008)	54 surveys mailed to rural hospice organizations in Montana and Nevada; 27 surveys returned	70%	Massage therapy (59%) Guided imagery (48%) Music therapy (48%)	Lack of qualified personnel; insufficient knowledge of dissemination of services; lack of funding; lack of staff time
Van Hyfte et al. (2013)	108 online surveys to hospice organizations in Illinois; 31 surveys returned	90%	Pet therapy (64%) Music therapy (61%) Massage therapy (54%)	Lack of funding and staff; lack of time to provide services

over longer periods of time due to learned strategies of coping. The results of these studies demonstrate the usefulness of acupuncture in hospice and palliative care settings. In the future, it would be interesting to investigate the outcomes of acupuncture combined with the other supportive interventions used by nurses in this study.

Standish et al. (2008) conducted a literature review of acupuncture randomized controlled clinical trials (RCT) among hospice and palliative care patients. Twenty-seven RCTs were found to address specific symptoms and conditions that are common to hospice and palliative care patients (e.g., nausea and vomiting, dyspnea, pain, and dry mouth). Of these 27 studies, 23 reported statistically significant results that favored the use of acupuncture for managing these symptoms and conditions.

Despite growing interest and evidence, acupuncture is widely underutilized in the United States (Leng, 1999; Standish et al., 2008). As was discussed earlier, Demmer's (2004) national survey of integrative medicine therapies offered in hospice and palliative care settings in the United States found that as little as 1% of these organizations offered acupuncture as an integrative medicine therapy to patients. This is in contrast to 59% of hospices and palliative care services in the United Kingdom offering acupuncture as an integrative medicine service to patients in 2013. Seventy-three percent of these organizations offered acupuncture alongside other hospice and palliative care services, while only 23% offered a dedicated acupuncture clinic for patients (Leng, 2013).

The research support investigating acupuncture therapy in hospice and palliative care has greatly expanded over the last 20 years. Acupuncture has been found to be beneficial for a multitude of symptoms across numerous randomized controlled trials (Standish et al., 2008) and to demonstrate positive effects for a range of treatment diagnoses that include not only cancer, but also chronic obstructive pulmonary disease (COPD) and cystic fibrosis. Acupuncture treatments gain additional support in that the research studies identified earlier consisted of medium sample sizes, many of which were over 40 participants. Additionally, acupuncture may be a more cost-effective option for treating common symptoms identified by hospice and palliative care patients (e.g., nausea, vomiting, dyspnea) with fewer side effects (Standish et al., 2008). However, despite the numerous RCTs demonstrating the effectiveness of acupuncture, there is a lack of consistency within the research methodology. Many experiments ranged in style and protocol of needles, such as differing depth and size of the needle, techniques (acupressure versus body acupuncture) as well as ranges in electric voltage used during treatment. In addition, few studies matched participants based on problem symptoms or external factors such as current diagnosis or medications. Consistent and well-designed clinical trials are needed in order to better assess the effectiveness of needle protocols and techniques for specific symptoms with hospice and palliative care patients.

Biofield Therapies (Therapeutic Touch, Healing Touch, and Reiki)

The goal of therapeutic touch (TT) and healing touch (HT) is to rebalance a patient's energy system through the use of compassionate intent and hand movements. Most HT research has suggested beneficial effects such as reduction of anxiety and depression, emotional and mental clarity, immune system enhancement, increased sense of well-being, pain control, relaxation, and spirituality (Hutchinson, 1999). Reiki is an additional energy-healing intervention, which has gained popularity among palliative care cancer patients for assisting with relaxation, anxiety, stress, and perceptions of pain (Burden, Herron-Marx, & Clifford, 2005).

While energy-healing interventions are gaining popularity, there is a lack of research examining the effects of these interventions in hospice and palliative care patients. Henneghan and Schnyer (2013) conducted a literature review to evaluate the use of biofield therapies (TT, HT, and Reiki) to manage common symptoms that occur in patients at the end of life. However, they found insufficient evidence of the use of these therapies specifically to end-of-life care. As a result, they expanded their search criteria to include the use of biofield therapies in related patient populations (patients with cancer, elderly patients, and patients experiencing pain). A total of 30 studies were included; however, only one-third of those studies were randomized controlled trials. Evidence from related patient populations supported the use of biofield therapies in relieving pain, improving quality of life and well-being, and reducing psychological symptoms of stress.

As stated previously, there is a paucity of current research that investigates the use of biofield therapies within end-of-life care. These interventions may be equally as effective for hospice and palliative care patients, as the above-mentioned studies have demonstrated a reduction in symptoms of pain in populations of older adults as well as cancer patients, which suggests that these interventions may be applicable to hospice and palliative care patients.

Hypnotherapy

Hypnotherapy is well recognized as an effective psychotherapeutic approach among hospice and palliative care patients to assist with pain control, chemotherapy side effects, nausea, relaxation, and emotional and psychological distress (Douglas, 1999; O'Connell, 1985; Peynovska, Fisher, Oliver & Mathew, 2005). Hypnotherapy consists of three stages: induction (e.g., progressive muscle relaxation), a deepener (e.g,. the word "now"), and therapy, which begins once the patient is in a trance state. During the trance state the hypnotherapist teaches the patient how to enhance the mind's receptivity to therapeutic suggestions, such as relaxation, calmness, and well-being (Douglas, 1999; Peynovska et al., 2005; Plaskota et al., 2012).

Case studies of hypnotherapy in hospice and palliative care patients have found hypnosis to be effective for managing pain, side effects from chemotherapy, nausea, vomiting, shortness of breath, phobias, anxiety, and depression, and enhancing relaxation and sleep (O'Connell, 1985; Rajasekaran, Edmonds, & Higginson, 2005). Finlay and Jones (1996) reported that 11 out of 52 palliative care patients who engaged in hypnotherapy reported improved coping skills, less anxiety and panic attacks, an increase in positive attitude with fewer negative thoughts, improved sleep, and a decrease in the use of sedative-hypnotic medications. Peynovska et al. (2005) conducted a trial of hypnotherapy as a supplemental therapy for hospice patients in the United Kingdom. After only two hypnotherapy sessions, most patients (19 out of 20) reported a decrease in pain and anxiety, an increase in relaxation, less fatigue and more energy, the ability to cope more effectively, and more refreshing sleep; however, there were no significant changes related to depression symptomology. Moreover, Plaskota et al. (2012) examined the use of hypnotherapy for the treatment of anxiety among palliative cancer care patients. They found a significant reduction in anxiety as measured by the Hospital Anxiety and Depression Scale (HADS) after two hypnotherapy sessions. Following the completion of four hypnotherapy sessions, patients reported a significant

decrease in depressive symptoms and an increase in sleep quality. This study was consistent with Liossi and White (2001), who conducted the only randomized controlled trial of hypnotherapy, which was compared to standard care. Findings from this study demonstrated that advanced cancer patients ($n = 50$) randomized to the hypnotherapy group demonstrated improved overall quality of life and lower levels of anxiety and depressive symptoms than the standard care patient group. These studies demonstrate the effectiveness of hypnotherapy for both psychological and physical concerns among hospice and palliative care patients.

The research on hypnotherapy demonstrates consistent findings of beneficial outcomes and positive responses by patients. Hypnotherapy interventions are associated with positive health outcomes such as decreased anxiety, improved sleep quality, increases in overall well-being, reduction of pain, and relaxation. However, despite the overall consistency of beneficial outcomes found in the existing literature, it would be irresponsible to suggest that the current findings alone could convey direct causation. At this time, there have been very few controlled experiments testing the efficacy of hypnotherapy (our review finding only one). Most of the literature consists of case studies with small sample sizes. Also, the current research has multiple variables that go unaccounted for in the methodology of the study. For example, the current research primarily focuses on cancer patients, and there is little if any research comparing hypnotherapy across multiple diagnoses. Along these same lines, very few studies controlled for severity of symptoms or time elapsed following diagnosis. Causes for concern within the experimental design arise also due to factors of age, in that there were typically wide sample ranges, which increase risk of cohort effects in the data. Finally, no study identified in the review had a long-term follow-up (greater than 4 months) to examine if positive effects remained following treatment condition.

Massage Therapy with and without Aromatherapy

Massage therapy is one of the most common and popular integrative medicine therapies offered to hospice and palliative care patients (Demmer, 2004). Research suggests that massage therapy may be beneficial for the physical and emotional distress caused by pain, which greatly impacts quality of life

(Kutner et al., 2008). Additionally, massage therapy may promote relaxation, and reduce muscular tension and fatigue (Meek, 1993; Wilkinson, Barnes, & Storey, 2008).

Kutner et al. (2008) conducted a large ($n = 380$) multi-site (15 US hospice organizations) randomized controlled trial to evaluate massage therapy versus simple touch. Massage therapy was found to have immediate and beneficial effects on pain and mood when compared to simple touch. However, it was unclear whether these effects lasted for hours or days. Additionally, Downey et al. (2009) conducted a randomized controlled trial among hospice patients to measure treatment effects of massage therapy and guided meditation ($n = 167$). Patients were randomized into three conditions: therapeutic massage; guided meditation; or attention control condition (friendly visits from hospice volunteers). Compared to other studies, Downey et al. (2009) found no significant effects on patients' quality of life or pain distress for either massage or meditation when compared to the control condition after 10 weeks of enrollment. Downey and colleagues suggest that receiving visits from trained hospice volunteers, which is a standard component of hospice care, demonstrates benefits equal to those of massage therapy or guided meditation.

Massage therapy often includes the use of aromatherapy. Aromatherapy consists of the use of essential oils in order to promote relaxation, calmness, balance, and to rejuvenate the mind, body, and spirit (Styles, 1997). One common essential oil used in aromatherapy is lavender, which has been suggested to have clinical effects on psychological and physiological issues (Cavanagh & Wilkinson, 2002). Aromatherapy as a stand-alone integrative medicine service is a fairly inexpensive and easy to administer service for hospice and palliative care patients (Louis & Kowalski, 2002). A study conducted by Louis and Kowalksi (2002) examined the use of lavender aromatherapy with a sample of hospice patients who were diagnosed with advanced cancer ($n = 17$). Patients received a 60-minute session and were monitored on 3 separate days over the course of 1 week. Results indicated a small but positive change in anxiety, blood pressure and pulse, depression, pain, and sense of well-being.

Studies have demonstrated that the use of essential oils with massage therapy has a significant effect on decreasing anxiety (Corner, Cawley, & Hildebrand, 1995). Wilkinson, Aldridge, Salmon, Cain, and Wilson (1999) conducted a study with

palliative care patients ($n = 87$) who were randomly assigned to traditional massage or aromatherapy massage (Roman chamomile essential oil). Patients in each group received a total of 3 massages over the course of 3 weeks. They found a statistically significant reduction in anxiety for both groups following each massage, as well as improvement in physical symptoms and quality of life. This study demonstrated that massage therapy with or without essential oils is an effective integrative medicine service for psychological and physical concerns, with beneficial effects lasting up to 1 week.

While many studies have confirmed the immediate effects of aromatherapy massage on anxiety (Corner et al., 1995; Wilkinson, Aldridge, et al., 1999) the long-term benefits are relatively unknown. As a result, Soden, Vincent, and Craske (2004) conducted a randomized controlled trial of aromatherapy massage in a hospice population ($n = 42$) in order to examine the long-term effects of aromatherapy massage on pain scores, sleep quality, anxiety and depression, and overall quality of life. Patients were randomized to one of three groups: (1) massage with lavender essential oil and an inert carrier oil; (2) massage with an inert carrier oil only; (3) control group (no massage). They found no significant long-term benefits of aromatherapy massage in decreasing anxiety, improving pain control, or enhancing quality of life. However, it was found that sleep quality improved significantly in the standard massage group and the aromatherapy massage group. This study also demonstrated no significant results for decreasing depression scores in the aromatherapy massage group; however, there were significant reductions in depression scores in the massage-only group.

A more recent randomized controlled trial was conducted in four United Kingdom cancer centers and a hospice (Wilkinson et al., 2007). A total of 288 advanced cancer patients with clinical depression and anxiety were randomized into aromatherapy massage or treatment as usual. As other studies have suggested (Corner et al., 1995; Wilkinson et al., 1999), initial short-term effects were found for those in the aromatherapy massage group, with a decrease in clinical depression and anxiety at 6 weeks post-randomization. However, there were no significant improvements found at 10 weeks post-randomization. Interestingly, those patients who received aromatherapy massage self-reported improvement in anxiety at both 6 and 10 weeks post-randomization. The results of these studies suggest that there may be immediate benefits to receiving aromatherapy massage (up to 2 weeks), but that the benefits are not long term.

Finally, aromatherapy was compared to cognitive behavioral therapy (CBT) for emotional distress in palliative cancer care patients ($n = 39$). Serfaty, Wilkinson, Freeman, Mannix, & King (2012) conducted one of the only studies that has compared a conventional and gold standard psychotherapy treatment for depression to an integrative medicine therapy. Findings indicated that patients in both groups demonstrated significant mood improvements. However, between-group comparisons demonstrated a significant trend toward greater improvement of depression with CBT. Once again, these results suggest that short-term effects and benefits may be gained with aromatherapy massage, but the development of new coping skills via CBT may have longer lasting effects for patients with depression.

Overall, the literature on the effectiveness of massage therapy with or without aromatherapy is quite mixed. Wilkinson, Barnes, et al. (2008) conducted a systematic review of the massage therapy literature among cancer patients. After reviewing 1325 papers, only 10 RCTs met the inclusion criteria for their review. Four of the 10 studies that used pain as an outcome measure found a nonstatistical trend toward improvement. All 10 RCTs demonstrated that massage therapy or aromatherapy massage might provide short-term benefits for psychological well-being. The literature remained mixed regarding the improvements on anxiety and depression. Finally, the data were inconclusive in regard to whether massage therapy improved quality of life, as one study suggested an improvement in quality of life while another study demonstrated no improvement.

Strengths of the massage therapy literature rest on its high volume of previous research using fairly large sample sizes and controlled experimental designs, often consisting of control group and multiple experimental conditions. Studies have shown immediate benefits of massage therapy for physical symptoms such as pain. However, the existing literature does not show many significant improvements in the short-term reduction of anxiety, emotional well-being, or quality of life. In addition, long-term effects on psychological outcomes also fail to support its effectiveness, which may suggest that traditional psychotherapy approaches may deliver long-standing effects for issues related to depression

and anxiety. The bulk of the research on massage therapy solely examines cancer patients, thus making it even more troublesome to attempt to extrapolate research findings to patients enrolled in hospice and palliative care. Additionally, there are currently no massage therapy protocols; thus, each study differed in the duration of the massage, frequency per week, total number of massages, and type of massage (i.e., foot massage, full body).

Music Therapy

Music therapy can include both live music and passive music–based experiences (listening to pre-recorded music) and has been shown to increase pain control, physical comfort, and relaxation (Krout, 2001). Additionally, hospice and palliative care staff members greatly value the inclusion of music therapy as an integrative medicine service for patients (O'Kelly, 2007). A certified music therapist conducts the therapy in order to address the physical, psychological, spiritual, and social needs of patients (Starr, 1999).

Hilliard (2005) conducted a review of the literature ($n = 11$ studies) and found that anxiety, energy and fatigue, mood, pain, physical comfort, relaxation, spirituality, time and duration of treatment, and quality of life were significantly and positively affected by the use of music therapy. Additionally, Horne-Thompson and Grocke (2008) conducted a randomized controlled trial to examine the effectiveness of a single music therapy session in reducing anxiety in patients who were terminally ill. A total of 25 patients were randomized to either the music therapy group ($n = 13$) or the control group ($n = 12$), which consisted of a one-time visit from a volunteer. Those patients in the music therapy group reported a significant difference in anxiety levels compared to the control group. Additional findings included a decrease in pain, tiredness, and drowsiness, suggesting that a single session of music therapy may provide a stimulating or uplifting experience for patients.

However, as with other integrative medicine modalities, the results are mixed in regard to the effectiveness of music therapy for alleviating physical and psychological symptoms. Bradt and Dileo (2010) conducted a thorough literature review in order to examine the effects of music therapy with standard hospice care versus standard care alone or standard care combined with other therapies. A total of five studies ($n = 175$ participants) met the criteria for inclusion. The results of this review found that there is not sufficient evidence to conclude a beneficial effect of music therapy on quality of life for patients at the end of life due to the small sample sizes of studies and a lack of randomized controlled trials. Similar results were established in a more recent review of the literature conducted by Korczak, Wastian, and Schneider (2013), who also found the results of music therapy to be inconclusive. Music therapy has been shown to produce slight benefits within hospice and palliative care, specifically in improving patient mood and decreasing tiredness. Benefits have also been shown in increasing familial communication during care. However, much of the research published examining music therapy contains methodological concerns within the research designs. Most of the data are given by case descriptions, and the controlled trials often have very small samples. There is very little experimental control for duration and frequency of treatment. Additionally, there are no studies that measured outcomes during follow-up sessions; however, despite mixed results, music therapy is increasingly offered as an integrative medicine service to patients in the hopes that it will alleviate pain and suffering while improving quality of life (Table 31.4).

LIMITATIONS TO THE IMPLEMENTATION OF INTEGRATIVE MEDICINE SERVICES IN HOSPICE AND PALLIATIVE CARE ORGANIZATIONS

Integrative medicine therapies provide care that is patient-centered and healing-oriented. Despite mixed results, acupuncture, biofield therapies (healing touch, therapeutic touch, Reiki therapy), hypnotherapy, massage therapy, and music therapy may be beneficial for hospice and palliative care patients in the areas of anxiety, depression, pain management, relaxation, sleep quality, quality of life, and well-being. Integrative medicine therapies hold promise to as an addition to standard hospice and palliative care.

However, one of the biggest barriers to offering these services is a lack of understanding on how to implement, deliver, and fund integrative medicine services. According to most hospice and palliative care organizations (97%), less than 5% of the total operational budget is dedicated to integrative

medicine services (Demmer, 2004). Integrative medicine services are typically made possible through general hospice funds (33%), donations (24%), volunteers (21%), grants (8%), fundraisers (7%), and memorial funds (3%) (Demmer, 2004). Further complicating funding problems is the lack of third-party reimbursements for integrative medicine therapies. The vast majority of integrative medicine therapies are ineligible for insurance reimbursement in the United States. As a result, the lack of funding is noted to be the greatest obstacle (55%) for delivery of these services in the United States and is consistent across site-specific studies (Kozack et al., 2009; Olotu et al., 2014; Running et al., 2008; Van Hyfte et al., 2013). As such, a majority of hospice and palliative care organizations (85%) utilize volunteers (Demmer, 2004) in order to deliver integrative medicine services. While volunteers are essential to hospice and palliative care organizations, the sole utilization of volunteers often interrupts continuity of care due to vacations, school schedules, lack of supervisors, and so on (Lewis et al., 2003). Furthermore, paid staff members often report a lack of knowledge regarding integrative medicine and how to implement these services. Many organizations lack staff time and qualified personnel in order to provide specific therapies that may be beneficial to patients. In Demmer's (2004) study, only 31% of organizations offering integrative medicine services had an assessment process in place in order to identify which patients might benefit.

Finally, while the integrative medicine literature is growing in end-of-life care, there remains a lack of randomized controlled trials and a lack of longitudinal studies to demonstrate the long-term beneficial effects of many of these services due to the frailty and short duration in life span of this population. Additionally, few studies report effect sizes, and as a result it is difficult to determine if the magnitude of the differences found between integrative medicine therapies or treatment as usual are not due simply to chance.

FUTURE DIRECTIONS

Hospice and palliative care organizations are frequently requesting more education on integrative medicine for not only patients and families, but also staff members (Demmer, 2004). There are few studies or other educational offerings that describe the implementation of integrative medicine programs in hospice and palliative care (Lewis et al., 2003).

Table 31.4. Summary Table of Integrative Medicine Treatment Modalities

TREATMENT	DESCRIPTION OF TREATMENT	PROS OF THE TREATMENT IN HOSPICE AND PALLIATIVE CARE	CONS OF THE TREATMENT IN HOSPICE AND PALLIATIVE CARE	COMMON SYMPTOMS ADDRESSED BY THE TREATMENT	APPROXIMATE # OF RANDOMIZED CONTROLLED TRIALS OF THIS TREATMENT
Acupuncture	Insertion of small needles into target points in the body	Interest in the treatment is growing; cost-effective; few side effects	Few patients have previous experience with the treatment	Dyspnea, nausea, pain, vomiting,	27
Biofield therapies	Rebalance a person's energy system through the use of compassionate intent and hand movements	Interest in the treatments is growing; cost-effective; few side effects	No research examining this intervention specifically in end of life	Anxiety, depression, pain, immune system deficiencies, spiritual concerns	10
Hypnotherapy	Therapeutic process that consists of three stages: induction (progressive muscle relaxation), a deepener (e.g. word "now"), and therapy during the trance state	Interest in the treatment is growing; cost-effective, few side effects	Lack of randomized controlled trials that examine the effectiveness of hypnotherapy	Anxiety, depression, dyspnea, nausea, pain, relaxation and sleep, vomiting	1
Massage therapy	The use of pressure on the body by hand with or without the use of aromatic oils	Most common and popular integrative medicine services; cost-effective, few side effects	Lack of short- and long-term benefits for managing symptoms	Anxiety, depression, muscular tension and fatigue, pain, relaxation, sleep	10
Music therapy	Includes both live and passive music–based experiences (listening to pre-recorded music)	Highly valued as an integrative service by hospice and palliative care staff; cost-effective, few side effects	Very slight improvement in symptoms	Anxiety, energy and fatigue, pain, relaxation,	5

Additionally, more data are needed in determining the cost and efficacy of delivering integrative medicine services at the end of life and what modalities bring the most comfort and are most desired by patients (Kozak et al., 2009). Educational interventions for hospice and palliative care administrators may prove useful in order to provide knowledge on how to design and structure integrative medicine services, as well as bill for these services when appropriate (Running et al., 2008). Additional research may also bolster fundraising for integrative medicine services. Hospice and palliative care organizations (85%) feel that integrative medicine services are "important or very important" for patients. However, it is difficult for integrative medicine services to be offered in this population without adequate funding, support from staff and administrators, and knowledge on how to implement these services.

REFERENCES

American Association of Retired Persons (AARP) and National Center for Complementary and Alternative Medicine (2011). *Complementary and alternative medicine: what people aged 50 and older discuss with their health care providers.* US Department of Health and Human Services, National Institutes of Health Annual Survey Report, pp. 1–14.

Bercovitz, A., Sengupta, M., Jones, A., & Harris-Kojetin, L. D. (2011). Complementary and alternative therapies in hospice: the national home and hospice care survey: United States, 2007. *CDC National Health Statistics Reports, 33,* 1–20.

Bradt, J. & Dileo, C. (2010). Music therapy for end-of-life care. *Cochrane Database Syst Rev, 20,* 1–32.

Burden, B., Herron-Marx, S., & Clifford, C. (2005). The increasing use of reiki as a complementary therapy in specialist palliative care. *Int J Palliat Nurs, 11*(5), 248–253.

Cavanagh, H. M. A. & Wilkinson, J.M. (2002). Biological activities of lavender essential oil. *Phytother Res, 16,* 301–308.

Chochinov, H. M., Wilson, K. G., Enns, M., & Lander, S. (1998). Depression, hopelessness, and suicidal ideation in the terminally ill. *Psychosomatics, 39,* 366–370.

Chochinov, H. M. (2002). Dignity conserving care: a new model for palliative care. *JAMA, 287,* 2253–2260.

Corner, J., Cawley, N., & Hildebrand, S. (1995). An evaluation of the use of massage and essential oils on the wellbeing of cancer patients. *Int J Palliat Nurs, 1,* 67–73.

Demmer, C. (2004). A survey of complementary therapy services provided by hospices. *J Palliat Med, 7*(4), 510–516.

De Faye, B. J., Wilson, K. G., Chater, S., Viola, R. A., & Hall, P. (2006). Stress and coping with advanced cancer. *Palliat Support Care, 4,* 239–249.

Downey, L., Diehr, P., Standish, L.J., Patrick, D.L., Kozak, L., Fisher, D., et al. (2009). Might massage or guided meditation provided "Means to a better end"? Primary outcomes from an efficacy trial with patients at the end of life. *J Palliat Care, 25*(2), 100–108.

Douglas, D.B. (1999). Hypnosis: useful, neglected, available. *Am J Hosp Palliat Care, 16*(5), 665-670.

Dusek, J. A., Finch, M., Plotnikoff, G., & Knutson, L. (2010). The impact of integrative medicine on pain management in a tertiary care hospital. *J Patient Safety, 6*(1), 48–51.

Ernst, E. (2001). Complementary therapies in palliative cancer care. *Cancer, 91*(11), 2181–2185.

Ewing, G., Todd, C., Rogers, M., Barclay, S., & McCabe, J. (2004). Validation of a symptom measure suitable for use among palliative care patients in the community: CAMPAS-R. *J Pain Symptom Manage, 27*(4), 287–299.

Faily, J. & Oneschuk, D. (2007). Acupuncture in palliative care. *Support Care Cancer, 15,* 1003–1007.

Finlay, I. G. & Jones, O.L. (1996). Hypnotherapy in palliative care. *J R Soc Med, 89,* 493–496.

Ford, G. (1998). Evolution and development of hospice and specialist palliative care services. *Clin Oncol, 10,* 50–55.

Henneghan, A. M., & Schnyer, R. N. (2013). Biofield therapies for symptom management in palliative and end-of-life care. *Ame J Hospice Palliat Med, 32*(1), 90–100.

Hilliard, R. E. (2005). Music therapy in hospice and palliative care: A review of the empirical data. *Evid-Based Compl Alt Med, 2*(2), 173–178.

Horne-Thompson, A., & Grocke, D. (2008). The effect of music therapy on anxiety in patients who are terminally ill. *J Palliat Med, 11*(4), 582–590.

Hutchinson, C. P. (1999). Healing touch: an energetic approach. *Am J Nurs, 99*(4), 43–48.

Kliger, B., Homel, P, Harrison, L. B., Levenson, H. D., Kenney, J. B, & Merrell, W. (2011). Cost savings in inpatient oncology through an integrative medicine approach. *Am J Managed Care, 17*(12), 779–784.

Korczak, D., Wastian, M., & Schneider, M. (2013). Music therapy in palliative setting. *GMS Health Technol Assess, 9,* 1–6.

Kozak, L. E., Kayes, L., McCarty, R., Walkinshaw, C., Congdon, S., Kleinberger, J., Hartman, V., & Standish, L. J. (2009). Use of complementary and alternative medicine (CAM) by Washington State hospices. *Am J Hospice Palliat Care, 25*(6), 463–468.

Krout, R. E. (2001). The effects of sing-session music therapy interventions on the observed and self-reported levels of pain control, physical comfort, and relaxation of hospice patients. *Am J Hospice Palliat Care, 18*(6), 383–390.

Kutner, J. S., Smith, M. C., Corbin, L., Hemphill, L., Benton, K., Mellis, B. K., Beaty, B., . . . Fairclough, D. L. (2008). Massage therapy vs. simple touch to improve pain and mood in patients with advanced cancer: a randomized trial. *Ann Intern Med, 149*(6), 369–379.

Leng, G. (1999). A year of acupuncture in palliative care. *Palliat Med, 13*, 163–164.

Leng, G. (2013). Use of acupuncture in hospices and palliative care services in the UK. *Acupuncture Med, 31*, 16–22.

Lewis, C. R., de Vedia, A., Reuer, B., Schwan, R., & Tourin, C. (2003). Integrating complementary and alternative medicine (CAM) into standard hospice and palliative care. *Am J Hospice Palliat Care, 20*(3), 221–228.

Lim, J. T., Wong, E.T., & Aung, S.K.H. (2011). Is there a role for acupuncture in the symptom management of patients receiving palliative care for cancer? A pilot study of 20 patients comparing acupuncture with nurse-led supportive care. *Acupuncture Med, 29*, 173–179.

Liossi, C., & White, P. (2001). Efficacy of clinical hypnosis in the enhancement of quality of life of terminally ill cancer patients. *Contemp Hypnosis, 18*(3), 145–160.

Louis, M. & Kowalski, S. D. (2002). Use of aromatherapy with hospice patients to decrease pain, anxiety, and depression and to promote an increased sense of well-being. *Am J Hospice Palliat Care, 19*(6), 381–386.

Maizes, V., Rakel, D., & Niemiec, C. (2009). Integrative medicine and patient-centered care. *Explore, 5*(5), 277–289.

Meek, S. S. (1993). Effects of slow stroke back massage on relaxation in hospice patients. *J Nurs Scholarship, 25*, 17–21.

National Hospice and Palliative Care Organization. (2014). Retrieved from http://www.nhpco.org/.

National Palliative Care Research Center. (2012). *Why is palliative care research needed?* Retrieved from http://www.npcrc.org/about/about_show.htm?doc_id=374985.

Nelson, J. P. (2006). Being in tune with life: complementary therapy use and well-being in residential hospice residents. *J Holistic Nurs, 24*, 152.

O'Connell, S. (1985). Hypnosis in terminal care: discussion paper. *J R Soc Med, 78*, 122–125.

O'Kelly, J. (2007). Multidisciplinary perspectives of music therapy in adult palliative care. *Palliat Med, 21*, 235–241.

Olotu, B. S., Brown, C. M., Lawson, K. A., & Barner, J. C. (2014). Complementary and alternative medicine utilization in Texas hospices: prevalence, importance, and challenges. *Am J Hospice Palliat Care, 31*(3), 254–259.

Peynovska, R., Fisher, J., Oliver, D., & Mathew, V. M. (2005). Efficacy of hypnotherapy as a supplement therapy in cancer intervention. *Eur J Clin Hypnosis, 6*, 3–7.

Plaskota, M., Lucas, C., Evans, R., Cook, K., Pizzoferro, K., & Saini, T. (2012). A hypnotherapy invervention for the treatment of anxiety in patients with cancer receiving palliative care. *Int J Palliat Nurs, 18*(2), 69-75.

Rajasekaran, M., Edmonds, P. M., & Higginson, I. L. (2005). Systematic review of hypnotherapy for treating symptoms in terminally ill adult cancer patients. *Palliat Med, 19*, 418–426.

Robert Wood Johnson Foundation, Task Force on Palliative Care; Last Acts Campaign. (1998). Precepts of palliative care. *J Palliat Med, 1*, 109–112.

Running, A., Shreffler-Grant, J., & Andrews, W. (2008). A survey of hospices use of complementary therapy. *J Hospice Palliat Nurs, 10*(5), 304–312.

Serfaty, M., Wilkinson, S., Freeman, C., Mannix, K., & King, M. (2012). The ToT study: helping with touch or talk (ToT): a pilot randomised controlled trial to examine the clinical effectiveness of aromatherapy massage versus cognitive behaviour therapy for emotional distress in patients in cancer/palliative care. *Psychol Oncology, 21*, 563–569.

Simms, T. J. (2007). A perspective on the end of life: hospice care. *Topics Adv Pract Nurs eJournal*. Retrieved from http://www.medscape.com/viewarticle/549702.

Soden, K., Vincent, K., & Craske, S. (2004). A randomized controlled trial of aromatherapy massage in a hospice setting. *Palliat Med, 18*, 87–92.

Standish, L. J., Kozak, L., & Congdon, S. (2008). Acupuncture is underutilized in hospice and palliative medicine. *Am J Hospice Palliat Med, 25*(4), 298–308.

Stiefel, F., Die Trill, M., Berney, A., Olarte, J. M., & Razavi, A. (2001). Depression in palliative care: a pragmatic report from the expert working group of the European association for palliative care. *Support Care Cancer, 9*(7), 477–488.

Starr, R. J. (1999). Music therapy in hospice care. *Am J Hospice Palliat Care, 16*(6), 739–742.

Styles, J. L. (1997). The use of aromatherapy in hospitalized children with HIV disease. *Compl Ther Nurs Midwifery, 3,* 16–21.

Van Hyfte, G. J., Kozak, L. E., & Lepore, M. (2013). A survey of use of complementary and alternative medicine in Illinois hospice and palliative care organizations. *Am J Hospice Palliat Med, 31*(5), 553–561.

Wilkinson, S., Aldridge, J., Salmon, I., Cain, E., & Wilson, B. (1999). An evaluation of aromatherapy massage in palliative care. *Palliat Med, 13,* 409–417.

Wilkinson, S., Barnes, K., & Storey, L. (2008). Massage for symptom relief in patients with cancer: systematic review. *J Adv Nurs, 63*(5), 430–439.

Wilkinson, S., Love, S. B., Westcombe, A. M., Gambles, M. A., Burgess, C. C., Cargill, A., . . . Ramirez, A. J. (2007). Effectiveness of aromatherapy massage in the management of anxiety and depression in patients with cancer: a multicenter randomized controlled trial. *J Clin Oncol, 25*(5), 532–539.

32

COMPLEMENTARY AND ALTERNATIVE MEDICINE AND INTEGRATIVE THERAPIES IN LONG-TERM AND RESIDENTIAL DEMENTIA CARE SETTINGS

Jo-Anne Rayner and Michael Bauer

INTRODUCTION

John: I took fish oil for years. I never took it here.
 I don't know really why I stopped.
Leonie: It is really good for you, fish oil!
Interviewer: Would you ask your doctor, to take it, to
 go back on it again?
John: I would take it now for my own back. It seems to
 be an open thing—fish oil, you want it or you don't.
 You know. But I found them very good.
Interviewer: What did you take it for?
John: Oh, um, just, you know, sort of um . . .
Leonie: I get osteoarthritis, in my foot. I probably
 wouldn't have if I had continued (soft laugh).

Consider the extract of a conversation between John and Leonie (pseudonyms), who were participating in a focus group discussion in 2010. John and Leonie are permanently living in a long-term care facility (referred to as residential aged care) in Victoria, Australia, and they were discussing their previous

use of nutritional supplements, a form of complementary and alternative medicine (CAM). Both these residents have a form of arthritis—a chronic, debilitating, and painful disease for which they had used CAM before they lived in the aged care facility. Unpublished findings from research undertaken by the authors exploring the use of CAM by people living in aged care facilities indicates that prior to moving into a facility, many older people, like John and Leonie, were active participants in their own health care, using both conventional medical treatments and CAM, often to treat the same conditions (Rayner & Bauer, n.d.). However, once living in residential aged care facilities (RACFs), their use of CAM stopped immediately or declined dramatically. Older people, once they had moved into an RACF, became increasingly reliant on family members or the facility staff to assist with the continuation or instigation of CAM use, such as arranging a massage or some acupuncture. Some used CAM covertly, without the knowledge of the staff and in particular the doctor providing medical management in the facility. This research with older people living in residential aged care facilities, some of whom had dementia in the early stages, would suggest that there are a number of factors that impact the use of CAM in institutional settings, including lack of evidence to support use; staff acceptance and adoption of therapies; the care options available to residents; and the cost of therapies.

There is increasing evidence of the use of CAM by older Australians living in the community to maintain quality of life (Adams et al., 2009; McLaughlin et al., 2012a; McLaughlin et al., 2012b; Sarris et al., 2010; Xue et al., 2007; Xue et al., 2008; Zhang et al., 2007; Zhang et al., 2008), particularly for the management of chronic conditions (Armstrong et al., 2011; Braun et al., 2010). However, little is known about residents' use of CAM in RACFs (Bauer & Rayner, 2012a) either for health maintenance or the treatment of conditions generally, or more specifically for the management of the psychological and behavioral symptoms (BPSD) of dementia. The Australian and international evidence does not provide many answers, as most research into the use of CAM by older people involves those living in the community. Although older people living in the community, including those with dementia, may be in receipt of some formal care services to enable them to continue to live in their own homes, they are more in control of the choices they make and what they can do. Older people living in residential care facilities, on the other hand, especially those with dementia, are a unique group in respect to CAM use, in that they are dependent on care staff for the provision of most of their care needs, including the use of CAM.

This chapter will focus on the Australian experience. We will define CAM and briefly describe the patterns of CAM use in Australia, focusing on older people—those aged 65 years and older. We will outline the aging of the Australian population and the increase in chronic illnesses that are associated with older age, including dementia. This will provide a background and context for the final section of this chapter, which will draw on Australian and international studies and focus on the use of CAM and integrative therapies in long-term care settings, including dementia care settings. This section of the chapter will include a discussion on the use of an increasing number of "therapies" commonly used in these settings that are often referred to as CAM.

COMPLEMENTARY AND ALTERNATIVE MEDICINE (CAM)

Defining CAM is an issue raised often in the literature; some argue that it is defined in terms of what it isn't, rather than the intrinsic quality that it brings to health and healing (Willis & Rayner, 2015). Terms such as *complementary*, *alternative*, and *integrative* are often used synonymously, despite having specific meanings, and the literature reveals the use of multiple and diverse modalities, medicines, and practices, including practitioner-based therapies, self-medication with over-the-counter and Internet-purchased supplements and herbs, in combination with conventional medical treatments. A literature review on the use of CAM in residential aged care (Bauer & Rayner, 2012a) points to the fact that there is no clear or common definition of CAM.

In this chapter, CAM is defined as "a group of diverse health care systems, practices, and products that are not presently considered to be part of conventional medicine" (National Centre for Complementary and Alternative Medicine [NCCAM], 2002), self-administered or delivered by a variety of practitioners. The most mainstream CAM modalities include, but are not limited to, naturopathy, chiropractic, osteopathy, Western herbal medicine, traditional Chinese medicine (TCM), and massage, as well as vitamins and dietary supplements.

TRENDS IN COMPLEMENTARY AND ALTERNATIVE MEDICINE USE IN AUSTRALIA

Australians are some of the largest consumers of CAM worldwide (Harris et al., 2012; Xue et al., 2007; Zhang et al., 2008). The National Institute of Complementary Medicine (NICM) reports that two in every three Australians use some form of CAM each year (NICM, 2014) and many use it on a daily basis (Swift et al., 2007). The most recent nationally representative prevalence survey conducted in 2005 (Xue et al., 2007) found that 69% of Australian adults reported using CAM; and 58% of older people participating in this survey reported using some form of CAM, with herbal medicines accounting for 19% of their consumption (Zhang et al., 2008).

The bulk of CAM used in Australia, including use by older people, is self-prescribed products such as vitamin and mineral supplements as a form of clinical nutrition (35.4%) and herbal medicines (19%) (Zhang et al., 2007), purchased over the counter from pharmacies, supermarkets, health food stores, and increasingly via the Internet (Zhang et al., 2008; Xue et al., 2007). However, despite CAM use being dominated by self-prescription, 60% of older people participating in the national prevalence survey reported visiting a CAM practitioner (commonly a chiropractor, naturopath, or acupuncturist) in 2005 (Zhang et al., 2007), with visits to practitioners almost equaling the number of consultations with medical practitioners in the same year (Xue et al., 2008), especially among Australians who have private health insurance. The number of CAM practitioners in Australia nearly doubled in the decade 1995–2005, with industry revenue estimated at AUD$3.5 billion in 2008 (Australian Bureau of Statistics [ABS], 2008). This revenue is forecast to grow to AUD$4.6 billion in 2017–2018 (NICM, 2014). As CAM products and consultations with most practitioners are not subsidized by the Australian health system,[1],[2] consumers have substantial out-of-pocket expenses. In 2010, out-of-pocket expenditure for CAM use for chronic illness was estimated at AUD$91 million (Spinks et al., 2013). For individuals on limited incomes, such as older people, the cost of using CAM may explain the reduced prevalence of use among the very old (Adams et al., 2009; Walkom et al., 2013).

The characteristics of older CAM users in Australia are consistent with the international literature (Cheung et al., 2007; McMahon & Lutz, 2004; Ness et al., 2005; Singh & Levine, 2006). Older women are more likely to use CAM compared to men, especially women with post-secondary education and higher household incomes (Xue et al., 2007; Zhang et al., 2008). Older CAM users differ from younger users, in that they are less likely to have private health insurance and are more likely to rate their health as only fair or poor rather than good or excellent. Responding to increased consumer demand for and use of CAM in Australia, private health insurance provides refunds for the services of some CAM practitioners. Health insurance refunds are limited and do not include refunds for CAM products because of financial constraints—these are "for-profit" organizations.

In Australia, as elsewhere (Bailey et al., 2013; Metcalfe et al., 2010), CAM is used for the maintenance of health and well-being, and to treat chronic diseases (Armstrong et al., 2011; Braun et al., 2010). However, CAM is not typically used at the exclusion of or as an alternative to conventional medicine, or because people want to avoid consulting medical practitioners. CAM users, especially those with chronic conditions, are more likely to supplement their medical treatments with CAM and regularly visit their medical practitioner, more than non-CAM users (Lin et al., 2014; Sarris et al., 2010; Zhang et al., 2007). Compared to younger people, older people are more likely to use CAM in conjunction with conventional medicine (Zhang et al., 2007). The use of CAM in combination with conventional medicine has generated considerable debate among medical doctors, with references to CAM as including "treatments on the margins," and notions of evidence, risk, accountability, and regulation (Dwyer, 2011). Yet, research conducted by the Australian National Prescribing Service (NPS) found that many Australian medical practitioners are unaware of the adverse effects of the most commonly used CAM or their potential interactions with conventional medicines, and that they did not routinely ask patients about CAM use (NPS, 2008). Many users of CAM report that they do not disclose their use to medical doctors, often because they are not asked, but also because of the negative responses they have received in the past (Lin et al., 2014; Spinks et al., 2013; Zhang et al., 2008). While older people are more likely to discuss their CAM use with their medical practitioner (Zhang et al., 2007) compared to younger people, the following quotes from Lin and colleagues (2014) illustrate the difficulties they often face:

"My doctor knows I follow CAM but does not want to know about it . . . and is not interested in hearing what my CAM [provider] has to say" (Female, 63 years).

"My doctor says I can't discuss with him: 'I know nothing about that. I don't know'" (Female, 85 years).

"I mentioned CAM to my doctor, he said he had trouble keeping up with traditional [conventional bio] medicine and had no time to study CAM, so I don't speak about it anymore" (Male, 60 years).

[1] Medicare is the Australian Universal Health Insurance Scheme, which covers 85% of all medical service costs and hospitalization in the public hospital system. Medicare does not cover the costs associated with CAM—medicines or services provided by therapists.
[2] The Pharmaceutical Benefits Scheme is a program of the National Government that provides subsidised prescription drugs to Australians.

Interestingly, in Australian there has been a growth of integrated practitioners who incorporate both CAM and conventional medicine in a medical practice (Rayner et al., 2011).

The use of CAM among older Australians reflects a trend in CAM use in industrialized countries more generally, which is explained by factors including dissatisfaction or poor outcomes associated with conventional medicine; a need for more control in decisions; the perceived naturalness of CAM (Iedema & Velijanova, 2013); and the personalized nature of the interactions with CAM practitioners, coupled with individually tailored interventions (Willis & Rayner, 2015). Conventional medical treatments used in the management of chronic health conditions related to aging provide only limited relief (Adams et al., 2009; Armstrong et al., 2011; Cartwright 2007; Cheung et al., 2007; Schnabel et al., 2014), and there is a growing trend in Western industrialized countries like Australia for individuals to take individual responsibility for their health (Hurd Clarke & Bennett, 2013).

THE AGING OF THE AUSTRALIAN POPULATION AND DEMENTIA

The population of Australia is approximately 23 million (ABS, 2013a) and Australians have one of the highest life expectancies in the world—79.9 years for men and 84.3 years for women (ABS, 2013b). The Australian population is aging rapidly—the number of people aged 65 years and older tripled between 1973 and 2013, and there was a sixfold increase in the number of people aged 85 years and over in the same period (ABS, 2013a). Over the next two decades, the population is expected to grow to 28.8 million, with growth strongest among the older age groups (Australia Institute of Health and Welfare [AIHW], 2014). Older people are also more likely to have multiple (five or more) long-term chronic conditions (ABS, 2010), an increased use of medicines, and a higher demand for all medical services, including services that offer CAM (Willison & Andrews, 2004). While many older Australians have good health, one in five report short- and long-term chronic health conditions that can impact on well-being and quality of life (AIHW, 2014), and as the population ages and the number of people with chronic illnesses increases, the demand for residential aged care services is likely to increase. Currently, nearly 169,000 older people live in RACFs, a rise of 20% over the past decade, particularly among people aged 85 years and older (AIHW, 2014). Older people living in RACFs are generally highly dependent on care, and many (63%) have a moderate to severe form of dementia.

Dementia is the fourth leading cause of burden of disease in Australia and is heavily concentrated in the oldest age groups (AIHW, 2014). An estimated 332,000 Australians have dementia, and due to the aging of the population this number is projected to increase to 900,000 by 2050 (AIHW, 2012). Dementia has no known cure and is treated medically using pharmacological interventions (drugs) to slow the progression of the disease and to manage the behavioral and psychological symptoms as they appear. Many pharmacological interventions are known to provide only modest benefits however (de Medeiros & Basting, 2014). A wide range of non-pharmacological treatments, such as CAM, are used for treating the cognitive impairment associated with dementia; however, the evidence for the effectiveness of many of these is limited.

THE USE OF COMPLEMENTARY AND ALTERNATIVE MEDICINES IN LONG-TERM AND RESIDENTIAL AGED CARE

There are an increasing number of international studies examining the clinical efficacy of specific CAM treatments and interventions for older people in the long-term care environment, particularly for the management of dementia, but the evidence for many is limited. Very little research into the use of CAM in long-term and residential aged care has been undertaken in Australia. Small and pilot studies of the use of CAM integrated into care in long-term care demonstrate that with careful preparation, collaboration, and evidence, an alternative model of care can be effective and sustainable in improving quality of life (Evans et al., 2015).

A review undertaken by the authors (Bauer & Rayner, 2012a) to determine existing patterns of CAM use among older people living in RACFs (nursing homes and assisted living) and how residents view CAM as a treatment option revealed only five research papers published between 2001 and 2010, two of which were Australian research (Henry, 2001; Webber, 2003). This review found great diversity in the CAM modalities offered as routine care in aged care facilities, generally to enhance well-being, promote health, and reduce pain. None gives us any indication of the prevalence of CAM use by older people living in aged care, or the motivations for and satisfaction with use, despite an increasingly large number of frail older people living in long-term care settings. As a consequence, very little is known about individual preferences for CAM use or the barriers to older people using CAM as a healthcare option in residential aged care. The protagonists for CAM use in residential aged care facilities are commonly nurses. The review also highlighted barriers to implementing CAM more broadly, including a lack of knowledge among staff, negative attitudes to CAM, fear of litigation and issues about medical responsibility, despite residents' reports of satisfaction with the modalities offered. The authors' own research (focus groups and interviews with residents, family members, and staff in aged-care facilities in Victoria, Australia) shows that residents officially and unofficially use various forms of CAM for pain relief and to improve health and well-being and that they would like to use it more, but access to CAM and cost are substantial barriers (Rayner & Bauer, n.d.).

While there are an increasing number of studies exploring the use of specific CAM modalities to manage the behavioral and psychological symptoms of dementia (BPSD), few show any meaningful benefit. A systematic review of non-pharmacological approaches in the treatment of some of the BPSD associated with dementia (Hulme et al., 2010) included 16 different interventions, seven of which would be considered CAM (see Table 32.1). The CAM modalities included aromatherapy, massage, acupressure, vitamin, mineral, and natural product supplementation, herbal medicine, yoga, and transcutaneous electrical nerve stimulation (TENS). The following section will briefly review the evidence available supporting the use of these CAM modalities for use in residential aged care facilities.

CLINICAL NUTRITION: VITAMINS, MINERALS, AND NATURAL HEALTH PRODUCTS

Nutritional supplements such as vitamins, minerals, amino acids, and metabolites have been shown to augment conventional medications, improve

Table 32.1.   Dementia Symptoms and CAM Interventions

DEMENTIA SYMPTOMS	CAM INTERVENTIONS
Reduced cognition	Transcutaneous electrical nerve stimulation (TENS); herbal medicines; acupressure; clinical nutrition
Reduced ability to perform activities of daily living	Aromatherapy
Behavioral and psychological	Aromatherapy; massage; TENS; phytomedicines/herbal medicines; yoga; reflexology; acupressure
Sleep disturbance	Aromatherapy; massage; acupressure
Pain	Massage; reflexology

Source: Hulme et al. (2010)

the symptoms of some disorders, and to reduce medication side effects. As such, they may have merit for use in long-term aged care, as older people with impaired cognition often have poor nutritional status (Ulger et al., 2010); and malnutrition has been found to be high among long-term aged care residents (Banks et al., 2007; Gaskill et al., 2008; Woods et al., 2009), particularly deficiencies in micronutrients such as the B group vitamins, vitamin D, zinc, calcium, and magnesium (Kjeldby et al., 2013; Woods et al., 2009). However, the evidence to support the use of nutritional supplements such as vitamins, minerals, and natural health products such as fish oils for people with dementia in long-term facilities is limited, conflicting, and inconclusive (Allen et al., 2013; Gestuvo & Hung, 2012; Harvey, 2011; Li et al., 2014). Excessive nutritional supplementation has also been associated with increased risk of adverse effects and interactions with conventional medications among older people living in the community (de Sousa Silva et al., 2014; Nahin et al., 2009).

PHYTOMEDICINES/HERBAL MEDICINES

A recent systematic review found herbal medicine use to be common among older people living in the community (de Sousa Silva et al., 2014), with nationally representative studies finding 19% and 20% of older people in Australia (Zhang et al., 2007) and North America (Wu et al., 2011), respectively, using herbal medicines on a regular basis. Only a small number of studies report on the use of specific herbal medicines among older people living in aged care; however, some phytomedicines (or herbal medicines, as they are more commonly known) are thought to stimulate the central nervous system and therefore have a role in psychogeriatrics. *Ginseng* is used to improve cognitive function, *Gingko biloba* is purported to enhance cognition and memory and has been indicated for use in Alzheimer's and age-associated dementia, and *Valerian* is a safe herbal sedative. *Saffron* and *Sage* have also been used in Ayurvedic medicine to improve cognition and reduce agitation in individuals with moderate Alzheimer's disease. *Gingko biloba* is the best studied herbal medicine for memory-related disorders like dementia; however, a Cochrane review (Birks & Grimley Evans, 2009) found no evidence of clinically significant benefit for people with dementia or other cognitive impairment. Little or no high-quality evidence was found to support other herbal medicines used to improve cognition or memory retention, such as *Acetyl-L-carnitine* (Hudson & Tabet, 2003), *Ginseng* (Geng et al., 2010), *Brahmi* or *Gotu kola* (Harvey, 2011). Herbal medicines can have adverse effects, and can interact with a number of medications that many older adults commonly take, in particular for chronic conditions (Lui & Chang, 2006). A third of older adults attending a memory disorders clinic in Canada using herbal products were at risk of an herbal product–conventional drug interaction (Dergal et al., 2002).

AROMATHERAPY

Aromatherapy, the use of pure essential oils from fragrant plants, is probably one of the most popular CAM modalities used in aged care and has been used to try to reduce disturbed behaviors, to promote sleep, and to stimulate motivational behavior of people with dementia. Lavender oil is thought to have modest efficacy in reducing agitation in dementia (Holmes et al., 2002; Lin et al., 2007); and lemon balm (*Melissa officinalis*) has been found to be safe and efficacious in improving cognition and reducing agitation in people with mild to moderate dementia (Akhondzadeh et al., 2003). However, the evidence for overall benefits of using essential oils for people with dementia remains equivocal, due to the absence of high-quality randomized placebo-controlled trials (Forrester et al., 2014).

MASSAGE, REFLEXOLOGY, AND THERAPEUTIC TOUCH

Massage and therapeutic touch have been suggested as alternatives or supplements to other treatments used to manage behaviors associated with dementia, such as anxiety and agitation, and there is the suggestion that these therapies may counteract cognitive decline. However, there is a paucity of high-quality research on the use of massage to manage the behaviors of older people with dementia living in long-term care facilities (Moyle et al., 2012). While a Cochrane review (Viggo Hansen et al., 2006) found very limited reliable evidence to support hand massage and touch as interventions for problems associated with dementia, the authors did recommend these therapies as alternatives to, or as complements to, other interventions. Sleep disturbances occur frequently in people with dementia, often increasing as the dementia progresses, and pain can be difficult to diagnose when there is dementia. Massage and reflexology have been suggested as non-pharmacological interventions to treat sleep disturbances and pain in long-term care residents. A number of small studies have shown some reduction in pain associated with massage (Sansone & Schmidtt, 2000) and reflexology (Hodgson & Anderson, 2008), but the methodological quality of papers is limited.

ACUPUNCTURE/ACUPRESSURE/ TRANSCUTANEOUS ELECTRICAL NERVE STIMULATION (TENS)

Acupuncture and acupressure have been used to manage a number of the symptoms associated with dementia, for example to assist in the quality of sleep (Kwok et al., 2013) and to reduce agitation (Yang et al., 2007. The effectiveness of these interventions is uncertain, due to the absence of any suitable randomized placebo-controlled trials (Peng et al., 2007). TENS is commonly used for pain control across many settings, and has more recently been used in the treatment of dementia. A Cochrane review (Cameron et al., 2003) found that the use of TENS can produce significant but short-lived improvements in some memory and cognitive functions. Further research is recommended for all modalities.

OTHER "THERAPIES" USED AS CAM IN RESIDENTIAL AGED CARE

Increasingly, possibly in an attempt to gain legitimacy and therefore therapeutic value, as well as to attract funding subsidies, a broad range of activities used in RACFs for the management of dementia has become labeled as CAM. The use of these therapies poses some challenges to the traditionally accepted definition and nomenclature of CAM (Bauer et al., 2012b). These "therapies" are used to assist in maintaining the well-being and quality of life of older people and to reduce agitation and increase engagement in people with dementia living in RACFs.

We have named these activities "therapies" and broadly grouped them (Table 32.2) as *physical*, which includes "exercise therapies" such as tai chi (Cheng et al., 2012), outdoor activities (Connell et al., 2007), and dance (Guzman-Garcia et al., 2013); *cultural*, which includes art, drama, and music therapies (Peisah et al., 2011), humor or "laughter therapy" (Goodenough et al., 2012), and "video game therapy" (Ryder-Jones et al., 2012); *psychological* interventions such as "validation therapy" (Livingston, et al., 2005); *sensory*, including a range of multisensory interventions and environments such as Snoezelen© (Cruz et al., 2013) and "garden or horticultural therapy" (Detweiler et al., 2012); *spiritual* therapies like prayer (Ceramidas, 2012); as well as other activities such as "pet therapy" (Kaldy, 2013) and "doll therapy" (Higgins, 2010). The literature suggests that many of these therapies may have some therapeutic value, insofar as they improve the well-being and quality of life of older people.

Music, with and without dance, is used increasingly to promote the quality of life of people in residential aged care and seems to have a positive impact on a range of behavioral and psychological symptoms of dementia, including a reduction in

Table 32.2. Dementia Symptoms and Therapies

DEMENTIA SYMPTOMS	THERAPIES
Reduced cognition	Reminiscence, music, light, Snoezelen/multisensory stimulation, art, validation
Reduced ability to perform activities of daily living	Reminiscence, Tai Chi/exercise, dance, Snoezelen/multisensory stimulation, validation
Behavioral and psychological	Validation, music, emotional-oriented, multisensory/Snoezelen, art, dance, horticultural, light, doll, pet, prayer
Sleep disturbance	Outdoor activities, light, gardening/horticulture
Reduced quality of life	Dance, music, art, storytelling, humor, horticulture, Tai Chi/exercise
Pain	Humor

agitation, aggression, wandering, restlessness, and irritability (Hulme, et al, 2010; Janata, 2012; Sung et al., 2006).

The benefits of physical activity on cognition have been studied for over 40 years, and a number of studies report the use of exercise-based therapies such as tai chi (Chang et al., 2010; Deschamps et al., 2009) and yoga (Fan & Chen, 2011) to promote physical and mental well-being among older people, including those with dementia. Multisensory interventions, such as Snoezelen, for the management of dementia-related behaviors have become increasingly popular in Australia and elsewhere (Bauer et al., 2012b), with little evidence of efficacy (Chung & Lai 2009). While there is little robust evidence to support the use of most of these "therapies," as individual studies have major methodological weaknesses that limit their generalizability as therapeutic interventions (de Medeiros & Basting, 2014), many provide opportunities to improve the quality of life and are options that pose no risk; thus they may be options that help address many of the challenges of caring for older people in residential and long-term care.

SUMMARY

The use of CAM by older people has been shown to be common in many industrialized countries, particularly for the treatment of the chronic conditions associated with old age; however, most of the research on the prevalence of CAM and the reasons for its use has been conducted with community-dwelling older people. In this chapter we have presented some examples of the use of CAM in residential aged care and have highlighted some of the issues that need greater clarity and understanding. CAM has become big business, driven by consumer demand, integrated within conventional medicine and distributed by multinational companies. While the popularity of CAM continues, definitional debates are evident across the spectrum of CAM used in residential aged care, and there is a lack of robust evidence to support the efficacy of use overall.

IMPORTANT CONSIDERATIONS

The high use of CAM among adults in many industrialized countries, coupled with the aging of these populations and the increased costs associated with providing care to people who can no longer care for themselves, requires rigorous research into alternative therapeutic interventions such as CAM, which may enhance the quality of life for older people. The increasing use of CAM needs to be acknowledged and respected, and definitional debates about what constitutes CAM need to be resolved. There is currently a paucity of research into the use of CAM in residential aged care, especially in Australia, including prevalence rates, preferences, costing, satisfaction, and effectiveness. CAM use must have an evidence base, especially when used as a therapeutic intervention among vulnerable groups.

DISCLOSURE STATEMENT

Both authors have no conflicts to disclose.

REFERENCES

Adams, J., Sibbritt, D., & Young, A.F. (2009). A longitudinal analysis of older Australian women's consultations with complementary and alternative medicine (CAM) practitioners, 1996–2005. *Age Ageing, 38*, 93–99.

Akhondzadeh, S., Noroozian, M., Mohammadi, M., Ohadinia, S., Jamshidi, A., & Khani, M. (2003). *Melissa officinalis* extract in the treatment of patients with mild to moderate Alzheimer's disease: a double-blind, randomised, placebo controlled trial. *J Neurol Neurosurg Psychiatry, 74*, 863–866.

Allen, V. J., Methven, L., & Gosney, M. A. (2013). Use of nutritional complete supplements in older adults with dementia: systematic review and meta-analysis of clinical outcomes. *Clin Nutrition, 32*, 950–957.

Armstrong, A., Thiebout, S., Brown, L., & Nepal, B. (2011). Australian adults' use of complementary and alternative medicine in the treatment of chronic illness: a national study. *Aust NZ J Public Health, 35*(4), 384–390.

Australian Bureau of Statistics. (2008). Australian Social Trends –Complementary Therapies. ABS, Canberra July 2008. Available at: http://www.abs.gov.au/AUSSTATS/abs@.nsf/Lookup/4102.0Chapter5202008

Australian Bureau of Statistics. (2010). *Disability, ageing and carers, Australia: summary of findings, 2009*. ABS Cat. no. 4430.0. Canberra: ABS.

Australian Bureau of Statistics. (2013a). *Australian demographic statistics, June 2013*. ABS Cat. no. 3101.0. Canberra: ABS.

Australian Bureau of Statistics. (2013b). *Deaths, Australia, 2012*. ABS Cat. no. 3302.0. Canberra: ABS.

Australian Institute of Health and Welfare. (2012). *Dementia in Australia*. Cat. no. AGE 70. Canberra: AIHW.

Australian Institute of Health and Welfare. (2014). *Australia's health 2014*. Australia's health series No. 14. Cat. no. AUS 178. Canberra: AIHW.

Banks, M., Ash, S., Bauer, J., & Gaskill, D. (2007). Prevalence of malnutrition in adults in Queensland public hospitals and residential aged care facilities. *Arch Gerontol Geriatr, 9*(Suppl.), 39–43.

Bailey, R. L., Gahche, J. J., Miller, P. E., Thomas, P. R., & Dwyer, J. T. (2013). Why US adults use dietary supplements. *JAMA Internal Medicine, 172*(5), 355–361.

Bauer, M., & Rayner, J. (2012a). Use of complementary and alternative medicine in residential aged care. *J Alt Compl Med, 18*(11), 1–5.

Bauer, M., Rayner, J, Koch, S., & Chenco, C. (2012b). The use of multi-sensory interventions to manage dementia-related behaviours in the residential aged care setting: a survey of one Australian state. *J Clin Nurs, 21*, 3061–3069.

Birks, J., & Grimley Evans, J. (2009). Ginkgo biloba for cognitive impairment and dementia. *Cochrane Database Syst Rev, 1.* Art. no.: CD003120. doi: 10.1002/14651858.CD003120.pub3.

Braun, L. A., Tiralongo, E., Wilkinson, J. M., Spitzer, O., Bailey, M., Poole, S., & Dooley, M. (2010). Perceptions, use and attitudes of pharmacy customers on complementary medicines and pharmacy practice. *BMC Compl Alt Med, 10*, 38.

Cameron, M., Lonergan, E., & Lee, H. (2003). Transcutaneous electrical never stimulation (TENS) for dementia. *Cochrane Database Syst Rev, 3.* Art. no.: CD004032. doi: 10.1002/14651858. CD004032.

Cartwright, T. (2007). "Getting on with life": The experiences of older people using complementary health care. *Social Sci Med, 64*, 1692–1703.

Ceramidas, D. M. (2012). Faith-based cognitive behavioral therapy: easing depression in the elderly with cognitive decline. *J Christian Nurs, 29*(1), 42–48.

Chang, Y-K., Nien, Y-H., Tsai, C-L., & Etnier, J. L. (2010). Physical activity and cognition in older adults: the potential of tai chi chuan. *J Aging Phys Activ, 18*, 451–471.

Cheng, S. T., et al. (2012). Leisure activities alleviate depressive symptoms in nursing home residents with very mild or mild dementia. *Am J Geriatr Psychiatry, 20*(10), 904–908.

Cheung, C. K., Wyman, J. F., & Halcon, L. L. (2007). Use of complementary and alternative therapies in community-dwelling older adults. *J Alt Compl Med, 13*, 997–1006.

Chung, J. C. C., & Lai, C. K. Y. (2009). Snoezelen for dementia. *Cochrane Database Syst Rev, 1.* Art. no.: CD003152. doi: 0.1002/14651858.

Connell, B. R., Sanford, J. A., & Lewis, D. (2007). Therapeutic effects of an outdoor activity program on nursing home residents with dementia. *J Housing Elderly, 21*(3–4), 194–209.

Cruz, J., Marques, A., Barbosa, A., Figueiredo, D., & Sousa, L. X. (2013). Making sense(s) in dementia: a multisensory and motor-based group activity program. *Am J Alzheimers Dis, 28*(2), 137–146.

de Medeiros, K., & Basting, A. (2014). "Shall I compare thee to a dose of Donepezil?": Cultural arts interventions in dementia care research. *Gerontologist, 54*(3), 344–353.

Dergal, J. M., Gold, J. L., Laxer, D. A., Binns, M. A., Lanctôt, K. L., Freedman, M., & Rochon, P. A. (2002). Potential interactions between herbal medicines and conventional drug therapies used by older adults attending a memory clinic. *Drugs Aging, 19*(11), 879–886.

Deschamps, A., Onifade, C., Decamps, A., & Bourdel-Marchasson, I. (2009). Health-related quality of life in frail institutionalized elderly: effects of a cognition-action intervention and tai chi. *J Aging Phys Activ, 17*(2), 236–248.

de Sousa Silva, J. E., Santos Souza, C. A., da Silva, T. B., Gomes, I. A., Brito Gde, C., de Souza Araujo, A. A., de Lyra-Junior, D. P., da Silva, W. B., & da Silva, F. A. (2014). Use of herbal medicines by elderly patients: a systematic review. *Arch Gerontol Geriatrics, 59*(2), 227–233.

Detweiler, M. B., Sharma, T., Detweiler, J. G., Murphy, P. F., Lane, S., Carman, J., Chudhary, A. S., Halling, M. H., & Kim, K. Y. (2012). What is the evidence to support the use of therapeutic gardens for the elderly?" *Psychiatry Investig, 9*(2), 100–110.

Dwyer, J. M. (2011). Is it ethical for medical practitioners to prescribe alternative and complementary treatments that may lack evidence?—No. *Med J Australia, 195*(2), 79.

Evans, R., Vihstadt, C., Westrom, K., & Baldwin, L. (2015). Complementary and integrative healthcare in a long-term care facility: a pilot study. *Global Adv Health Med, 4*(1), 18–27.

Fan, J. T., & Chen, K. M. (2011). Using silver yoga exercises to promote physical and mental health of elders with dementia in long-term care facilities. *Int Psychogeriatrics, 23*(8), 1222–1230.

Forrester, L. T., Maayan, N., Orrell, M., Spector, A. E., Buchan, L. D., & Soares-Weiser, K. (2014). Aromatherapy for dementia. *Cochrane Database Syst Rev, 2.* Art. no.: CD003150. doi: 10.1002/14651858.CD003150.pub2.

Gaskill, D., Black, L. J., Hassall, S., Sanders, F., Isenring, E. A., & Bauer, J. D. (2008). Malnutrition prevalence and nutrition issues in residential aged care facilities. *Australas J Ageing, 27*, 189–194.

Geng, J., Dong, J., Ni, H., Lee, M. S., Wu, T., Jiang, K., Wang, G., Zhou, A. L., & Malouf, R. (2010). Ginseng for cognition. *Cochrane Database Syst Rev, 12.* Art. no.: CD007769. doi: 10.1002/14651858. CD007769.pub2.

Gestuvo, M. K., & Hung, W.W. (2012). Common dietary supplements for cognitive health. *Aging Health, 8*(1), 89–97.

Goodenough, B., Low, L-F., Casey, A-N., Chenoweth, L., & Fleming, R. (2012). Study protocol for a randomized controlled trial of humor therapy in residential care: the Sydney Multisite Intervention of Laughter Bosses and Elder Clowns (SMILE). *Int Psychogeriatrics, 24*(12), 2037–2044.

Guzman-Garcia, A., Hughes, J., James, I., & Rochester, L. (2013). Dancing as a psychosocial intervention in care homes: a systematice review of the literature. *Int J Geriatr Psychiatry, 28*(9), 914-924.

Harris, P. E., Cooper, K. L., Relton, C., & Thomas, K. J. (2012). Prevalence of complementary and alternative medicine (CAM) use by the general population: a systematic review and update. *Int J Clin Practice, 66*(10), 924–939.

Harvey, K. (2011). Caution with complementaries for cognitive impairment. *Aust Prescr, 34*(1), 19–21.

Henry, P. R. (2001). Update on care: using complementary therapies in residential services. *Geriatrician, 19*, 27–28.

Higgins, P. (2010). Using dolls to enhance the wellbeing of people with dementia in residential care. *Nursing Times, 106*(39), 18–20.

Hodgson, N. A., & Anderson, S. (2008). The clinical efficacy of reflexology in nursing home residents with dementia. *J Alt Compl Med, 14*(3), 269–275.

Holmes, C., Hopkins, V., Hensford, C., MacLaughlin, V., Wilkinson, D., & Rosenvinge, H. (2002). Lavender oil as a treatment for agitated behaviour in severe dementia: a placebo controlled trial. *Int J Geriatr Psychiatry, 17*(4), 305–308.

Hudson, S. A., & Tabet, N. (2003). Acetyl-l-carnitine for dementia. *Cochrane Database Syst Rev, 2.* Art. no.: CD003158. doi: 10.1002/14651858.CD003158.

Hulme, C., Wright, J., Crocker, T., Oluboyede, Y., & House, A. (2010). Non-pharmacological approaches for dementia that informal carers might try or access: a systematic review. *Int J Geriatr Psychiatry, 25*, 756–763.

Hurd Clarke, L., & Bennett, E. V. (2013). Constructing the moral body: self-care among older adults with multiple chronic conditions. *Health, 17*, 211.

Iedema, R., & Velijanova, I. C. (2013). Lifestyle science: self-healing, co-production and DIY. *Health Sociol Rev, 22*(1), 2–7.

Janata, P. (2012). Effects of widespread and frequent personalized music programming on agitation and depression in assisted living facility residents with Alzheimer-type dementia. *Music Medicine, 4*, 8–15.

Kaldy, J. (2013). Alternative therapies for a new era of health care. *Consult Pharm, 28*(2), 84–90.

Kjeldby, I. K., Fosnes, G. S., Ligaarden, S. C., & Farup, P. G. (2013). Vitamin B6 deficiency and disease in elderly people: a study in nursing homes. *BMC Geriatrics, 13*, 13.

Kwok, T., Leung, P. C., Wing, Y. K., Wong, B., Ho, D. W., Wong, W. M., & Ho, F. (2013). The effictiveness of acupuncture on sleep quality of elderly with dementia: a within-subjects trial. *Clin Interv Ageing, 8*, 923–929.

Li, M-M., Yu, J-T., Wang, H-F., Jiang, T., Wang, J., Meng, X-F., Tan, C-C., Wang, C., & Tan, L. (2014). Efficacy of vitamins B supplementation on mild cognitive impairment and Alzheimer's disease: a systematic review and meta-analysis. *Curr Alzheimer Res, 11*(9), 844–852.

Lin, P. W., Chan, W. C., Ng, B. F., & Lam, L. C. (2007). Efficacy of aromatherapy (Lavendula angustifolia) as an intervention for agitated behaviours in Chinese older persons with dementia: a cross-over randomized trial. *Int J Geriatr Psychiatry, 22*(5), 405–410.

Lin, V., Canaway, R., & Carter, B. (2014). Interface, interaction and integration: how people with chronic disease in Australia manage CAM and conventional medical services. *Health Expectations.* doi: 10.1111/hex.12239.

Livingston, G., Johnston, K., Katona, C., Paton, J., & Lyketsos, C. G. (2005). Systematic review of psychological approaches to the management of neuropsychiatric symptoms of dementia. *Am J Psychiatry, 162*(11), 1996–2012.

Lui, J., & Chang, D. (2006). Vascular dementia. *J Compl Med, 5*(2), 14–22.

McLaughlin, D., Lui, C-W., & Adams, J. (2012a). Complementary and alternative medicine use among older Australian women: a qualitative analysis. *BMC Compl Alt Med, 12*, 34.

McLaughlin, D., Adams, J., Sibbritt, D., & Lui, C-W. (2012b). Sex differences in the use of complementary and alternative medicine in older men and women. *Australas J Ageing, 31*(2), 78–82.

McMahon, S., & Lutz, R. (2004). Alternative therapy use among the young-old (ages 65 to 74): An evaluation of the MIDUS database. *J Appl Gerontol, 23*(2), 91–103.

Metcalfe, A., Williams, J., McChesney, J., Patten, S. B., & Jette, N. (2010). Use of complementary and alternative medicine by those with a chronic illness and the general population: results of a national population based survey. *Compl Alt Med, 10*, 58.

Moyle, W., Murfield, J., O'Dwyer, S., & van Wyk, S. (2012). The effect of massage on agitated behaviours in older people with dementia: a literature review. *J Clin Nurs, 22*, 601–610.

Nahin, R. L., Peccha, M., Welmerink, D. B., Sink, K., DeKosky, S. T., Fitzpatrick, A. L., & Ginkgo Evaluation of Memory Study Investigators. (2009). Concomitant use of prescription drugs and dietary supplements in ambulatory elderly people. *J Am Geriatr Soc, 57*(7), 1197–1205.

National Institute of Complementary Medicine (NCIM). *Information for consumers.* Retrieved December 15, 2014, from http://www.nicm.edu.au/health_information/information_for_consumers/understanding_cm.

National Center for Complementary and Alternative Medicine (NCCAM), 2002. What is Complementary and Alternative Medicine (CAM)?, May 2002, USA. Last Modified 02 October 2002. http://nccam.nih.gov/health/whatiscam/

National Prescribing Service (NPS). (2008). *Complementary medicines information use and needs of health professionals: general practitioners and pharmacists.* Sydney: NPS. Retrieved from http://www.nps.org.au/about-us/what-we-do/our-research/complementary-medicines/cms-health-professionals-research.

Ness, J., Cirillo, D. J., Weir, D. R., Nisly, N. L., & Wallace, R. B. (2005). Use of complementary medicine in older Americans: results from the Health and Retirement Study. *Gerontologist, 45,* 516–524.

Peisah, C., Lawrence, G., & Reutens, S. (2011). Creative solutions for severe dementia with BPSD: a case of art therapy used in an inpatient and residential care setting. *Int Psychogeriatr, 23*(6), 1011–1013.

Peng, W., Wang, Y., Zhang, Y., & Liang, C. M. (2007). Acupuncture for vascular dementia. *Cochrane Database Syst Rev, 2.* Art. no.: CD004987. doi: 10.1002/14651858.CD004987.pub2.

Rayner J., & Bauer, M. (n.d.). *The use of complementary and alternative medicine (CAM) in Victorian residential aged-care facilities.* Focus groups conducted with older people with dementia and staff about the use of CAM. Unpublished.

Rayner, J., Willis, K., & Pirotta, M. (2011). What's in a name: integrative medicine or simply good medical practice? *Fam Pract, 28,* 655–660.

Ryder-Jones, C., Bullock, A., & Anderson, L. (2012). Wii can make a difference. *Austr J Dementia Care, 1*(1), 10–11.

Sansone, P., & Schmidtt, L. (2000). Providing tender touch massage to elderly nursing home residents: a demonstration project. *Geriatr Nurs, 21*(6), 303–308.

Sarris, J., Robins Wahlin, T-B., Goncalves, D. C., & Byrne, G. J. (2010). Comparative use of complementary medicine, allied health, and manual therapies by middle-aged and older Australian women. *J Women Aging, 22*(4), 273–282.

Schnabel, K., Binting, S., Witt, C. M., & Teut, M. (2014). Use of complementary and alternative medicine by older adults: a cross-sectional survey. *BMC Geriatr, 14,* 38.

Singh, S. R., & Levine, M. A. H. (2006). Natural health product use in Canada: analysis of the National Population Health Survey. *Can J Clin Pharmacol, 13*(2), e240–e250.

Spinks, J., Hollingsworth, B., Manderson, L., Lin, V., & Canaway, R. (2013). Costs and drivers of complementary and alternative medicine (CAM) use in people with type 2 diabetes or cardiovascular disease. *Eur J Integr Med, 5,* 44–53.

Sung, H. C., Chang, A. M., & Abbey, J. (2006). The effects of preferred music on agitation of older people with dementia in Taiwan. *Int J Geriatr Psychiatry, 21,* 999–1000.

Swift, W., Stollznow, N., & Pirotta, M. (2007). The use of alcohol and medicines among Australian adults. *Austr N Z J Public Health, 31*(6), 529–532.

Ulger, Z., Halil, M., Kalan, I. I., Yavuz, B. B., Cankurtaran, M., Gungor, E., et al. (2010). Comprehensive assessment of malnutrition risk and related factors in a large group of community-dwelling older adults. *Clin Nutrit, 29*(4), 507e11.

Viggo Hansen, N., Jorgensen, T., & Ortenblad, L. (2006). Massage and touch for dementia. *Cochrane Database Syst Rev, 4.* Art. no.: CD004989. doi: 10.1002/14651858.CD004989.pub2.

Walkom, E., Loxton, D., & Robertson, J. (2013). Cost of medicines and health care: a concern for Australian women across the ages. *BMC Health Services, 13,* 484.

Webber, G. (2003). Complementary therapies in dementia care: Which therapies are used in South Australian nursing homes? *Counterpoints, 3,* 61–71.

Willison, K., & Andrews, G. J. (2004). Complementary medicine and older people: past research and future directions. *Compl Ther Nurs Midwifery, 10,* 80–91.

Willis, K., & Rayner, J. (2015). The nexus between the social and the medical: how can we understand the proliferation of complementary and alternative medicines for enhancing fertility and treating infertility? In Nicola K. Gale & Jean V. McHale (Eds), *The Routledge handbook of complementary and alternative medicine: perspectives from social science and law* (pp. 110–125). London: Routledge.

Woods, J. L., Walker, K. Z., Juliano-Burns, S., & Strauss, B. J. (2009). Malnutrition on the menu: nutritional status of institutionalised elderly Australians in low-level care. *J Nutrition, 13*(3), 693–698.

Wu, C-H., Wang, C-C., & Kennedy, J. (2011). Changes in herb and dietary supplement use in the US adult population: a comparison of the 2002 and 2007 National Health Interview Surveys. *Clin Therapeut, 33*(11), 1749–1758.

Xue, C., Zhang, A., Lin, V., da Costa, C., Story, D. (2007). Complementary and alternative medicine use in Australia: a national population-based survey. *J Alt Compl Med, 13*(6), 643–650.

Xue, C. C., Zhang. A. L., Lin, V., Myers, R., Polus, B., & Story, D. (2008). Acupuncture, chiropractic, and osteopathy use in Australia: a national population survey. *BMC Public Health, 8*, 105.

Yang, M. H., Wu, S. C., Lin, J. G., & Lin, L. C. (2007). The efficacy of acupressure for decreasing agitated behaviour in dementia: a pilot study. *J Clin Nurs, 16*(2), 308–315.

Zhang, A. L., Story, D. F., Lin, V., Vitetta, L., & Xue, C. (2008). A population survey on the use of 24 common medicinal herbs in Australia. *Pharmacoepidemiol Drug Safety, 17*, 1006–1013.

Zhang, A. L., Xue, C. C., Lin, V., & Story, D. F. (2007). Complementary and alternative medicine use by older Australians. *Ann NY Acad Sci, 1114*, 204–215.

33

THERAPEUTIC GARDENS AND EXPRESSIVE THERAPIES

Theresa L. Scott and Nancy A. Pachana

INTRODUCTION

Human understandings of the importance of the aesthetics of plants and gardens date back to antiquity and the elaborate ancient gardens of Persia (Turner, 2005). For centuries, people have sought out gardens as a place to relax and enjoy the aesthetics of nature, but only recently has the therapeutic benefit of gardens been the focus of scientific analysis. It is only during the last quarter century or so that the systematic study of nature as therapy began in earnest and resulted in the establishment of horticulture as an evidence-based therapy for a variety of populations and conditions.

Research confirms the relaxation and restorative effects of being in nature: either gardening in one's home garden, wandering through a public garden, or simply being around plants indoors (Scott, Masser, & Pachana, 2014a, 2014b). Contact with nature promotes emotional, physical, social, mental, and spiritual well-being, according to a growing body of research. Contact with nature through gardens enhances well-being for individuals across all stages of development, from childhood to older adulthood (Bhatti, 2006; Butterfield & Relf, 1992). In particular for older adults, their home gardens provide an outlet for engagement and activity that may support positive aging. Social benefits accrue for older adults who garden in community garden settings (Scott, Masser, & Pachana, 2014b). For older adults in residential aged-care settings, gardening presents opportunities not just for leisure, but also for enhanced social, psychological, and physiological well-being. Gardens and plants provide the impetus for social exchange through a shared appreciation of the aesthetics of nature. For people living with physical or mental illness, gardens and gardening activities can provide a retreat, and may be a soothing distraction from their illnesses (Pachana, Kidd, & Alpass, 2000; Townsend, 2006).

Therapeutic gardening, social and therapeutic horticulture, and *horticultural therapy* are all terms that are used to describe a process, either active or passive, of using contact with nature to positively impact an individual's well-being. The goal of this chapter is to provide evidence in support of the vitalizing and rehabilitative effects of therapeutic gardens and horticultural therapy in later life. The first section provides a brief history of gardening as therapy, including an overview of the main theoretical explanations and seminal studies. The second section focuses on social and therapeutic horticulture—using gardens and horticulture as a means of achieving well-being in later life. In addition, we explore the use of other forms of expressive therapy—animal-assisted therapy and music therapy—to enhance older adults' psychosocial well-being. The therapeutic effects of music and of nature and animals are said to arise from our evolutionary experiences, that is, because our brains are wired to respond positively to nature and animals, and to respond to and process music.

DEFINITIONS

Therapeutic gardens is the term often used to describe a variety of therapeutic spaces that can include certain natural and non-natural features (as shown in Table 33.1) that provide a sense of restoration or relief from anxiety, or positively affect a set of defined health outcomes (Cooper-Marcus & Barnes, 1999). There are many different types of therapeutic gardens based on their use (as shown in Table 33.2), although a therapeutic garden could be designed with several uses in mind. Therapeutic gardens have been included in healthcare settings to treat a range of populations and conditions and to positively affect patient well-being—including hospitals, psychiatric facilities, rehabilitation centers, day-care centers and nursing homes, schools, community centers, and institutions.

Table 33.1.   The Features of Therapeutic Gardens, Including Example Natural and Non-Natural Elements

FEATURES	ELEMENTS
Natural	Flourishing plants: familiar, non-toxic, non-injurious, tactile, aromatic
	Plantings that attract biodiversity, e.g., birds and insects, etc.
	Ornamental plantings, flowers, shrubs, and grasses
	Edible plantings, e.g., vegetables, herbs
	Trees with foliage that moves easily in breeze
	Perennial and annual plants to create an awareness of changing seasons
	Soil
	Sunlight, shade, fresh air, breezes
	Precipitation, moving water
Non-natural	Shaded areas, e.g., pergolas, umbrellas, gazebo, patio
	Comfortable seating in shaded areas: tables, chairs, and benches
	Raised planter beds
	Bird bath to attract birds
	Water features, fountains, water supply, and hose
	Landscape lighting
	Ramps and sealed paths, smooth and meandering paths
	Wind chimes

Table 33.2. Therapeutic Gardens Meeting the Needs of Special Populations

CATEGORY	DESCRIPTION	DESIGN CONSIDERATIONS
Enabling gardens	Outpatient units and residential facilities for people with developmental disabilities, brain injury, mental disability	Easily accessible
Vocational gardens	Sheltered workshops, vocational residential centers, juvenile detention centers, prisons	Use of the garden is directed at employment of the client
Healing gardens	Healthcare facilities, acute care and sub-acute care hospital units, managed care/residential care nursing facilities, hospices	Designed with an awareness of issues of mobility, e.g., wide paths to cater to wheelchairs, raised beds, hanging planters
Restorative gardens	Psychiatric hospitals and outpatient units, psychogeriatric units	Designed to contrast interior space, e.g., creating a sense of "getting away," meandering paths that invite exploration, consider patient monitoring and views of garden through window for those unable to go outside
Sensory gardens	Vocational and recreational gardens for people with visual and/or hearing impairment	Aromatic, non-toxic plants, no nuisance or injurious plantings, e.g., thorns, spikes
Wandering gardens	Dementia care units, adult day-care programs, nursing care homes	Designed for way-finding, e.g., simple layout, looping paths, visibility from inside (balance need for privacy with need to monitor for safety); nontoxic, nostalgic familiar plantings, and aromatic plants to invite reminiscence
Restoration gardens	Public and private gardens usually not affiliated with health care	Designed for contemplation restoration, e.g., seating in quiet spaces, semi-private spaces "enclosed" by greenery
Community gardens	Shared gardening on public allotments, particularly important for older, disabled, disadvantaged, socially isolated or marginalized individuals living in urban areas	Signs to stimulate conversation

Horticultural therapy is a term used to describe the purposeful use of plants in activities designed to improve or maximize an individual's social, cognitive, psychological, and physiological functioning. Horticultural therapy is usually facilitated by a trained horticultural therapist to achieve specific treatment goals in a wide variety of settings, including hospitals, rehabilitation centers, residential care facilities, psychiatric care facilities, and special education programs (AHTA, 2014). It can include various forms of activity connected with nature: hands-on propagation and potting up plants, flower arranging, viewing photos or pictures of natural scenes, observations of unusual plants or natural curiosities, and "smell and tell" sessions. In addition, horticultural therapy can be accommodated in smaller, indoor spaces, such as one's home, and on an ongoing basis, therefore encouraging repeat interactions and increased socialization between participants.

Animal-assisted therapy, pet therapy, and *companion animals* are terms often used interchangeably to describe therapeutic interactions with domesticated pets, farm animals, and marine animals, to positively impact an individual's health and psychosocial well-being and cognitive functioning (LaJoie, 2003). Animal-assisted therapy is more than just petting animals, although therapy may include such activities—therapy needs to be goal directed, individualized to the patient, and have documented progress (Chandler, 2005). In particular, for older adults, companion animals provide important social support and buffer the negative effects of loneliness, stress, illness, and depression (Pachana, Massavelli, & Robleda-Gomez, 2011). Animal-assisted therapy is suitable for persons with dementia and is an effective non-pharmacological treatment to help manage the behavioral and psychological symptoms of the disease (Filan & Llewellyn-Jones, 2006).

Music therapy is a research-based practice and profession in which music is used within a therapeutic relationship to actively support the mental health and well-being of people across ages and cultures, regardless of musical skill or abilities (Australian Music Therapy Association). Music therapy can include singing, creating, listening to, or moving to, music. Research supports the therapeutic effectiveness of music therapy in a wide variety of healthcare and educational settings. In particular for older adults, music therapy has been used to successfully treat depression and anxiety, and to recreate memories and enhance well-being for people with dementia.

HISTORY: GARDENING AS THERAPY

Historically, gardens and plants have been used as remedies for restoration, as far back as 2000 B.C. in Mesopotamia (Turner, 2005). The earliest documented use was in ancient Egypt, when court physicians prescribed a "walk in the palace garden" for those royals suffering from mental fatigue and illness (Lewis, 1976). An appreciation of the aesthetics of gardens and engaging the senses of visitors was intrinsic to the design of the Paradise gardens of ancient Persia around 500 B.C., which included fragrant and flowering plants, running water, and shade to provide cooling temperatures.

During the Middle Ages (to ca. 1500) gardens were used to provide food and pharmaceuticals, and for recuperation. Throughout Western Europe, monastic gardens included flowers, medicinal herbs, fruit orchards, vegetable beds, and fish ponds, which provided monks with their livelihood and enabled them to care for the sick and poor—as part of their charitable duty.

In the late eighteenth and nineteenth centuries, hospitals and asylums included gardens for their patients as a soothing distraction from their illnesses (Ulrich, 2002). Male patients were employed in the gardens and kitchens of asylums for economic purposes—to reduce the costs of caring for patients. The cheerfulness with which the patients went about their duties and the calming influence these duties had on them led to the recognition of the garden and grounds as a therapeutic instrument; male patients were later directed to be engaged as much as possible in the garden to "promote happiness" (Conolly, 1847).

The positive effect of plant-based activities on returned servicemen was the catalyst for much further investigation of the rehabilitative and restoration effects of nature. Patients in 1940s and 1950s veterans' hospitals—established by the US government to care for wounded servicemen—showed remarkable improvements in emotional, mental, and physical health after working with plants in the hospitals' gardens.

However, functional efficiency, medical technology, and the introduction of antibiotics resulted in the emergence of the starkly institutional hospital setting in the early 1900s (Ulrich, 2002). The emotional needs of patients and the therapeutic value of nature were then largely overlooked (Ulrich, 2002) until the early 1970s, when one of the earliest systematic analyses of the benefits of gardening was conducted by Kaplan (1973); this was followed by other seminal studies in the late 1970s and early 1980s of the healing benefits of plants (Langer & Rodin, 1976) and views of nature in healthcare settings (Ulrich, 1984).

THEORETICAL EXPLANATIONS OF PEOPLE–PLANT RELATIONSHIPS

Several theories have been proposed to account for the relationship between human contact with natural elements and increased well-being.

Biophilia Theory

One reason for the vitalizing effect of nature and natural elements, according to biophilia theory, is that humans have an "innate tendency to focus on life and life-like processes" (Wilson, 1984, p. 1). Biophilia theory suggests that humans have an inborn affinity with the natural world, arising from our evolutionary history when our ancestors roamed the savannahs. During evolution, verdant environments would have provided a safe haven to shelter from predators, to rest and recover; therefore the theory suggests that all humans have evolved to prefer and to respond positively to natural environments and their elements, such as trees, plants, water, and wildlife. Over millions of years, repeated experiences in natural environments thus encoded humans with a behavioral response—attraction to natural environments (Wilson, 1993).

The aesthetic experience of nature is fundamental to the theory, which proposes that our emotional health and well-being are dependent upon having access to nature, or at least to views of nature. Theorists argue in support of the logic of this theory. That is, the brain evolved in a biocentric world, not a machine-regulated one, and therefore it would be difficult to believe that all learning rules in that environment would be erased in a few thousand years (Wilson, 1993). Indirect support for the theory comes from cross-cultural studies that consistently show people's preference for, and positive responses to, park-like environments compared to man-made

environments (Kaplan, Kaplan, & Wendt, 1972), and to scenes of natural environments compared to those of man-made environments (Ryan, Weinstein, Bernstein, Brown, Mistretta, & Gagné, 2010). Further support for the theory is suggested by the empirical evidence relating to "biophobia": humans' innate fear response to certain living stimuli such as snakes, which would have constituted risks throughout human evolution, and the absence of such a fear response to more contemporary dangers such as electric wires (Wilson, 1993).

Stress Reduction Theory

A closely related theory is Ulrich and colleagues' stress reduction theory—a psycho-evolutionary explanation for why being in natural environments or even viewing (unthreatening) nature promotes recovery from stress. The theory proposes that, based on evolutionary experience, humans have been advantaged to recover from stress in natural environments. That is, humans have inherited the capacity to restore and to recover from states of continued heightened stress in nature. Natural environments tend to be less perceptually demanding than many urban environments and therefore have more positive effects on people, according to the theory (Ulrich & Parsons, 1992).

Support for the theory is demonstrated through studies that show people's heart rate and blood pressure vary, such that they show a relaxation response to views of natural environments, but not to views of urban environments, after exposure to a stressor. Ulrich and colleagues randomly assigned participants recovering from exam stress to view videotapes of either nature settings or built settings that contained no natural elements (Ulrich, Simons, Losito, & Fiorito, 1991). Those viewing nature settings experienced significantly shorter and more positive recovery, compared to those viewing a built environment, as determined by physiological and self-report measures.

Attention Restoration Theory

In some ways similar to stress reduction theory, Kaplan and Kaplan's (1989) attention restoration theory provides a psychophysiological explanation for the link between natural environments and human well-being. Whereas Ulrich (1984) emphasized recovery from stress, Kaplan and Kaplan (1989) emphasized recovery from attention fatigue and directed attention by spending time in nature. Directed attention—a key concept of the theory—describes the state of effortful attention that is fundamental when a task requires conscious and sustained attention and active suppression of irrelevant information. The theory proposes that because individuals expend a great deal of mental effort to inhibit potential distractions and attend to their daily tasks, mental fatigue follows. Spending time in nature is said to allow people a break from periods of prolonged mental effort and concentration and the capacity to recover focused attention (Kaplan & Kaplan, 1989). Furthermore, according to research, interactions with nature can enhance concentration, improve attention and memory, and reduce anxiety because natural environments and their elements require effortless attention and act as a distraction (Kaplan & Kaplan, 1989). For example, wandering through a garden, tending to houseplants, or simply admiring a flower requires effortless attention, providing a separation from prolonged mental activity, a break from mental fatigue, and an opportunity to recharge. Studies showed that leisure activities in natural settings, such as parks and nature reserves, had important restorative effects for individuals who frequented them (Kaplan & Kaplan, 1989), and people recovered from stress and regained a contemplative state of being from visits to natural environments such as parks and forests (Hansmann, Hug, & Seeland, 2007).

PSYCHOLOGICAL AND PHYSIOLOGICAL HEALTH BENEFITS OF CONTACT WITH NATURE

Classic Case Study Examples

One of the earliest and most influential studies to demonstrate the physiological and psychological healing benefits derived from observation of nature was the empirical study of Ulrich, published in 1984. The retrospective study examining the recovery of postoperative gall-bladder patients took place during a time when the procedure was more invasive and patients' recovery stays were necessarily much longer. The hospital records of patients were examined and 23 pairs ($n = 46$) were retrospectively matched on all health and demographic variables, such as gender, age, socioeconomic status, and health behaviors (e.g., history of smoking); they

differed only in the type of window view that they saw from their hospital bed, either trees or the wall of a brick building. Results showed that compared to patients with the brick wall view, patients with the nature view had significantly shorter hospital stays, fewer postoperative complications and negative evaluative comments from nurses, and took fewer strong analgesics to manage pain. This study was one of the first to provide reliable empirical evidence for the healing benefit of contact with nature and was the catalyst for much further research and the later acceptance of the stress-reducing qualities of nature to improve clinical outcomes.

As well as the restorative properties of merely observing nature, an earlier study conducted by Langer and Rodin (1976) provides evidence to suggest that active participation in caring for potted plants delivers additional benefits. Specifically, the care of a potted plant may provide the stimulus for interaction and engagement for older adults in long-term residential care settings. Langer and Rodin (1976) compared two groups of older adults residing in nursing homes. Each group was given a potted plant, with one group being given the responsibility for the care of it and the other being informed that staff would take responsibility for all care. There was significant improvement relating to increased well-being and enhanced sociability in the group who were permitted to make choices about the care of the potted plants, compared to the control group who had no such choice or responsibility for the plants.

These studies show that a potted plant or a window view of nature, such as a tree or garden, have significant positive effects on mood and anxiety and compensate for the loss of direct contact with nature (Ulrich, 1984), and can therefore provide a soothing, peaceful distraction for people who are infirm or who spend lengthy periods of time indoors. The results have implications for older adults who are bed-bound or who reside in long-term care settings, where they may have limited access to the outdoors.

SOCIAL AND THERAPEUTIC HORTICULTURE

As well as the aesthetic experience of nature, participation in gardening—whether in one's own garden or in group gardening programs—provides older adults with an outlet for meaningful engagement, self-expression, and mental stimulation.

Home Gardens

Whereas simply *being* in view of a garden or nature leads to enhanced well-being, research suggests that *doing* gardening may be in accord with components of successful aging theory, such as activity and meaningful engagement (Lampinen et al., 2006). In particular, for retired older adults, gardening may become a part of everyday homemaking and an important leisure pursuit. Older adult gardeners obtain identity benefits such as accomplishment and enhanced self-esteem through their efforts at cultivating fruit and vegetables, or planting a tree that encourages wildlife and biodiversity (Scott, Masser, & Pachana, 2014b).

Home gardens provide access to fresh air and sunshine, restoration, and relaxation. Furthermore, for older adults actively engaged in maintaining the aesthetics of their home gardens, gardening provides an outlet for regular physical activity (Park, Lee, Son, & Shoemaker, 2012). Participation in gardening activities was identified as having a direct relationship with reduced feelings of anxiety and depression for older adults (Patterson & Chang, 1999). Regular, moderate- to heavy-intensity gardening reduced the risk of morbidity and mortality in a group of mid- to older-aged men with cardiovascular disease (Wannamethee, Shaper, & Walker, 2000).

Generally, advanced age is correlated with a reduction in many kinds of activities that require physical exertion (Lawton, 1987); however, unlike other active leisure pursuits such as tennis or hiking, cessation of gardening is not an inevitable consequence of aging because passive involvement—watering or wandering through a garden—is possible. Furthermore, older adults who reported that they compensated for losses in functioning by adapting their time in activities, downsizing their gardening area, or seeking assistance with tasks that they could no longer accomplish themselves managed to retain this important leisure activity and still derived satisfaction from their engagement (Scott, Masser, & Pachana, 2014b).

Community Gardens

In addition to the restorative and healthy aging benefits of gardening activities, there is evidence to suggest that social benefits accrue for people who garden in communal gardening settings. Group-based gardening activities provide healthy recreation, access to social partners, and the opportunity for social interaction through shared enjoyment of gardening (Hawkins, Thirlaway, Backx, & Clayton, 2011; Kingsley & Townsend, 2006; Scott, Masser, & Pachana, 2014b), which is especially important for disenfranchised and socially isolated older adults. As well, community gardening provides opportunities for social identification (with other gardeners and neighbors) and enhanced self-esteem (from the tangible rewards of group gardening, such as vegetables, fruits, and herbs).

Group gardening activities facilitate social connection, and promote social cohesion and a shared sense of identity (Kingsley & Townsend, 2006), which has important implications for older adults in residential care settings, many of whom spend a lot of time in their own rooms alone (Hauge & Heggen, 2007). Being around other people and being actively engaged in life's activities are key to well-being at any age, especially for older adults who reside in long-term care settings, where the incidence of depression and anxiety is high and often goes undiagnosed (Terisi, Abrams, Holmes, Ramirez, & Eimicke, 2001). Participation in a communal gardening group enhanced social connectedness and promoted social and emotional well-being for a group of participants experiencing anxiety and depression symptoms (Townsend, 2006).

Continuity of identity is an important factor in maintaining self-esteem and aging well, according to theory (Atchley, 1998). If older adults must leave their gardens, for example to relocate to a retirement home or a residential care setting, it is vitally important that they have some access to a garden, or at least some contact with nature. Even regular visits to a park resulted in positive improvements in mood for a group of older adults (Godbey & Blazey, 1983).

Healthcare Settings

The traditional view that the physical environment has little influence on the health outcomes of patients if the medical care provided is outstanding has been challenged in research since the seminal studies of the health-giving effects of simply viewing nature (see Ulrich, 1984). The link between simply viewing nature and increased well-being is evident in controlled studies that manipulate aspects of the visual environment of healthcare settings, where people usually experience an amount of anxiety, such as dental waiting rooms and psychiatric units (Katcher & Wilkins, 1993; Pachana, McWha, &

Arathoon, 2003). By including plants, flowers, aquariums, or even wall murals of nature, these environments can have a calming or healing effect on patients (Dijkstra, Pieterse, & Pruyn, 2006).

The construction of an indoor conservatory-style garden resulted in positive feedback from patients and their families in an inpatient psychogeriatric setting (Pachana, McWha, & Arathoon, 2003). Within non-clinical samples, the positive effect of exposure to posters of plants, real plants, or artificial plants on patients' experience of stress was examined in two hospital radiology department waiting rooms (Beukeboom, Langeveld, & Tanja-Dijkstra, 2012). Patients' experience of stress was significantly lower in the "real plants" and "posters of plants" conditions, compared to a "no-plants" control condition (Beukeboom et al., 2012).

Healing gardens in healthcare settings cater to the psychological and physiological needs of specific populations by providing a reduction in stress levels and relief from physically and emotionally draining experiences, trauma, and illness (Cooper-Marcus & Barnes, 1995). The healing effects emerge from passive experiences such as wandering through the garden and viewing the garden from within or through a window, but might also include activities such as cultivating flowers, herbs, and vegetables. The gardens usually include natural features, such as a variety of nontoxic, tactile, and fragrant plants and flowers that are designed to encourage biodiversity, and non-nature-based elements such as comfortable seating and shaded areas (see Table 33.1). As such, the gardens provide important sensory experiences, such as visual, olfactory, and auditory stimulation, which are important to institutionalized older adults whose indoor living environment may be quite static and hospital-like.

Residential Aged-Care Settings

Therapeutic gardens in residential care facilities promote well-being and encourage socialization through a shared appreciation of the aesthetics of nature. They stimulate the senses, as well as social interaction through mutual admiration of the garden's elements and recalling flowers or past gardens (Heath & Gifford, 2001; Yee Tse, 2010). The therapeutic effects of horticulture extend beyond the bounds of the outdoors and direct access to gardens; simply introducing a "sense of nature" into an austere corridor space of residential aged-care facilities can positively impact well-being. Introducing

a multisensory gardening installation—including plants, audio of birdsong, aromatherapy of garden scents, and wall murals of trees—into the indoor environment of residential aged-care facilities was an effective way to improve aesthetics, increase novelty and, in turn, social exchange for residents and staff, according to recent research (Scott, Pachana, & Masser, 2014a). Being tasked with the care of a potted plant has important therapeutic benefits such as enhanced self-esteem and purpose, which is particularly important for older adults who are living in a long-term care environment where responsibilities and choice are usually removed (Langer & Rodin, 1976).

Outdoor gardens may provide residents of long-term care facilities with access to social partners, increased social interaction, and improved overall morale. Including healing gardens in residential care settings will have additional feedback effects on residents because the garden will encourage visitors and provide a pleasant meeting place. However, if access to the outdoors is not possible, even views through a window to the outdoor garden have significant psychological and physiological healing benefits (Ulrich, 1984).

Barriers to Inclusion of Therapeutic Gardens

The benefits of including healing gardens in residential aged-care settings are numerous and include opportunities for social interaction, access to fresh air, sunshine, and subsequently increased vitamin D absorption, and exercise. However, barriers to their inclusion or use exist. These might include a lack of space or finance necessary to install or upkeep such gardens. Also, design considerations are crucial to reduce the risk of falls, and enable free access to all residents, whether physically limited or very frail. Staff motivation and commitment to a maintenance program are important so that the garden thrives, and staff awareness of the garden's potential impact upon residents' well-being is vital to its ongoing use. Despite the substantial evidence for their effectiveness, gardens are often considered desirable, but not achievable, by administrators (Ulrich, 2002), one reason being financial constraints. However, the ongoing maintenance of many varieties of large trees is negligible and, as noted, even views of trees have important therapeutic effects.

An alternative and cost-effective way to introduce the benefits of contact with nature is to include horticultural therapy. Furthermore, because residents with physical and/or cognitive limitations can readily engage in horticultural therapy activities, they are ideally suited to use in residential aged-care settings. Horticultural therapy activities provide residents with meaningful recreational activities and facilitate socialization among residents. Significant effects were found for residents of a Japanese nursing home who took part in an 8-week program that included potting up and caring for plants in a regular group setting. After the 8-week intervention period, residents showed significant improvements in measures of loneliness, social interactions, and overall life satisfaction (Yee Tse, 2010).

MEETING THE NEEDS OF SPECIAL POPULATIONS

People with Depression

Depression is a serious health concern, and is one of the most disabling of mental health conditions in later life (Fiske, Wetherell, & Gatz, 2009). Depression is sometimes misunderstood as an inevitable part of aging, and is often unrecognized in the older adult population (Cahoon, 2012). People experiencing depression suffer with low mood, reduced interest in activities, and low behavioral activation, which in turn may lead to social isolation. Being around other people, being active, and being engaged in pleasant and valued activities are key protective factors (Deiner, Suh, Lucas, & Smith, 1999), and gardening activities provide a means to attain these.

Participating in group gardening activities led to positive improvement in well-being for people experiencing depression, anxiety, and social isolation (Gonzalez, Hartig, Patil, Martinsen, & Kirkevold, 2011; Townsend, 2006). As well as the experience of the restorative benefits of nature, community gardening led to increased feelings of social cohesion and connectedness for participants (Townsend, 2006). Active (sowing seeds, planting, and cultivating) and passive (sitting and observing, listening to birdsong) participation in a 12-week therapeutic horticulture intervention resulted in significant improvement in mental health for a group of clinically depressed persons—an effect that was sustained at 3-month follow-up (Gonzalez et al., 2011). Regular visits to a botanical garden were found to promote well-being, and in fact the relaxation effects were most acutely experienced for those with the highest depression scores across a group of older adults (Kohlleppel, Bradley, & Jacob, 2002).

Regular exercise is one protective factor to offset increased risk of depression and increase resilience in later life. Physical inactivity, which leads to increased risk of depression as well as some cancers, type 2 diabetes, and heart disease, is highest among older adults. Spending time gardening in one's own garden or in community garden settings not only offers recreation and access to fresh air and sunshine, but also presents opportunities for manageable and enjoyable physical activity (Wannamethee, Shaper, & Walker, 2000).

Other psychological factors that are associated with resiliency in later life include a positive self-concept and a sense of mastery or self-efficacy, all of which have been reported by older adult gardeners as being among the benefits of their regular gardening activities. For example, tending to fruit, vegetable, and herb gardens, and encouraging biodiversity (Scott, Masser, & Pachana, 2014b), or in their contributions toward environmentalism in gardening groups (Townsend, 2006). However, it is important that older adults are either supported in their efforts to continue to garden if some tasks become unmanageable as they age, or that they downsize their gardening areas, because watching one's garden deteriorate can lead to feelings of powerlessness and depression (Bhatti, 2006).

People with Physical Limitations

Healing gardens that are designed to meet the needs of wheelchair-bound, or very frail, older people are especially beneficial as they provide a place of restoration. In one Swedish study, care home residents who had a high frequency of hospital visits benefited substantially from visits to an outdoor garden as measured by their increased levels of concentration (Ottosson & Grahn, 2005). In particular, for those residents who had "low tolerance" of other residents and were identified as being "unhelpful" in usual group activities, time spent in the garden led to substantial improvements in their stress levels, as measured by changes in heart rate and blood pressure. Therapeutic gardens therefore may be an important non-pharmacological alternative to managing agitation in people with dementia residing in nursing homes.

People with Dementia

Studies of people living with dementia show improved outcomes, such as increased morale, improved mood, and positive affect from being in a garden (Cohen-Mansfield, 2001), and as compared to other parts of the facility (Cox, Burns, & Savage, 2004). Memory can be stimulated as well, by being exposed to the sights and smells of nature, such as plants, flowers, birds, water, and insects (Hartig, Mang, & Evans, 1991). Importantly for residents with dementia, healing gardens provide a safe area in which to wander or pace when looping paths are built into the design (Burgess, 1989). If space and financial constraints prohibit the inclusion of an outdoor garden, introducing elements of nature—for example, potted plants and flowers, an aquarium, atrium, or audio of birdsong—into the indoor environment is a highly achievable way for care facilities to capitalize on the therapeutic effects of nature.

Horticultural therapy activities, such as planting seeds, are more effective than traditional activities, such as games and craft, at engaging people with dementia residing in nursing homes. Participants of one study spent more time engaged in horticultural therapy activities compared to traditional activities (Gigliotti, Jarrott, & Yorgason, 2004). Furthermore, compared to their baseline observations, participants' time "spent doing nothing" was significantly lower, and they displayed more positive affect during the horticultural therapy intervention period (Gigliotti, Jarrott, & Yorgason, 2004).

Horticultural therapy has been used as a non-pharmacological intervention to manage agitation in residents with dementia. One study involved the recreation of natural environments during residents' bath time—a normally stressful occasion for staff, and for residents with dementia (Whall et al., 1997). The multisensory intervention included audio, such as birdsong, a babbling brook, and small animal sounds; visuals of large and bright nature pictures; and food such as pudding. The intervention resulted in a significant decrease in agitation for the treatment group compared to a control group—who received usual care at bath time (Whall et al., 1997). In another study, an enhanced environment relating to gardens—artificial plants, nature scenes, and comfortable bench seating—had a positive effect on the exit-seeking behaviors of residents with dementia, and led to a significant decrease in agitation

(Cohen-Mansfield & Werner, 1998). Participants were observed stopping and sitting for longer periods of time at the enhanced corridor, compared to other locations in the home.

Based on the evidence to date, the inclusion of a therapeutic garden or natural elements indoors—with due consideration to the needs of staff and residents—is highly recommended for enhancing well-being for people living in long-term care settings. At least, horticultural therapy activities should be included as a complementary and expressive therapy for people with dementia because of their direct impact on residents' engagement and quality of life outcomes.

ANIMAL-ASSISTED THERAPY

Animal-assisted therapy also draws on the bond between humans and the natural world that is the result of our evolutionary history. According to biophilia theory, our innate love of life and living things helps to explain people's affiliation with animals and the health and well-being benefits of direct contact with them. For example, even observing an aquarium of fish in a dental waiting room—an environment that is usually associated with increased anxiety—resulted in significant decreases in blood pressure for patients (Katcher, Segal, & Beck, 1984).

Companion animals have also been a part of human experience for thousands of years (Pachana, Massavelli, & Robleda-Gomez, 2011). Increasing numbers of aged-care facilities recognize the therapeutic benefits of introducing companion animals, such as dogs, cats, fish, and birds (and even llamas, donkeys, and goats) into their facilities (Pachana, Massavelli, & Robleda-Gomez, 2011). Upon entering a residential care facility, older adults experience a series of losses, including the loss of home and familiar surroundings, and the loss of relationships—with people and with their pets. Direct contact with companion animals may help compensate for this loss to some extent. Studies of animal-assisted therapy in nursing homes show that residents express more social behaviors when dogs and cats are present—an effect that is present whether the animals are visiting or living at the facility. Quiet interactions with pet dogs can lower blood pressure and increase neurochemicals that are associated with relaxation and bonding (Odendaal & Meintjes, 2003).

Companion Animals

Pet ownership mitigates loneliness in older adults who are living alone in their own homes. Several studies have shown that older adults living alone were less likely to report loneliness if they reported an attachment to a pet (Krause-Parello, 2012; Krause-Parello, & Gulick, 2013; Stanley, Conwell, Bowen, & Van Orden, 2014), and pet ownership offset the relationship between loneliness and depressed mood for older adults (Krause-Parello, 2012) and between loneliness and ill health (Krause-Parello, 2008). The reasons include that companion animals provide an outlet for giving and receiving unconditional love, identity, a sense of purpose, and responsibility for another living being.

Residential Care Facilities

Animal-assisted activities and therapy programs have been used in residential care facilities to alleviate depressive symptoms and to increase quality of life. Residents reported feeling happier and less anxious and lonely after a visit from a companion animal (Cole & Gawlinski, 1995). Having an animal to look after and relate to resulted in decreased symptoms of anxiety and depression, and perceptions of increased quality of life, for a group of cognitively intact institutionalized older adults (Colombo, Buono, Smania, Raviola, & De Leo, 2006).

People with Dementia

There is growing interest in the therapeutic effects of animal-assisted therapy with people with dementia, in particular to manage the behavioral and psychological symptoms that are an expression of the disease. Behavioral and psychological symptoms of dementia (BPSD) include physical and verbal aggression, agitation, apathy, delusions, and hallucinations, and are a major source of distress for the person with dementia and his or her caregivers (Lowery & Warner, 2009). Research in this area is often difficult to design and perform (Wilson & Barker, 2003) and therefore the number of rigorously controlled studies and studies that use physiological parameters is limited. However, there is mounting empirical evidence from several small-scale studies to suggest that animal-assisted therapy may be an appropriate psychosocial treatment for BPSD and in some cases an alternative to medication.

The presence of pets stimulates positive interactions among people with dementia. In observational studies, residents smiled, laughed, and were more socially communicative in the presence of a visiting dog (Churchill, Safaoui, McCabe, & Baun, 1999; Kongable, Buckwalter, & Stolley, 1989) and became less hostile to their caretakers. In one study, the inclusion of aquariums in a dementia-specific unit's dining rooms led to decreased agitation, increased appetite, and, in turn, increased nutrition and weight gain. The intervention led to increased health for residents and a decrease in the need for, and costs of, nutritional supplements (Edwards & Beck, 2002).

There are, on occasions, objections raised regarding safety and cleanliness in relation to the introduction of animals into dementia-specific units; however, these concerns are mitigated if therapy animals are carefully chosen (Tedeschi, Fitchett, & Molidor, 2005). Even substituting robotic pets for live pets has been found to significantly lower agitation for people with dementia living in long-term care settings (Libin & Cohen-Mansfield, 2004; Tamura et al., 2004). Furthermore, live therapy animals are put through rigorous safety trainings before being introduced into homes by a facilitator (Tedeschi, Fitchett, & Molidor, 2005).

MUSIC THERAPY

Music therapy is another sensory experience and therapeutic modality for older adults. Recognition of the therapeutic value of music has a long history, dating back to ancient Greece, when music was thought to cure diseases of the mind. The first music therapy intervention and experimentation can be traced back to the early 1800s; by the 1950s, music therapy was acknowledged as an organized field of research and practice (American Music Therapy Association, 2014). Recent systematic reviews suggest that music therapy, administered by a certified professional, is an effective treatment for people with severe mental disorders (Gold, Solli, Krüger, & Lie, 2009; Maratos, Gold, Wang, & Crawford, 2008). As a therapeutic intervention, music has a strong and growing evidence base that supports its effectiveness in a variety of settings, including communities, hospitals, and nursing homes, and to address a range of physical, social, emotional, and cognitive needs in an individual (American Music Therapy Association, 2014).

The term music therapy is widely used in the literature to describe a range a music-related activities and interventions. Music therapists, who are trained or experienced to work with clients to treat a range of conditions and disorders, and to improve symptoms and global functioning, deliver clinical music therapy. Techniques used in music therapy can be broadly classified as "receptive" (e.g., listening to music) and "active" (e.g., re-creating, improvising, or composing music). Music therapy approaches are grounded in diverse traditions such as behavioral, psychoanalytic, educational, and humanistic models of therapy. The agent of change is the music as well as the therapy (Bruscia, 1998). However, participants do not have to be musically trained to react to, or benefit from, music therapy. In addition to clinical music therapy, group activities that are organized around music, such as listening to music, or piano playing, or involvement in sing-alongs, can lead to positive benefits for older adults in residential care settings. Music can enhance memory because memories can be embedded in a familiar song. Furthermore, participants can continue to derive benefits from music therapy, despite declining cognition and severe dementia.

Music is a medium for emotional expression. Either listening to or creating music is used as the catalyst to insight into therapeutically relevant issues, feelings, memories, and associations for individuals (Gold, Solli, Krüger, & Lie, 2009), and provides an outlet for expression of these issues (American Music Therapy Association, 2014). For people with depression, who usually have difficulty sustaining treatment, music is a motivating force for engagement in therapy sessions. One meta-analysis found that levels of uptake were high and dropout levels were rare across studies of participants with depression taking part in music therapy sessions (Maratos, Gold, Wang, & Crawford, 2008). Music therapists may use an active or receptive approach to treatment, or a combination of the two, when working with people with depression. Receptive techniques can include listening to music for relaxation, reminiscence, reflection, or mood elevation; active techniques may include writing lyrics, composing music, or improvisation.

Depression and Anxiety

One study found that music therapy was effective for older adults with depression, even when it was self-administered; treatment could be assigned to participants in a similar way that homework is assigned in cognitive behavior therapy (Hanser & Thompson, 1994). Treatment included guided imagery, drawing and painting to music, and facial massage and progressive relaxation to music, for an average of 3.25 hours per week, across 8 weeks. The home-based program plus a weekly session with a therapist was compared to the home-based program alone, and to a wait-list control group. Participants in both music conditions showed significant improvements in tests of depression, stress, and mood, which were maintained over a 9-month follow-up period (Hanser & Thompson, 1994).

The effect of music therapy on stress, anxiety, and depression levels was examined with a group of nursing home residents. In this randomized controlled trial, the intervention group received 10 weeks of daily music-based sessions, of 90 minutes duration, including listening to music, singing and playing percussion instruments, while the control group (no music) received daily regular activities (Mohammadi, Shahabi, & Panah, 2011). Results showed significant differences in the mean scores of anxiety, stress, and depression between the control and intervention group post-intervention. That is, music therapy significantly decreased levels of anxiety, stress, and depression for nursing home residents receiving treatment compared to a control group. Even listening to music through headphones had a positive influence on people's experience of anxiety and agitation because music allows an individual to shut out unwanted noise (Devlin & Arneill, 2003).

Music can also motivate older adults to be more physically active. A music-facilitated exercise program for people with Parkinson's disease resulted in improved motor function and quality of life for participants (Clair, Lyons, & Hamburg, 2012). In another study, the addition of music to an exercise program increased motivation and improved capacity in a clinical sample of older adults participating in a cardiac rehabilitation program (Ziv & Lidor, 2011).

Music making is a social experience. Group sessions that involve music—either listening to, or singing—provide relational experiences. The positive effects of shared music activities on mental health have been demonstrated in several studies, including choir singing (Dingle, Brander, Ballantyne, & Baker, 2013) and listening to music and songs (Mohammadi, Shahabi, & Panah, 2011; Olson, 1984). Kicking and stamping to music improved circulation and increased tolerance and strength for a group of nursing home residents taking part in sing-along sessions (Palmer, 1983). Sing-along sessions not only encouraged memory recall, but also promoted social interaction and appropriate social behavior among nursing home residents. Group participation in listening to piano playing enhanced positive feelings of well-being and facilitated reminiscence for older participants. Furthermore, the positive reactions to the music were found whether participants were familiar or unfamiliar with the pieces (Olson, 1984).

People with Dementia

A recent review of the literature suggests that interventions with music, including group and individual music activities and directed therapy, were a noteworthy support to the management of BPSD (Raglio et al., 2012). For example, music can have a calming effect on agitation and disruptive behaviors of people with dementia, whether it is background music during periods of non-activity (Ziv, Granot, Hai, Dassa, & Haimov, 2007), listening to classical music, individually or group preferred music, or singing along to favorite songs (Zare, Ebrahimi, & Birashk, 2010). Hearing a familiar piece of music can also help improve memory and language for people with dementia, an effect that is partially explained by the parts of brain that respond to music being close to the part of brain that is responsible for memory. Compared to usual care, listening to familiar songs in twice-weekly music therapy sessions, across 8 consecutive weeks, led to a significant improvement in language ability and a significant decrease in irritability for a small sample of patients with dementia (Suzuki, Kanamori, & Watanabe, 2004). In another, longer intervention, a group of residents with moderate to severe dementia took part in several different music therapy activities, including listening to familiar folk songs and attending music concerts. Participants took part in the sessions once a week for 2 years, and their outcome measures were compared to a non-music therapy group (Takahashi & Matsushita, 2006). Outcome assessments included cognition, and cortisol and blood pressure levels. Differences were found between the music therapy and non-music therapy groups, such that music therapy led to significant lowered levels of blood pressure and overall better physical and mental health for participants compared to the control group. Participation in group music therapy activities, such as listening or singing and dancing along to music, increased a sense of belonging, self-esteem, and depressive symptoms for people with early to moderate-stage dementia (Cooke, Moyle, Shum, Harrison, & Murfield, 2010).

SUMMARY

Gardens and horticulture-based activities, domesticated animals, and music have been used to positively affect older adults' well-being and to improve social, psychological, physical, and vocational adjustment across a variety of settings and populations. Activities can be varied to accommodate all ages and abilities. Therapeutic benefits may be derived from hands-on activities, such as propagating plants, singing along to or re-creating songs, or petting a dog or cat; and from passive involvement, such as touching or smelling aromatic plants, viewing a garden through an open window, or hearing nature through an audio recording of birdsong. The importance is on the multisensory experience and engaging all of the senses in different ways, such as listening to birdsong through a recording while admiring a tree through a mural or window.

The International Psychogeriatric Association's (IPA) Task Force on Mental Health Services in Long Term Care Facilities advocates explicit focus on quality of care that promotes quality of life for residents as a primary objective (Gibson, Carter, Helmes, & Edberg, 2010). If we are to address the quality of life needs of the projected increased numbers of residents in long-term care facilities, and in particular those with dementia, over the next few decades, physical and social environmental design must be an important guiding principle—making small environmental adjustments can lead to significant improvements in quality of life. Complementary and alternative therapies and activities that incorporate music, animals, and nature are pleasurable and meaningful experiences that result in high levels of engagement, increased interpersonal contact and sociability, and improvements in overall psychological well-being.

DISCLOSURE STATEMENT

The authors declare that there are no conflicts of interest to disclose.

REFERENCES

AHTA (American Horticultural Therapy Association). (2014). *Definitions and positions*. Retrieved from http://ahta.org.

American Music Therapy Association. (2014). *Facts about music therapy*. Retrieved from http://www.musictherapy.org/.

Atchley, R. C. (1989). A continuity theory of normal aging. *Gerontologist, 29*(2), 183–190.

Australian Music Therapy Association, retrieved from http://www.austmta.org.au/

Beukeboom, C. J., Langeveld, D., & Tanja-Dijkstra, K. (2012). Stress-reducing effects of real and artificial nature in a hospital waiting room. *J Alt Compl Med, 18*(4), 329–333. doi: 10.1089/acm.2011.0488.

Bhatti, M. (2006). "When I'm in the garden I can create my own paradise": homes and gardens in later life. *Sociol Rev, 54*(2), 318–341.

Bruscia, K. E. (1998). *Defining music therapy*. Gilsum, NH: Barcelona Publishers.

Burgess, C. W. (1989). Horticulture and its application to the institutionalized elderly. *Activities Adapt Aging, 14*(3), 51–61.

Butterfield, B., & Relf, D. (1992). National survey of attitudes toward plants and gardening. In D. Relf (Ed.), *The role of Horticulture in Human Well-being and Social Development: A National Symposium*, 211-212. Portland: Timber Press.

Cahoon, C. G. (2012). Depression in older adults. *Am J Nurs, 112*(11), 22.

Chandler, C. K. (2005). *Animal assisted therapy in counseling*. New York: Routledge.

Churchill, M., Safaoui, J., McCabe, B. W. & Baun, M. M. (1999). Using a therapy dog to alleviate the agitation and desocialization of people with Alzheimer's disease. *J Psychosoc Nurs, 37*, 16–22.

Clair, A. A., Lyons, K., & Hamburg, J. (2012). A feasibility study of the effects of music and movement on physical function, quality of life, depression, and anxiety in patients with Parkinson disease. *Music Medicine, 4*(1), 49–55.

Cohen-Mansfield, J., & Werner, P. (1998). The effects of an enhanced environment on nursing home residents who pace. *Gerontologist, 38*(2), 199–208.

Cohen-Mansfield, J. (2001). Nonpharmacologic interventions for inappropriate behaviors in dementia: a review, summary, and critique. *Am J Geriatr Psychiatry, 9*(4), 361–381.

Cole, K. M., & Gawlinski, A. (1995). Animal assisted therapy in the intensive care unit: a staff nurse's dream come true. *Nurs Clin N Am, 3*, 529–536.

Colombo, G., Buono, M., Smania, K., Raviola, R., & De Leo, D. (2006). Pet therapy and institutionalized elderly: a study of 144 cognitively unimpaired subjects. *Arch Gerontol Geriatrics, 42*(1), 207–216. doi: 10.1016/j.archger.2005.06.011.

Conolly, J. (1847). *The construction and government of lunatic asylums and hospitals for the insane*. London: Churchill (pp. 78–79).

Cooke, M., Moyle, W., Shum, D., Harrison, S., & Murfield, J. A. (2010). Randomized controlled trial exploring the effect of music on quality of life and depression in older people with dementia. *J Health Psychol, 15*, 765–776.

Cooper-Marcus, C., & Barnes, M. (1999). *Healing gardens: Therapeutic benefits and design recommendations*. NY, EE. UU.: John Wiley & Sons.

Cooper-Marcus, C., & Barnes, M. (1995). *Gardens in healthcare facilities: uses, therapuetic benefits and design recommendations*. Concord, CA: The Center for Health Design.

Cox, H., Burns, I., & Savage, S. (2004). Multisensory environments for leisure: promoting well-being in nursing home residents with dementia. *J Gerontol Nurs, 30*(2), 37–45.

Deiner, E., Suh, E., Lucas, R., & Smith, H. (1999). Subjective well-being: three decades of progress. *Psychol Bull, 125*(2), 276–302.

Devlin, A. S., & Arneill, A. (2003). Health care environments and patient outcomes: A review of the literature. *Environment & Behavior, 35*(5), 665–694. doi: 10.1177/0013916503255102

Dijkstra, K., Pieterse, M., & Pruyn, A. (2006). Physical environmental stimuli that turn healthcare facilities into healing environments through psychologically mediated effects: systematic review. *J of Advanced Nursing, 56*, 166–181. doi: 10.1111/j.1365-2648.2006.03990.x

Dingle, G. A., Brander, C., Ballantyne, J., & Baker, F. A. (2013). "To be heard": the social and mental health benefits of choir singing for disadvantaged adults. *Psychol Music, 41*(4), 405–421.

Edwards, N. E., & Beck, A. M. (2002). Animal-assisted therapy and nutrition in Alzheimer's disease. *Western J Nurs Res, 24*, 697–712.

Filan, S. L., & Llewellyn-Jones, R. H. (2006). Animal-assisted therapy for dementia: a review of the literature. *Int Psychogeriatrics, 18*(4), 597–611. doi: 10.1017/S1041610206003322.

Fiske, A., Wetherell, J. L., & Gatz, M. (2009). Depression in older adults. *Ann Rev Clin Psychology, 5*(1), 363–389. doi: 10.1146/annurev.clinpsy.032408.153621.

Gibson, M. C., Carter, M. W., Helmes, E., & Edberg, A. K. (2010). Principles of good care for long-term care facilities. *Int Psychogeriatrics, 22*(07), 1072–1083.

Gigliotti, C. M., Jarrott, S. E., & Yorgason, J. (2004). Harvesting health: effects of three types of horticultural therapy activities for persons with dementia. *Dementia, 3*(2), 161–180.

Godbey, G., & Blazey, M. (1983). Old people in urban parks: an exploratory investigation. *J Leisure Res, 15*(3), 229–244.

Gold, C., Solli, H. P., Krüger, V., & Lie, S. A. (2009). Dose–response relationship in music therapy for people with serious mental disorders: systematic review and meta-analysis. *Clin Psychology Rev, 29*(3), 193–207.

Gonzalez, M. T., Hartig T., Patil G. G., Martinsen, E. W., & Kirkevold, M. (2011). A prospective study of group cohesiveness in therapeutic horticulture for clinical depression. *Int J Mental Health Nurs, 20*, 119–129.

Hague, S. & Heggen, K. (2007). The nursing home as a home: a field study of residents' daily life in the common living rooms. *J Clin Nursing, 17*, 460–467.

Hanser, S. B., & Thompson, L. W. (1994). Effects of a music therapy strategy on depressed older adults. *J Gerontology, 49*(6), 265–269.

Hansmann, R., Hug, S. M., & Seeland, K. (2007). Restoration and stress relief through physical activities in forests and parks. *Urban Forestry Urban Greening, 6*(4), 213–225.

Hartig, T., Mang, M. & Evans, G. (1991). Restorative effects of natural environment experiences. *Environ Behav, 23*, 3–26.

Hawkins, J., Thirlaway, K. J., Backx, K., & Clayton, D. A. (2011). Allotment gardening and other leisure activities for stress reduction and healthy aging. *HortTech, 21*, 577–585.

Heath, Y., & Gifford, R. (2001). Post-occupancy evaluation of therapeutic gardens in a multi-level care facility for the aged. *Activities Adapt Aging, 25*(2), 21–43.

Kaplan, R. (1973). Some psychological benefits of gardening. *Environ Behav, 2*, 145–162.

Kaplan, R., & Kaplan, S. (1989). *The experience of nature: a psychological perspective.* Cambridge, UK: Cambridge University Press.

Kaplan, S., Kaplan, R., &Wendt, J. S. (1972). Rated preference and complexity for natural and urban visual material. *Percept Psychophysics, 12*, 354–356.

Katcher, A., & Wilkins, G. (1993). Dialogue with animals: its nature and culture. In S. R. Kellert & E. O. Wilson (Eds.), *The biophilia hypothesis* (pp. 173–197). Washington, DC: Island Press.

Katcher, A., Segal, H., & Beck, A. (1984). Comparison of contemplation and hypnosis for the reduction of anxiety and discomfort during dental surgery. *Am J Clin Hypnosis, 27*(1), 14–21.

Kingsley, J. Y., & Townsend, M. (2006). "Dig In" to social capital: community gardens as mechanisms for growing urban social connectedness. *Urban Policy Research, 24*(4), 525–537. doi: 10.1080/08111140601035200.

Kohlleppel, T., Bradley, J. C., & Jacob, S. (2002). A walk through the garden: can a visit to a botanic garden reduce stress. *Hort Technology, 12*(3), 489–492.

Kongable, L. G., Buckwalter, K. C., & Stolley, J. M. (1989). The effects of pet therapy on the social behavior of institutionalized Alzheimer's clients. *Arch Psychiatr Nurs, 3*, 191–198.

Krause-Parello, C. (2008). The mediating effect of pet attachment support between loneliness and general health in older females living in the community. *J Commun Health Nurs, 25*(1), 1–14.

Krause-Parello, C. A. (2012). Pet ownership and older women: the relationships among loneliness, pet attachment support, human social support, and depressed mood. *Geriatr Nurs, 33*(3), 194–203.

Krause-Parello, C. A., & Gulick, E. E. (2013). Situational factors related to loneliness and loss over time among older pet owners. *Western J Nurs Res, 35*(7), 905–919.

LaJoie, K. R. (2003). *An evaluation of the effectiveness of using animals in therapy.* Unpublished doctoral dissertation, Spalding University, Louisville, KY.

Lampinen, P., Heikkinen, R. L., Kauppinen, M., & Heikkinen, E. (2006). Activity as a predictor of mental well-being among older adults. *Aging Mental Health, 10*(5), 454–466. doi: 10.1080/13607860600640962.

Langer, E. J. & Rodin, J. (1976). The effects of choice and enhanced personal responsibility for the aged: a field experiment in an institutional setting. *J Personal Social Psychol, 134*, 191–198.

Lawton, M. P. (1987). Activities and leisure. In M. P. Lawton & G. Maddox (Eds.), *Ann Rev Gerontol Geriatrics*, Vol. 5. New York: Springer.

Lewis, C.A. (1976). The evolution of horticulture therapy in the US. Paper presented at the *Fourth Annual Meeting of the National Council for Therapy and Rehabilitation through Horticulture.* September 6, 1976, Philadelphia.

Libin, A., & Cohen-Mansfield, J. (2004). Therapeutic robocat for nursing home residents with dementia: preliminary inquiry. *Am J Alzheimers Dis, 19*(2), 111–116.

Lowery, D., & Warner, J. (2009). Behavioural and psychological symptoms of dementia (BPSD): the personal and practical costs of dementia. *J Integrated Care, 17*(2), 13–19. doi: 10.1108/14769018200900010.

Maratos, A., Gold, C., Wang, X., & Crawford, M. (2008). Music therapy for depression. *Cochrane Database Syst Rev, 1.* Art. no.: CD004517. doi: 10.1002/14651858.CD0045 17.pub2.

Mohammadi, A. Z., Shahabi, T., & Panah, F. M. (2011). An evaluation of the effect of group music therapy on stress, anxiety, and depression levels in nursing home residents. *Can J Music Ther, 17,* 55–68.

Odendaal, J. S. J., & Meintjes, R. A. (2003). Neurophysiological correlates of affiliative behaviour between humans and dogs. *Veterinary J, 165,* 296–301.

Olson, B. K. (1984). Player piano music as therapy for the elderly. *J Music Ther, 21*(1), 35–45.

Ottosson, J., & Grahn, P. (2005). Measures of restoration in geriatric care residences: the influence of nature on elderly people's power of concentration, blood pressure and pulse rate. *J Housing Elderly, 19*(3–4), 227–256. doi: 10.1300/J081v19n03_12.

Pachana, N. A., Kidd, J. L., & Alpass, F. (2000). Impact of physical disability on pursuit of gardening activities in mid-aged women. *Aust J Rehabil Counsel, 6*(2), 75–85.

Pachana, N. A., McWha, J. L., & Arathoon, M. (2003). Passive therapeutic gardening. *J Gerontol Nursing, 29*(5), 4–10.

Pachana, N. A., Massavelli, B. M., & Robleda-Gomez, S. (2011). A developmental psychological perspective on the human–animal bond. In C. Blazina, G. Boyra, & D. S. Shen-Miller (Eds.), *The psychology of the human-animal bond* (pp. 151–165). New York: Springer. doi: 10.1007/978-1-4419-9761-6_9.

Palmer, M. (1983). Music therapy in a comprehensive program of treatment and rehabilitation for the geriatric resident. *Activities, Adaptation & Aging, 3*(3), 53–59.

Park, S.-A., Lee, K.-S., Son, K.-C., & Shoemaker, C. (2012). Metabolic cost of horticulture activities in older adults. *J Japan Soc Horticult Sci, 81*(3), 295–299. doi: 10.2503/jjshs1.81.295.

Patterson, I., & Chang, M., (1999). Participation in physical activities by older Australians: A review of the social psychological benefits and constraints. *Austr J Ageing, 18,* 179–185.

Raglio, A., Bellelli, G., Mazzola, P., Bellandi, D., Giovagnoli, A. R., Farina, E., . . . Trabucchi, M. (2012). Music, music therapy and dementia: a review of literature and the recommendations of the Italian Psychogeriatric Association. *Maturitas, 72*(4), 305–310. doi: 10.1016/j.maturitas.2012.05.016.

Ryan, R. M., Weinstein, N., Bernstein, J., Brown, K. W., Mistretta, L., & Gagné, M. (2010). Vitalizing effects of being outdoors and in nature. *J Environ Psychol, 30*(2), 159–168.

Scott, T. L., Masser, B. M., & Pachana, N. A. (2014a). Multi-sensory installations in residential aged-care facilities: increasing novelty and encouraging social engagement through modest environmental changes. *J Gerontol Nurs, 40*(9), 20–31. doi: 10.3928/00989134-20140731-01.

Scott, T. L., Masser, B. M., & Pachana, N. A. (2014b). Exploring the health and wellbeing benefits of gardening for older adults. *Ageing Society,* 1–25, available on CJO2014. doi: 10.1017/S0144686X14000865.

Stanley, I. H., Conwell, Y., Bowen, C., & Van Orden, K. A. (2014). Pet ownership may attenuate loneliness among older adult primary care patients who live alone. *Aging Mental Health, 18*(3), 394–399.

Suzuki, M., Kanamori, M., & Watanabe, M., et al. (2004). Behavioral and endocrinological evaluation of music therapy for elderly patients with dementia. *Nursing Health Sci, 6,* 11–18.

Takahashi, T., & Matsushita H. (2006). Long-term effects of music therapy on elderly with moderate/severe dementia. *J Music Ther, 43,* 317–333.

Tamura, T., Yonemitsu, S., Itoh, A., Oikawa, D., Kawakami, A., Higashi, Y., ... & Nakajima, K. (2004). Is an entertainment robot useful in the care of elderly people with severe dementia? *The Journals of Gerontology Series A: Biological Sciences and Medical Sciences, 59*(1), M83–M85.

Tedeschi, P., Fitchett, J., & Molidor, C. (2005). The incorporation of animal-assisted interventions in social work education. *J Fam Social Work, 9*(4), 59–77.

Teresi, J., Abrams, R., Holmes, D., Ramirez, M., & Eimicke, J. (2001). Prevalence of depression and depression recognition in nursing homes. *Social psychiatry and psychiatric epidemiology, 36*(12), 613–620.

Townsend, M. (2006). Feel blue? Touch green! Participation in forest/woodland management as a treatment for depression. *Urban Forestry Urban Greening, 5,* 111–120. doi: 10.1016/j.ufug.2006.02.001.

Turner, T. (2005). *Garden history, philosophy and design, 2000 BC–2000 AD.* New York: Spon Press.

Ulrich, R. S. (1984). View through a window may influence recovery from surgery. *Science, 224* (4647), 420–421.

Ulrich, R. S. (2002). Health benefits of gardens in hospitals. Paper presented at *Plants for*

People Conference, International Exhibition Floriade, 2002.

Ulrich, R., & Parsons, R., (1992). Influences of passive experiences with plants on individual wellbeing and healt, In D. Relf (Ed.), *The role of horticulture in human wellbeing and social development* (pp. 93–105). Portland, OR: Timber Press.

Ulrich, R. S., Simons, R. F., Losito, B. D., & Fiorito, E. (1991). Stress recovery during exposure to natural and urban environments. *J Environ Psychol, 11*(3), 201–230.

Wannamethee, S., Shaper, A., & Walker, M. (2000). Physical activity and mortality in older men with diagnosed coronary heart disease. *Circulation, 102*(12), 1358–1363.

Whall, A., Black, M., Groh, C., Yankou, D., Kupferschmid, B., & Foster, N. (1997). The effect of natural environments upon agitation and aggression in late stage dementia patients. *Am J Alzheimers Dis, 5*(12), 216–220. doi: 10.1177/153331759701200506.

Wilson, C. C., & Barker, S. B. (2003). Challenges in designing human–animal interaction research. *Am Behav Scientist, 47,* 16–28.

Wilson, E. O. (1984). *Biophilia.* Cambridge, MA: Harvard University Press.

Wilson, E. O. (1993). Biophilia and the conservation ethic. In S. R. Kellert & E. O. Wilson (Eds.). *The biophilia hypothesis.* Washington, DC: Island Press.

Yee Tse, M. M. (2010). Therapeutic effects of an indoor gardening program for older people living in nursing homes. *J Clin Nurs, 19,* 949–958.

Zare, M., Ebrahimi, A. A., & Birashk, B. (2010). The effects of music therapy on reducing agitation in patients with Alzheimer's disease, a pre–post study. *Int J Geriatr Psychiatry, 25,* 1309–1310.

Ziv, G., & Lidor, R. (2011). Music, exercise performance, and adherence in clinical populations and in the elderly: a review. *J Clin Sport Psychol, 5*(1), 1–23.

Ziv, N., Granot, A., Hai, S., Dassa, A., & Haimov, I. (2007). The effect of background stimulative music on behavior in Alzheimer's patients. *J Music Ther, 44,* 329–343.

Epilogue

FOLLOWING this comprehensive review of recent advances in research in CAIM, we can say that scientific evidence in understanding some CAIM practice and implementation is advancing, but it still lags behind those in Western medicine. At the same time, mainstream Western medicine has struggled with understanding, accepting, and documenting the effects and the mechanisms of CAIM interventions. An integration of CAIM and mainstream Western medicine has the potential to improve both of these treatment modalities. On the research front, funding CAIM research has been limited compared to that of mainstream Western medicine. The major push for the use of CAIM has come mostly from the general public that uses CAIM extensively, and the current cost burden of CAIM is mostly funded by out-of-pocket individual expenses because most medical insurance companies do not pay for CAIM. On a global level, CAIM could help to prevent major diseases of aging and thereby reduce the cost of chronic disease and end-of-life care around the world.

In the future, we can hope that government funding agencies will be better able to appreciate the potential cost and burden savings by gaining a better understanding of how CAIM may advance care for patients and families and how to use resources most efficiently. At present, there are insufficient data on the prevalence, effectiveness, efficacy, safety, and health economic benefits of most CAIM treatments. Patients, health providers, and other stakeholders are unable to access reliable and rigorous evidence on CAIMs. When considering future directions for this field, it is important to consider the most recent strategic plan from the National Center for Complementary and Integrative Health (NCCIH) entitled "Exploring the Science of CAM: Third Plan 2011–2015." This plan has five main objectives: (1) to advance research on mind and body interventions, practices, and disciplines; (2) to advance research on CAIM natural products;

(3) to increase understanding of real-world patterns and outcomes of CAIM use and its integration into health care and health promotion; (4) to improve the capacity of the field to carry out rigorous research; and (5) to develop and disseminate objective, evidence-based information on CAIM interventions.

The chapters in this book point to recommendations for future CAIM trials and clinical utilization. The field needs to achieve consensus on the appropriate methods of evaluation of the efficacy of CAIM interventions. It is not entirely clear that the traditional research methods of evaluation that have been used up to this point are capturing all benefits of the CAIM interventions. Perhaps, some blend of mainstream medicine and alternative measures of outcome should be included in the studies. However, CAIM trials should aim to replicate the highest scientific standards, which means adequate blinding, allocation concealment, randomization, complete outcome data presentation, and thorough reporting. CAIMs trials should utilize adequate control groups. Controls groups for holistic treatments should have similar elements to active groups; control groups for biologically based treatments can use placebo. Randomized clinical trials must include treatment and prevention of all major mental and physical disorders in older adults in order to build a comprehensive evidence for such practices. Other approaches to improved quality of research would include agreements on the "gold standard" tools and measures for the evaluation of outcomes across studies, as well as examination of the targets for CAIM interventions, identifying subpopulations who respond to the interventions (moderators), and the mechanisms by which they respond (mediators) that are employed by mainstream medicine.

This high standard of evidence might influence regulatory bodies such as the FDA to be involved in the regulation of CAIM practices. In addition, care must be taken to ensure the reliability, safety, and consistency of CAIM supplements. It is important that doctors and patients are utilizing the same preparations, which are free from toxins or other potentially harmful ingredients. Researchers must disclose conflicts of interest, matching current trends in pharmaceutical trials.

In conclusion, neuropsychiatric disorders in older adults, such as mood, anxiety, sleep, chronic pain, and cognitive disorders, are among the most common reasons for older adults to use CAIM therapies. As evidenced by the chapters in this book, the use of CAIM therapies in older adults is promising, and the body of empirical research is growing rapidly. However, the quality of the research within this field is highly variable, making firm conclusions difficult. This methodological diversity is reflected in the chapters of this book and the field in general. This book represents a first attempt to bring together an interdisciplinary team of authors in order to enrich our mutual understanding of the field to date. Overall, we recommend the continuation of high-quality research to establish efficacy and safety. With the established safety of various natural products, clinicians could offer important information for those patients who are less comfortable with mainstream medicine and who prefer alternative "natural" therapies, as well as the ability to offer advice on drug–CAIM interactions and direction with respect to evidenced-based CAIM indications. In conclusion, it is clear that CAIM use is significant in older adult populations and will likely increase; thus empirical research is essential.

Index

massage therapy (*Cont.*)
   National Health Interview Survey data, 124
   neck pain studies, 128*t*
   outcomes of, 127, 132
   safety and adverse effects, 125–126
   shoulder pain studies, 128*t*–129*t*
Master Resilience Trainer (MRT) course (US Army), 309
Matsumoto, K., 85*t*
Matsutani, L. A., 129*t*
Mayer, J. M., 150*t*
Mayo Clinic website, 302
MBCT. *See* mindfulness-based cognitive therapy
MBIs. *See* mindfulness-based interventions
MBSR. *See* mindfulness-based stress reduction
McBride, S., 311*t*
McCaddon, A., 63
McCarty, R. L., 131*t*
McCleery, J., 417
MCI. *See* mild cognitive impairment
McNeill, G., 357*t*, 360
MDD. *See* major depressive disorder
meaning-enhancement therapy, 261*t*, 264–265
mechanisms of aging
   biomarkers for, 13*f*
   cellular senescence, 10*f*, 12, 13*f*
   chronic inflammation, 10*f*, 12, 13*f*
   compression of morbidity focus, 7
   epigenetic alterations, 10*f*, 11, 13*f*
   genomic instability, 10–11, 10*f*, 13*f*
   loss of proteostasis, 10*f*, 11–12, 13*f*
   mind-body practices effects, 13–14
   mitochondrial dysfunction, 10*f*, 12, 13*f*
   natural product's effect on, 16
   nutritional intervention's effect on, 15–16
   physical activity's effect on, 14–15
   telomere attrition, 10*f*, 11, 13*f*
Medical Expenditure Panel Survey, 123, 141
medical marijuana. *See* Cannabis sativa (cannabis) use
meditation. *See also* specific forms of meditation
   Alzheimer's disease and, 216
   chiropractic incorporation of, 154
   dementia and, 468–469, 471*t*
   description, 216, 220–221
   forms of, 8, 13–14, 216, 220, 231, 244
   goals of, 220
   impact on inflammatory pathways, 13
   for low back pain, 445–446
   sleep and, 221
   stress/aging, impact on, 220
   strokes and, 232
   telomeres and, 220–221
Mediterranean dietary pattern
   cognitive decline and, 351, 377
   components, 377
   late-life depression and, 343, 349
   longevity and, 39
   meta-analysis of epidemiological trials, 8–9
"MedlinePlus Guide to Healthy Web Surfing, and Evaluating Health Information" (MedlinePlus), 296
MedlinePlus® portal, 296
"Meet Me at MOMA" program, 287
Megame program, 325
Meier, M. H., 114
melatonin
   Alzheimer's disease and, 404, 417
   in cognitively impaired older adults, 417
   in cognitively intact older adults, 417–418

   dementia and, 457–458, 464*t*, 470*t*
   insomnia and, 405*t*–409*t*
   side effects/drug interactions, 418
Melton, I. J., 228
memory and memory loss. *See also* Alzheimer's disease; cognitive decline; cognitive decline, lifestyle factors; cognitive decline, lifestyle interventions; cognitive function; dementia; memory training programs
   alternative nostril breathing and, 241
   Ayurvedic herbs for, 176*f*, 177
   creative arts and, 283, 285–287
   DBT breathing and, 243
   East-West approach, 182, 183
   endocannabinoids and, 112–114
   estrogen and, 102–103.105
   ginseng and, 53–54
   MBSR program and, 266
   meditation and, 221, 232
   neural plasticity and, 228–229
   neurodegeneration and, 202*f*
   plant adaptogens and, 197, 202, 203*t*, 205, 207
   PLIE exercise program and, 232
   PS-DHA study, 64–65
   SAMe study, 66
   subjective memory impairment (SMI), 371–372, 377
   tai chi and, 220
   testosterone and, 10104
   Women's Health Initiative study, 100
   yoga and, 234*f*
memory training programs (MTPs). *See also* cognitive training
   in classrooms, in small groups, 322–323
   for mild cognitive impairment, 328, 329*t*, 330–331
   mnemonic strategies, 322–323
   for normal aging, 326–328
   peer led/exportable programs, 323–324
   transferability/generalizability of, 331
Memory-Impacting Factors (memory mnemonic technique), 324*t*
menopause
   bipolar disorder and, 102
   depression and, 100
   estrogen fluctuation, 99
Meserve, B. B., 151*t*
metabolomic regulatory level, 198
Metchnikoff, Elie, 75
Michaleff, A. Z., 150*t*
mild cognitive impairment (MCI)
   amnestic, 371
   CoCoA study, 361
   cognitive training in, 322, 325, 328, 329*t*, 330–332, 333*t*
   exercise efficacy in, 8
   HRV and, 249
   in multiple domains, 371
   non-amnestic, 371
   overweight/obesity and, 374
   potential conversion to AD, 372
military service-related trauma, 247
Miller, J., 153*t*
Miller, L., 266
mind-body practices, 215–223. *See also* breathing practices; meditation; qi gong; tai chi; yoga
   breathing methods used in, 245
   clinical evidence for, 8
   for coping/stress reduction, 215–223
   effects on mechanisms of aging, 13–14
   efficacy levels for, 6
   genetic effects of, 244

World Wide Web. *See* Internet resources for CAIM interventions

Würtzen, H., 348*t*, 484*t*

Yale-Brown Obsessive-Compulsive Scale (Y-BOCS), 248

Yang, L., 129*t*, 130*t*, 131*t*

Yang, X. F., 129*t*

years lived with disability (YLD), 6

Yen, C. H., 91*t*

YLD. *See* years lived with disability

yoga, 6, 8, 227–234. *See also* breath-focused yoga; high-frequency yoga breathing

  Alzheimer's disease and, 216

  anxiety/mood disorders and, 391, 395

  biodirectional feedback loops in, 242

  breath-focused, 243, 246

  brief benefits summary, 234*f*

  cancer survivors and, 218, 479, 480*t*–483*t*, 490–491

  dementia and, 218, 232–233

  description, 217–218

  diabetes and, 233

  forms of, 217

  Hatha yoga, 217, 263

  hypertension and, 217–218, 230

  immune/stress response systems and, 217–218

  impact on aging mechanisms, 14

  for insomnia, 413*t*–414*t*

  insomnia and, 218

  laughter yoga, 395

  low back pain and, 218, 446

  mental component, 229

  mood disorders and, 466

  for mood/anxiety disorders, 390*f*

  osteoarthritis and, 442*t*

  osteoporosis and, 230

  PMR comparison, 263

  RCTs challenges, 216

  relaxation response and, 14

  rheumatoid arthritis and, 218

  Silver yoga program, 231, 262, 395

  sleep and, 218

  for sleep disorders, 218, 420–421

  sleep disorders and, 420–421, 466

  spiritual benefits of, 261*t*, 262–263

  stroke and, 231–232

  tai chi's parallels with, 218

  Thai massage incorporation of, 126

  unipolar depression and, 393*t*

  VRBPs and, 245

yogic breathing (*pranayama*), 217

yogic meditation, 13–14

Yokoyama, W., 46*t*, 50

Youn, J., 327*t*, 333*t*

Yuan, S. L., 129*t*

Zaharoni, H., 88*t*

Zehnder, F., 330

Zhang, L. P., 131*t*

Ziegenfuss, T., 43*t*

zinc

  dose ranges/side effects, 363*t*

  effects on mechanisms of aging, 16

  late-life depression and, 342–343

  for mood/anxiety disorders, 390*t*

Zinke, K., 327*t*, 333*t*

Printed in the USA/Agawam, MA
May 7, 2018

674572.006